Stuttering

An Integrated Approach to Its Nature and Treatment

SIXTH EDITION

Stuttering

An Integrated Approach to Its Nature and Treatment

SIXTH EDITION

Barry Guitar, PhD

Professor Emeritus
Department of Communication Sciences and Disorders
University of Vermont
Burlington, Vermont

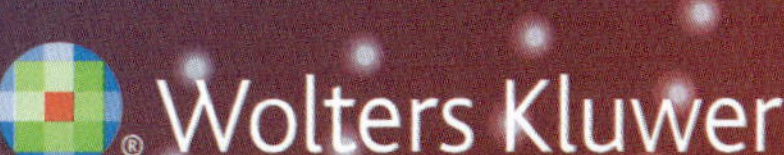

Philadelphia • Baltimore • New York • London
Buenos Aires • Hong Kong • Sydney • Tokyo

Acquisitions Editor: Lindsey Porambo
Senior Development Editor: Amy Millholen
Editorial Coordinator: Varshaanaa SM
Editorial Assistant: Parisa Saranj
Marketing Manager: Danielle Klahr
Production Project Manager: Justin Wright
Manager, Graphic Arts & Design: Stephen Druding
Art Director: Jennifer Clements
Manufacturing Coordinator: Margie Orzech
Prepress Vendor: Straive

Sixth Edition

9 8 7 6 5 4 3 2 1

Printed in Mexico

Cataloging-in-Publication Data available on request from the Publisher

ISBN: 978-1-9751-8215-1

shop.lww.com

QUADM1123

Preface

As *Stuttering: An Integrated Approach to Its Nature and Treatment* reaches its sixth edition, we have strived to retain features that the previous editions' readers have found helpful and made some changes we believe can make it even better.

As we have done for each new edition, we have made additions, deletions, and other changes to bring to you the latest research and treatment approaches dealing with stuttering and related disorders. Using updates from colleagues and library resources, including powerful search engines, such as Ovid MEDLINE and Google Scholar, is vital because research, especially on the neurology of stuttering, as well as clinical research on treatment, is moving at a rapid pace. Although we have tried to be as current as possible, we still advise you to turn to the most recent literature to keep abreast of the newest developments in research and to turn to more popular sources, such as webcasts and stuttering support group outlets, to gain insights from the powerful of voices of people as they share their personal journeys.

In keeping with efforts to stay current, we have included a brand-new chapter by Naomi Rodgers. Her chapter "Treatment of Adolescents: Advanced Stuttering" (Chapter 16) brings new perspectives to stuttering therapy with teens, acknowledging how important it is to let clients take the lead in deciding when to start therapy and to determine the pace of treatment. Dr. Rodgers' extensive experience with teens is reflected in the guidance and recommendations she makes and enriched by her own experience as a teen who stuttered.

Another change in this new edition is the use of gender-inclusive pronouns (they and them and themselves, in place of he or she or hers or his or herself or himself). This change reflects our effort to respect individuals' gender identity and convey an accepting attitude toward all individuals no matter what gender they were born with or what gender they have chosen.

As research on the nature of stuttering has progressed, it is clearer that differences in brain function in many who stutter may be permanent and even some of the learned behaviors may be difficult to unlearn. Thus, another change that we hope readers of earlier versions of this book will notice is an increasing emphasis on incorporating acceptance as an important component of treatment. This is especially true of therapy for school-age stutterers, adolescents, and adults. As you will see in the treatment chapters, individuals who stutter are guided to make peace with their stuttering, learn to be open with others about their stuttering, and reduce the tension and struggle that they have used to try not to stutter. This approach makes stuttering a minor problem that is no longer associated with shame, embarrassment, and fear. Some of us even look forward to moments of stuttering so that we can handle them smoothly and openly as well as experience the feeling of triumph that accompany a stutter well-handled—or not handled at all but still not allowed to take away the importance of what we are saying.

Although we are emphasizing acceptance as particularly important for older individuals who stutter, we see stuttering in young children as a different issue. In my experience and according to my clinical data, early indirect or direct treatment of stuttering—rather than acceptance of it—is effective in eliminating stuttering or nearly so. Children younger than age 6, before they enter their first year of school, respond well to a parent- or caregiver-based program of therapy managed by a dedicated stuttering clinician. Although we agree that clinicians need to stay alert for signs that a child's feelings of shame, embarrassment, and fear that might in fact be triggered by a focus on fluency, we believe working on fluency does not make such feelings inevitable.

Thus, we give wings to this new edition of our stuttering textbook, with hope that it will help many who stutter and many who work with them!

Barry Guitar
Professor Emeritus, University of Vermont

Acknowledgments

I want to begin by thanking my clients and my students, who—over the last 6 decades—let me help them learn about the nature and treatment of stuttering. As much I as I may have taught them, they have taught me.

Thank you also to my colleagues at the University of Vermont and around the world who were invaluable in helping me understand research, treatment, and the goodness of other people.

Huge applause for my friends and editors at Wolters Kluwer. These heroes include Amy Millholen, Senior Development Editor, and Varshaanaa Muralidharan, Editorial Coordinator, who have been generous with their time, endlessly patient, and deeply insightful. Lindsey Porambo, Acquisitions Editor, has been most benevolent in supporting this sixth edition, as well as responsive to issues that have come up as I have worked on this textbook. I would like also to bestow great thanks to all the staff at Wolters Kluwer who have taken this book through its many stages of production.

Immeasurable thanks to Bot Roda, a gifted illustrator, who has the ability to transform my scrap art into vivid compositions that more than capture what I want to convey to the reader! He is amazing!

Many thanks to Lydia Sack—a former student and now a full-fledged stuttering therapist—for developing new quiz questions for Lippincott Connect and for creating an entirely new feature: Suggested Answers to Study Questions at the end of each chapter, for teachers to use with their classes. And thanks to Lydia and to Dunra Kazenski for their very valuable help with many other digital assets on the website.

In this sixth edition, we are indeed fortunate to welcome Naomi Rodgers who has written an outstanding new chapter on Treatment of Adolescents who Stutter: Advanced Stuttering. She is internationally known as an expert in working with this sometimes puzzling and always entertaining group of individuals who stutter.

As in each of the preceding five editions, Rebecca McCauley and Charles Barasch have given their valuable time and energy to reading every word and every punctuation mark of every chapter and suggesting changes that have made this edition sing.

I also thank my Tibetian Terrier, Deano (named after the famous Dr. Dean Williams), who has taken me on many walks and nuzzled my face to keep me happy and healthy.

And finally, I am endlessly indebted to my wife, Carroll, who has used her many talents to find, organize, and attach more than a thousand references—many of them hot off the press—for this edition. Moreover, she has managed the permissions, videos, and my time, allowing us to break a bottle of champagne over the bow of this sixth edition.

Contents

Section II Assessment of Stuttering

Section III Treatment of Stuttering

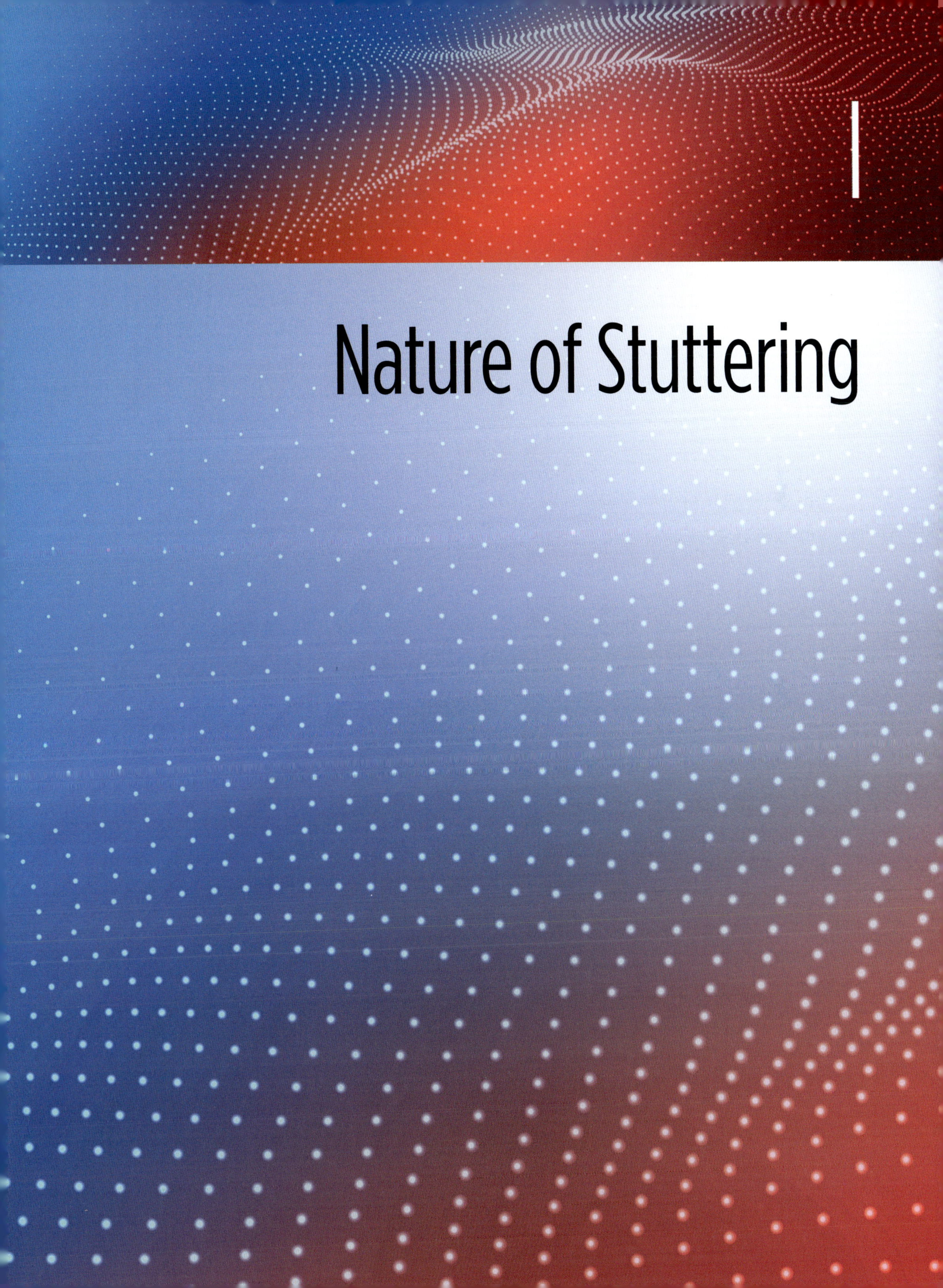

I

Nature of Stuttering

1

Introduction to Stuttering

Chapter Outline

Chapter Objectives

After studying this chapter, readers should be able to:

- Describe factors that may (1) predispose a child to stutter, (2) precipitate stuttering, and (3) make stuttering persistent
- Name and describe the core behaviors of stuttering
- Name and describe the two major categories of secondary stuttering behaviors
- Name and describe different feelings and attitudes that can accompany stuttering
- Describe the elements of the International Classification of Functioning, Disability, and Health (ICF) system that are most relevant to stuttering
- Discuss the age range types of stuttering onset, and explain why the onset of stuttering is often difficult to pinpoint
- Describe the meanings of the terms "prevalence" and "incidence," and give current best estimates of each of these characteristics for stuttering

- Give an estimate of the percentage of children who recover without treatment, and describe factors that predict this recovery
- Give an estimate of the sex ratio in stuttering at onset and in the school-age population
- Explain what is meant by "anticipation," "consistency," and "adaptation" in stuttering
- Explain some relationships between stuttering and language, and suggest what they mean about the nature of the disorder
- Describe several speaking conditions under which stuttering is usually reduced or absent, and suggest why this may be so
- Give a brief, simple description of what stuttering is, possible causes, and influences on it

Key Terms

Adaptation: The tendency for speakers to stutter less and less (up to a point) when repeatedly reading a passage

Anticipation: An individual's ability to predict on which words or sounds they will stutter

Attitude: A feeling that has become a pervasive part of a person's beliefs

Avoidance behavior: A speaker's attempt to prevent stuttering when they anticipate stuttering on a word or in a situation. Word-based avoidances are commonly interjections of extra sounds, like "uh," said before the word on which stuttering is expected

Block: A disfluency that is an inappropriate stoppage of the flow of air or voice and often the movement of articulators as well

Consistency: The tendency for speakers to stutter on the same words when reading a passage several times

Core behaviors: The basic speech behaviors of stuttering—repetitions, prolongations, and blocks

Developmental stuttering: A term used to denote the most common form of stuttering that develops during childhood (in contrast to stuttering that develops in response to a neurological event or trauma or emotional stress)

Disfluency: An interruption of speech—such as a repetition, hesitancy, or prolongation of sound—that may occur in both individuals who are developing typically and those who stutter

Escape behavior: A speaker's attempts to terminate a stutter and finish the word. This occurs when the speaker is already in a moment of stuttering. An example is when the speaker is struggling to say "Boston" and says "BBBB....uh....Boston," using the "uh" to break out of the stutter

Fluency: The effortless flow of speech

Heterogeneity: Differences among various types of a disorder

Incidence: The percentage of people who have stuttered at some time in their lives

Persistent: Stuttering that the child does not spontaneously recover from during early childhood

Prevalence: The percentage of people who stutter, when a survey is made at any particular time

Prolongation: A disfluency in which sound or air flow continues but movement of the articulators is stopped

Repetition: A sound, syllable, or single-syllable word that is repeated several times. The speaker is apparently "stuck" on that sound or syllable and continues repeating it until the following sound can be produced

Secondary behaviors: A speaker's reactions to their repetitions, prolongations, and blocks in an attempt to end them quickly or avoid them altogether. Such reactions may begin as random struggle but soon turn into well-learned patterns. Secondary behaviors can be divided into two broad classes: escape and avoidance behaviors

Typical disfluency: An interruption of speech in a typically developing individual

PERSPECTIVE

No one is sure what causes stuttering, but it is an age-old problem that may have its origins in the way our brains evolved to produce speech and language. Its sudden appearance in some children is triggered when they try to talk using their emerging speech and language skills. The many variations and manifestations of stuttering are determined by an individual's brain structure and function, learning patterns, personality, and temperament. Stuttering also provides lessons about human culture: the variety of responses that stuttering provokes in cultures around the world is a reflection of the many ways in which human groups deal with individual differences. In the last few years in some cultures, particularly in the United States, stuttering is viewed as part of human diversity, rather than a curse that must be completely eradicated.

This description of stuttering makes it seem like a very complicated problem—one that will take a long time to learn about. It's true that you could spend a lifetime and still not know everything there is to know about stuttering. But you don't need to understand everything in order to help people who stutter. If you read this book critically and carefully, you will get a basic understanding of stuttering and a foundation for evaluating, treating, and supporting people who stutter and their families. And once you start meeting and working with people who stutter, your understanding and ability will expand exponentially.

If you continue to work with stuttering, you will soon outgrow this book and begin to make your own discoveries. You will experience the satisfaction of helping children, adolescents, and adults regain an ability to communicate easily. Someday you may even write about your therapy procedures and measure their effectiveness. Those of us who have spent many years engaged in stuttering research and treatment and working with the stuttering community all began where you are right now, at the threshold of an exciting and rewarding profession that can have a major impact on others' lives.

The Words We Use

In any field—whether it's education, medicine, or speech-language pathology—words may be used in specific ways. Definitions of many of the specialized terms used in our field are provided in the Key Terms list at the beginning of each chapter. But some words and phrases deserve to be discussed at the beginning.

People Who Stutter

Until recently, it was common practice to refer to people who stutter as "stutterers." In fact, some of us who stutter refer to ourselves as stutterers and feel some pride in this term. It reminds me that a friend of mine who has Parkinson's disease is happy to call himself a "parkie" and even "a mover and shaker." However, many people prefer not to be labeled "a stutterer" and prefer instead to be called "a person who stutters." They feel, and rightly so, that this captures the reality that stuttering is only a small part of who they are.

Adults who stutter often say that changing the way they think of themselves—as people who happen to stutter but with many more important attributes—was one of the most significant things they did to break free of the bonds of stuttering. Such reports remind us that clients are far more than people who stutter. They are people, each with a huge array of characteristics, only one of which happens to be that they stutter. This way of thinking enables us to help both our clients and their families. When we use the phrase "child who stutters" rather than "stutterer," families listen beyond the sounds of stuttering to the thoughts and feelings that their children are communicating. It helps everyone view disfluencies in perspective as only a small part of the whole child.

Some authors abbreviate "people who stutter" as "PWS." Personally, I feel that substituting an acronym that highlights stuttering is not really different from using "stutterer." In fact, it may be even more demeaning. So, I won't employ "PWS" as an acronym. However, I know that the language in this book would grow stale and cumbersome if I were to use "person who stutters" over and over. So, I often refer to the "adult…," "child…," or "adolescent" you are working with. I also may use the honorific that I use for myself, "stutterer."

That term, "stutterer," is coming back to into more common use in the stuttering community. Self-help groups, especially those associated with the National Stuttering Association, have embraced an attitude of Stuttering Pride. This is in step with a world-wide shift in attitude by those with disabilities. Many individuals and groups with challenges, such as hearing impairment and movement disorders, are seeing themselves as "differently abled" rather "disabled." They are proud rather than ashamed of their differences and how they respond to them. This view also applies to treatment of stuttering, insofar as many stutterers feel they were humiliated by therapies that stressed fluency at any cost, because they could not achieve that perfection. Increasingly, clients choose their own goals, often with clinicians' guidance, to continue to stutter as they do now but feel more comfortable and open; to continue to stutter, but in an easier way; or to obtain as much fluency as possible. They may begin with some goals and then discard them and choose others. Clinicians need to be accepting and encouraging of clients' own choices; part of a clinician's role is to help the client—a child, an adolescent, an adult—gain freedom from others' judgments and from their own doubts, and then soar.

Disfluency

In our literature, "**disfluency**" is used to denote interruptions of speech that may be either normal or abnormal. That is, it can apply to pauses, repetitions, and other hesitancies in individuals who are typical speakers. It can also apply to moments of stuttering. This makes it a handy term to use when describing the speech of young children whose diagnosis is unclear.

When someone's speech hesitancies are unequivocally not stuttering, I'll use the term "**typical disfluency**." I won't use the older term for the abnormal hesitations in stuttering—"dysfluency" with a "y"—because it can easily be mistaken for "disfluency" when you see it on the page and because the two are indistinguishable when spoken.

OVERVIEW OF THE DISORDER

This section previews the next few chapters on the nature of stuttering and gives me a chance to reveal my own slant on the disorder. I think this may be helpful for anyone, but especially for those readers who have not had a course in stuttering and who may, therefore, know very few details of its nature.

Do All Cultures Have Stuttering?

Stuttering is found in all parts of the world and in all cultures and races. It is indiscriminate of occupation, intelligence, and income; it affects both sexes and people of all ages, from toddlers to the elderly. It is an old curse, and there is evidence that it was present in Chinese, Egyptian, and Mesopotamian cultures more than 40 centuries ago (Van Riper, 1982). Moses was said to have stuttered (Garfinkel, 1995) and to have used a trick typical of many of us who stutter—getting his brother to speak for him. I did something similar when I was asked to read a prayer aloud in Sunday school.

What Causes People to Stutter?

The cause of stuttering is still something of a mystery. Scientists have yet to discover exactly what causes stuttering in each individual, but they have many clues. First, there is strong evidence that stuttering often has a genetic basis—that is, something is inherited that makes it more likely a child will stutter. This genetic "something" has to do with the way a child's brain develops its neural pathways for speech and language. For example, the neural pathways for talking may be less dense and less well developed in those who stutter. The neural pathways show less connectivity among the many brain regions that need to cooperate to produce fluent speech. This could impede the rapid flow of information needed to sequence the movements of many muscles as precisely as needed for fluent speech. What's more, the commands to muscles must be coordinated with the many components of language, including word choice, syntax, and semantics. The pathways may also be vulnerable to disruption by other brain activity, such as that connected with emotions. Isn't it amazing that most of us learn to talk at 200 syllables per minute, using huge vocabularies and complicated syntax to suit what we say to every particular situation!

Another clue about the nature of stuttering is that most stuttering begins in children between ages 2 and 5. Thus, the onset of stuttering occurs at about the same time that many typical stresses of early childhood are occurring. One child may begin to stutter during a dramatic growth in vocabulary and syntax. Another's stuttering may first appear when the family moves to a new home. Still another child may start soon after a baby brother or sister is born. Many different factors, acting singly or in combination, may precipitate the onset of stuttering in a child who has a neurophysiological predisposition, or inborn tendency, for stuttering.

Once stuttering starts, it may disappear within a few months or it may get gradually worse. When it gets worse, learned reactions may be an important factor in its severity. Playmates at school or adults who don't know how to correctly respond may cause children to become highly self-conscious about their stuttering. Children will quickly learn that by pushing hard, they can get traction on a word that has been stuck. They may find that an eye blink or an "um" said quickly before trying to say a hard word may avoid stuttering temporarily. By the time children become teens, learned reactions influence many of the symptoms. They have learned to anticipate stuttering and may thrash around in a panic when they speak, trying to escape or avoid it. By adulthood, their fear of stuttering and their desire to avoid it can permeate their lifestyle. Adults who stutter often cope with it by limiting their work, friends, and fun to those situations and people that put few demands on speech. Figure 1.1 provides an overview of many of the contributing factors in the evolution of stuttering. In this and the subsequent four chapters, I'll describe in detail our current understanding of these influences.

Can Stuttering Be Cured—and Does It Even Need to Be?

As implied above, it often cures itself. Many young children who begin to stutter stop stuttering without treatment. For others, early intervention may be needed to help the child develop typical fluency and prevent the development of a chronic problem. Once stuttering has become firmly established, however, and the child has developed many learned reactions, a concerted treatment effort is needed. Good treatment of mild and moderate stuttering in preschool and early elementary school children may leave them with little trace of stuttering, except perhaps when they are stressed, fatigued, or ill. Most of those who stutter severely for a long time or who are not treated until after puberty achieve only a partial remission of stuttering problems. Some of these people are able to stutter more easily and to be less bothered by their stuttering. Some, however, will not improve, despite our best efforts. And remember, for teens and adults, the goals of therapy and even the choice to undertake therapy should be chosen by the client in consultation with the clinician, and these goals may change over the course of therapy. Some clients may want to learn to communicate effectively but continue to stutter. For myself, I enjoy have a little bit of stuttering still remaining in my speech. Every time I catch a stutter and resist the urge to push and struggle, but, instead, choose to be present in the moment of stuttering, allowing it to relax and end slowly and loosely, I feel a triumph over my old feelings of being out of control when I stuttered.

Repeated embarrassment with stuttering leads to negative feelings and attitudes about communication
I wish talking were easier
Hey... uh...l-l-lets go... uh... p-p-play v...v...v... well... uh... video games
Yo! B-B-BILLY! how cccome you talk so f-f-funny?
Age 18
Age 8
Now stop and start over
Environmental influences such as criticism of speech or stressful events combine with neurodevelopmental factors to make stuttering more severe and chronic
I wo... wo... wonder what sssschool will be... be... like
Billy, we're going to be moving tomorrow!
Age 6
Mmm... mommy's sock
Age 3
Speech and language acquisition and other developmental influences precipitate disfluencies
Genetic and congenital influences predispose the child to stuttering
Mommy's sock
Mommy sock
Sock
Start

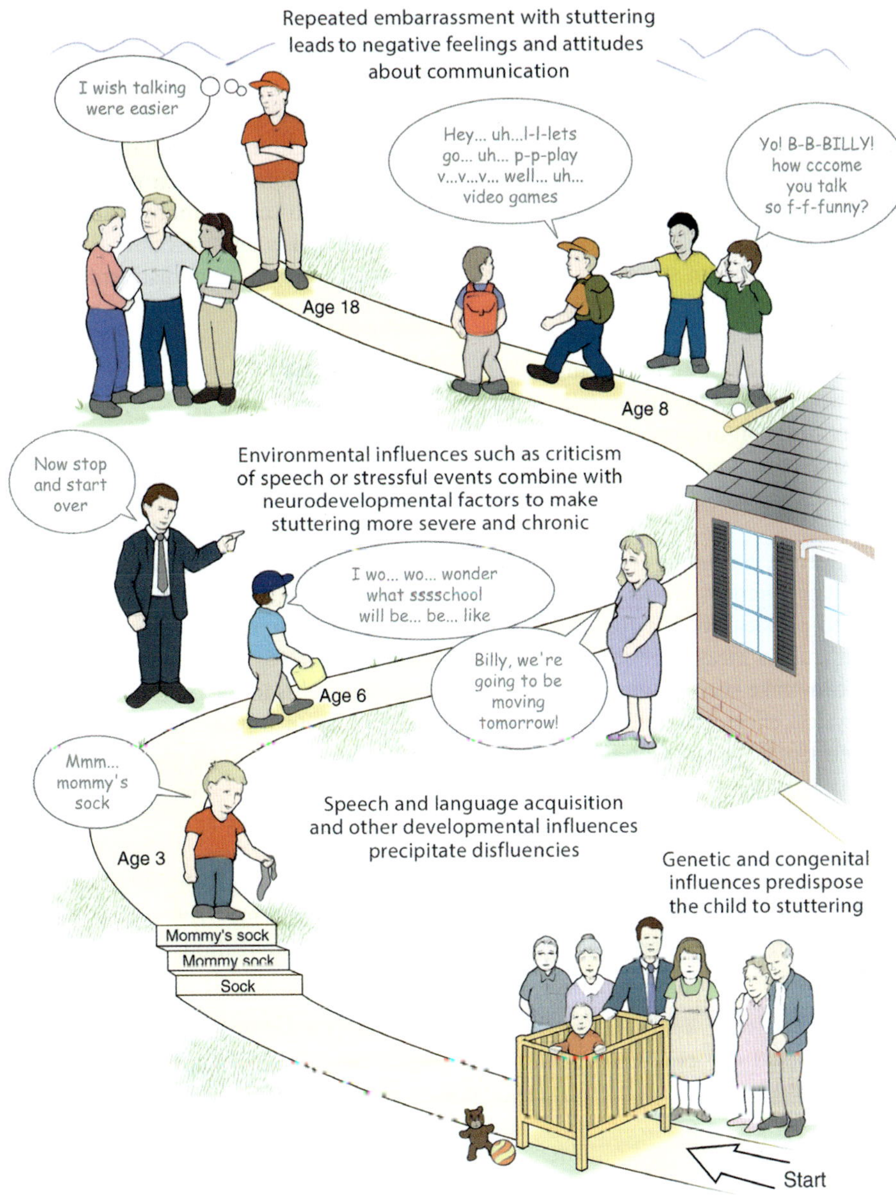

Figure 1.1 Factors contributing to the development of stuttering

DEFINITIONS

Fluency

By beginning with a definition of fluency rather than stuttering, I am pointing out how many elements must be maintained in the flow of speech if a speaker is to be considered fluent. It is an impressive balancing act. Little wonder that everyone slips and stumbles from time to time when they talk. Although it's incorrect to say that everyone stutters, every fluent person will still experience times when they are more or less smooth, or fluent, in their speech production.

Fluency is hard to define. In fact, most researchers have focused on its opposite, disfluency. (As I mentioned earlier in this chapter, I use the term disfluency to apply both to stuttering and to typical hesitations, making it easier to refer to hesitations that could be either typical or abnormal.) One of the early fluency researchers, Goldman-Eisler (1968), showed that typical speech is filled with hesitations. Other researchers have acknowledged this and expanded the study of fluent speech by contrasting it with disfluent speech. Dalton and Hardcastle (1977), for example, distinguished fluent from disfluent speech by differences between the two: the presence of extra sounds, location and frequency of pauses, the rhythmic pattern of speech, intonation and stress in speech, and rate of speech. Inclusion of intonation and stress in this list may seem unusual. It could be said that speakers who reduce stuttering by using a monotone are not really fluent. We would argue that it is not their fluency but the "naturalness" of their speech that is affected. Nonetheless, both aspects will be of interest to the clinician working to help clients with all areas of their communication.

Starkweather (1980, 1987) suggested that many of the variables that determine fluency reflect temporal aspects of speech production. These include such variables as pauses, rhythm, intonation, stress, and rate that are controlled by when and how fast we move our speech structures. So, our temporal control of the movements of these structures determines our fluency. Starkweather also noted that the rate of information flow, not just sound flow, is an important aspect of fluency. Thus, a person who speaks without hesitations but has difficulty conveying information in a timely and orderly fashion might not be considered a fluent speaker. For example, they may have a disorder known as cluttering, which will be described in Chapter 8.

In his description of fluency, Starkweather (1987) also included the effort with which a person speaks. By effort, he means both the mental and physical work a speaker exerts when speaking. This is difficult to measure, but it may turn out that trained listeners can make such judgments reliably. Moreover, mental and physical effort may reflect important components of what it feels like to be a person who stutters (Tichenor & Yaruss, 2019).

The American Speech-Language-Hearing Association adds the dimensions of "continuity" and "smoothness" to the list of variables mentioned previously (www.ASHA.org/practice). Once you're on the practice page, click "enter the practice portal," then see a link on the left side of the page that says "clinical topics." Once there, choose "fluency disorders" and you'll find a description of fluency. The term "continuity" suggests speech that is flowing without interruptions by irrelevant elements. "Smoothness" also suggests that speech flows like a calm river. I will discuss aspects of fluency again when I relate some of the elements of fluency, such as rate and naturalness, to various therapy approaches.

Table 1.1 lists and describes the important variables that distinguish fluency from disfluency.

Stuttering

General Description

At first, stuttering may appear to be complex and mysterious, but much of it is based on human nature and can be easily understood if you think about your own experiences. In some ways, it is like a problem you might have with a cell phone.

Imagine that you have a cell phone with intermittent problems, such as not holding a charge, dropping calls, and dropping words in the middle of a conversation. The listener may say, in an impatient voice, "What did you say? I can hardly hear you." Then momentarily the connection may clear up and you feel relief, only to be followed by exasperation when the call gets noisy again or is completely dropped (Fig. 1.2).

Compare this with the interruptions in communication caused by stuttering. The typical behaviors of stuttering—repetitions, prolongations, and blocks—often interfere with

TABLE 1.1 Characteristics of Fluent Speech compared to Disfluent Speech in Speech Disorders (ie, Stuttering)

Variable	Characteristic of Fluent Speech	Characteristic of Disfluent Speech in Fluency Disorders
Continuity	Smooth and continuous production of intended (expected) words, without inappropriate pauses or other interruptions.	Choppy flow of speech, marred by (1) inappropriate pauses; (2) repetitions of sounds, syllables, words, or phrases; (3) prolongations of sounds; and/or (4) moments of being unable to finish words that were started (blocks).
Effort	Ordinary, expected movements to produce speech that do not distract from the message.	Moments when the exertion or struggle of speaking interrupts the smooth flow of speech and may distract from the message.
Rate	Speed of speaking that accommodates listener comprehension, meets expectations, and sounds natural.	Speaking too fast, especially in bursts (this may be more common in the disorder of "cluttering" than in developmental stuttering) or speaking too slowly in an unnatural way that may be the speaker's attempt to avoid stuttering.
Rhythm	Speaking with the stress pattern, which is natural to the language being. English, for example, is a stress-timed language so that key words in a sentence get stress and others don't.	Speaking in a monotone so that each word has equal stress. This may be a way in which the speaker avoids stuttering, but it distracts from the speaker's message.

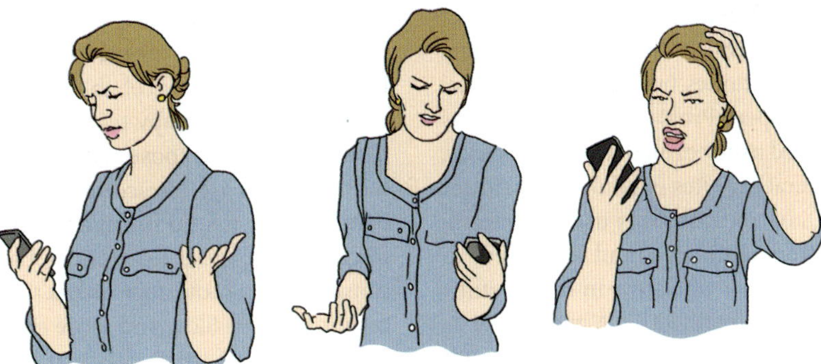

Figure 1.2 Stuttering can be like having a cell phone that doesn't always work.

the smooth flow of information and effective communication. It's not unusual, in my experience, for a listener to respond to my stuttering by asking, "What did you say?"

Returning to the cell phone analogy: When you realize the listener isn't hearing you, you might resort to talking louder or slower or just giving up and calling back later. Similarly, speakers who are stuttering usually react to their repetitions, prolongations, or blocks by trying to force words out or by using extra sounds, words, or movements in their efforts to become "unstuck" or to avoid getting stuck. Sometimes they just give up and say "Never mind."

If your cell phone calls were often hard to understand and calls were often dropped, you would probably develop some bad feelings about your phone. The first time it happened, you would be surprised. Then, as it happened more and more, surprise would give way to frustration. If you frequently had poor connections, dropped calls, and not holding a charge, you would begin to anticipate problems and become afraid they would happen whenever you tried to make an important call.

People who stutter go through many of the same feelings—surprise, frustration, dread. These feelings—in combination with the actual difficulty in speaking—may cause people who stutter to limit themselves in school, in social situations, and at work. This might be similar to your responses to a troublesome cell phone. After months of problems, you would probably use a landline, e-mail, or other forms of communication. You at least have the option of buying a new phone—an option not enjoyed by the person who stutters.

Another aspect of any description of stuttering involves specifying what it is not. For example, an important distinction must be made between the stuttering behaviors just described and typical hesitations. Children whose speech and language are developing typically often display repetitions, revisions, and pauses—which are not stuttering. Neither are the brief repetitions, revisions, and pauses in the speech of most nonstuttering adults when they are in a hurry or uncertain. Chapter 7 describes the differences between typical disfluency and stuttering in more detail to prepare you for the task of differential diagnosis of stuttering in children.

A distinction should also be made between stuttering and certain other fluency disorders. Disfluency resulting from brain damage or disease or psychological trauma differs from stuttering that begins in childhood. In addition, stuttering differs from cluttering, another fluency disorder, which is characterized by speech that seems rapid and is often unintelligible, often with more typical than stuttering-like disfluencies and words that seem underarticulated (Scaler Scott, 2020). These other fluency disorders may be treated somewhat differently than stuttering, although some of the same techniques that clinicians use with stuttering are also useful with these disorders. These other disorders are discussed in Chapter 8.

Core Behaviors

I have adopted the term "**core behaviors**" from Van Riper (1971, 1982a), who used it to describe the basic speech behaviors of stuttering: repetitions, prolongations, and blocks. In most cases I have observed, repetitions and prolongations are the first signs of stuttering, and blocks usually, but not always, appear later.

Repetitions are the core behaviors observed most frequently among children who are just beginning to stutter. Repetitions consist of a sound, syllable, or single-syllable word that is repeated several times. The speaker is apparently "stuck" on that sound and continues repeating it until the following sound or syllable or word can be produced. In children who have not been stuttering for long, single-syllable word repetitions and part-word repetitions are much more common than multisyllabic word repetitions. Moreover, children who stutter will frequently repeat a word or syllable more than twice per instance, li-li-li-li-like this (Bloodstein et al., 2021; Yairi, 1983; Yairi & Lewis, 1984). You can see a very vivid example of this in a 2-and-a-half-year-old child named Ashley, described in the Case Examples section at the end of this chapter and shown in a video clip available on Lippincott Connect. After starting with a repetition of the sound "da," Ashley tries to say the cat's name "Cookie." Watch her start to say it and then become mired down in endless repetitions of the first syllable "Co-". She then gives up and just finishes with "...knocked the plant down."

Prolongations of voiced or voiceless sounds also appear in the speech of children beginning to stutter. They usually appear somewhat later than repetitions (Van Riper, 1982b), although both Johnson et al. (1959) and Yairi (1997a) reported that prolongations—as well as repetitions—may be present at onset. I use the term prolongation to denote those stutters in which sound or air flow continues but movement of the articulators appears to be stopped. Prolongations as short as half a second may be perceived as abnormal, but in rare cases, they may last as long as several minutes in adults who stutter severely (Van Riper, 1982b). In contrast to my use of the term, earlier writers include stutters with no sound or airflow as well as stopped movement of the articulators in their definitions of prolongations (eg, Van Riper, 1982a; Wingate, 1964).

Repetitions and sound prolongations are usually part of the core behaviors of more advanced stutterers, as well as of children just beginning to stutter. Sheehan (1974) found that repetitive stutters occurred in every speech sample of 20 adults who stuttered. Indeed, 66% of their stutters were repetitions. Although many of their stutters were also prolongations, as defined above, how many is not clear, because Sheehan's definition of prolongations seems to differ from mine.

Blocks are typically the last core behavior to appear. However, as with prolongations, some investigators (Johnson et al., 1959; Van Riper, 1982b; Yairi, 1997a) have observed blocks in children's speech at or close to stuttering onset. Blocks occur when a person inappropriately stops the flow of air or voice and often the movement of their articulators as well. As I suggested earlier, blocks may be a learned behavior. As I describe in the chapter on learning (Chapter 5) blocks result from physical tension. This tension (a co-contraction of muscles paired to result in smooth movement) can be a response to the fear that a child or adult may experience when they anticipate or experience the terrifying feeling of not being able to control what is happening to their mouth when they try to speak. Because blocks are mostly learned, they can be unlearned. However, because blocks are often learned under conditions of high emotion, they may be somewhat resistant to unlearning. Blocks may involve tension at any level of the speech production mechanism—respiratory, laryngeal, or articulatory. There is some evidence and much theorizing that inappropriate muscle activity at the laryngeal level characterizes many blocks (Conture et al., 1977; Freeman & Ushijima, 1978; Kenyon, 1942; Schwartz, 1974). Others disagree (Smith et al., 1996).

As stuttering persists, blocks often grow longer and more tense, and tremors may become evident. These rapid tremor oscillations, most easily observable in the lips or jaw, occur when a stutterer has blocked on a word or sound. The individual closes off the airway, increases air pressure behind the closure, and squeezes their muscles particularly hard (Van Riper, 1982b). You can duplicate these tremors by trying to say the word "by" while squeezing your lips together hard, not letting the sound out, and building up air pressure behind the block.[1] Imagine this happening to you unexpectedly while you were trying to talk.

Blocks are rewarded by the feeling of relief (whew!) experienced by the speaker when the word finally pops out. Because blocks are probably learned, I strongly advocate—when I discuss therapy techniques—that stutterers end their blocks slowly and loosely. This has two effects. (1) Slow and loose endings are rewarded by the good feeling that accompanies being able to finish a word. The reward increases the frequency of these slow and loose endings, and may even cause them to move forward in time, creating slow and loose beginnings. (2) Slow and loose endings help you feel like you are in charge of your speech at the end of a stutter, and this reduces the fear you feel as you approach a stutter because you expect to show the stutter that you are the boss.

People who stutter differ from one another in how frequently they stutter and how long their individual core behaviors last. Research indicates that a person who stutters does so on average on about 10% of the words while reading aloud, although individuals vary greatly (Bloodstein et al., 2021). Many people who stutter mildly do so on fewer than 5% of the words they speak or read aloud, and a few with severe stuttering stutter on more than 50% of the words. The durations of core behaviors vary much less, averaging around 1 second, and are rarely longer than 5 seconds (Bloodstein et al., 2021).

Secondary Behaviors

People who stutter dislike stuttering, to put it mildly. They react to their repetitions, prolongations, and blocks by trying to end them quickly if they can't avoid them altogether. Such reactions may begin as a random struggle to get the word out, but soon turn into well-learned patterns. I divide **secondary behaviors** into two broad classes: escape behaviors and avoidance behaviors. I make this division, rather than follow the traditional approach of dealing with secondary behaviors as "starters" or "postponements," for example, because my treatment procedures focus on the principles by which secondary behaviors are learned.

The terms "escape" and "avoidance" are borrowed from behavioral learning literature. Briefly, **escape behaviors** occur *when a speaker is stuttering and attempts to terminate the stutter* and finish the word. Common examples of escape behaviors are eye blinks, head nods, and interjections of extra sounds, such as "uh," which are often followed by the termination of a stutter and are, therefore, reinforced. ***Avoidance behaviors***, on the other hand, *are learned when speakers anticipate stuttering and do something to try to keep from stuttering.* To avoid stuttering and the negative experience that it entails, they often resort to behaviors they have used previously to escape from moments of stuttering—eye blinks or fillers like "uh," for example. But they employ these behaviors before attempting to say the word that they expect to stutter on. Or, they may try something different, such as changing the word they were planning to say.

In many cases, especially at first, avoidance behaviors may prevent the stutter from occurring and provide highly rewarding emotional relief from the increasing fear that a

[1]If you can't get a tremor going by squeezing your lips, try pushing your index finger down on your desk as hard as you can. Your finger should "jiggle" in a tremor when you are pushing really hard.

stutter will occur.[2] Soon these avoidance behaviors become strong habits that are resistant to change. The many subcategories of avoidances (eg, postponements, starters, substitutions, and timing devices such as hand movements timed to saying the word) are described in Chapter 7.

When trying to decide if a secondary behavior is an escape or avoidance, just remember that an escape behavior occurs only after a moment of stuttering has begun, and an avoidance behavior occurs before the moment of stuttering begins.

Feelings and Attitudes

Individuals' feelings are usually as much a part of the disorder of stuttering as their speech behaviors. Feelings may precipitate stutters, just as stutters may create feelings. In the beginning, children's positive feelings of excitement (eg, at seeing a grandmother they haven't seen in many months) or negative feelings of fear (like fear of a big dog) may result in repetitive stutters that they hardly notice. Then, as they stutter more frequently, they may become frustrated or ashamed because they can't say what they want to say—even their own name—as smoothly and quickly as others. These feelings—which are associated with stuttering itself—make speaking harder, as frustration and shame may increase physical tension and impede fluent speech. Feelings that result from stuttering may include not only frustration and shame but also anticipatory fear of stuttering again, guilt about not being able to help oneself, and hostility toward listeners as well.

Attitudes are feelings that have become a pervasive part of a person's beliefs. As people who stutter experience more and more stuttering, they begin to believe that they generally have trouble speaking, just as you might believe that cell phone or your cell phone service is a lemon if you continue to have trouble calling. Adolescents and adults who stutter usually have many negative attitudes about themselves that are derived from years of stuttering experiences (Blood et al., 2001; Daniels et al., 2012; Gildston, 1967; Rahman, 1956; Rodgers et al., 2020; Wallen, 1960). After reviewing many years' worth of studies, Bloodstein et al. (2021) indicate that even very young children may have negative attitudes toward communication and these attitudes become even more negative in stutterers as they grow and have more negative experiences.

Stutterers often project their attitudes on listeners, believing that listeners think they are stupid or nervous. Often this is understandable: a history of listeners' negative reactions may contribute directly to speakers' attitudes. Research has shown that most people, even classroom teachers and speech-language pathologists, stereotype people who stutter as tense, insecure, and fearful (eg, Boyle, 2017; MacKinnon et al., 2007; Turnbaugh et al., 1979; Walden & Lesner, 2018; Woods & Williams, 1976). Such listener stereotypes can affect the way individuals who stutter see themselves, which can make helping clients revise their negative attitudes about themselves a major focus of treatment.

The three components of stuttering—core behaviors, secondary behaviors, and feelings and attitudes—are depicted in Figure 1.3. The core behavior is the individual's block on the "N" in "New York." The secondary behaviors consist of postponement devices such as "uh," "well," and "you know" and substitution of "the Big Apple" for "New York." These secondary behaviors are avoidances. Feelings and attitudes are depicted as the individual's thoughts that they won't succeed in saying the word fluently and the individual's belief that listeners will think they are dumb because they stutter.

Functioning, Disability, and Health

Some time ago, the World Health Organization (WHO, 1980) adopted the International Classification of Impairment, Disabilities, and Handicaps to describe the consequences of various diseases and disorders. A number of authors have applied this framework to stuttering (Curlee, 1993; McClean, 1990; Prins, 1991, 1999; Yaruss, 1998, 1999). More than a decade ago, WHO changed its taxonomy to the International Classification of Functioning, Disability, and Health (ICF) (2001). Even more recently, they have devised a version that is specific to children and youth—the ICF-CY (WHO, 2007). In the following paragraphs, I will suggest ways in which this system may be applied to stuttering.

The taxonomy begins with "Functioning and Disability," wherein body structures and body functions are considered. Structures that are dysfunctional in stuttering, as brain imaging studies have shown, are cortical and subcortical structures, such as white matter tracts that may be critical for coordinating planning, execution, and sensory feedback for speech. Functions that differ in stuttering are the dysfunctions in the smooth flow of speech that characterize the disorder. The ICF system becomes more useful when "Activity and Participation" are considered. Individuals who stutter may be affected to a greater or lesser extent in two of the ICF activity areas, "Speaking" and "Conversation." These are domains in which stuttering is noticeable. A third area, "Interpersonal Interactions," may also be affected if speaking and conversation are restricted by the stuttering to the extent that the person who stutters refrains from fully engaging with others, thereby affecting their participation in different social roles (eg, being a student or a family member).

A new and important section of the latest ICF system is titled "Contextual Factors." One component of this section is the "Environment." This is particularly relevant to individuals who stutter because people in the environment may range from unsupportive (eg, a home with great stress or classmates who tease a child) to highly supportive (eg, a family that is accepting of the child and encouraging of their participation). Also, under "Contextual Factors" is the category of "Personal Factors." These are the attributes of a person who stutters—their character and personality.

---

[2]Some stutterers become so skilled at avoiding that they seem never to stutter and develop what has been called "covert stuttering." In other words, they are stutterers, but they never stutter because they avoid so much.

Core Behavior
"I WENT TO
N.... N.... NEW YORK"
Secondary Behavior
"I WENT TO.... UH....
WELL.... YOU KNOW....
UH.... UH....
THE BIG APPLE"
Feelings and Attitudes
"Where did you go
last weekend?"
Oh no, I'll never
get this word out.
She'll think I'm
really dumb.

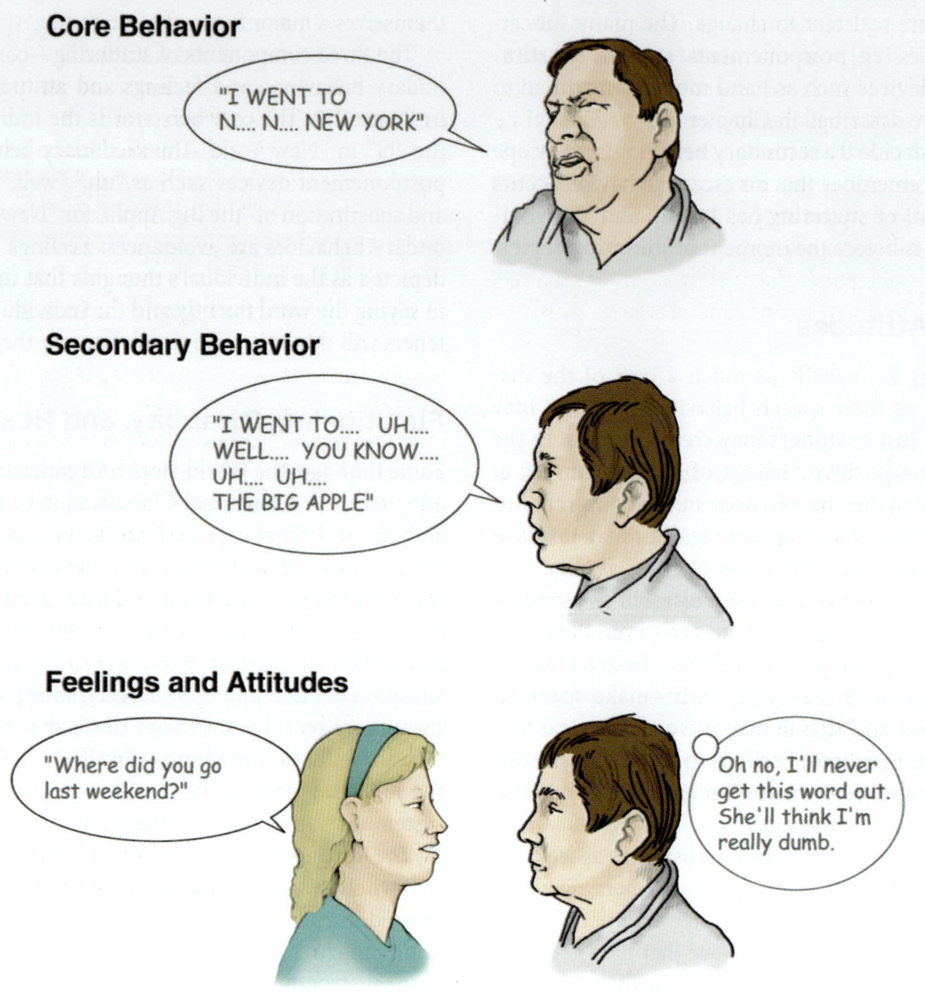

Figure 1.3 Components of stuttering: core behaviors, secondary behaviors, and feelings and attitudes.

Consider the influence of environmental and personal factors on two individuals who stutter. The first is the successful former CEO of General Electric, Jack Welch, who authored *Jack: Straight from the Gut.* His assertive temperament and early acceptance of his stuttering by his family were no doubt important in helping him succeed in the high-pressure world of corporate boardrooms. From an early age, Welch refused to let stuttering stand in the way of his goals (Welch & Byrne, 2001). In contrast, actor James Earl Jones initially reacted to his stuttering in a vastly different way. When he was 6 years old, he was so traumatized by his stuttering that he pretended he was mute so he wouldn't have to speak. Only later, with the support of someone in his environment—a high school English teacher—did he begin to learn that he could overcome his stuttering by facing difficult situations and practicing reading aloud in front of an audience (Jones & Niven, 1993).

Other examples of men who had stuttered severely since childhood but obtained excellent college educations, were highly successful in business, and used their wealth to help others include Malcolm Fraser, who was a cofounder of the National Auto Parts Association and created the Stuttering Foundation of America, and Walter Annenberg, who established a media empire and later the Annenberg Foundation, a large philanthropic organization.

In all four cases, their functioning may have been impaired, but environmental and personal factors enabled them to overcome potential limitations in the domains of speaking and interpersonal interactions. You can see in this classification system why clinicians play a vital role in the lives of children and adults who stutter. They can influence environmental factors by helping families, teachers, and entire schools become supportive of the individuals who stutter and facilitative of increased fluency. And they can help build the personal attributes of each client through counseling, insightful listening, educating, and caring.

Perhaps the most famous face of stuttering since the 2020 U.S. election is President Joe Biden. In an insightful article about Biden, journalist John Hendrickson (2020) described Biden's verbal ducks and dodges because of stuttering in debates and campaign speeches, often mistaken for mental lapses, such as when Biden couldn't say Obama's name and substituted "my boss" which the media trumpeted as "Biden Forgets Obama's Name." In an interview with Biden, Hendrickson learned of Biden's more severe stuttering in high school and his successful self-therapy, reading aloud while using a mirror in the privacy of his bedroom. Biden, as president, has gained strength as an inspiring speaker. He has commented that the renowned empathy he shows to Americans and to people all over the world is a result of his stuttering. He says that the struggle he has had with his speech has provided him with the ability to understand others' pain.

THE HUMAN FACE OF STUTTERING

Before I delve deeper into the basic facts about stuttering, I'd like to touch briefly on the personal side of the problem. Some of you may never have had a friend or acquaintance who stutters or may never have worked with a stutterer in treatment, so I will present several examples of what stuttering can be like. Even if you are familiar with stuttering, these brief sketches, which portray four individuals who differ in age and in their accommodations to stuttering, may expand your sense of what stuttering is like for the person who experiences it. I will present these case studies in the next few pages. You may also visit *Lippincott Connect* to watch video clips of these different levels of stuttering.

BASIC FACTS ABOUT STUTTERING AND THEIR IMPLICATIONS FOR THE NATURE OF STUTTERING

This section relates some of the best-known "facts" about stuttering. These are established research findings that pertain to when and where stuttering occurs and how variable it is, in the population and in individuals. As I discuss these findings, I will point out what they suggest about the nature of stuttering. Thus, as you read the rest of this chapter, you will become increasingly aware of my perspective on the nature and treatment of stuttering.

Much has been made of the "**heterogeneity**" of stuttering. A number of authors have suggested that stuttering is not one disorder, but many. Researchers have proposed various divisions of the disorder, such as Van Riper's (1982) four "tracks" of stuttering development and St. Onge's (1963) triad of speech-phobic, psychogenic, and organic stutterers. There are also suggestions of different brain anomalies in some subtypes of individuals who stutter (eg, Ajdacic-Gross et al., 2018; Foundas et al., 2004). My approach is to focus on the majority of people who stutter—those whose stuttering begins during childhood without an apparent link to psychological or organic trauma. This most common type of stuttering has been called "**developmental stuttering**," because symptoms usually emerge gradually as a child develops, especially during the period of intense speech and language acquisition. I simply call it "stuttering." In denoting similar fluency problems that are associated with psychological issues, brain damage, cognitive impairment, and cluttering, I refer to their assumed etiology, such as "disfluencies associated with brain damage."

Note, however, that even within the group of individuals whose stuttering begins in early childhood during rapid speech and language development, there is a great deal of variability in the behaviors we call stuttering and in how these behaviors come and go as the child progresses toward persistence or recovery.

Onset

Imagine yourself in your doctor's office with an annoying cold that just won't go away—runny nose, sore throat, and cough. She asks you to describe when the first signs of your illness

Case Examples

A Young Preschool Child: Borderline Stuttering

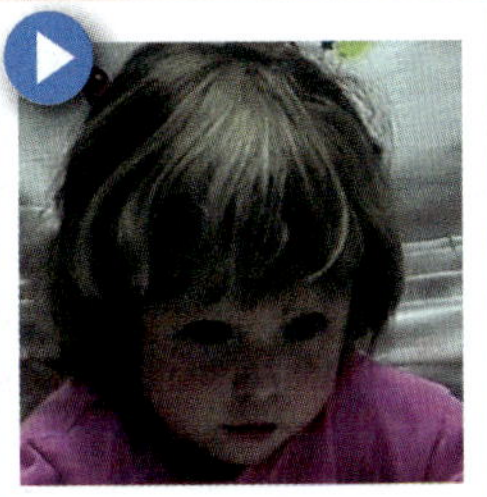

Ashley was a happy, outgoing child who was advanced in her language development; she spoke in well-formed sentences when she was 18 months old. Then suddenly, when she was 21 months old, she began to stutter. Her stuttering took the form of multiple repetitions, most often at the beginnings of sentences. For example, she would say "I-I-I-I want some water" or "Ca-ca-ca-ca-can you lift me up?" Despite the fact that she would sometimes repeat a syllable 10 or more times before getting the word out, she didn't show obvious signs of frustration when she stuttered. She continued to develop language rapidly, talk copiously, and socialize easily.

About 6 months after she started stuttering, her parents contacted a speech-language pathologist who evaluated Ashley. The evaluation indicated that Ashley's language development was advanced for her age, that her phonological development was also advanced, and that she stuttered on 4% of the syllables she spoke. (This means that when a few minutes of her speech were analyzed and the number of syllables she spoke was counted, Ashley stuttered on 4% of those syllables.)

continued

Ashley's parents told the clinician that they had no idea why Ashley started stuttering. She was happy, secure, and talkative; no big event occurred around the time of stuttering onset; and she didn't have any relatives who stuttered.

For a description of Ashley's treatment and its outcome, turn to Chapter 11.

Discussion

The two segments in this video show Ashley talking about a picture (a cat named Cookie knocking a plant off a shelf) that the clinician has previously described to her. In the first segment, the clinician elicits Ashley's response by asking "What happened to Cookie, again?" Ashley's response is "Cat....nn... de-de-de .... Coo-Coo-[approximately 15 repetitions of this syllable and then she gives up trying to say the cat's name]....knocked the plant down." In the second segment, the clinician says "Let's take another one. Tell me. Remember?" Ashley replies "Then Coo-Coo-Coo-Coo-Cookie knocked the plant down."

These segments are a pretty good illustration of what stuttering can be like when it first starts in a preschool child. What are the primary core behaviors that Ashley shows? Repetitions? Prolongations? Blocks?

When we are trying to determine whether a child needs immediate and direct treatment for stuttering, it is often helpful to assess the child's emotional reaction to her stuttering. Can you tell from the video whether Ashley is frustrated or embarrassed by her stuttering? What do you see in the video that gives you clues about this?

An Older Preschool Child: Beginning Stuttering

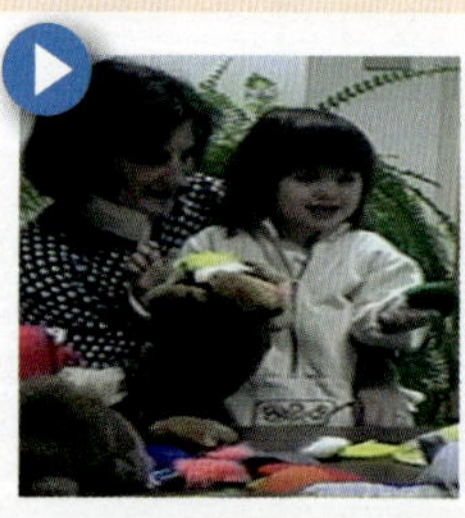

Katherine developed speech and language normally, speaking her first word at about 1 year and beginning to combine words at 15 months with complete fluency. When she was 3, after a particularly hectic Christmas holiday, she began to stutter. Her first disfluencies were easy part- and whole-word repetitions, but she soon began to tense her articulators, momentarily blocking the flow of speech until the word "popped out." Sometimes, when she was completely stuck for several seconds, she responded by hitting her parents or crying out. She also showed much less interest in talking and using new words and phrases.

Her parents soon brought her to a speech and language clinic for an evaluation. Katherine was found to be stuttering on 21% of the syllables she spoke—a very high percentage for any child. Her overall severity was assessed with the Stuttering Severity Instrument (Riley, 1994), which rated it as severe. Her receptive language was found to be far above average for her age. Her expressive language was found to be typical for her age, but it was likely that she was inhibited in expressing herself because of her stuttering. Her phonological development was found to be appropriate for her age.

For a description of Katherine's treatment, see Chapter 12.

Discussion

In Segment 1, Katherine responds to a question from her mother by saying "O-O-O-O...an...an...an...OK now...I think he is still hungry...[unintelligible]...a leaf." This may be an example of a child getting stuck on an attempt to say a word ("OK") and then, finding herself in a block, changing the word she tries to say (from "OK" to "and"). Then she is able to say the original word and go on.

In Segment 2, still with her mother, she is stuck on the first sound of the word "OK," then she seems to be able to move on to the "kay" but gets stuck there too, and so she doubles back to the "o" and finally finishes the word by pushing out of the stutter on "o" and then having a slight stutter on the first sound of "kay." Whew! You can see how much work this 3-year-old must do just to get a few words out. No wonder she doesn't seem as expressive as she did before her stuttering started.

In Segment 3, Katherine is playing with the clinician and says, "uh...nnnnn...ne...ne...nnnn...na...now, what is this?" The "uh" might be Katherine's way of getting ready for the stutter she anticipates on "now."

In Segment 4, Katherine is playing with both of her parents and says "Lo-look what I made. Oh... uh...bbbbb...buh...bbbbb...buh..." The first stutter is a part-word repetition ("lo-look") that is so mild it might be considered a typical disfluency in another context. But the second stutter (on a word beginning with "b") is quite a long stutter in which Katherine struggles heroically to produce the word but is interrupted by the door opening before she can finish. How would you describe this last stutter? Repetition? Prolongation? Block? What emotions do you think she's feeling? Why do you think so?

continued

A School-Age Child: Intermediate Stuttering

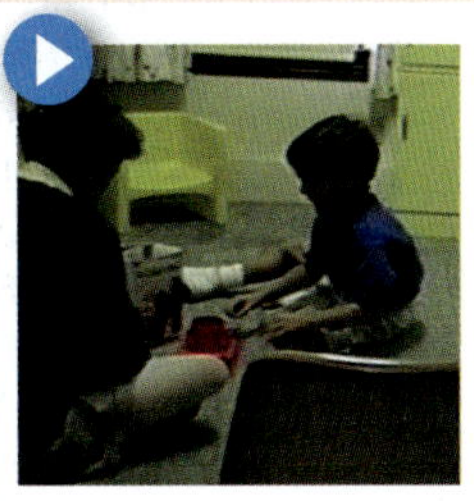

David was the second of three children in a family with no history of speech or language disorders. His speech was developing normally until age 4, when he began to show excessive part-word and whole-word repetitions. After several months, when David's stuttering had not decreased, his mother took him to his pediatrician who assured her it would resolve on its own.

When David was almost 6, his stuttering was growing steadily more severe, and he was avoiding talking in many situations. His mother then decided to consult a speech-language pathologist at a university clinic, who evaluated David. In the evaluation, David was stuttering on 8% of his syllables spoken; many stutters were tightly squeezed blocks with evident struggle behavior.

David's subsequent treatment and his current status as a 20-something-year-old are described in Chapter 13.

Discussion

In this video, you can see how stuttering may be more complicated as children grow older and become more self-conscious. In the video for the first child, Ashley's moments of stuttering seemed to pop up out of the blue and surprise her. In the video for the second child, Katherine's stuttering was a little more predictable to her, but it was mostly confined to those few words on which she got blocked. Now we will see that David's stuttering affects more of his entire speech pattern and is characterized by much avoidance and struggle.

In Segment 1, showing him talking with his mother, David's style of speaking is hesitant, with many stops, "ums," false starts, and changes in direction. He says something like "and then...it like that...and then...then put...um the same a-mount of...of...of...of ...um... [then some unintelligible words, after which he seems to give up on the sentence and begins counting]." As you can imagine, it's hard to assess what percentage of syllables are stuttered when David avoids saying the words on which he expects to stutter.

Segment 2 shows a block on the word "whoever," preceded by several words that seem to postpone David's attempt on this word. He says "and then ...uh ...whoever gets um ...um the four, four... an, an ... um ... um these [unintelligible word]." Do you think he expects to stutter on "whoever?" What are the cues that tell you so? What escape behaviors does David use as he struggles with this block?

In Segment 3, David has another block with a few avoidance behaviors before the stutter and escape behaviors during it. He says "He ... [unintelligible word] ... he goes home automatically because ... um ... because he-he has done the shortcut an-an he goes all the way home." Can you describe the avoidance and escape behaviors David shows in this clip?

An Adult: Advanced Stuttering

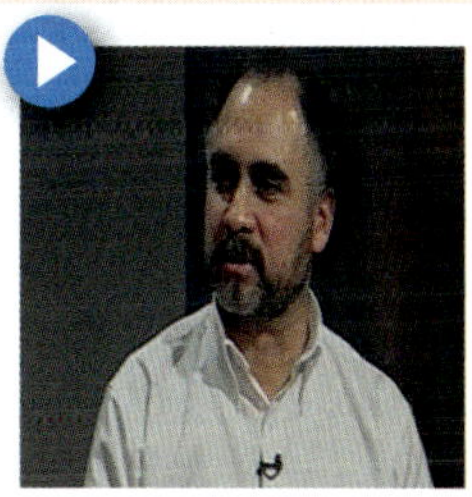

Sergio is a 44-year-old musician who has stuttered since he was 3 years old. Eight of his maternal aunts and uncles stuttered, suggesting a genetic origin to his problem. His stuttering began as multiple repetitions of one-syllable words and parts of words. Much of his speech was fluent, but whenever he was excited or hurried, Sergio's stuttering flared up, sending his parents into a state of alarm and concern for his future. At first, his father's solution for Sergio's stuttering was hitting him on the head with his knuckles when he blocked. When this failed and Sergio developed physically tense prolongations and blocks that occurred regularly in his speech, his parents took him to various therapists, including a hypnotist and a psychotherapist who prescribed tranquilizers. None of these seemed to have more than a temporary effect, and Sergio's stuttering grew steadily worse. During his elementary and junior high school years, he was frequently ridiculed for his stuttering, even by teachers, and Sergio found himself an outcast among his peers.

This changed, however, soon after "Beatlemania" swept through America. Sergio bought a guitar and taught himself to sing "I Want to Hold Your Hand" and other Beatles songs. As a result, his popularity with schoolmates shot up, even though his stuttering continued to worsen. He had so much difficulty speaking in class, and his teachers were so unsympathetic, that he finally dropped out of school and pursued a vagabond lifestyle as a singer and songwriter.

As he traveled, working various jobs by day and singing at night, Sergio continued to stutter severely, with one happy exception. When he was performing with his band, not only did he sing fluently, but he also spoke to the audience easily, announcing each number and making casual, funny comments

continued

between songs. As a result of his constant battle with stuttering, Sergio developed a wide variety of avoidances. He dodged making phone calls, and whenever he received calls, he used elaborate facial grimaces and starter sounds to fight his way through stutters.

Discussion

The telephone is a difficult situation for most people who stutter, and Sergio is no exception. Segment 1 shows Sergio talking about his past experiences on the phone when he had long silent blocks, and Segment 2 is a phone call Sergio made more recently. On both clips you'll see a mix of avoidance and escape behaviors that are now well entrenched in Sergio's speech pattern after years of stuttering. There are also some straightforward stutters without escape and avoidance behaviors that are witness to Sergio's attempts to stutter in a simpler way. See if you can identify the types of stutters that Sergio has on both segments, as well as his particular escape and avoidance behaviors, more of which are seen in Segment 2.

appeared and what they were like at onset. It is quite likely you won't remember exactly when your symptoms first occurred and exactly what they were like, especially if they came and went over the course of a week or two before they became persistent. This is the problem with determining the onset of stuttering. Parents are asked to recall exactly when the child's stuttering started and what it was like when they first noticed it; thus, some of our information on onset—especially from older studies—may be inaccurate. The description of stuttering onset given here is relatively brief. More details are given in Chapter 7 when I describe the differences between typical disfluency and the beginning stages of stuttering.

Let's first consider the question of how old children are, on average, when they begin to stutter. In the earliest studies (eg, Milisen & Johnson, 1936), researchers asked parents a year or more after the onset of stuttering had occurred to recall the age of stuttering onset in their children. The average age of onset, taken from nine pre-1990 studies summarized in Bloodstein et al. (2021), was roughly 4 years. After 1990, led by Ehud Yairi and his colleagues at the University of Illinois, researchers were careful to interview parents of children who began to stutter within the previous 12 months. In other words, they only included children whose stuttering had begun no more than a year before, so that parents' memories would be relatively fresh. Bloodstein et al. (2021) list six studies conducted after 1990 in which parents were interviewed closer to onset than in earlier studies. The average age of onset in these newer studies is about 33 months (2 years, 9 months). Thus, the newer studies are getting a more accurate picture of the age of onset, the age of onset is getting younger, or both. The current consensus is that the onset of stuttering typically occurs just before age 3, and most onsets occur between ages 2 and 3.5 years (Bloodstein et al., 2021; Yairi & Ambrose, 2005, 2013). Some older children—up to about age 12—may begin to stutter, but these are much rarer cases. Stuttering onset in adolescents and adults is likely to be a different form of disfluency—psychogenic or neurogenic—that I will discuss in Chapter 8, "Atypical Disfluency."

Next, let's look at the first signs of stuttering, as reported by parents. Most early reports of stuttering onset (eg, Bluemel, 1932) indicated that simple, relaxed repetitions of syllables and words were the typical first signs of stuttering. However, some early studies (eg, Taylor, 1937) and the carefully conducted interviews by Yairi (1983) found that, in many cases, parents described prolongations and blocks, along with signs of struggle, as the first stutters shown by their child. Yairi and Ambrose (2013) suggest that syllable and single-syllable word repetitions are by far the most common behavior that parents report as the first signs of stuttering. No matter what the first signs of stuttering are, excessive numbers of syllable repetitions seem to be a universal indicator of the presence of stuttering in a child. It is generally agreed that if children have more than 2 syllable repetitions per instance of disfluency, it is a sign that they may be stuttering (Yairi & Ambrose, 2005). Here is an example of clearly excessive syllable repetitions: "I-I-I-I-I-I-I don't want that."

Last, there is the question of whether onset is sudden, intermediate, or gradual. In other words, do parents notice very evident disfluencies seen in the course of a day or two, or do they realize only after several weeks of milder disfluencies that their child is having a problem? Remember our example of getting a cold and trying to remember the onset? No doubt some colds come on suddenly, with sore throat and runny nose appearing overnight and getting worse quickly. Other colds tiptoe into your life, with a sore throat that comes and goes and later turns into a runny nose and cough.

In contrast to the earliest reports on stuttering always having a gradual onset, Yairi and Ambrose (2005) found in their sample of 163 children many cases (41%) in which onset was reported to be sudden, with another group (32%) reported as intermediate, and a third group (27%) as gradual. Studies by Buck et al. (2002) and by Reilly et al. (2009) also found that about 50% of parents reported a sudden onset of their child's stuttering. These figures may be influenced by how attentive to their child's speech these parents were. Almost certainly, parents who had relatives who stuttered would have been more likely to recognize stuttering sooner.

Prevalence

The term "**prevalence**" is used to indicate how widespread a disorder is at any particular time. Information about the prevalence of stuttering tells us how many people "currently" stutter, that is, when the data were gathered. Why is this important? Studies of prevalence can tell us if there is more stuttering now that there was 30 years ago. Or less. We can also compare cultures to see if some cultures appear to have more stuttering—and then explore why this might be so. Sometimes this information may help us understand causal factors, as well as provide leads for prevention and treatment. Accurate, up-to-date information on the prevalence of stuttering, however, is difficult to obtain. Many differences in how the data are collected have a strong effect on the results of any particular study. For example, age of the individuals studied can have a huge effect because many preschool children may be stuttering at a particular time, but then natural recovery from stuttering—which happens largely during the preschool years—may cause many of those children to become fluent by the time they are in elementary school. Other differences in methodology that will affect the prevalence data are (1) the definition of stuttering used (highly disfluent typical speakers may be counted by mistake); (2) how reliable the listeners are (are they trained?); and (3) the culture from which the sample is taken (some cultures are relatively blasé about stuttering and may not count disfluencies that other studies in other cultures would count).

Beitchman et al. (1986) assessed the prevalence of speech and language disorders in kindergarten children, using a representative sample (reflecting the population as a whole). They retested children who failed the initial screening as well as a random sample of children who passed. The prevalence of stuttering in this sample of kindergarten children was 2.4%. Although this is only one study's finding, the care with which the data were collected increases its credibility.

Bloodstein et al. (2021) reviewed many studies of school age children throughout the world and suggested that these studies showed that the prevalence of stuttering throughout the school years is about 1%. If the 2.4% prevalence among kindergartners noted above is valid, a considerable number of recoveries must take place between kindergarten and the upper grades. This finding is confirmed in Zablotsky et al.'s (2019) study of the prevalence of developmental disabilities that found a prevalence of stuttering in 2.73% between ages 3 and 5 years but 1.43% between ages 12 and 17.

Studies of prevalence over the entire life span are limited. Craig et al. (2002) used telephone surveys to assess the life span prevalence of stuttering in Australia and found that the overall prevalence (from preschool to over 50 years) was a little less than 0.75%. They also found that children from ages 2 to 10 showed a higher prevalence, about 1.5%. Prevalence dropped to near 0.50% in individuals older than that. As Bloodstein et al. (2021) urge, more prospective studies are needed that track children from the beginning of speech to the end of secondary school. And, of course, studies should also be done that include careful assessment of stuttering in preschool, school age, adolescent, adult and elderly populations, all done by the same researchers using careful definitions of stuttering and in-person assessments.

Incidence

The **incidence** of stuttering is an index of how many people have stuttered at some time in their lives. Data on incidence can be useful for comparing stuttering in different cultures, in different countries, in different eras. Like the data on prevalence, incidence figures are not clear-cut because different researchers have used different definitions of stuttering and methods for obtaining their data. Some researchers only report stuttering that lasted 6 months or more, not wanting to include shorter episodes of disfluency. Others reported any speech behaviors that informants or parents considered to be stuttering. Because many preschool children recover from stuttering, studies of children will show a higher incidence than studies of adults, who may not remember stuttering, even though they may have stuttered for a brief period. Many studies have considered only individuals who have stuttered at least 6 months and reported a value of 5% for incidence (eg, Andrews & Harris, 1964).

A review of studies of incidence (since 2000) by Yairi and Ambrose (2013) considered the 5% figure to be low. For example, studies by Dworzynski et al. (2007) in the United Kingdom and by Reilly et al. (2009) in Australia suggested that the incidence figures for individuals who have stuttered at some time in their lives is likely to be at least 8%. Bloodstein et al. (2021) considered all recent studies and focused on those with very careful methodology such as ensuring that parent reports are supplemented by expert evaluation of the children's speech. They suggested that the lifetime incidence of stuttering is between 8% and 10%.

Recovery From Stuttering

Recovery from stuttering without treatment, also referred to as "spontaneous" or "natural" recovery, has long been a puzzling issue. Putting aside the important question about why some children recover without treatment, there is debate about what percentage of children recover naturally.

Reviews of early research reported findings that range from 20% to 80% natural recovery (Andrews et al., 1983; Bloodstein et al., 2021). This wide range results from different methodologies used by different studies. Some asked large numbers of adults if they ever stuttered when they were children. This method, which is called "retrospective," may be affected by faulty memories, poor definitions of stuttering, and the inclusion of individuals who may have stuttered for only very brief periods.

Recent research has proceeded more carefully, using "prospective" methodology—done by first identifying a group of children close to the onset of their stuttering and then following them for several years without offering treatment and assessing how many recover and how many persist. Those who persist are then referred for therapy. Several studies using this methodology have been published. Yairi and Ambrose (1999) followed a group of 84 children for a minimum of

4 years after the onset of their stuttering and determined that over this span of time, 74% had recovered without treatment. Kloth et al. (1999) followed 23 children for 6 years and discovered that 70% had recovered. Mansson (2000) identified 51 children between the ages of 3 and 5 who started to stutter and found that 71% recovered within 2 years. When the follow-up continued for another few years until the children were 8 or 9 years old, recoveries were up to 85%. Mansson's data were closely approximated by a later study by Dworzynski et al. (2007). These researchers studied 14,000 pairs of twins, some of whom were found to be stuttering between the ages 2 and 7. Repeated questionnaire assessments completed by parents indicated that by age 7, 87.55% of the children who had been stuttering earlier had recovered. Recent reviews, including Yairi and Ambrose (2013), estimated the percentage of children who recovered from stuttering at 85% or higher. Whether these recoveries were completely "natural" is unclear. Some of the children may have received some form of treatment, direct or indirect.

Recovery Versus Persistence of Stuttering

Haven't we already talked about recovery? Yes, but in this section, we will discuss one of the most fascinating aspects of childhood stuttering: *Why* do some children recover from their stuttering and others keep on stuttering? What factors predict which children will recover and which will persist? Several studies have compared children who recover and those who persist, to determine what might characterize these two groups. Research at the University of Illinois (Yairi & Ambrose, 2005) over the past 30 years indicated that there are several factors that are useful for indicating the likelihood that a child's stuttering will persist rather than disappear naturally. You may wish to follow up on this brief overview by reading the article (Yairi & Ambrose) that describes these findings in detail. The following factors appeared to be among the most important predictors found by Yairi and Ambrose:

Family history: When a child's family includes individuals whose stuttering persisted, there is increased risk of persistence.

Gender: Boys have a greater risk of persistence. However, girls typically recover more quickly; therefore, if a girl doesn't recover fairly soon after onset, she may well persist in stuttering.

Age at onset: Children who begin to stutter "later" have a greater risk of persistence. Onsets occur most frequently between ages 2 and 3.5 years, so children with onset after 3.5 years are more at risk.

Trend of stuttering frequency and severity: Children whose stuttering (defined as part-word repetitions and single-syllable word repetitions, prolongations, and blocks) is not decreasing in frequency and severity over a period of a year after onset are at more risk of persistence.

Duration since onset: The longer the child continues to stutter beyond a year after onset, the greater the risk of persistence, especially for girls.

Duration of stuttering moments: Continued presence of more than one repetition unit, especially more than three (li-li-li-li-like this) is a sign of increased risk. Also, continued rapid repetitions are a sign of increased risk. Children who recover tend to have fewer repetition units (li-like this) and slower repetitions (li...like this).

Continued presence of sound prolongations and blocks: The percentage of prolongations and blocks at onset doesn't predict persistence, but if prolongations and blocks do not decrease as stuttering goes on, the child is more likely to persist.

Phonological skills: Children whose phonological skills are below the norms have a greater risk for continued stuttering.

Many other studies examined factors associated with recovery. A longitudinal study by Brosch et al. (1999) followed a group of 79 stuttering children for several years. The group that persisted in stuttering had a significantly larger proportion of left-handed children. Because this was a preliminary report, caution should be exercised in considering this factor as critical to recovery. Nonetheless, the factor of laterality may be one of the additional genetic factors that influence recovery; replication of this work is critical. Brosch et al. (2002) also reported that acoustic measures of these children's fluent speech before stuttering onset and at several points after stuttering were related to persistence of stuttering. For example, more variability in measures of voice onset time appeared to be related to persistence.

In the study by Kloth et al. (1999) described earlier, results indicated that children who recovered had a more mature speech motor system (as defined by less variability of articulatory rate), a slower speaking rate, and a mother whose interaction style was nondirective and whose language was less complex. Rommel et al. (2000) assessed the speaking environments of 71 children identified as stuttering soon after onset and followed them for 3 years. The mothers of those who recovered naturally compared to the mothers of those who persisted used less complex syntax and a smaller number of different words when talking to their children.

Recent research on this topic has focused on neurodevelopment, particularly of white matter tracts connecting areas of the brain that must coordinate to provide the timing and sequencing for fluent speech. The findings of a neuroimaging study of white matter tracts throughout the brain in children who stutter by Chang et al. (2015) may shed new light on the persistence of stuttering. Younger children who stuttered showed many deficits in white matter nerve tracts throughout the brain (compared to control children), suggesting a lack of efficient connectivity, including in the sensorimotor areas related to speech. Strikingly, older children who stuttered (children with persistent stuttering) continued to show less development of white matter tracts than their age-matched controls. However, the older control children's white matter tracts were more developed compared to the younger control children. This developmental change was not as present in the older stuttering children, compared to their controls. This may indicate that persistence of stuttering (vs recovery) is related to lack of maturation of the white matter pathways connecting areas related to speech production.

If this finding about problems in the development of neural pathways is supported in future studies, we may find that there are many possible reasons for lack of maturation in the white matter tracts in children who persist in stuttering. Researchers looking at a number of related disorders have noted, interestingly enough, that the duration of breast-feeding in infancy correlates with presence or persistence of some disorders (Tanoue & Oda, 1989). Following this lead, Mahurin-Smith and Ambrose (2013) compared 17 children who persisted in stuttering with 30 children who recovered and found that the duration of breast-feeding in the persistent children was less than that in the recovered children (especially so in boys). Their explanation of this finding was that the fatty acids in human milk have been shown to enhance neural development and influence the expression of certain genes.

Another study of factors that appear to predict recovery from stuttering was conducted by Leech et al. (2017). They studied language growth in both syntax and vocabulary and found that greater syntax growth, but not vocabulary growth, was related to recovery from childhood stuttering. This finding gives rise to the hope that work on syntactic development in children who are stuttering will aid in their recovery. Some members of this group of researchers and others comprise the Purdue University Stuttering Project that has published much work on factors related to recovery versus persistence of stuttering. A newer publication by some members of this group (Walsh et al., 2018) gives an excellent summary of their current findings on this topic. Two years later, Walsh et al. (2020) suggested that analysis of stuttering in 4- to 5-year-old children indicates that those children who had greater stuttering-like-disfluency scores (part-word repetitions, blocks, prolongations and broken words) were more likely to persist in stuttering.

Pulling many of these studies together, Singer et al. (2020) conducted a meta-analysis of 11 studies of persistence and recovery and found that the following variables were predictive of persistence: child is older at onset of stuttering, child has higher frequency of stuttering-like disfluencies, child has lower accuracy in producing speech sounds, child has lower expressive and receptive language skills, child is male, and child has a family history of persistent or recovered stuttering. Note that this last finding is in contrast with earlier evidence that only children with a family history of **persistent** stuttering were likely to be persistent.

In a study just published as this chapter was being written, Walsh et al. (2021) also found that a combination of many variables can predict persistence. This group of researchers were working from a multifactor view of stuttering (Smith & Weber, 2017) that suggests the development of stuttering is not determined by a single factor but by many variables interacting together and combined in unique ways for each individual child. By looking at many factors in each of 52 children ages about 3.5 to 5.5 years—and following these children for several years to determine recovery versus persistence—they were able to suggest which variables were most predictive for this group of children. Best predictors were as follows:

Family History of Stuttering (whether or not the family member recovered)
Poorer Performance on Test of Articulation/Phonology
Higher Frequency of Stuttering-Like Disfluencies
Lower Accuracy on a Nonword Repetition Task

Surprisingly, they found that some old favorites were *not* predictive of persistence. These included sex of the child, age of onset of stuttering, and the duration of the amount of time that the child had been stuttering. No doubt future studies will provide other unexpected predictors or nonpredictors. In the chapter on diagnosis and evaluation of preschoolers who stutter I will give more details on the procedures these researchers recommend for assessment. I strongly recommend reading the Walsh et al. publication to get a full understanding of how various combinations of factors predict various outcomes.

In summary, early studies of recovery reported wide variations in results. Their findings depend on many factors—among them, the accuracy with which stuttering is differentiated from typical disfluency, whether the study is retrospective or longitudinal, and the size of the group studied. The most careful studies are longitudinal (prospective) assessments of children who are identified soon after the onset of stuttering and are followed for several years (eg, Mansson, 2005; Leech et al., 2017; Walsh et al., 2021). In these studies, a high percentage of the children who began to stutter recover without formal treatment. Many factors have been suggested as associated with recovery. These include having less effect of emotion on speech motor control, having effective processing of linguistic information, having greater growth of density of white matter tracts compared to children who persist, showing greater growth in syntax, having relatives who stuttered, having an early onset of stuttering (some studies dispute this), showing a decrease in frequency and severity of stuttering in the year after onset, having a slower speech rate, having a more stable speech-motor system, having a mother who has a nondirective interaction style and uses less complex language when speaking to the child, being right-handed, having less severe stuttering as the child grows, having good phonological, language, and nonverbal skills, and being female (some studies dispute this). We now consider this last variable, the sex factor, in more detail.

Sex Ratio

Studies of the sex ratio in stuttering were first published in the 1890s and have been published every decade since. With this steady stream of information, we ought to have reliable data on this phenomenon. In fact, we do. The results from studies of people who stutter at many ages and in many cultures put the ratio at about three male stutterers to every one female stutterer. There is strong evidence, however, that the ratio increases as children get older. For example, Yairi (1983) reported that of 22 children who were 2 and 3 years of age and whose parents believed they were stuttering, 11 were boys, and 11 were girls. In a larger study of 87 children between 20 and 69 months, Yairi and Ambrose (1992b) found a male:female ratio of 2.1:1 overall, although the 20 youngest subjects, those under 27 months, showed a 1.2:1 ratio.

A review by Bloodstein et al. (2021) indicated that the male to female sex ratio is about 3:1 for school children in the United States. They also cite studies that show about the same ratio in Egypt and India. There is also evidence that the sex ratio increases as children get older. Evidence of the increasing male to female ratio was provided by several studies. Kloth et al. (1999) found a male to female ratio of 1.1:1 ratio near onset, which rose to 2.5:1 six years later. Mansson (2000) found a male to female ratio of 1.65:1 at the initial screening (age 3), which rose to a ratio of 2.8:1 two years later. The nearly even sex ratio among very young children who stutter and the gradually increasing proportion of boys who stutter may be a consequence of several factors. West (1931) presented data indicating that the change in sex ratio was the result of an increasing proportion of boys beginning to stutter in the late preschool and early school-age years. However, more recent data indicate that girls begin to stutter a little earlier than boys (Yairi, 1983; Yairi & Ambrose, 1992b) and recover earlier and more frequently (Andrews et al., 1983; Yairi & Ambrose, 1992b, 1999; Yairi, Ambrose, & Cox, 1996). A study in Australia (Reilly et al., 2013), however, is the lone finding that suggests boys recover more frequently than girls. This study only followed children from age 2 to age 4, so that if many girls recovered after age 4, they were missed.

Why do more boys stutter than girls? Recent reviews suggest boys are much more vulnerable to disorders of communication (Adani & Cepanec, 2019). Bloodstein et al. (2021, p. 214) comment that "The sex ratio has been attributed to nature (sex-linked patterns of genetic transmission, sex differences in constitution, physical maturation) or nurture (speech and language development, differences in parental attitudes and expectations with regard to boys and girls). The first set of factors are more likely explanations than the latter."

As a side note to the sex-ratio issue, females who stutter and don't recover by adulthood may be an interesting subpopulation to study. They may have inherited a stronger predisposition to stutter, may have been subjected to strong environmental pressures on their speech, or both (Andrews et al., 1983). Alternately, they may lack the "recovery factor" that most young female stutterers appear to have, or they may have inherited additional factors that interact with stuttering to inhibit recovery. Further research is needed and readers of this text should consider contributing to it.

Variability and Predictability of Stuttering

Another important piece of background information about stuttering is how it varies in some ways, yet is surprisingly predictable in other ways. This predictability is an important clue to its nature. As we trace the research on stuttering's variability, we will see how this information reflects changing theoretical perspectives on the disorder.

Before the 1930s, stuttering had been commonly regarded as a medical disorder. Lee Edward Travis, the first person trained as a PhD to work with speech and hearing disorders, established a laboratory at the University of Iowa in 1924 to study stuttering from a neurophysiological perspective. He hypothesized that stuttering was the result of an anomalous or inefficient organization of the brain's two cerebral hemispheres. To Travis and his fellow researchers, the variability of stuttering behaviors was seen as part of a larger, somewhat heterogeneous organic disorder, and an unimportant part at that. To their research, stutterers' brain waves, heart rates, and breathing patterns were far more relevant that stuttering behaviors. But as this decade progressed, psychologists at Iowa and elsewhere began taking a keen interest in behavioral (rather than neurophysiological) approaches to the study of all human disorders, which spilled over into research on stuttering. Scientists who had been trying to understand the neurophysiology of stuttering gradually began trying to examine the social, psychological, and linguistic factors that govern its occurrence and variability (Bloodstein et al., 2021).

Anticipation, Consistency, and Adaptation

Before describing these interesting findings, I'll briefly explain these terms that are best understood in the context of someone who stutters reading a passage several times. "**Anticipation**" refers to an individual's ability to predict the words or sounds on which they will stutter (Johnson & Solomon, 1937; Knott et al., 1937; Milisen, 1938; Van Riper, 1936). "**Consistency**" is the tendency for people to stutter on the same words when they read a passage more than once (Johnson & Inness, 1939; Johnson & Knott, 1937). "**Adaptation**" is the finding that when speakers read a passage several times, they gradually stutter less and less over the course of five or six readings (Johnson & Knott, 1937; Van Riper & Hull, 1955).

These studies were usually carried out by the experimenter giving an individual who stutters a passage and asking them to read it aloud. Before reading it aloud, however, the individual is asked to read it to themselves and mark the words they expect to stutter on. The experimenter then marks the words actually stuttered on and compares that with the individual's marked copy to see how much they have accurately *anticipated* which words they will stutter on. Then the experimenter has the individual read the passage again and, using a copy of the passage on which the previously stuttered words were marked, marks those words that were stuttered on in both readings. This assesses how *consistent* the individual is in their stuttering. And thirdly, the experimenter has the individual read the passage six consecutive times and observes whether the individual *adapts* to the reading task and stutters less and less with each reading.

These findings, called anticipation, consistency, and adaptation, respectively, changed some assumptions about the disorder. Stuttering, it seemed, was not simply a neurophysiological disorder. It showed characteristics of a learned behavior, as well. In other words, the behaviors demonstrated by these studies could best be explained by the hypotheses that subjects had learned which words they might stutter on, the learning caused them to stutter on many of the same words, and lessening of stuttering with repeated readings of a passage were similar to decreasing behaviors via conditioning. The work of Wischner at the Universities of Iowa and Illinois in the 1950s (eg, Wischner, 1950) studying anticipation, consistency, and adaptation was instrumental (no pun intended) in helping researchers realize that much of stuttering behavior was learned.

These studies not only changed existing views of stuttering but also opened the door to new treatment possibilities. The reason was this: If much of stuttering is learned, it may be unlearned. The challenge was to determine how much is learned and how to help people who stutter develop new responses. Many of the treatment approaches we discuss later in the book use principles of learning to help clients acquire more fluent speech, especially young children. Learning, especially learning to reduce the strong emotion yoked to stuttering, can also help older children and adults reduce the tension and avoidance of their old stuttering responses and speak with milder stuttering or none. Remember this. Learning principles will be critical to your clinical work.

Language Factors

One of the many stuttering researchers at the University of Iowa, Spencer Brown, pushed investigations of the predictability of stuttering into the realm of language. In seven studies completed over a stretch of 10 years, Brown found correlations between stuttering and seven grammatical factors during reading aloud. These findings were reported in a remarkable series of papers Brown published from 1935 to 1945 (Brown, 1937, 1938a, 1938b, 1938c, 1943, 1945; Brown & Moren, 1942; Johnson & Brown, 1935). Brown showed that most adults who stutter do so more frequently on:

consonants
sounds in word-initial position
speech in a larger context (vs on isolated words)
nouns, verbs, adjectives, and adverbs (vs articles, prepositions, pronouns, and conjunctions)
longer words
words at the beginnings of sentences
stressed syllables

The findings strongly suggest that stuttering is highly influenced by these linguistic factors.

Later investigators applied Brown's hypotheses to the speech of children who stutter. An advantage in studying language factors in children's stuttering is that the loci (places where stuttering occurs in speech) and frequency of stuttering might be less influenced by responses learned from years of stuttering and more by innate language processing characteristics. Indeed, researchers discovered that although stuttering in elementary school children follows the same linguistic patterns as adult stuttering, the loci and frequency of stuttering in preschool children are different. Stuttering in these very young children occurs most frequently on pronouns and conjunctions, not on nouns, verbs, adjectives, and adverbs (common stuttering targets for adults). For these children, stuttering occurs not as repetitions, prolongations, or blocks of sounds in word-initial positions but as repetitions of parts of words and single-syllable words in sentence-initial positions (Bloodstein et al., 2021; Bloodstein & Gantwerk, 1967). This led researchers to hypothesize that in its incipient stage (ie, when it first starts), stuttering is located at the beginning of syntactic units (sentences, clauses, and phrases), as if the task of linguistic planning and preparation were a key ingredient in the recipe for stuttering (Bloodstein et al., 2021).

Conture (2001) and others (eg, Byrd et al., 2007) have focused particular attention on the phoneme or sound selection component of linguistic planning in individuals who stutter.

Findings that recovery from stuttering may be associated with good phonological skills, a slower speech production rate, and a stable speech-motor system suggest that some individuals who begin to stutter may recover by overcoming a linguistic planning delay by relying on strengths in related language areas or by slowing their rates of speech production to compensate for such deficits. We will revisit these methods of dealing with stuttering when we discuss treatment approaches.

Researchers at Purdue University have conducted interesting experimental and theoretical work that implicates language factors, among others, as part of their characterization of stuttering as a "multifactorial dynamic disorder." For example, Smith and Weber (2017) suggest that the speech of stutterers become more variable and less stable as language becomes more complex—even their fluent speech. They suggest that as children grow and use longer and linguistically complex sentences, the tendency for their speech motor control to break down increases. This, combines with other stresses and pressures, results in early stuttering that becomes more severe in many children as they grow.

Purdue studies of persistent versus recovered stuttering children has also revealed that those with slower *growth* of expressive syntax are more likely to be persistent in stuttering than those children who showed substantial growth of expressive syntax between ages 4 years and 9 months and ages 7 years and 11 months (Leech et al., 2017). Another association between stuttering and language has been found by Walsh et al. (2018). Their results suggest that the effectiveness of neural networks in the brain associated with processing linguistic information is related to recovery from stuttering.

In summary, there are strong links between language and stuttering—not only in expressive language, as might be expected, but also in receptive language. As mentioned in the section describing onset, stuttering usually first appears when children are going through the most intense period of language acquisition (Bloodstein et al., 2021). It is also clear that deficits in language (including phonology) often accompany stuttering and may predict its persistence (Yairi & Ambrose, 1999, 2005). Future studies may also confirm what several researchers have suggested that even stutterers who show no clinically significant language disorders may have subtle subclinical language or phonological deficits that may contribute to their stuttering (eg, Byrd et al., 2007). More information about the influence of language factors on stuttering will be found in the next two chapters.

Fluency-Inducing Conditions

One of the researchers at the University of Iowa, Oliver Bloodstein, wrote his PhD dissertation on "Conditions Under Which Stuttering Is Reduced or Absent" (Bloodstein, 1948, 1950). In studying the speech of stutterers in 115 conditions, Bloodstein found that stuttering is markedly decreased in many of them. Some of these conditions are speaking when alone, when relaxed, in unison with another speaker, to an animal or an infant, in time to a rhythmic stimulus or when singing, in a different dialect, while simultaneously writing, and when swearing. In later studies, reviewed in Andrews et al. (1982), additional conditions were found to reduce stuttering. These conditions included speaking in a slow prolonged manner, speaking under loud masking noise, speaking while listening to delayed auditory feedback, shadowing another speaker (repeating what they say immediately afterward), and speaking when reinforced for fluent speech.

Various explanations have been proposed to account for the impact of these conditions. Most are compatible with the idea that stuttering has a substantial learned component and is affected by such external stimuli as communicative pressure. Recent brain imaging studies—reviewed in Chapters 2 and 3—indicate that cortical and subcortical networks for speech and language are impaired in people who stutter. This may make it difficult for a speaker to orchestrate rapid and coordinated production of phonological and lexical items, syntax, intonation, and other subcomponents of spoken language. Thus, many conditions may induce fluency by providing timing cues, reducing rate, lowering stress on vulnerable pathways, or marshalling attentional resources to overcome the limitations of the neurological system of a person who stutters.

As you might imagine, many findings of increased fluency in specific conditions have led clinician-researchers to try to use these conditions to provide therapy. None have been particularly successful in long run.

One of the best-known stories of induced fluency is Demosthenes' use of pebbles in his mouth to cure his stuttering. It must have worked for him because he subsequently became one of the most famous orators in ancient Athens. Something like that worked for me when I was in high school and stuttered severely. I would surreptitiously slip hard candies into my mouth whenever I had to talk in class and wanted to become more fluent. However, in those days, you weren't allowed to chew gum or suck on candies in class and I was eventually exposed and made to spit them out. Didn't my teachers know about Demosthenes?

An Integration

Modern research on stuttering has taken a long and complex journey from Travis's laboratory in Iowa in 1924. Yet, in many ways, those early findings are not irrelevant. Travis's theory of stuttering, which viewed it as a problem of coordinating the two sides of the brain for speech, has reemerged as a view of stuttering as a problem of coordinating multiple brain networks for speech and integrating them with networks for language, cognition, and emotion. This juggling act breaks down in all speakers when the resources needed to process language, cognition, or emotion momentarily drain available central nervous system capacities, leaving too little capacity for the intricacies of rapid, smooth speech production. The result is typical disfluency. Those individuals who stutter appear to have even more than this typical trouble managing the needed multiple neural networks for speech production under conditions of high demand. They have inherited or acquired a more vulnerable speech production system—one that is less able to deal with the norm of rapid, smooth speech under a wide variety of conditions, perhaps because the neural pathways used to produce speech are not as efficient as they need to be.

In those children who recover naturally from stuttering, this vulnerable speech production system may heal itself and become more resistant to disruption. Because of the great neural plasticity of the very young (especially young girls), some children's brains will spontaneously develop new, more efficient pathways for speech, and these children will become entirely fluent. Others may recover because they learn to compensate by speaking more slowly or finding other ways to marshal their resources to overcome disfluency.

Children who persist in stuttering may have important neurodevelopmental differences from those who recover.

The parts of their brains used in speech and language production—and the interconnections among these parts—may develop more slowly and less completely. Thus, they will have difficulty producing the lightning-fast sensorimotor coordination needed for fluent speech. When their speech breaks down again and again, they are flooded with feelings of frustration and embarrassment, depending on temperament and reactivity. These emotions can cause children to tense their muscles during stutters and try to escape the moment of stuttering by squeezing and pushing out words, blinking their eyes and nodding their head. Anticipatory fears gradually develop as children stutter more frequently on certain words (eg, their names) and in certain situations (eg, meeting new people). These highly learned reactions—which are influenced by an individual's personality and the responses of people around the individual—become part of children's stuttering patterns and influence the way they think and feel about speaking.

This view is essentially the model of stuttering presented in this book. To state it more formally, stuttering is an inherited or congenital neurodevelopmental disorder of neural pathways in the brain that first appears when a child is learning the complex and rapid coordinations of speech and language production. Children who do not recover but persist in stuttering are those who may have more extensive deficits in these neural networks. They may also have more sensitive temperaments or other vulnerabilities. As stuttering persists, they learn maladaptive responses to their disfluencies. This learning is influenced by their biological temperament, developing social and cognitive awareness, and the response of people in their environment.

The next few chapters expand on this theme and prepare you to use this information in diagnosis and treatment.

SUMMARY

- Stuttering appears in all cultures and has been a problem for humankind for at least 40 centuries.
- It is characterized by a high frequency or severity of disruptions that impede the forward flow of speech.
- It begins in childhood and often becomes more severe as children grow to adulthood unless they recover with or without formal treatment.
- Core behaviors of stuttering are repetitions, prolongations, and blocks. Secondary behaviors are the result of attempts to escape or avoid core behaviors and include physical concomitants of stuttering, such as eye blinks, or verbal concomitants, such as word substitutions.
- Feelings and attitudes can also be important components of stuttering that reflect the individual's emotional reactions to the experience of being unable to speak fluently and to listener responses to their stuttering. Feelings are immediate emotional reactions and include fear, shame, and embarrassment. Attitudes crystallize more slowly from repeated negative experiences associated with stuttering. An example is the belief that listeners think you are stupid when they hear you stuttering.
- Stuttering begins between 18 months of age and puberty, but most often between ages 2 and 5 years, with a peak just before age 3. Its first appearance may be either a gradual increase in easy repetitions of words and sounds or a sudden onset of multiple repetitions, sometimes with prolongations or blocks as well.
- Prevalence of stuttering is about 1%. Incidence is about 5%. Recovery rate without professional treatment may be above 80% of children who ever stuttered. The male to female ratio in schoolchildren and adults is about 3:1 but may be lower, close to 1:1, in very young children who start to stutter. More girls recover during early childhood, increasing the proportion of males with the disorder after the preschool years.
- Many people who stutter are able to predict the words they will stutter on in a reading passage before reading it aloud (anticipation), and most tend to stutter on many of the same words each time in repeated readings of a passage (consistency). Stuttering frequency decreases for most stutterers when they read a passage several times (adaptation).
- Stuttering occurs more frequently in certain grammatical contexts. The nature of these grammatical contexts differs somewhat for adults and children.
- A variety of conditions reduces the frequency of stuttering. Their effects may be attributable to changes in speech pattern, reductions in communicative pressure, or both. Research on these fluency-inducing conditions suggests that stuttering may be decreased by conditions that reduce the demands on speech motor control and language formulation functions.
- Cortical and subcortical neural networks for speech and language may be slow to develop in children who stutter, particularly those whose stuttering becomes chronic. In addition to slow development of networks, these children also have poorer functional *connectivity* among different neural networks used for the coordinated stages of speech production.
- Many of these children who persist in stuttering develop cognitive, emotional, and behavioral responses to their stuttering. This can make the problem more difficult to treat and cause social, occupational, and academic difficulties for these individuals.

STUDY QUESTIONS

1. What might make some children's core behaviors progress from repetitions and prolongations to blocks?
2. What are the differences between core and secondary behaviors in stuttering?
3. From what other kinds of hesitations in speech should stuttering be distinguished?
4. What are some feelings and attitudes people who stutter might have, and what is their origin? Are these feelings and attitudes ever experienced by people who don't stutter?
5. What is the age range for the onset of stuttering (the youngest and oldest ages at which onset is commonly reported)? Why might it occur at that time?
6. What is the difference between "incidence" and "prevalence"?
7. What problems do researchers encounter when they try to determine how many stutterers recover without treatment?
8. Why might the ratio of male to female stutterers change with age?
9. In what ways is stuttering predictable? In what ways does it vary?
10. Why is it difficult to answer the question, "What is the cause of stuttering?"
11. The International Classification of Functioning, Disability, and Health (ICF) indicates that with some conditions, interpersonal interactions may be affected. How might stuttering affect these interactions?
12. How can stuttering treatment help change factors affecting the individual in the ICF area called "Contextual Factors"?
13. How would you describe the etiology of stuttering to a parent who has had limited education and is not used to discussing abstract concepts?

SUGGESTED PROJECTS

1. Enlist the help of an adult who stutters, and have him teach you to stutter. Then ask him to go with you while you use some voluntary stuttering in public. Write a report (no more than a page) of what feelings you experienced and how people reacted to you.
2. Use an internet search engine like Google to find an online discussion group of people who stutter and clinicians. Join the group and observe what issues they discuss.
3. Attend a support group for people who stutter.
4. Listen to some preschool children talking and note their typical disfluencies. Then listen to elementary school children talking, and compare their disfluencies to those of the preschool children.
5. If you are a fluent speaker, record your own speech in a conversation with someone and observe the types of disfluencies you hear. Do they differ from stuttering? In what ways?
6. Conduct a search on the internet for resources that guide you to critically evaluate websites (eg, https://www.library.georgetown.edu/tutorials/research-guides/evaluating-internet-content). Using that format, critically evaluate a website you find when searching for "stuttering" sites with your search engine.

SUGGESTED VIEWING

The King's Speech. This film depicts King George VI of England, who stuttered severely but found a great deal of help from his Australian speech therapist, Lionel Logue. The movie provides an excellent depiction of the emotions surrounding stuttering. It begins with a severe stuttering episode when he has to give a speech to a large audience before he becomes King. The reactions of listeners vividly capture what stutterers go through every day.

When I Stutter. This is a documentary about stuttering produced by a speech-language pathologist, John Gomez. It is a compelling depiction of the experiences endured by people who stutter and their inspiring stories of coping. We see one man stuttering severely and then, with the help of a stuttering therapist over several months, confronting his fears and learning to speak more easily. The testimony of many stutterers about their fears, their agonizing experiences, and about how they compensated with their creative talents is deeply moving. In the spirit of full disclosure, you should know that the author of your textbook plays a bit part in this movie.

My Beautiful Stutter. This powerful film captures the bravery and the suffering of kids and teens at a camp for young people who stutter. The movie depicts the experiences of young people who stutter as they spend 2 weeks at a camp where bonding and acceptance are the watchwords of the day. We follow them as they speak to an audience of friends about their traumatic experiences back home and at school and learn to be proud rather than ashamed of their speech. Most viewers (including me) will have tears in their eyes as they watch these kids (and sometimes their parents) confront their past and prepare for a new future. One of the main messages of the movie is that yes, gaining fluency is good, but learning that Stuttering is OK is everything.

SUGGESTED READINGS AND VIEWING

Bloodstein, O. (1993). *Stuttering: The search for a cause and cure.* Allyn and Bacon.

This book is part history and part analysis, written with charm and clarity. Bloodstein covers early treatments for stuttering; the burgeoning of research in the 1930s, 1940s, and 1950s; and more recent findings in the realm of neurophysiology. His own orientation on the learning-environmental basis of stuttering comes through, but he gives good coverage of other possible factors as well. Bloodstein is particularly good at conveying the excitement that accompanies research.

Bobrick, B. (1995). *Knotted tongues: Stuttering in history and the quest for a cure.* Simon and Schuster.

A highly readable account of various treatments for stuttering throughout the ages and of famous people who stutter.

Campbell, P., Constantino, C., & Simpson, S. (Eds.) (2019). *Stammering pride and prejudice: Difference not defect.* J&R Press.

If you have the view that stuttering is something to be fixed, that it must be overcome and replaced with fluency, you should read this book. It reflects a powerful movement among people who stutter and their advocates that stuttering is something to be proud of and that people who stutter just have a different way of talking. This is an edited book with poems, stories, and essays that espouse that view, but it also discusses the possibility that many individuals who stutter want to speak more easily—that is, still stutter, but stutter in a looser, more comfortable way.

Helliesen, G. (2002). *Forty years after therapy: One man's story.* Apollo Press.

An autobiography of someone who stuttered severely and was treated by Charles Van Riper, the world-renowned stuttering clinician. This book presents a unique view of stuttering therapy from the client's viewpoint.

Hendrickson, J. *Video: "I stutter. But I need you to listen."* https://www.youtube.com/watch?v=m0E_wMIwfSI

This Youtube video is a moving description of someone quite successful—he's a senior editor at Atlantic magazine—who continues to stutter severely. After explaining and describing the phenomenon of stuttering, John talks about his decision to stutter openly, to say every word he intends to, and rely on the listener's ability to stay with him as he talks. The visual special effects accompanying his life story are impressive. There is one error in his description of the elements of stuttering. Can you find it?

Murray, F. P. (n.d.). *A stutterer's story.* Stuttering Foundation of America (www.stutteringhelp.org).

An autobiography depicting the long struggle of someone who stuttered severely and spent his life searching for answers. The author describes his acquaintance with many of the pioneers of stuttering therapy.

Rabinowitz, A., & Chien, C. (2014). *A boy and a jaguar.* Houghton Mifflin Harcourt.

A children's book that tells the true-life story of Alan Rabinowitz who stuttered severely and could only talk fluently to animals. Rabinowitz learned to manage his stuttering effectively and later was called the "Indiana Jones of wildlife conservation." This book received the American Library Association's Schneider Family Book Award.

St. Louis, K. (Ed.) (2001). *Living with stuttering: Stories, basics, resources, and hope.* Populore Publishing Company.

The life stories of 25 people who stutter and how they have coped with their stuttering.

2

Primary Etiological Factors in Stuttering

Chapter Outline

Chapter Objectives

After studying this chapter, readers should be able to:

- Describe the evidence supporting genetic inheritance of stuttering from (1) family studies, (2) twin studies, and (3) adoption studies
- Explain how genetic studies are done and what has been found about how chromosomes and genes are associated with stuttering
- Explain why congenital and early childhood factors are thought to contribute to a predisposition to develop stuttering and what some of these factors may be
- Describe the ways in which brain functions in stuttering individuals differ from those of nonstuttering individuals
- Describe the ways in which brain structures in stuttering individuals differ from those of nonstuttering individuals
- Describe changes in the brain that are associated with improvements in fluency as the result of treatment

Key Terms

Adoption studies: Investigations of stuttering in siblings who were adopted soon after birth and placed with different families. A higher incidence of stuttering among biological relatives than adoptive family members provides evidence of a genetic basis of stuttering rather than an environmental basis

Anomaly: A difference from the normal structure or function

Concordance (in twins): If one twin has a condition, such as stuttering, the other twin also has the condition

Congenital factor: A physical or psychological trauma that occurred at or near birth that may predispose an individual to develop stuttering

DNA: These letters stand for deoxyribonucleic acid—a double-stranded molecule passed on from a mother and a father to a child containing the "instruction book" for inheriting traits

Family studies: Examination of family trees of individuals who stutter to determine the frequency and pattern of the occurrence of stuttering in relatives. These studies can answer questions such as whether males or females are more likely to have children who stutter and whether persistent stuttering (as opposed to natural recovery) is a trait that is inherited

Gene: A segment of DNA that contributes to an individual's traits, such as height and weight

Genetic linkage studies: Because two or more genes connected with a disorder are physically close to each other on a chromosome, they are often inherited together in individuals who have that disorder. By comparing genes and chromosomes of family members who do have the disorder with those who don't, these disorder-related genes can be identified

Recovery (from stuttering): Stuttering that disappears within a year or two after onset from natural causes rather than from treatment. Also called natural recovery or spontaneous recovery.

Persistent stuttering: Stuttering that persists for several years after onset, beyond the time at which natural recovery is likely to occur

Predisposition: A susceptibility to developing a condition

Twin studies: Research on the co-occurrence of stuttering of both members of a twin pair if one twin stutters; questions such as whether identical twins show more concordance than fraternal twins can be answered, shedding light on the extent of a genetic basis of stuttering

Whole brain intrinsic network connectivity: Connectivity among networks throughout the whole brain can be compared between those who stutter and those who do not. Looking for inter-connecting networks is in contrast with looking only at specific areas of the brain—a localizationist approach

WHAT DO WE KNOW ABOUT CONSTITUTIONAL FACTORS IN STUTTERING?

We know a lot, but there is much more to be learned. Let's start with what we do know about factors inside the person—aspects of their constitutional makeup—that influence their stuttering. Knowing this will help you counsel people who stutter and reassure parents of children who stutter to help them understand that stuttering is not their fault. You will also be able to explain that, despite the biological basis of stuttering, much of the handicap of stuttering can be overcome. Think of the many famous and successful people, like Emily Blunt, James Earl Jones, Bruce Willis, Carly Simon, Elvis Presley, and President Joe Biden, who have stuttered and have not let stuttering hold them back.

In addition to putting this knowledge of constitutional factors to clinical use, you may be interested in contributing to the science of stuttering yourself. Information in this chapter can be helpful to future researchers who may find new and more effective interventions based on what they discover. As you read about the information that I present here, keep your creative portals open; that way, you may come up with new ideas that could solve remaining riddles related to the causes of stuttering. I have created a video that will outline the stages you may go through as you come up with a research idea and carry it through from developing a plan to making the relevant measurements to writing up the results and presenting your findings to an audience. Titled "Process of Research," it can be found on Lippincott Connect the Chapter 2 videos.

In this chapter, I will give you an overview of the heredity of stuttering and the possible influence of childhood brain injury and trauma on the disorder. Then, I will describe how differences and deficits in specific areas of the brain and the networks that connect them may be associated with stuttering. Figure 2.1 gives a quick impression of the areas we will cover. The chapters that follow will help you understand how all these details

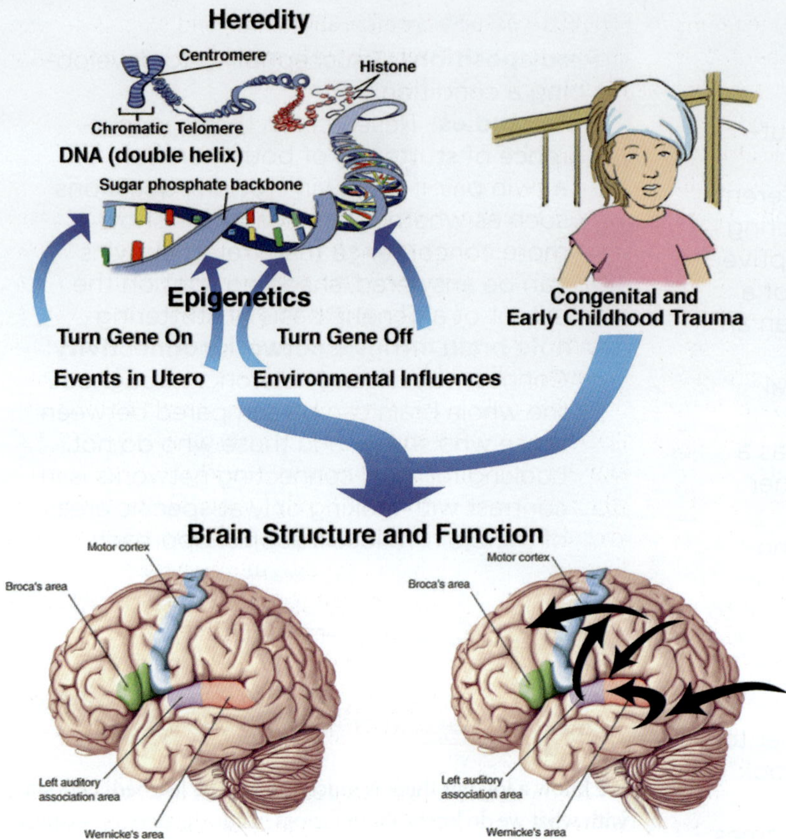

Figure 2.1 Constitutional factors in stuttering.

about heredity and brain structure and function may lead to the speech production difficulties that result in stuttering.

HEREDITARY FACTORS

Remember when you realized you were beginning to resemble your parents in some ways? Or that you look like your sister or brother? Obviously, many traits that make parents and children so similar are inherited. It wasn't until the mid-1800s that we began to understand how this works. Two individuals contributed a vast amount to our understanding of heredity. One was the Augustinian monk, Gregor Mendel, whose experiments in breeding varieties of peas gave rise to his insights about genetic inheritance in people. He established the principle that each parent in a breeding pair contributes equally to the genetic makeup of the offspring, and Mendel developed the understanding of dominant and recessive traits (see Fig. 2.2 and related text for more on genes). Another major contributor to the science of genetics was Charles Darwin. Darwin is quite relevant to the topic of this book because he is thought to have inherited stuttering from his ancestors, including his famous grandfather, Erasmus Darwin (Thomson, 2009).[1] Charles Darwin's theory of evolution (natural selection) suggested that while specific characteristics (such as height and skin color) could be inherited by one generation from another, variations in how those characteristics expressed themselves produced slight differences in members of a species. These differences favored some individuals more than others, depending on the environment. The most useful traits for surviving in the species' environment will be passed on to future generations because those individuals possessing them would thrive and reproduce most successfully. For example, deer that can run at astonishing speeds can escape predators and thereby survive to produce more offspring. Thus, deer have evolved to be fast runners.

Let's go back to stuttering. The idea that stuttering is inherited because it often runs in families is a fact long recognized by researchers (eg, Bryngelson, 1935). For many years, researchers debated about what this meant. Some suggested that the appearance of stuttering in several generations of a family must mean that it is caused by an inherited neurological difference or **anomaly**. Others disagreed, countering that religious beliefs often run in families too but aren't inherited. Some researchers argued that stuttering develops in response to a critical attitude toward normal disfluency that has been handed down from one generation to the next (Johnson et al., 1959). Children whose parents were critical of their typical disfluencies would grow afraid of speaking because of their critical remarks and would "hesitate to hesitate" (Johnson, 1944, p. 457). This would start a spiral of more hesitations leading to greater criticism, greater fear, more disfluencies, and so on.

[1]Erasmus Darwin was a famous British physician, natural philosopher, physiologist, slave-trade abolitionist, inventor, and poet. He was known to have had a severe stutter, but obviously, it didn't hold him back.

For many years, researchers aligned themselves with one side of the argument or the other: Is stuttering inherited or are just critical attitudes passed down? Currently, however, there is broad agreement that stuttering is frequently inherited (Bloodstein et al., 2021; Frigerio-Domingues & Drayna, 2017; Kraft & Yairi, 2012; Yairi & Ambrose, 2005, 2013). In other words, for many people who stutter, one or both of their parents or some other close ancestor had some **predisposition** to stuttering that was transmitted in their genes. Current thinking may be due to new strong evidence about heredity in stuttering but is probably also due to the rise of less deterministic views of heredity. Research has shown, for a number of inherited disorders, that genes do not work alone. Stuttering, asthma, migraine headaches, and many other disorders are seen as the result of heredity and environment acting together, with elements of chance thrown in (Kidd, 1984). The interaction between heredity and environment is something we commonly encounter.

For example, a few summers ago, I grew all my tomato plants from the same seed packet, giving them an identical heredity. But I planted some near Burlington, in a relatively warm environment (for Vermont), and I planted others in the Northeast Kingdom of Vermont, which has a colder, cloudier summer environment. As you might guess, by mid-August, the tomatoes near warmer, sunnier Burlington were plump and red, while those in the Northeast Kingdom were smaller with many shriveled blossoms, showing that environment had a strong differential effect on heredity. And so it is with stuttering.

A child in one family may inherit genes predisposing them to stutter, but their environment may be so low-key that stuttering never develops. A different child, inheriting similar genes, may grow up in a culture that favors rapid speech and a fast-paced lifestyle and may begin to stutter at age 3.

In this chapter, I review four approaches to the study of heredity and stuttering: family studies, twin studies, adoption studies, and genetic studies. These different ways of gathering evidence all suggest that for many individuals, stuttering is partly attributable to heredity. These methods complement each other because no single method can provide all the information we want and because they can provide converging insights into what is really going on when we think about how genetics is involved in stuttering. The insights we gain from these studies are vital in counseling individuals and families about the nature of their or their child's stuttering.

The studies that I review are a good example of the increasing rigor of science as it progresses. Investigations of heredity in family studies were often casual in the 1930s, using only parents' reports to determine if a child was stuttering and not using control groups (children who had no family history of stuttering) in their studies. Twin studies and adoption studies had tighter methodology and strongly suggested what portion of stuttering was the result of heredity and what portion was from environmental factors. Genetic studies that actually examined participants' DNA were more rigorous still and were often able to pinpoint exact genes and chromosomes that were related to stuttering. We'll begin with the most casual studies.

Family Studies

Table 2.1 summarizes the studies that I discuss here. I will begin by describing research from early studies. These provide the first clear evidence that stuttering has a strong genetic component. However, as you'll see, these studies had several weaknesses (these weaknesses are detailed in Felsenfeld, 1997; Yairi et al., 1996). Here is a quick summary of these weaknesses. First, researchers only studied families with stuttering and did not use closely matched control families. Second, their subjects were adults who stuttered—who were asked about their family history of stuttering. This excluded subjects (children) who had begun to stutter and then recovered while still young. Another weakness in several early studies is that parent reports of children's speech—rather than observation by the experimenters—were used to determine whether a child stuttered or not. Relying solely on parent reports might introduce some errors. Now, let's look at some of those pioneering studies, which are interesting despite their flaws.

The first two among those early reports on the genetics of stuttering were published by a group of researchers in Newcastle, England (Andrews & Harris, 1964; Kay, 1964). They compared the family histories of older children who stuttered with those of children who didn't. They found good evidence for inheritance of stuttering. Children who stuttered had far more relatives who stuttered. The researchers also found that certain aspects of stuttering were different in males and females. Males were more likely to stutter, but females who stuttered were more likely to have relatives who stuttered. This means that something about boys makes them more vulnerable to stuttering. And something about girls makes them more resistant to stuttering so that in order to develop stuttering, girls need to inherit more genetic material (ie, more stuttering relatives passing on a tendency to stutter).

Ten years after the Newcastle studies, researchers at Yale University confirmed these early findings that males are more vulnerable to stuttering and females are more resistant (Kidd, 1977; Kidd et al., 1973, 1978). Kidd (1984) concluded that these patterns were best explained by an interaction between the environment and a combination of several genes.

A decade later, researchers at the University of Illinois (Ambrose et al., 1993) studied the family histories of children who had just been diagnosed with stuttering. These younger children were a mix of children who would later recover from their stuttering and children who would persist. They found, like the earlier studies, that the children who stuttered had far more stuttering relatives than control children and more stuttering relatives were male. Unlike past studies, however, these researchers found that male and female children who stuttered had similar chances of having relatives who stuttered.

TABLE 2.1 Summary of Family Studies of Stuttering

Authors, Date	Major Findings	Implications
Andrews and Harris (1964) and Kay (1964)	Children who stuttered had more relatives who stuttered than children who didn't. More males than females stuttered. Females who stuttered were more likely to have relatives who stuttered.	Stuttering seems to be inherited. Males are more susceptible to stuttering. Females who stutter are likely to have more genetic "loading" in order to overcome female resistance to stuttering.
Kidd (1977), Kidd et al. (1973, 1978)	More males stuttered than females; females who stuttered had more relatives who stuttered. This team developed statistical polygenetic model of stuttering.	This study confirmed findings by Andrews and colleagues that stuttering is often inherited. They suggested that stuttering is best explained by interaction of several genes and environment.
Ambrose et al. (1993, 1997)	This study used very young children just after onset, thus a mix of persistent and those who may recover. The authors found that male and female children had equal chance of having relatives who stutter and that females are more likely to recover. Persistence runs in families.	This study confirmed earlier studies indicating that stuttering is often inherited. Children who stutter from families with persistent stuttering are more likely to persist.
Viswanath et al. (2004)	These researchers suggested that persistent stuttering and recovered stuttering may be two different disorders.	It may be possible someday to predict if a child will recover from stuttering.
Nandhini Devi et al. (2018)	This team found that when stuttering occurred in families in which the parents were genetically related to each other, more family members stuttered.	This is further evidence that stuttering has a genetic component.

Thus, the inheritance of stuttering was supported. But unlike Kay (1964), they found no evidence that females needed more "stuttering genes" to account for their stuttering.

Four years later, the Illinois group published another study of children who were assessed soon after the onset of their stuttering (Ambrose et al., 1997). They followed the children for 36 months and categorized them into those who completely recovered from stuttering and those whose stuttering persisted for more than 36 months after initial evaluation. The researchers found strong evidence that recovery is far more frequent among females. A second finding was that persistence tended to run in families. In other words, children who did not outgrow their stuttering were likely to come from families in which relatives who had stuttered also persisted in their stuttering. Conversely, children who recovered were likely to come from families in which relatives who initially stuttered also recovered when they grew older. Further analysis of their data led the authors to propose that persistent and recovered stuttering are transmitted by the same major gene or genes but that those individuals whose stuttering persisted had additional genetic factors that affected recovery. The authors conclude their study by discussing the possible role of environmental factors that interact with genetic factors that should be considered in understanding the nature of stuttering. They also consider the effect of these findings on treatment of the disorder.

Viswanath et al. (2004) give a different view of the genetics of persistence and recovery. Their studies of family members of persistent stutterers led them to hypothesize that persistent and recovered stuttering are two genetically different disorders, meaning that two or more different genes are involved. Other aspects of their work confirmed that stuttering is inherited through a dominant gene (a gene related to stuttering can come from *just one* parent rather than requiring one from each parent). They also found, like other studies, that males are more susceptible and that if a parent (rather than a more distant relative) stutters, inheritance is more likely.

As suggested by Ambrose et al. (1997), **family studies** have clinical relevance as well as giving us a window into the nature of stuttering. As a clinician, you can ask families whether they have relatives who have stuttered and then find out if these relatives recovered. If they did, the preschool children you are evaluating have a good chance of recovering themselves. If children had relatives who stuttered, you can inform the parents about the likelihood that their children's stuttering was inherited. This may relieve their guilt that they may have caused the stuttering by something they did or didn't do. As an example of this, I have a friend whose parents both stuttered. They originally met at a stuttering therapy center in New York City and made improvements to their speech, but they continued to stutter noticeably throughout their lives. Their first child, my friend, began to stutter at age 4, but neither parent was willing to talk with him about their stuttering or his. His stuttering persisted and he grew up thinking it was unmentionable. But when he had children and one of them began to stutter, he did some reading and talked to professionals. This led him to conclude that he was not to blame. His son hadn't imitated him nor had he caused his son's stuttering by something he did or didn't do. Thus, unlike his parents, he felt comfortable talking openly about his own stuttering to his son and reassuring his son that stuttering was okay. His son has grown up with only a mild stutter and no self-consciousness about it.

Let's go back to the researchers in Illinois for a moment. They examined a number of genetic and seemingly nongenetic factors that might predict recovery or persistence and thereby might be useful in deciding which children are in immediate need of treatment. In an early study, Yairi et al. (1996) found that predictors of recovery include (1) good phonology, language, and nonverbal skills; (2) family members who had recovered from stuttering; and (3) early age of onset of stuttering. Some of the factors that impede recovery, such as problems in phonology or language, might be determined by other genes accompanying a gene related to the initial onset of stuttering. In another study, a few years after the initial study (Yairi & Ambrose, 1999), the Illinois group expanded this list of factors; this larger list, which includes eight factors, was presented in Chapter 1 in the section titled "Recovery Versus Persistence of Stuttering." In addition to the three factors just mentioned, attributes that predict recovery include (4) being female, (5) decreasing severity and frequency of stuttering during the period after onset, (6) currently having stuttered less than a year, (7) having fewer repetition units (li-like this) and slower repetitions (more time between iterations, li......like this), and (8) decreasing number of prolongations and blocks (if they occur at all).[2]

While we are on the topic of family studies, Yairi et al. (1996) suggested that future family studies (1) look for subgroups of stutterers that may have different genetic etiologies, (2) examine family members who don't stutter to find factors that may resist stuttering, and (3) search for environmental factors that may interact with genetic factors to precipitate or maintain stuttering.

In fact, Subramanian and Yairi (2006) did conduct a study of family members that turned up a factor that may have helped them resist stuttering. The task was finger tapping at comfortable and at very fast rates. Three groups were studied: stutterers, their fluent family members, and a control group. In the fast-tapping condition, the stutterers tapped faster than either the family-member group or the control group, but they also had greater variability, suggesting instability in this motor task. However, in the fast-tapping condition, the *family-member* group had the *slowest* tapping rate and showed *little variability*. The implication is that even though the family-member group may have had genetic material underlying stuttering, they were able to resist the pressure to tap far beyond their natural rate. Thus, they may have been fluent speakers because they were also able to resist speaking faster than their natural rate. This finding is discussed further in the section on Nonspeech Motor Control in Chapter 3: Sensorimotor, Emotional, and Language Factors in Stuttering.

One interesting family study looked not only at the number of stuttering relatives that subjects had but also whether there was more stuttering in *consanguineous* families. That is, in families where the parents were genetically related to each other, Nandhini Devi et al. (2018) studied a sample of 74,544 children between ages 2.5 and 16 years in the state of Tamil Nadu, India. The prevalence of stuttering in this sample was relatively low (0.46% of these children stuttered), and 56% of those who stuttered had relatives who stuttered. Family aggregation of stuttering (multiple family members stuttered) was higher in families where the parents were related, being first or second cousins, for example.

Twin Studies

The twin studies I discuss are summarized in Table 2.2. **Twin studies** of stuttering have shown that the disorder occurs much more often in both members of identical (monozygotic) twin pairs than in both members of fraternal (dizygotic), same-sex twin pairs (Andrews et al., 1991; Felsenfeld et al., 2000; Howie, 1981; Luchsinger, 1944; Seeman, 1937). To use the vocabulary of genetics, there is higher ***concordance*** of stuttering in identical than in fraternal twins. This supports the hypothesis that stuttering is inherited, but it doesn't reveal exactly what is inherited.

In addition to providing evidence of genetic factors in stuttering, twin studies demonstrate that heredity does not work alone. In one of the twin studies, although there was higher concordance for stuttering among identical twins, some identical twin pairs were discordant (Howie, 1981). Specifically, Howie found that in 6 of the 16 identical twin pairs, 1 twin stuttered but the other didn't. This means that even though both members of the twin pair had the same genetic inheritance, something else must have been operating. This may not be surprising when one learns that genes must interact with the environment to produce their effects (eg, Gibson, 2008; LeDoux, 2002). A gene might not express itself in stuttering unless, for example, there is some kind of prenatal or postnatal stress on the child. In the case of stuttering, where there may be several genes working together to produce a chronic disorder, the situation is even more complex because several genetic tendencies may need to interact with different aspects of the child's internal and external environment to create stuttering. No wonder more than a third of the pairs were discordant (6/16 or 37.5%) in the Howie study.

[2]Remember that, in Chapter 1, we reported on studies that showed that certain aspects of the stuttering in children 4 to 5 years old predicted persistence versus recovery.

TABLE 2.2 Summary of Twin Studies of Stuttering

Authors, Date	Participants	Major Findings	Implications
Howie (1981)	30 pairs of same-sex twins, in each of which at least one twin stuttered	Findings included 62.5% concordance in identical twin pairs and 23% in fraternal twin pairs In 6 of 16 identical twin pairs, one twin stuttered and the other didn't, implicating nongenetic factors	This study provided evidence for inheritance of stuttering but also evidence for nongenetic factors
Andrews et al. (1991)	3,810 unselected twin pairs	Findings included 71% of variance attributed to genetic factors and 29% attributed to individual's fetal and postpartum environment	Evidence for inheritance was provided
Felsenfeld et al. (2000)	1,567 pairs and 634 individuals from Australian Twin Registry	70% of variance attributed to "additive genetic effects"; 30% attributed to environment	Evidence for inheritance was provided by this study. Similar findings as in previous studies were obtained
Ooki (2005)	1,896 twin pairs	Findings included 80% variance attributed to genetic factors in males and 85% in females	Slightly more genetic effect in females may be related to their natural resistance to stuttering
Dworzynski et al. (2007)	950 twins who recovered from stuttering; 150 twins who persisted	Regarding concordance among recovered twins, findings included 40% concordance for identical twins vs 20% for fraternal twins. Regarding concordance among twins with persistent stuttering, findings included 19% concordance for identical twins vs 0% for fraternal in persistent twins	Suggests that persistent stuttering may be the result of multiple genes being inherited; that is, concordance may be less likely in persistently stuttering fraternal twins if more than one gene must be inherited
van Beijsterveldt et al. (2010)	105,000 total twin pairs For categorization, parents described speech characteristics	Concordance higher in identical vs fraternal twins in terms of whether they are categorized as "probably stuttering" and as "high nonfluency"	Strong evidence for higher concordance in identical twins using a judicious categorization process
Fagnini et al. (2011)	22,316 pairs of twins. 9% of males and 5% of females reported stuttering	Significantly greater concordance was obtained for monozygotic twins compared with dizygotic twins. It was estimated that 70% of variance in stuttering was due to heredity	This large sample provided strong evidence of a hereditary factor for stuttering
Rautakoski et al. (2012)	1,728 total twins	Of the 2.3% of total twins who said they had stuttered at one time, 28% said they continued to stutter Concordance rates indicated that whereas 82% of variance were due to additive genetic effects, 18% were due to nonshared environmental factors	This study provides further evidence of the major influence of genes on stuttering and a minor influence of twins' nonshared environment

An estimate of the relative proportions of genetic and environmental influences was suggested in a later study involving 3,810 unselected (from Australian Twin Registry) twin pairs (Andrews et al., 1991). Analyses of stuttering in these 3,810 unselected twin pairs estimated that 71% of the variance (the probability of whether or not one would stutter) was accounted for by genetic factors and 29% was accounted for by the individual's environment (including factors influencing the fetus, such as maternal stress), as well as factors after birth (such as family conversational style or serious childhood illness). Felsenfeld et al. (2000) followed this with a study of a new sample of 1,567 twin pairs and 634 individuals from the same Australian Twin Registry. They found 17 monozygotic and 8 dizygotic twin pairs who were concordant for stuttering and 21 monozygotic and 45 dizygotic twins who were discordant for stuttering. Statistical analyses estimated that "additive genetic effects" (the effects of different genes working together) accounted for 70% of the variance and that an individual's unique environment accounted for 30% of the variance. These proportions are essentially the same as those found by Andrews et al. (1991) and support the now-common assumption that genes and environment interact to set the stage for stuttering.

Five years after the study by Felsenfeld et al., Ooki (2005) studied 1,896 twin pairs, also comparing concordance in identical and fraternal twins. Using sophisticated statistical techniques, Ooki determined that the proportion of genetic influence on stuttering in males was 80% and 85% in females. It is interesting that the females' rate of stuttering showed slightly more genetic influence than the males'. Perhaps, this echoes the evidence that females have some resistance to stuttering. For a female to develop stuttering, more genetic influence is needed—an idea that had been previously raised by Andrews and Harris (1964) and Kay (1964).

Dworzynski et al. (2007) discovered interesting differences between a group of twins who recovered from stuttering (n = 950) and a group who persisted (n = 150). In the recovered group, concordance for stuttering was 40% for identical twins and 20% for fraternal twins. However, in the persistent stuttering group of twins, the concordance was 19% for identical twins and 0% for fraternal twins—meaning that every member of a fraternal twin pair who persisted in stuttering had a sibling who did not. This suggests that the genetics of **persistent stuttering** are complex. What makes them complex? Well, as we noted previously, the family studies of Ambrose et al. (1997) indicated the possibility that while recovered and persistent stuttering are transmitted by the same major gene(s), persistent stuttering itself may have additional genetic factors that make recovery more difficult (or recovered stutterers may have genetic factors that facilitate recovery). The findings of Dworzynski et al. (2007) may support this supposition because there is so little concordance in the persistent fraternal twin group—meaning that to get concordance, the same array of multiple genes (the "additional genetic factors") must be transmitted. This is far less likely in fraternal twins.

van Beijsterveldt et al. (2010) conducted a twin study using a very large participant pool: 105,000 twin pairs at age 5. They reduced the usual problem of parent identification of their children as stuttering by asking parents merely to estimate the frequency of repetitions, prolongations, and blocks they observed in their children's speech. Children were categorized by the experimenters as "probably stuttering" or "high nonfluency," or as having typical speech. Concordance for probable stuttering was higher in identical twins, supporting the genetic/heritability hypotheses. It was notable that high nonfluency also appeared to be genetically based (see Barasch et al., 2000, for more on a commonality between stuttering and high levels of typical disfluency).

Fagnani et al. (2011) used a large participant pool (33,317) of adults from the Danish Twin Registry, employing questionnaires to ascertain whether they had ever stuttered. They found that 9% of the males and 4% of the females reported stuttering at some point in their past. There was significantly greater concordance in monozygotic twins, and the researchers estimated that 70% of the variance in stuttering probability was due to heredity and the other 30% was due to environment or environment-gene interaction. This matches the findings of Andrews et al. (1991) and Felsenfeld et al. (2000) but with a much larger sample. Similar findings were reported by Rautakoski et al. (2012), using self-report from adults in a study of 1,728 twins in Finland. They indicated that 82% of the variance could be attributed to additive genetic effects and 18% to nonshared environmental influences.

In summarizing the evidence from twin studies, Frigerio-Domingues and Drayna (2017) made this assessment: "First, monozygotic (MZ) twins consistently display a higher concordance for stuttering than dizygotic (DZ) twins, indicating strong evidence for a genetic component to this disorder. Second, the MZ twin concordance for stuttering is consistently <1, indicating that germ line genetic factors by themselves do not explain all of stuttering. Third, while heritability estimates from these studies have varied, many have produced estimates of high heritability, often exceeding .80" (p. 1). Heritability is a statistic that expresses how likely it is that traits of interest are from genetic rather than other factors and vary from zero to one.

In an interesting aside, Bloodstein et al. (2021) questioned the assumption that influence on stuttering that was not accounted for by genetic factors must be attributed to environmental factors. Research using animal models suggests that identical twins sometimes have discordance for certain traits *not* because of environmental influences but because of variations in the way two identical embryos develop. Some of these variations may be related to "epigenetics," which are non-DNA factors that are inherited and influence the expression of genes as effects on specific behaviors or phenotypes. Readers wishing to understand the latest developments in genetic research may wish to visit www.genome.gov. The link on that website called "Resources for Teachers" has good tools to help you understand genes.

TABLE 2.3 Summary of Adoption Studies

Authors, Date	Participants	Major Findings	Implications
Bloodstein (1961a) and Bloodstein et al. (2021)	13 adopted individuals who stuttered	Four of the 13 individuals studied reported having relatives who stuttered in adoptive families	Four is a larger number than would happen by chance. This may imply these four individuals had been influenced by adoptive family members who stuttered
Felsenfeld (1997)	No information on number of individuals	Preliminary data only summarized as from both biological and adoptive families	Data suggested stuttering in biological families was more predictive of stuttering in subject than stuttering in adoptive families

Adoption Studies

Adoption studies are summarized in Table 2.3. Because the birth records of adopted children are often difficult to obtain, studies of adopted stutterers are rare. Nonetheless, they can be helpful because they offer larger contrasts in environmental factors than seem to be available in twin studies, where family environments are somewhat shared. Bloodstein (1961a) interviewed 13 adopted stutterers about the presence of stuttering in their adoptive families (information about their biological families was not available). Four of the 13 reported having relatives who stuttered in their adoptive families, which is higher than would be expected by chance. This small sample, without data from biological families, supports the possibility that environmental factors may have an effect. If the relatives in the adoptive family were key figures, such as a parent or older sibling who was close to the child, this would be stronger evidence for the influence of the environment on stuttering. Unfortunately, this information is not available.

Felsenfeld (1997) reported some preliminary data on a small sample of adopted children who had speech disorders (primarily stuttering) and for whom data were available from both adoptive and biological families. These data indicated that a history of stuttering in the biological families was slightly more predictive of disorders in these children than was stuttering in the adoptive family.

Again, the evidence from family and twin studies suggests that both genetic and environmental factors influence whether or not a child will stutter and that genetic inheritance appears to contribute more strongly. Methods developed relatively recently allow more direct examination of the genetics of families with and without members who stutter; these will be discussed in the next section.

Genes

Genes are the basis of inheritance. They are sequences of **DNA** that determine traits—like your hair color, and whether you have the "Achoo" syndrome.[3] Genes ride on chromosomes that are wormlike strings of DNA contained in the nucleus of every cell. Figure 2.2 will give you a visual impression of these dynamos of heredity.

Genetic Linkage Studies

Genetic linkage studies can be difficult to understand. The Stuttering Foundation produced a video in 2013 in which one of the scientists, Dennis Drayna, explains his work in this area (https://www.youtube.com/watch?v=HK-TyKKW-ok; or Google "YouTube Dennis Drayna genes and stuttering"). Other videos can be seen by Googling "Genes and Stuttering."

Drayna and his colleagues at the National Institutes of Health have carried out genetic linkage studies using large numbers of families to try to isolate genes for stuttering (for an early overview, see Drayna, 1997). The term "genetic linkage" refers to the fact that the genes related to a disorder may

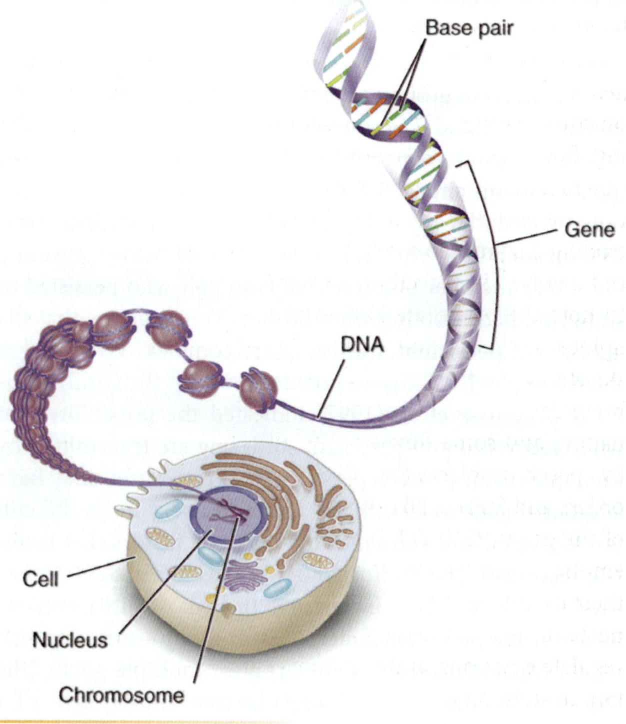

Figure 2.2 Chromosomes and gene.

[3]This syndrome is about sneezing when you look into bright light. If your father had this, you may also.

be physically close together (linked) on the chromosome when they are inherited. Genetic linkage analysis compares the chromosomes of family members who have a trait with those of family members who do not. In this way, the approximate chromosomal location of the stuttering gene or genes can be identified. Genetic linkage analysis is in accord with the view that stuttering, like most inherited disorders, is the result of more than one gene. To use the proper term, stuttering is thought to be "polygenic."

To begin their hunt for a stuttering gene, Drayna and his colleagues studied families in which there is more than one individual who stutters. They examined 68 families in North America and Europe and found evidence that genes on chromosome 18 may be related to stuttering in these families (Shugart et al., 2004—a research group that included Drayna). Because these are a set of genes that control intercellular communication, this finding suggests that such intercellular communication may be important among neurons involved in speech production and that when such communication goes wrong, the flow of information for speech production may be discoordinated, perhaps resulting in stuttering.

Several years after the Shugart study, Drayna, his students, and his colleagues joined with geneticists in Lahore, Pakistan, to continue the hunt for more stuttering genes. They chose Pakistan because tradition in that culture encourages marriage within families (cousins marrying cousins), and this produces a smaller degree of genetic variation that results in a greater concentration of genetic disorders. Kang et al. (2010)—again, a group that included Drayna—published a study in the prestigious *New England Journal of Medicine* that reported on 123 Pakistani individuals who stuttered as well as 270 individuals in the United States and England who stuttered. They also used a control group of 372 individuals in these three countries who didn't stutter. Mutations of three genes (the genes were called *GNPTAB*, *GNPTG*, and *NAGPA*) on chromosome 12 were found to be associated with stuttering. Some individuals showed mutations of gene *GNPTAB*, others had mutations on *GNPTG*, and still others had mutations on *NAGPA*. The work of all three genes is related to controlling enzymes in a cell's lysosome structure—the part of a cell involved in recycling cell waste products. It is important to note that there are known genetic disorders (eg, mucolipidoses) of this waste recycling process that affect joint, skeletal, and other body components. These disorders affect brain development, resulting in delays in movement coordination, and some forms of mucolipidoses are accompanied by speech problems (National Institute of Neurological Disorders and Stroke, 2011). Also important is the fact that one of the genes, *GNPTG*, is associated with motor control and emotional regulation by way of the gene's expression in (ie, their effects on) the cerebellum and the hippocampus. It is noteworthy that the hippocampus is affected because it helps regulate emotions, and emotion-related responses are important in stuttering.

Further exploring the findings described above, Lee et al. (2011) provided stronger evidence that mutations in one of these genes—*NAGPA*—may cause stuttering. The effect of the mutations is to diminish enzyme activity in cells. The authors caution that not enough is known (in 2011, anyway) about exactly how neuronal deficits affect speech to be able to explain how these mutations result specifically in stuttering. Nonetheless, one hypothesis about the underlying mechanism relating diminished enzyme activity in cells' lysosome structure was proposed by Budde et al. (2014). Through a meta-analysis of many studies of differences in individuals who stutter, they concluded that the diminished activity related to lysosomal processing may underlie incomplete myelination of white matter tracts important in speech motor control. The incomplete myelination hypothesis will be discussed again when I present findings on white matter tracts (the brain's connecting pathways) later in the chapter. Interestingly, for more than 70 years (beginning with Karlin, 1947), there have been hypotheses that incomplete myelination of nerve tracts, a factor that could lead to less efficient transmission of electrical impulses, contributes to stuttering. Another gene, *AP4E1*, was found by Raza et al. (2015) to be associated with stuttering and also involved in lysosomal processing.

There have been many genetic linkage studies in the last 30 years and, of course, more are being published every year. Rather than describe each study, I have created a table of these studies (Table 2.4) that summarizes this research.

More detailed summaries of the genetic research are given in Chapter 2 of Bloodstein et al. (2021). In addition, Frigerio-Domingues and Drayna (2017) reviewed findings related to the four genes described above (*GNTAB*, *GNPTG*, *NAGPA*, and *AP4E1*) and noted that because no other neurological deficits appear with stuttering when one of the genes is mutated, the pathology seems to be "limited to a small and specialized population of neurons" (p. 5). These authors go on to suggest that animal models would be extremely helpful in identifying these neurons. Indeed, as they point out, mice that have been given mutations of *GNPTAB* have shown stutteringlike vocalizations.

Mutations in *GNPTAB* also feature prominently in a study linking *genes* associated with stuttering and *brain areas* that appear to be dysfunctional in stuttering. Benito-Aragon et al. (2020), using neuroimaging and a mathematical process called "graph theory," suggested that mutations in the gene *GNPTG* may be associated with disruption in cortical networks that support auditory-motor integration for speech motor control. Problems in auditory-motor integration may be an important element in stuttering, as will become clear later in this chapter and also in Chapter 6—Theories About Stuttering. Benito-Aragon et al.'s findings suggested that the auditory-motor integration dysfunction is part of the basic neuropathology of stuttering, rather than the result of brain changes caused by years of stuttering.

If you wish to know the very latest on the genetics of stuttering, you can conduct a search using a research database

TABLE 2.4 Summary of Genetic Studies of Stuttering

Authors, Date	Participants	Major Findings	Implications
Cox and Yairi (2000)	Community of Hutterites in North Dakota	Chromosomes 1, 13, and 16 identified as possibly being the locus of genes related to stuttering	Early evidence that specific chromosomes related to some individuals' stuttering may have been found
Shugart et al. (2004)	68 families in North America and Europe	Evidence for stuttering related to genes associated with chromosome 18	These genes may be related to intercellular communication in speech production areas of the brain
Riaz et al. (2005)	44 Pakistani families	A locus on chromosome 12q may contain a gene related to stuttering in these families No evidence found for linkage on chromosome 18 as was suggested by Shugart et al. (2004)	Stuttering is probably a complex trait transmitted by non-Mendelian inheritance and can be caused by genes on different chromosomes, as seen in different studies
Kang et al. (2010)	123 individuals who stuttered in Pakistan	Mutations found in 3 genes on chromosome 12: *GNPTAB*, *GNPTG*, and *NAGPA*	These mutations affect recycling cell waste products, sometimes producing known genetic disorders such as problems with the joints and motor systems, and developmental delay Possible source of motor control and emotion effects in stuttering individuals
Raza et al. (2010)	Large, consanguineous Pakistani family with many individuals with persistent stuttering	Significant linkage found on chromosome 3q13.2-3q13.33	One individual with this genetic linkage did not stutter but may have outgrown childhood stuttering This study provides more evidence of inheritance of stuttering
Raza et al. (2012)	Family in Lahore, Pakistan, with 14 members who stuttered	Linkage found for several genes on chromosome 16q	Evidence for new locus for stuttering gene was provided by this study
Raza et al. (2013)	Family of 71 individuals in Cameroon, of whom 33 have persistent stuttering	No single locus for stuttering was found; instead, evidence found for linkage to loci on previously reported 3q and 15q and new finding of loci on 2p, 3p, 14q, and new region of 15q	Strong evidence for linkage at several loci was provided by this study
Han et al. (2014)	602 unrelated cases of persistent stuttering	*FOXP2* and *CNTNAP2* genes seen as important in verbal dyspraxia and specific language impairment (SLI) not found in stuttering individuals	Genetic neuropathological origins of stuttering differ from those in dyspraxia and SLI
Raza et al. (2015)	A large number of stutterers from Cameroon, Pakistan, and North America and matched controls	Variants of gene *AP4E1* found in stutterers were shown to be related to the product of formerly identified gene *NAGPA*	Findings suggest problems in intercellular communication (cf., Shugart et al., 2004)
Chen et al. (2015)	502 Chinese families with dyslexia and 502 without	Stuttering risk genes *GNPTAB* and *NAGPA* shown to be associated with dyslexia	Common genes associated with stuttering found in dyslexic families

TABLE 2.4 Summary of Genetic Studies of Stuttering (*Continued*)

Authors, Date	Participants	Major Findings	Implications
Raza et al. (2016)	1,013 unrelated individuals who stutter from around the world	Mutations in genes *GNPTAB*, *GNPTG*, and *NAGPA* were shown to be related to stuttering but also to serious mucolipidosis disorders Stuttering individuals did not show any mucolipidosis disorders	Mutations of these genes in stuttering are different from those in mucolipidosis These mutations are estimated to occur in 16% of stuttering individuals worldwide
Frigerio-Domingues and Drayna (2017)	A review study of the genes *GNTAB*, *GNPTG*, *NAGPA*, and *AP4E1*	This study points out that stuttering appears to be associated with mutations of these genes but no other neurological deficits co-occur with stuttering	Only a small and specialized group of neurons may be responsible for stuttering that occurs with these gene mutations
Benito-Aragon et al. (2020)	Analysis of the expression of mutation of *GMPTG* and neural networks connectivity deficits associated with stuttering	This study provided evidence that mutations in *GMPTG* affect neurotransmission in networks associated with auditory-motor integration	This is one of the first studies to show how mutation of a gene may directly affect networks that affect speech fluency

such as Ovid MEDLINE or PubMed, using the two terms "stuttering" and "genetics." Another approach—one *not* using families with many individuals who stutter—to studying genes is described in the next section.

A Genome-Wide Association Study

Genome-wide association studies examine the DNA of a large number of individuals who *have* a disorder and compare them with the DNA of a large number of individuals who *don't* have it. This comparison is hoped to reveal genetic differences between the two groups—the "haves" and the "have-nots"—thus pinpointing genes that may be responsible for the disorder. The difference between genome-wide association studies and linkage studies is that the genome-wide studies look at large populations and the linkage studies look within families, although both studies compare those who have a disorder with those who do not.

Kraft (2010) carried out a genome-wide association analysis of the genes of 84 persistent stutterers and 107 controls in which the DNA of a population of unrelated individuals is examined. She scanned the DNA of all of her participants, looking for "markers" that distinguished the DNA of stuttering participants. She didn't find a single gene that clearly characterized stuttering, supporting other findings that no single gene seems to be responsible for stuttering. Kraft's findings did identify 10 "candidate genes" that were statistically more likely to appear in the DNA of those who stuttered. These could work by influencing (1) neural development, (2) neural function, and (3) behavior. Some genes were associated with both neural development and neural function. Other candidate genes, in the behavior category, happened to be associated with other disorders, such as autism. Kraft points out that future research should look for combinations of genes that are related to stuttering.

CONGENITAL AND EARLY CHILDHOOD TRAUMA STUDIES

This section moves away from *heredity* as a causal factor in stuttering to *congenital and early childhood trauma* as alternative causal explanations of stuttering. These causal explanations can also be considered "constitutional" and may account for the many individuals who stutter who have no family history of stuttering or related disorders—no heredity of stuttering.

One of the first studies to look closely at stutterers who had no family history of stuttering—West et al. (1939)—examined a sample of 204 people who stuttered and found that 100 of them reported no family members who stuttered. Of these 100 who had no family members who stuttered, 85 reported **congenital factors** or other early childhood stressors that may have been related to the onset of stuttering. These stressors included infectious diseases, diseases of the nervous system, and injuries—all reported to have occurred just prior to stuttering onset, although the exact proximity to onset was not reported. Thus, these factors may have created some sort of trigger for the development of stuttering, but we don't know exactly how such stressors would result in the symptoms of stuttering.

A later study by Poulos and Webster (1991) found that 57 of the clients in a clinic sample of 169 adults and adolescents who stuttered reported no family history of stuttering. Of these without family histories, 37% reported congenital or early childhood factors that may have been associated with the onset of stuttering, whereas only 2.4% of the clients having a positive family history of stuttering reported such factors. The factors reported in this study included anoxia at birth, premature birth, childhood surgery, head injury, mild cerebral palsy, mild retardation, and experiencing intense fear.

A good example of intense fear triggering stuttering was provided in a story in the New York Times (Abi-Habib, 2022). A man named Raoul recalled his childhood experience during a bombing in Lebanon's civil war.

The journalist wrote: *One night as Raoul slept.... bombing started. His mother cried out for him, looking frantically until they found Raoul, then 5, crying while hugging a framed photo of the Virgin Mary that had fallen from the wall, praying for his life. He developed a stutter after that. [Raoul said,] "When I left Lebanon, I left. I only took my stutter with me."*

We have no information about his family history of stuttering, but it seems likely that he was fluent until he was traumatized by the bombing.

A study by Alm and Risberg (2007) examined a group of 32 individuals who stuttered to look for etiological subgroups. Twenty-three of the 32 (72%) who stuttered had family histories of stuttering. Seventeen of the 32 (53%) had sustained neurological lesions prior to onset of stuttering. Of note is the finding that seven of the nine individuals with no family history of stuttering (78%) reported preonset neurological lesions. This further supports the hypothesis that two different predispositions may contribute to stuttering: genetic inheritance and brain injury.

Two studies took the opposite approach to those described in the previous paragraphs: they looked at a brain-injured population and assessed whether it comprised more individuals who stuttered than in the general population. In the first, Böhme (1968) examined a sample of 313 individuals who had sustained brain damage at birth or in early childhood; 24% of those 313 developed stuttering (compared to 5% in the general population). Unfortunately, no information is given about family history of stuttering in those who developed it, but the implication drawn was that congenital or early childhood brain injury can often result in stuttering. In a similar study, Segalowitz and Brown (1991) surveyed more than 600 high school students to ascertain how many had experienced head injury during their childhoods. Of the students, 92 reported head injury, and, of those, 9 (about 10%) reported having been diagnosed with stuttering. However, it was not clear if the stuttering appeared after the head injury. The authors found that there was a significant relationship between having a head injury and being diagnosed with stuttering, particularly for those children who were unconscious for a period of time after the head injury. Again, there is no information as to whether some of the children who stuttered and had head injuries also had family histories of stuttering.

In a study that examined psychological trauma as an etiological factor in stuttering, Ozgür and Ozgür (2019) evaluated 64 stuttering children younger than age 18 at two clinics in Turkey. Only 21% were found to have family histories of stuttering, but a separate 31.3% were found to have experienced "life stressors" within a week of stuttering onset. These stressors include death of their mother, birth of a sibling, starting primary school, and moving to a new home. All diagnoses were made at either a psychiatric clinic or an ENT clinic where the two authors were employed. Thus, the subjects in this study were a special group and probably not representative of the general population of Turkey.

The fact that neurological or psychological traumas may be associated with childhood stuttering in those without family histories of stuttering is not surprising. Adult onset of stuttering is often associated with head injury, neurological disease, stress, or psychological trauma as I have described in Chapter 8, "Atypical Disfluency." Thus, mechanisms similar to those that precipitate adult onset may be involved in childhood stuttering in the absence of family history of stuttering, but this possibility raises as many questions as answers. Why would some children (and adults), but not others, begin to stutter as a result of intense fear or brain injury? Which brain structures and functions affected by head injury and neurological disease result in stuttering? How are they similar to and how do they differ from the effects of inheriting a predisposition to stutter?

In relation to the last question, a number of investigators have looked at whether individuals who stutter who have family histories of stuttering showed any differences in their stuttering behavior, such as severity, compared with those without family histories. Andrews and Harris (1964) and Kidd et al. (1980) found no differences in the stuttering of those with and without family histories of stuttering. However, Janssen et al. (1990) looked at a wider variety of speech- and language-related variables in several different age groups. They found several significant differences (as well as similarities) between the group with family histories of stuttering and the group without such histories. In terms of similarities, the groups did not differ significantly in responsiveness to treatment, reading ability, or speech-related anxiety. However, when stuttering behaviors were examined closely, those with family histories of stuttering showed more prolongations and blocks than those with no family history of stuttering, although the frequency of repetitions was the same for both groups. Another difference between the groups was that those with positive family histories for stuttering showed significantly longer durations of voiced segments of speech and significantly greater variability in length of unvoiced segments during fluent speech than those with no family history of stuttering. The authors interpreted this finding to suggest that the stutterers with positive family histories were slower and more variable in their fluent speech. What might this mean?

From these studies, we can conclude that individuals with family histories of stuttering have inherited greater neuromotor instability than those without family histories of stuttering—an instability that produces more prolongations

TABLE 2.5 Summary of Congenital and Early Childhood Factors in Stuttering

Authors, Date	Participants	Major Findings	Implications
West et al. (1939)	204 individuals who stuttered	One hundred of the 204 participants reported no family history of stuttering, and 85 reported congenital or early childhood factors, such as nervous system diseases and injuries	This study provided an early indication that congenital or early childhood factors may create predisposition for stuttering
Bohme (1968)	313 children who had sustained brain damage at birth or in early childhood	24% of those children developed stuttering (compared to 5% of all children). This early brain damage was associated with high percentage of stuttering. No information on family history of stuttering in these children	Early brain damage may be associated with stuttering. However, no information about family history of subjects and no information on long-term outcome make these findings more difficult to interpret
Poulos and Webster (1991)	169 individuals who stuttered	57 individuals reported no family history of stuttering. Of these, 37% reported congenital or early childhood events that might be related to stuttering predisposition. These included anoxia at birth, premature birth, head injury, experiencing intense fear. Only 2.4% of those with family history reported such events	This study provides further evidence that congenital and early childhood factors may predispose a child to stuttering
Segalowitz and Brown (1991)	600 high school students surveyed	92 of the 600 students reported head injury during childhood. 9 of them (~10%) reported stuttering, more often if child was unconscious for a period of time. No information was given on family history of stuttering	This study provides evidence that head injury with a period of unconsciousness may result in stuttering. Not known if family history of stuttering has an influence
Alm and Risberg (2007)	32 individuals who stuttered	78% of those with no family history of stuttering reported "neurological lesions" prior to the onset of stuttering	Genetic factors may explain only some of the causal factors in the onset of stuttering
Ozgur and Ozgur (2019)	64 stuttering children younger than age 18 who came to a psychiatric or ENT clinic	In this study, 21.9% had family history of stuttering; a separate 31.3% were found to have "life stressors" no more than 1 week prior to stuttering onset. Stressors included death of a mother, birth of a sibling, moving to a new home, and starting primary school	This study provides evidence that, in some cases, stressful experiences may trigger stuttering

and blocks and that may require the individual to speak more slowly to maintain fluency. This is not to say that those without family history of stuttering did not inherit the predisposition to stutter. Their family histories may contain other speech-related deficits (eg, articulation problems evident in my family history), and their underlying neuromotor anomalies may result in stuttering. Future research can try to answer this question: Do individuals who stutter but have no family history of stuttering have more family history of other speech and language disorders than the general population? Perhaps you would like to carry out this research yourself.

Table 2.5 summarizes the important findings regarding congenital and early childhood factors as possible etiologies of stuttering.

BRAIN FUNCTION AND STRUCTURE

Brain functions and structures are the link between what you've just been reading about—genetic predisposition or childhood trauma—and the behaviors of stuttering that we see and hear. In other words, when someone has a genetic predisposition for stuttering or has had childhood trauma, we ask: how does that affect the brain in a way that results in stuttering? Research on brain function and structure, comparing individuals who stutter with a control group of fluent speakers can help us answer that. For example, mutations in a particular gene may be found to affect areas of the brain that are vital in producing speech. Remember the findings reported in Benito-Aragon et al. (2020) that mutations in the gene *GNPTG* affect auditory-motor integration for speech? Read the following sections on brain function and structure to see what areas of the brain control auditory-motor integration.

In the following sections, I will review studies of brain function and brain structure in separate sections, even though they obviously influence each other. The influence goes both ways. Not only does an anomalous structure (such as less dense nerve fibers) result in slow or mistimed transmission of information, but the converse may be true as well: repeated dysfunctions in transmissions may cause changes in structures. As an example, read about how individuals who stutter may use right-hemisphere brain areas to compensate for deficits in speech-specialized left-hemisphere areas. Do you think that this change will affect the structures in right-hemisphere areas?

I will discuss brain function first because scientists, in the early days, had only the tools to study brain function, not brain structure. However, as I discuss function, you will need to consult Figure 2.3 to orient yourself to landmarks in the brain related to speech and language production.

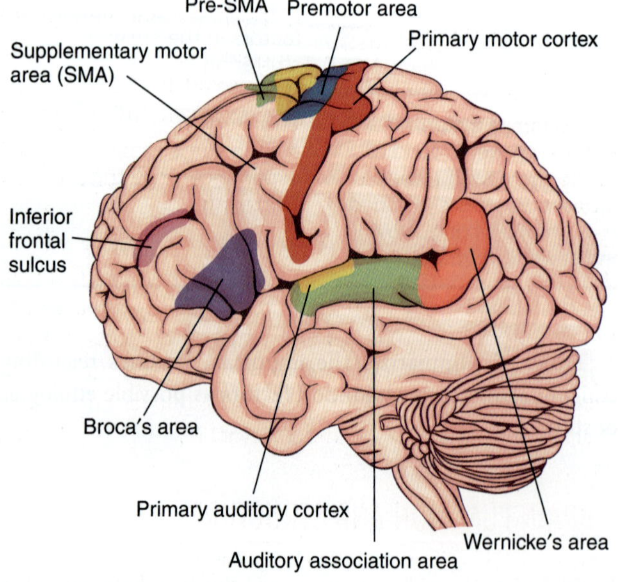

Figure 2.3 Areas in the left side of the brain that are thought to be involved in speech production.

Brain *Function* Differences in People Who Stutter Compared With People Who Do Not Stutter

Some of the earliest research on the brain and stuttering was conducted in the 1920s, as I described in Chapter 1. Because of the limited technology available at that time, brain function rather than brain structure was the target of researchers' questions. They could see that the brain wasn't working quite right, but they couldn't yet visualize the activity of brain nerve fibers and networks. As research into the causes of stuttering was heating up, scientists had a new tool—electroencephalography (EEG)—they could use to measure brain waves, which are the "signatures" of the electrical activity in the brain as it functions. EEG had been developed by Hans Berger, in part because of his fascination with mental telepathy (to read details on this surprising interest, see his biography in Wikipedia). By the late 1920s, Lee Edward Travis at the University of Iowa learned about EEG and used it to study the brains of people who stutter, as you will see in the following sections.

Cerebral Dominance for Speech

Both old and new studies have shown that individuals who stutter have greater activity in their right hemispheres than in their left hemispheres, during both fluent and stuttered speech—the reverse of the pattern shown by fluent typical subjects who show considerable left-hemisphere activity and little right-hemisphere activity during speech. Figure 2.4 shows this difference between adults who stuttered and those who didn't. The activity seen in the brains of adults who stuttered was often in the same location in the right hemisphere as the left-hemisphere areas most active in fluent speakers. These other hemisphere structures are usually referred to as "homologous" areas.

These findings about greater right-hemisphere activity (compared with left-hemisphere activity) suggest that left-hemisphere structures for speech and language in individuals who stutter may have developed more slowly or differently in ways that contribute to stuttering. Slower or different development may prompt these individuals' use of homologous right-hemisphere structures, which themselves may not be as suited for rapid speech production as left-hemisphere structures (Geschwind & Galaburda, 1985; Kent, 1984). This may result in stuttering, especially under the stress of increasing language demands and faster speaking as children develop, as well as because of interference with right-hemisphere processing from nearby right-hemisphere centers for emotion.

Electroencephalographic Studies

Samuel Orton and Lee Edward Travis (Orton, 1927; Orton & Travis, 1929; Travis, 1931) used EEG to measure brain waves in stuttering and nonstuttering subjects. Their hope

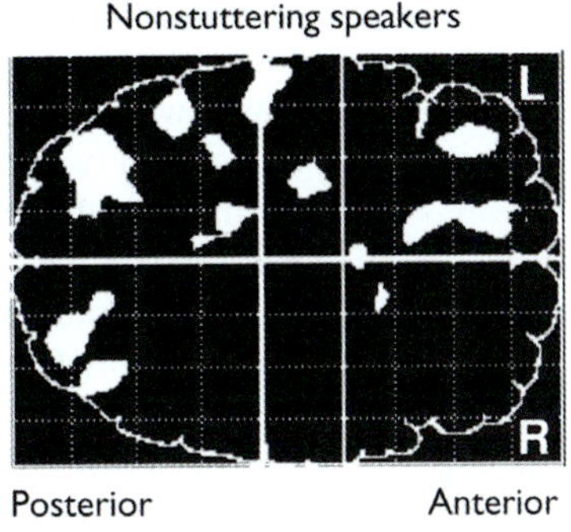

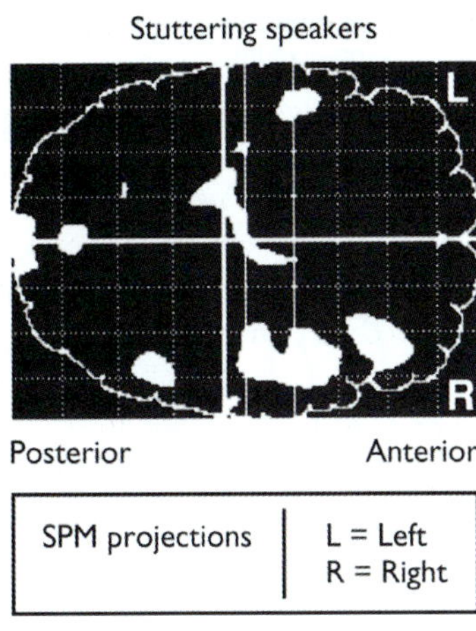

Figure 2.4 Positron emission tomography scans of brains of nonstuttering (*left*) and stuttering (*right*) adults while reading aloud. SPM, statistical parametric mapping. (From De Nil, L. F., Kroll, R. M., Kapur, S., & Houle, S. [1995, December]. *Silent and oral reading in stuttering and nonstuttering adults: A positron emission tomography study*. Paper presented at the Annual Convention of the American Speech-Language-Hearing Association, Orlando, FL. Reprinted with permission from Luc De Nil, PhD.)

was to find proof that the brains of stutterers didn't show the normal left-hemisphere dominance during speech and that this difference might account for the mistiming of signals sent from the brain to muscles of the speech production system. EEG studies are carried out by pasting electrodes to the surface of the scalp to measure the electrical activity of the brain lying several millimeters below. This procedure, like any assessment of the brain, was fraught with methodological quandaries and imprecise technology (Bloodstein, 1995; Bloodstein et al., 2021). For example, how faithfully would electrical activity on the scalp reflect the activity of brain cells several millimeters below? How do we know that the electrical activity recorded isn't created by muscle contractions during speech or even the result of the subject blinking their eyes or wiggling their nose? How do we know which part of the brain is active when we see the squiggles on the chart paper that represent electrical impulses? These sources of variability made it likely that the EEG studies by different scientists in different laboratories would produce widely different findings due to different methodologies and different interpretations of the data.

Despite these problems, many EEG studies of people who stutter and those who don't have been conducted. Some interesting findings have turned up. However, as with other experimental results, you should be cautious about accepting the results as final proof. Several EEG studies supported the notion that the brains of people who stuttered functioned differently, although other studies didn't find such differences. EEG studies by Douglass (1943), Ponsford et al. (1975), Travis and Knott (1937), Zimmerman and Knott (1974), many by Moore and his colleagues (eg, Moore & Haynes, 1980), and a study by Boberg et al. (1983) all showed in different ways that individuals who stuttered tended to have more activity on the right side of the brain during speech and especially during stuttering than did those who didn't stutter. This activity seemed to involve structures in the right hemisphere that were in locations similar to those in the left hemisphere that control speech and language (as I said earlier, homologous structures). One of those areas is called the right frontal operculum (see Fig. 2.5) and is in the same location in the right hemisphere that Broca's area[4] is in the left hemisphere (Fox, 2003). Although this was not exactly what Orton and Travis had predicted in their theory, it was close. Whereas the Orton-Travis theory hypothesized that individuals who stuttered lacked hemispheric dominance, findings from these EEG studies suggested that rather than lacking dominance, individuals who stutter may be more likely to have a right-hemisphere dominance for speech and language (whereas nonstutterers generally have left-hemisphere dominance for speech and language).

Cerebral Blood Flow Studies: A More Detailed Look at Different Areas of the Brain

In the 1970s and 1980s, researchers developed new technology that was more precise than EEG in detecting exactly where brain activity was occurring by measuring the amount of blood flowing to those areas. Cerebral blood flow (CBF) is usually detected by injecting a radioactive tracer into the bloodstream, which allows detecting and graphically illustrating the amount of radioactivity given off. The greater the amount of neural activity in an area, the greater the blood flow in that area and the greater the amount of radioactivity given off.

Interpretation of CBF and other brain imaging studies must take into account many different variables that can influence the results (Ingham, 2001). The temporal and spatial resolution of CBF is relatively poor. Subjects' gender, prior therapy, the tasks performed by the participant, and the exact techniques used for analysis can all influence the results (Lauter, 1995, 1997). Keep these factors in mind as you read about the research in this area.

[4]Broca's area has long been thought to link phonemic sequences to articulatory representations in the motor cortex, thus making it a key element in speech production. Some studies (eg, Flinker et al., 2015) have suggested that, instead of being a direct controller of motor speech behavior, it coordinates information across large-scale cortical networks beyond its boundaries to result, eventually, in the articulation of words.

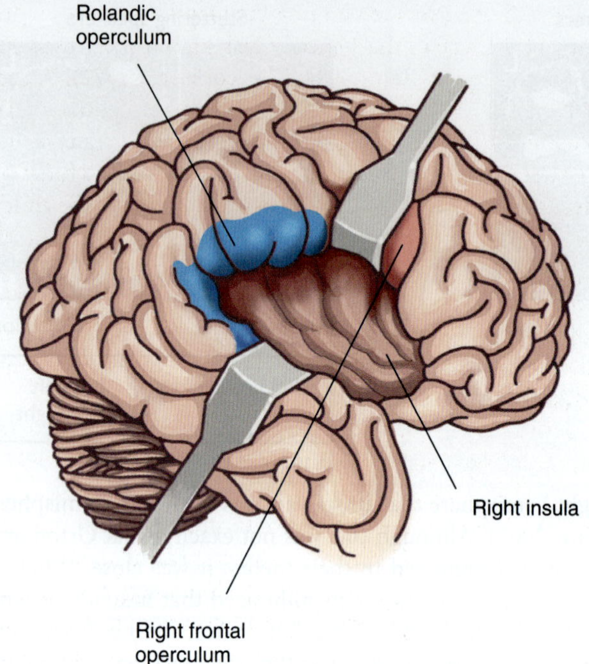

Figure 2.5 Areas overactive for stutterers compared to controls, during speech. These are areas in the right hemisphere that are homologous to areas in the left hemisphere that are active for typical speakers.

Wood et al. (1980) published the first study of CBF in stuttering, using only two participants. They found greater activity in the right-hemisphere region corresponding to Broca's area (the right frontal operculum, remember?) than in Broca's area (left hemisphere) itself during stuttering before treatment with the drug haloperidol.[5] After 2 weeks of treatment with haloperidol, both participants showed that the greater activity had shifted from right- to left-hemisphere speech areas. Pool et al. (1991) studied the brains of 20 adults who stuttered using single photon emission computed tomography scan, an improved technology that enabled scientists to view the brain from multiple angles and obtain better images of what was going on. The principal finding from this study was that the stuttering group showed less left-hemispheric dominance compared to controls in areas that are believed to be associated with language processing.

Positron Emission Tomography Studies and Beyond

In 1995, another CBF study took advantage of a new brain imaging tool, positron emission tomography, which allowed researchers to make more accurate inferences about where increased blood flow was occurring in the brain (Wu et al., 1995). A large team of researchers studied the brains of four adults who stuttered and a matched group of control participants in two conditions: reading aloud alone and reading in unison with someone else, which is called "choral reading." As you may remember from Chapter 1, when individuals who stutter read aloud along with someone else, they become more fluent. This research revealed that two important speech and language areas of the brain—Broca's area and Wernicke's area, both in the left hemisphere (see Fig. 2.3)—showed decreased activity (compared to their normal-speaking controls) when participants were stuttering under typical speaking conditions compared to when they were fluent during choral reading. Why might this be? Broca's area is responsible for coordinating the activity across a large number of cortical networks that eventually results in speech motor output. Wernicke's area is the storehouse for the sounds that form words—the phonological representations that are called upon before the motor commands are given (see Sussman, 2016). These functions may have been shifted away from Broca's and Wernicke's areas to right-hemisphere homologous areas in these stutterers when they were stuttering. Perhaps because choral reading provides external timing cues, it compensated for poorly timed speech, allowing fluency and the use of left-hemisphere typical-speech structures.

In November 1995, three different research groups using positron emission tomography brain imaging tools presented their findings at the annual convention of the American Speech-Language-Hearing Association in Orlando, Florida (De Nil et al., 1995; Ingham et al., 1995; Wu et al., 1995). As the presentations were given, the excitement in the room was palpable because so many of their findings were similar, although the groups were working entirely independently. Here at last was clear evidence that the brains of people who stutter worked differently than those of people who don't. Years of previous speculation and studies suggesting anomalous cerebral dominance, inadequate laterality, auditory processing problems, and language dysfunction in stuttering seemed to be confirmed. These findings and others are reviewed below, organized by the types of anomalies they suggest. I have chosen to describe the anomalies by whether they are overactivations or underactivations in various areas of the brain. Then, I describe two other sets of findings: those on brain changes after stuttering therapy and anomalies in the structure and functions of white matter nerve tracts that convey information.

Brain Overactivation During Stuttering

Many studies have shown that certain areas of the brain show higher levels of activation in those who stutter than in controls. Sometimes this is present during stuttering, but it has also been shown in fluent speech. Researchers have suggested that some of the overactivations may be important etiological factors (causing stuttering), while others may be compensatory (attempts by the brain to compensate for low activity in key areas by activating areas not usually used for speech).

[5]Early experiments with haloperidol had shown success using it to treat Tourette syndrome. It was then tried with children who stuttered and found to be helpful. Most later studies with adults had mixed results. Because haloperidol often has adverse side effects, such as constipation and increased sexual desire, it is no longer used for stuttering.

Overactivation of Right-Hemisphere Cortical Areas During Stuttering

A common finding by several of the brain research teams in 1995 and afterward is that individuals who stutter demonstrate high levels of activity in the right hemisphere when they are speaking, especially when they are stuttering, as illustrated in Figure 2.5.

The focus of this activity is greatest in right-hemisphere structures that are homologous to those in the left hemisphere used by speakers who don't stutter (Braun et al., 1997a, 1997b; De Nil et al., 2000; Fox et al., 1996, 2000; Neef et al., 2018; Weber-Fox et al., 2013). One active right-hemisphere area (right frontal operculum—part of the cortex covering the insula) may be compensating for an underactive Broca's area that is usually thought to be used in coordinating the many cortical networks that transform sensory representation of words to corresponding articulatory gestures in the motor cortex (Flinker et al., 2015). Another area in the right hemisphere commonly found to be active during stuttering is the right insula itself (Fox, 2003). In the left hemisphere, the insula may function as a connection between Wernicke's area (which may be important for phonological representations of words and auditory monitoring of one's own speech) and the coordinations that take place in Broca's area (Ingham et al., 2003). In the right hemisphere, the insula may be compensating for lack of activity of the left-hemisphere insula.

Continuing to search for evidence of hemispheric anomalies, Brown et al. (2005) conducted a "meta-analysis" comparing many brain studies that included people who stuttered and controls. A meta-analysis is a way of statistically analyzing a large number of studies on the same topic and summarizing what findings are common among them. Their analysis confirmed that a major abnormality in those who stutter was a general overactivation of right-hemisphere areas that are homologous to left-hemisphere areas active for speech production: the right frontal operculum, right Rolandic operculum, and right anterior insula (see Fig. 2.5). These findings of overactivity in right-hemisphere areas were confirmed in another meta-analysis (Budde et al., 2014). It should be noted that these researchers *also* observed that a common finding was overactivation in left-hemisphere areas related to motor control of speech compared to nonstuttering peers, perhaps as a result of the extra effort required to speak.

Researchers have considered two possible explanations for the overactivation of right-hemisphere structures during stuttering. One is that during embryonic development, the right side of the brain, instead of the left, becomes "wired" to be the primary speech and language area (eg, Geschwind & Galaburda, 1985). This may result in some difficulty speaking because right-hemisphere structures are not generally suited for the rapid processing of signals required for speech (such as the quick transitions in many consonant-vowel combinations). When a child with this right-hemisphere "wiring" for speech develops language beyond the single-word stage, stuttering may emerge as they try to produce multiword utterances at the typically fast speech rates used for longer sentences (Kent, 1984; Malecot et al., 1972). A second hypothesis is that the child who stutters initially tries to use left-hemisphere regions for speech and language, but the neural networks for speech and language fail to function adequately and result in stuttering. Only then does the child's brain begin to use right-hemisphere structures in a compensatory way to try to achieve more normal speech, similar to the way in which the brains of some individuals with aphasia employ right-hemisphere structures in a way that compensates for damaged areas in the left hemisphere (eg, Neef et al., 2018; Sommer et al., 2002; Weiller et al., 1995).

Several researchers have provided evidence in favor of the second (compensation) hypothesis. Braun et al. (1997a, 1997b) found that activations of right-hemisphere sensory areas were negatively correlated with stuttering; that is, these regions became more active as speech became more fluent. Moreover, researchers in Germany (Neumann et al., 2003) found that right-hemisphere activations were greater in participants who stuttered moderately compared to those who stuttered severely, suggesting that right-hemisphere activity may indeed be a way in which individuals could partially overcome dysfunctions in the left-hemisphere areas. In other words, the moderate stutterers used more compensatory right-hemisphere activity to reduce the severity of their stuttering.

It is possible, of course, that both hypotheses are correct—that some individuals develop right-hemisphere processing for speech and language before they begin to stutter, and others develop right-hemisphere processing after they begin to stutter, as a compensatory response. Still others may in fact process speech and language in both hemispheres simultaneously. Each of these options is probably inefficient and may create the dyssynchrony in processing assumed to result in stuttering. Future research examining changes in the processing of individuals who stutter as they develop from early childhood would be very helpful in sorting this out.

Overactivation in Midbrain Areas

The midbrain is situated beneath the cortex and is the top section of the brainstem. Researchers have reported unusually high levels of activity in midbrain structures that, via pathways to the cerebral cortex, may disrupt smooth speech movements. Specifically, some structures of the basal ganglia have been shown to be overactive in stutterers (eg, substantia nigra, subthalamic nucleus, red nucleus, globus pallidus) (Fox et al., 1996; Watkins et al., 2008).

A number of neuroscientists have developed models of stuttering based on the notion of basal ganglia circuit dysfunction. Alm (2004), Guenther (2016), and Chang and Guenther (2020) have proposed that the basal ganglia play an important role in stuttering because of their part in the cortico-basal ganglia-thalamocortical loop that provides

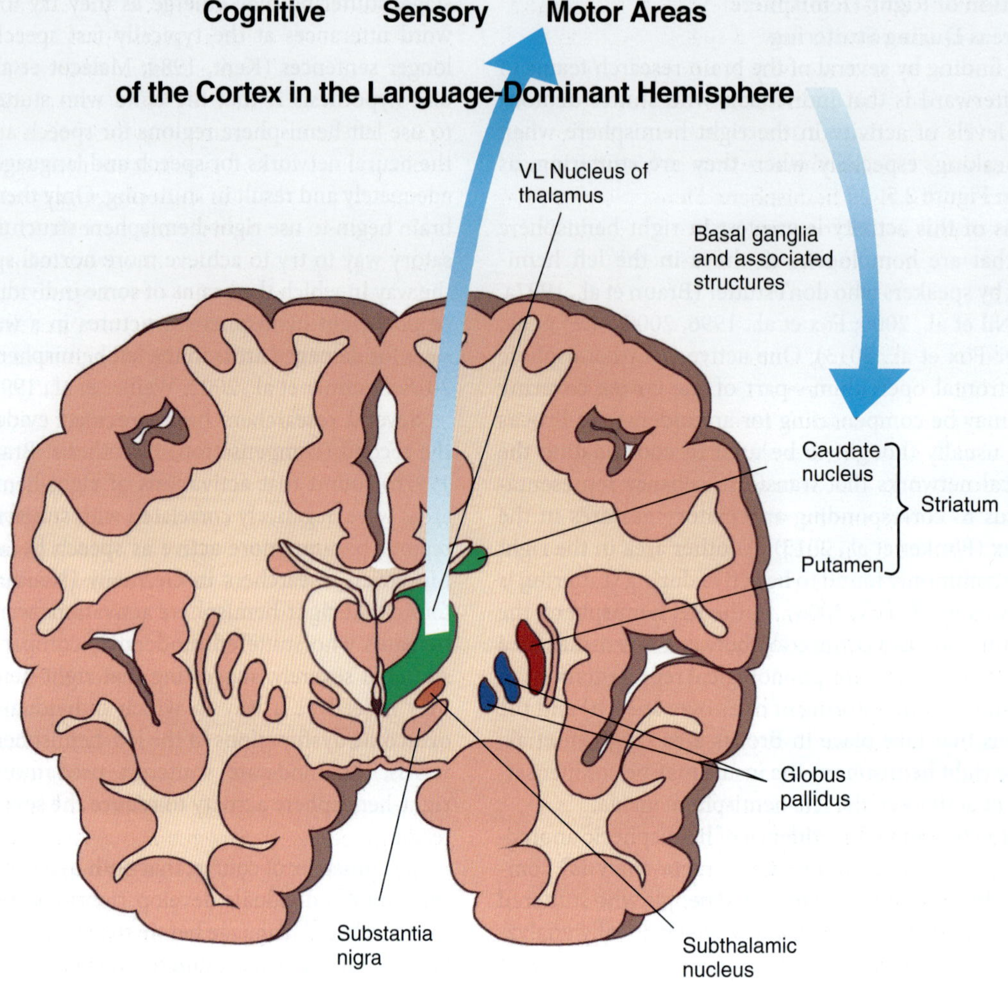

Figure 2.6 Hypothetical model of cortico-basal ganglia-thalamocortical loop. Information cycles from **cognitive, sensory, and motor cortex** areas to **basal ganglia** structures, then to **thalamus**, and back to **premotor and motor areas of the cortex**.

timing signals to the supplementary motor area (SMA) of the cortex to initiate motor programs for speech. This loop sends information about the desired syllable to be produced from cortical areas (such as pre-SMA and posterior inferior frontal sulcus) to structures of the basal ganglia (striatum and globus pallidus) where the timing information about when to initiate, sustain, or terminate the syllable is generated. This information is passed on to the thalamus, which sends it back to the premotor and motor cortices, especially to the SMA. In fluent speech, the SMA acts on this timing information from the basal ganglia/thalamus to generate the appropriate speech movements for the desired phonemic sequence. Figure 2.6 depicts this timing loop that is so important in speech production. In stuttering, Alm and other theorists propose that overactivation in the production of the neurotransmitter dopamine causes the timing information to be "muddled" so that the smooth production of syllables is disrupted. Details about these models of dysfunction in basal ganglia circuitry are given in Chapter 6, Theories of Stuttering. Brief videos depicting basal ganglia function are available on YouTube. They are called "2-Minute Neuroscience: Basal Ganglia" and "2-Minute Neuroscience: Basal Ganglia (Direct vs Indirect Pathways)."

Brain Underactivation During Stuttering

Several areas of the brain, including both motor and sensory centers, have been found to be underactive in stuttering. Because speech motor control involves the integration of motor and sensory information, it is not surprising that underactivation of *both* areas is sometimes reported in these studies.

Underactivation in Speech Motor Areas

Watkins et al. (2008) found that during speech production, individuals who stutter showed decreased activity compared to controls in areas related to using sensory and motor information and planning sequential movements: ventral premotor, Rolandic opercula, and sensorimotor cortex on both sides of the brain. This underactivity was in the same area of the brain as the structural differences found by Chang et al. (2008)—less dense white matter tracts connecting articulatory planning and sensory feedback areas. Thus, structural differences seem to result in functional deficits that presumably interfere with the smooth flow of speech. Watkins et al. point out that because underactivity is seen on both sides of the brain in their study, the deficits present serious problems. Earlier studies had shown that some stutterers have learned to compensate for left-hemisphere deficits by using homologous structures in the right hemisphere. Here, it is clear that successful compensation isn't occurring because underactivity is seen on both right and left sides of the brain.

Underactivation in Auditory Areas

Many brain imaging studies of stuttering have shown a lack of activity in the superior temporal lobe, including auditory association areas and Wernicke's area (Braun et al., 1997a, 1997b; De Nil et al., 2003; Fox et al., 1996, 2000). The meta-analysis by Brown et al. (2005) mentioned earlier indicated that a common finding among several of these studies was that auditory areas in both hemispheres were underactivated, suggesting that in individuals who stutter mechanisms for guiding their speech by self-hearing were not functioning properly. Budde et al. (2014) followed up the meta-analysis by Brown et al. and found that the 17 studies they analyzed showed that during speech, individuals who stuttered showed less activity in left auditory cortex than did controls. They also found that activity was reduced in both left and right auditory cortices when the stuttering individuals were stuttering compared to when they were fluent. Watkins et al. (2008) found in their study of adolescent and young adult stutterers that underactivity was notable in Heschl gyrus, a part of the auditory cortex that is important for processing speech sounds. Kikuchi et al. (2017) found heightened increased phase synchronization[6] in the right auditory cortex but *not* in the left auditory cortex, suggesting right-hemisphere compensation for deficits in left-hemisphere auditory function. Evidence of dysfunction in auditory areas during stuttering is especially pertinent in light of the many studies that have shown that stutterers may have difficulty performing auditory processing tasks (eg, Barasch et al., 2000; Kent, 1984; Molt, 1997) and that fluency can be induced by changing the way stutterers hear their own speech (eg, Brayton & Conture, 1978; Howell et al., 1987).

How does auditory self-monitoring affect fluency? It may provide a stimulus to synchronize or integrate the sequence of activities that run in parallel when speakers decide what they will say, select the linguistic elements for it, and execute the utterance. Thus, the asynchrony or timing disturbance that many researchers see as the basis of stuttering (eg, Etchell et al., 2014; Kent, 1984; Perkins et al., 1991; Van Riper, 1982a) may be caused by a paucity of signals that can help synchronize the sequence for speech output. Therapies (eg, Van Riper, 1973a) that emphasize the use of increased explicit attention to their speech by speakers may increase the amount of information available for synchronizing speech by focusing on another feedback modality. Specifically, therapies that focus on the use of slow speech, gentle onsets, and light articulatory contacts may help clients more easily use feedback to guide and synchronize their speech motor commands. Alm (2004), for example, suggested that in the case of dysfunction of internal timing cues from the basal ganglia, deautomatization of speech can provide for other structures (such as lateral premotor cortex) to generate timing cues.

Other functions besides monitoring one's own speech may also reside in the underactivated regions of the auditory cortex. For example, Wernicke's area may be important for storing the phonological representations of words (Caplan, 1987; Paulesu et al., 1993; Sussman, 2016). Activation of this region of the brain, therefore, may be a key stage in phonological planning for speech production. Lack of adequate activation during stuttering may reflect a deficit in the sequence of phonological selection, phonetic planning, and motor execution.

Connectivity Deficits in White Matter Tracts

In a study of adults who stutter, Chang et al. (2011) discovered structural connectivity deficits in white matter tracts in the left hemisphere that linked inferior frontal areas (these areas may be involved in programming speech movements) and premotor cortex (these areas may be involved in sensory guidance of speech movements). Moreover, deficits in functional connectivity in these tracts were found both for speech and nonspeech movements, which would help explain findings that show poorer performance among stutterers for tasks like repeating sentences (Walsh et al., 2015) and finger-tapping (Subramanian & Yairi, 2006). In addition, Chang et al. found heightened functional connectivity for stutterers compared to nonstutterers in the right hemisphere, which may have been a compensation for left-hemisphere deficits.

In one of the first multimodal neuroimaging studies of young children, Chang and Zhu (2013) compared both structural and functional connectivity in white matter tracts of 56 children 3-9 years old who stuttered versus their fluent peers. They found deficiencies in the networks connecting auditory-motor and basal ganglia-thalamocortical areas in the children who stuttered. These deficiencies were hypothesized to create problems in planning and carrying out speech movements. Findings of this study included evidence that girls who stutter showed higher connectivity in auditory-motor tracts than boys who stutter. In a later publication, Chang (2014) expanded on the sex differences in neuroimaging studies of boys and girls that may be important in our understanding of why girls are more likely to recover from stuttering than boys. Chang's review of research in this area makes it clear that girls' brains show better connectivity between motor and auditory regions, promoting development of speech and language. Therefore, they may be able to recover from stuttering more rapidly.

Table 2.6 presents two meta-analyses of brain imaging studies of stuttering that include many of the most relevant publications on brain function differences. As you will

[6]Phase synchronization is a sign a biological oscillator is working well. One example is when fireflies in an area recognize each other and flash simultaneously. In the auditory cortex such synchronization suggests effective functioning.

TABLE 2.6 Summary of Recent Meta-analyses of Studies of Brain Function Differences in People Who Stutter

Authors, Date	Participants	Major Findings	Implications
Brown et al. (2005)	Meta-analysis of eight studies focusing on both stuttering and control participants	"Neural signatures" of stuttering were described as overactivity in right-hemisphere areas homologous to speech areas in the left hemisphere; absence of activity in the auditory areas used to monitor one's own speech; and a high level of activity in an area of the cerebellum not activated in participants who did not stutter	The authors suggested that findings support an "efference copy" dysfunction in stuttering; in other words, the predicted sensory outcome of the motor plan for speech is typically compared with what the speech output actually is, and thus, errors can be detected and the motor plan can be corrected See Chapter 6 for a description of efference copy dysfunction (the "Reduced Capacity for Internal Modeling" theory)
Budde et al. (2014)	Meta-analysis of 17 studies, following up on Brown et al. (2005), using many more studies and participants and a more rigorous statistical meta-analysis	This study confirms the "neural signatures" found in Brown et al. meta-analysis The SMA, implicated in other studies, was found to be more active in individuals who stutter than in controls, especially during stuttered speech	This study suggested that continued meta-analyses of brain imaging studies of stuttering may lead to better models of stuttering and eventually to treatments that can be personalized to fit an individual's particular deficits

SMA, supplementary motor area.

remember, meta-analysis is a way of statistically analyzing a large number of studies on the same topic and summarizing what findings are common among them.

Brain *Structure* Differences in People Who Stutter Compared With People Who Do Not Stutter

Research on structural differences in brains of people who stutter began to proliferate after the year 2000. Several studies between 2000 and 2007[7] examined the brain anatomy of adults who stuttered by measuring the shape, size, and density of speech and language areas. The findings suggested that sensory, planning, and motor areas in the left hemisphere of these individuals developed differently from those in matched nonstuttering individuals. For example, white matter tracts, which convey information from sensory centers in the left hemisphere to motor execution areas of the left hemisphere, have been shown to be less dense than those in typical speakers. However, the same tracts were found to be denser in the right hemisphere of those who stuttered than in their left hemisphere. This is likely to be a consequence of the right hemisphere takeover of some typical left-hemisphere functions, when left-hemisphere speech areas fail to work effectively.

By 2008, neuroimaging researchers had developed techniques that were safe enough to use with children for the purposes of examining brain structures. In that year, two groups of investigators published studies of school-age children who had stuttered in their preschool years. One study of children who recovered from stuttering compared them to those who hadn't recovered and to a control group of age-matched children who had never stuttered (Chang et al., 2008). They showed that, compared to the control group, both recovered and persistent stutterers had reduced volumes of gray matter around Broca's area, the part of the brain that you will remember is associated with coordination of neural networks associated with motor control for speech. They also found reduced volume in bilateral temporal lobe areas that may be related to auditory perception of speech. The subgroup of children who persisted in stuttering (but not the subgroup who recovered) also showed less dense white matter tracts connecting areas associated with phonological representations of sounds to speech motor execution areas, the same deficit as discovered in adult stutterers, described earlier. This finding was reported again in a second 2008 study of slightly older children in that same year, indicating that this structural abnormality in the left hemisphere may well be a major factor in the disorder—and not the result of years of stuttering (Watkins et al., 2008).

[7]These include Beal et al. (2007), Foundas et al. (2001, 2004), Jancke et al. (2004), and Sommer et al. (2002).

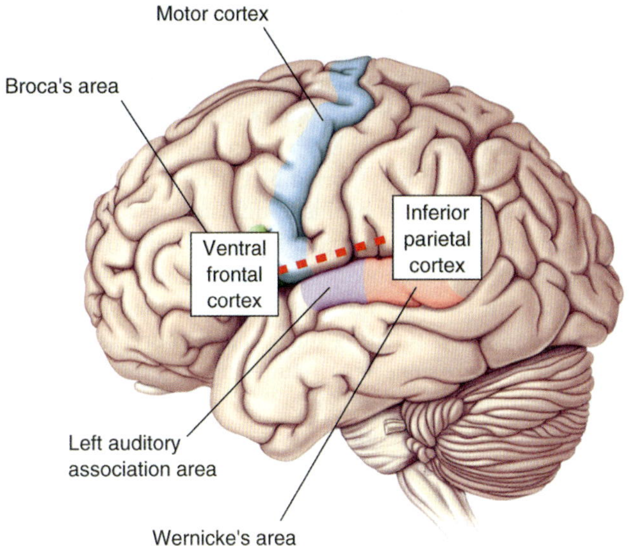

Figure 2.7 The superior longitudinal fasciculus III is a bidirectional pathway between the inferior parietal cortex (sensory integration) and the ventral frontal cortex (motor planning).

The 2008 findings of the two groups cited above were replicated by Cykowski et al. (2010), using more extensive brain imaging technology. They found that the most robust difference between adults who stutter and those who don't is in left-hemisphere white matter fiber tracts that communicate between the inferior parietal cortex (sensory integration) and the ventral frontal cortex (motor planning). As in earlier studies, the authors found that in individuals who stutter compared to individuals who don't, certain nerve fibers aren't structured as effectively to conduct impulses along the directional flow of the nerve bundle. This may be called reduced "connectivity" in white matter tracts. Thus, conduction is not as fast as it might be. The fiber tract implicated in Cykowski et al. is called the superior longitudinal fasciculus (SLF III). It is illustrated in Figure 2.7. This tract connects speech output planning areas of the ventral frontal cortex with sensorimotor integration areas of the inferior parietal lobe. Cykowski and his colleagues speculated that the etiology of the less efficient transport structure of the white matter tracts in individuals who stutter may be a result of reduced myelination of nerves in these pathways.

As mentioned earlier, this explanation is essentially a reprise of Karlin's (1947) hypothesis that "the basic cause for stuttering is a delay in the myelination of the cortical areas in the brain concerned with speech" (p. 319). Karlin pointed out that the myelin sheath surrounding nerves functions to insulate them. This insulation speeds the flow of electricity just as it does in the lines carrying electricity inside and outside your house. Incomplete myelination of some nerves results in slower transmission in those nerves, and thus, where many different nerves are working together in a network, the slow transmission in some nerves but not others could result in actions that are less well coordinated. Karlin further pointed out that myelination occurs earlier in girls than in boys (Flechsig, 1927), which may help explain the greater persistence of stuttering in boys.

An important effect of reduced myelination in these bidirectional nerve pathways may be that, in addition to slowing transmissions, without adequate insulation provided by the myelin sheath, these pathways may also be vulnerable to "cross talk" from high levels of activity in emotion and language processes. By cross talk, I mean the disruption of some pathways by activity in others. The term itself comes from discussions of electric transmission lines but seems relevant here. Vulnerability of poorly myelinated fibers to interference by emotional activity seems possible given the evidence that the left frontal cortex is active for positive emotional arousal (eg, Davidson, 1995; Machado & Cantilino, 2017) and the evidence reported by Johnson et al. (2010) and Choi et al. (2016) that stuttering may increase during positive emotional arousal, not just negative emotional arousal. Furthermore, emotion-related disorders (eg, pediatric bipolar disorder) are reported to be associated with decreased myelination in the SLF III (Pavuluri & Passaroti, 2008). Taking these finding together, increased stuttering during high levels of emotion may be the result of disruptions in neural transmission in poorly myelinated white matter tracts in speech areas of the brain. These disruptions then may cause mistiming of the signals that, in turn, result in discoordinated movements.

In addition to the effects of emotion on stuttering, the effects of language processing may sometimes overwhelm neural "transmission lines" because so much information must be passed back and forth at such high speeds (eg, longer sentences are spoken more quickly, as reported by Malecot et al., 1972 and others). Karlin (1947) pointed out that stuttering first appears when "sentence formation and flow of language has become more fully developed" (p. 319), implying that this increased demand of more developed language is too much for the pathways that are not fully myelinated, with stuttering as a result. Cykowski et al. (2010) also suggested that speech-language demands (such as the production of low-frequency or more complex words that require more careful monitoring) can put enough stress on the less myelinated fiber tracts to provoke stuttering.

Later studies have continued to support earlier findings about deficits in white matter nerve tracts in children who stutter. For example, Chang et al. (2015) used a technique called fractional anisotropy to analyze white matter fiber integrity. Fractional anisotropy is a means of assessing connectivity of white matter tracts; it reflects the diameter and density of axons and the extent of their myelination. Chang and her colleagues used this technique to study white matter nerve tracts throughout the brain in 37 children who stutter comparing them with 40 matched control children, all between ages 3 and 10 years. Their findings point to widespread white matter connectivity deficits in children who stutter, not only in left-hemisphere cortical areas linking premotor, motor, and auditory systems but also in areas outside the left hemisphere, affecting interhemispheric communication and cortical-subcortical pathways. These deficits would obviously hinder speech motor coordination in children who stutter.

Because Chang et al. (2015) studied so many children in such a wide age range, they could effectively compare the brains of younger children with those of older children in both the stuttering and nonstuttering groups. They found that white matter integrity increased with age in both groups. However, the children in the stuttering group showed less increase with age compared to the nonstuttering group. In addition, increases in white matter integrity were uneven and inconsistent in the stuttering group, compared to the nonstuttering group. White matter deficits shown by the analysis were significantly correlated with the age of the children in the stuttering group. This led the authors to surmise that there are continuing white matter deficits with persistent stuttering, because the older children had not recovered. In other words, "It is likely that [white matter] differences become more exaggerated with age as stuttering persists" (p. 705).

In this same study, Chang et al. (2015) also investigated whether children with more severe stuttering showed white matter integrity differences (from nonstuttering children) compared to children with less severe stuttering. They found that differences in white matter deficits did indeed differentiate the more severely stuttering children from the less severe children. Some of the areas that were deficient in the severe stutterers were connections with the laryngeal motor cortex. The authors noted that these poorer connections would involve white matter tracts linking the laryngeal motor cortex with surrounding cortical areas involved in the "integration of proprioceptive and tactile feedback from the orofacial, respiratory, and laryngeal regions during voice production" (quoted by Chang et al. from Simonyan & Horowitz, 2011, p. 203). Therefore, it would not be surprising if problems in integrating feedback during speech would result in severe stuttering, particularly laryngeal blocks.

The study by Chang et al. (2015) is clearly an important one because it was the first to show white matter deficits in many areas of the brain in young children who stutter, to suggest what might distinguish recovery from persistence, and to find connectivity differences that distinguish mild and moderate stuttering from severe stuttering. Another important study that compared more severely stuttering individuals (adults) with less severely stuttering individuals was conducted by Neef et al. (2018). They found that *increased* connectivity was present in the *right* (rather than left) frontal aslant tract (FAT). The right FAT may be related to executive function and inhibitory control in speech, whereas the left FAT appears to control speech initiation. Does this mean that the more severely stuttering subjects had left FAT areas that functioned poorly for speech initiation and they activated right-hemisphere areas in an attempt to compensate?

Neef et al. (2020) found laryngeal motor cortex structure deficits similar to those reported by Chang et al. (2015) discussed above. Using probabilistic diffusion tractography (a type of neuroimaging), they found that the ventral laryngeal motor cortex neural networks had less connectivity in stuttering subjects compared to fluent subjects. They also found that more severely stuttering subjects had poorer connectivity than less severe subjects. All stuttering subjects underwent intensive fluency-shaping therapy but showed no change in this connectivity as a result of treatment, despite increases in fluency. These findings support those of Chang et al. (2015) that the neural networks that control laryngeal function in stuttering show structural weakness.

Garnett et al. (2019), following up on Chang et al. (2015), also showed structural deficits (in white matter integrity) in children who stuttered compared to those who did not. In particular, white matter integrity was significantly lower in the arcuate fasciculus that connects left temporoparietal junction and posterior temporal gyrus. Deficits in white matter integrity were also found in the corpus callosum in fibers connecting bilateral motor regions in the children who stuttered. The authors suggested that these deficits interfered with integration of sensory feedback and speech movements, as well as limiting the ability of the left and right motor cortices to work together.

Whole Brain Intrinsic Network Connectivity

The imposing title of this section signals a new perspective on how brain differences in people who stutter are investigated. Much of the previous research described in this chapter has used a "localizationist" approach. In other words, researchers have looked at differences in structure and function in specific areas of the brain, such as speech motor and auditory processing areas in the left hemisphere. Whole brain studies examined activity in the entire cortex. Chang et al. (2017) reported on the study of 42 children who stuttered and 42 controls. Both groups were given repeated brain scans over a period of several years. Some of the children who stuttered were persistent in their stuttering, and others recovered over the span of the study. The brain scans used were termed "rsfMRI"—fMRI stands for functional magnetic resonance imaging, a technique to measure changes in blood flow that accompany brain activity. The "rs" means that the scans were done because they were done while the children were in a resting state, rather than speaking. Resting brain scans allow the natural interconnectivity (or lack thereof) of different networks to be viewed. This resting interconnectivity is termed "default mode network" or DMN. Without going into too much detail about the particular networks involved, the results can be summarized as follows.

One of the aberrant connections found was between the DMN and the posterior cingulate cortex, which is involved in attention. Because of the influence that dopamine can have on this connection, this finding was cited as some support for the hypothesis that stuttering is characterized by excess dopamine (Alm, 2004; Chang & Guenther, 2020; Guenther, 2016).

Some of the anomalous connections in the DMN—including those related to speech motor control—were found in children who stutter, whether they recovered or not.

Children who persisted in stuttering *also* tended to show abnormal connectivity in networks associated with attention and executive function.

Overall, stuttering was associated with abnormal connectivity in networks associated with attention, motor performance, perception, and emotion. This finding may help explain why there is such variability in stuttering (connectivity changes over time) and why stuttering may co-occur with other disorders such as attention deficit disorder and anxiety. This study (Chang et al., 2017) is probably the first of many that will follow, exploring abnormal connectivity in networks of individuals who stutter (Table 2.7).

TABLE 2.7 Summary of Studies of Brain Structure Differences in People Who Stutter

Authors, Date	Participants	Major Findings	Implications
Chang et al. (2008)	School-age children	Findings included reduced volume of gray matter around Broca's area and reduced volume in bilateral temporal lobe areas related to auditory perception, important because of the interface between speech production and perception Persistent stuttering was associated with less dense white matter tracts connecting areas for phonological representation of sounds to motor execution areas (replicated by Watkins et al., 2008)	This study provided clear indications that children who stutter show structural deficits in key areas related to speech production (not just adults who have been stuttering for years)
Cykowski et al. (2010)	Fourteen stuttering adults and 13 nonstuttering adults	Deficits in myelination of white matter tracts connecting sensory integration areas with motor planning areas in superior longitudinal fasciculus	This study found possible deficits in effective connectivity in areas related to speech production, which may lead to discoordination among many interconnecting pathways critical for smooth speech production This study also found a potential for interference with speech production by language overload and emotional arousal
Chang et al. (2015)	37 children who stuttered and 40 matched controls	Widespread white matter connectivity deficits were found in children who stutter compared to their matched controls. These deficits were found not only in left-hemisphere areas linking premotor, motor, and auditory systems but also affecting interhemispheric and cortical-subcortical communication	Children with persistent stuttering and children with more severe stuttering were more likely to show these white matter deficits
Chang et al. (2017)	42 children who stuttered and 42 controls Brain scans repeated over a period of years as children developed	Resting brain scans showed widespread anomalies in the connections between the resting networks and those associated with speech motor control, attention, executive function, perception, and emotion	This study helps to explain why stuttering can be so variable because connections varied over the course of development It also suggests why stuttering may co-occur with many other disorders such as those affecting attention and anxiety

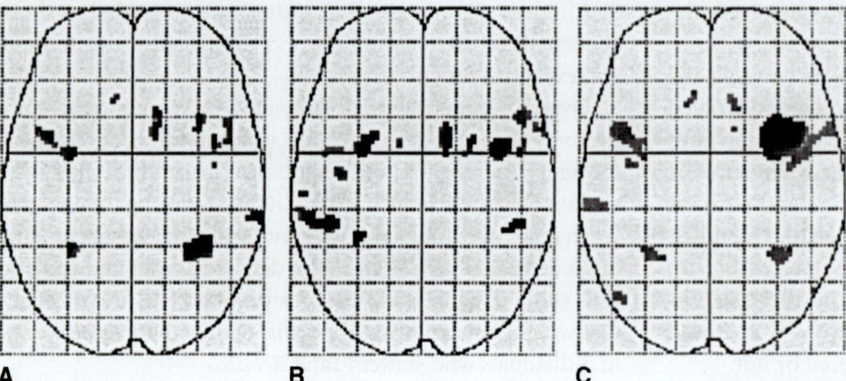

Figure 2.8 Overt reading: statistical parametrical maps of between-group comparisons (people who stutter vs people who do not stutter) **(A)** before therapy, **(B)** immediately after therapy, and **(C)** 2 years after therapy. (Reprinted from Neumann, K., Euler, H. A., von Gudenberg, A. W., Giraud, A. L., Lanfermann, H., Gall, V., et al. (2003). The nature and treatment of stuttering as revealed by fMRI: A within- and between-group comparison. *Journal of Fluency Disorders, 28*(4), 381–410. Copyright © 2003 Elsevier. With permission.)

Changes in Brain Activity After Treatment

Both short-term and long-term treatment outcome studies using brain imaging suggested that areas of the left hemisphere that were previously underactivated were reactivated after effective treatment and that right-hemisphere sites became more normally activated (ie, less overactivated) (Boberg et al., 1983; De Nil et al., 1998, 2003; Kroll et al., 1997, 1999; Moore, 1984; Neumann & Euler, 2010; Neumann et al., 2003, 2005; Wood et al., 1980). A chapter by Neumann and Euler (2010) has additional details about brain changes following treatment using the Kassel Stuttering Therapy program. This approach changes the client's speech pattern, using prolonged speech, easy onsets, and smooth transitions, all using computer-guided feedback. Neumann and Euler suggested that successful treatment activates left-hemisphere areas near those that were deficient before treatment.

Figure 2.8—from Neumann et al. (2003)—depicts the differences in brain activity in people who stutter (1) before treatment, (2) immediately after treatment, and (3) 2 years after treatment. It is evident that activity levels shift from greater in the right hemisphere to greater in the left hemisphere following treatment.

An fMRI study by Kell et al. (2009) compared the recovery processes of 13 male adults who stuttered and were given treatment with those of a fluent control group and a matched group of adult males who recovered on their own as adults, without treatment. These findings were reviewed in Neumann and Euler (2010) as noted above, but some of the details are of interest here. Those subjects who were still stuttering at the time of the fMRI scans showed right-hemisphere "compensation" (use of right-hemisphere structures for speaking), which was not very effective in generating fluency. However, after treatment, the same subjects showed generally increased left-hemisphere activation for speech. But the adults who had recovered unassisted from their stuttering had specific left-hemisphere activation very near to areas of white matter that are found to be dysfunctional in persistent stuttering. The gray matter area associated with unassisted recovery was Brodmann area 47/12—an area in the inferior frontal cortex thought to be important in linguistic processing and timing structure in music (eg, Levitin & Menon, 2003). In these individuals who recovered on their own, the white matter areas were functioning well. The authors suggested that this reflects plasticity in the adult brain, wherein the white matter anomalies repaired themselves as a part of the recovery process. Some of the authors who have studied stuttering therapy (eg, Kell et al., 2009) suggested that the effect of treatment may be to reestablish in the left-hemisphere mechanisms that integrate auditory feedback with proper timing for speech production, leading to increased fluency.

A publication by Ingham et al. (2018) reviewed a large number of studies of neural changes associated with recovery—both natural and after treatment. Among the treatments that this paper reviewed was the Modified Phonation Interval (MPI) approach that had been reported by Ingham et al. (2013, 2015). This approach teaches clients to change the length of the phonated portion of their utterances, inducing fluency. In the first of these papers, the authors reported that the brain change most related to successful treatment was increased activity in the left putamen, a structure critical for the regulation of movement. The left putamen has been identified in other research as one of the brain structures than normalizes after stuttering treatment (eg, Neumann & Euler, 2010).

The publication by Ingham et al. (2018) also reviewed the effects of various types of brain stimulation on stuttering. Readers are encouraged to read this paper to learn more about new approaches to treatment (see Suggested Readings for the full citation).

SUMMARY

- Stuttering appears to have a genetic basis in many individuals. However, twin studies and adoption studies confirm that genes must interact with environmental factors for stuttering to appear.
- Recent research identifies some genes associated with stuttering in some individuals. For some genes,

specific speech production deficits associated with those genes can be linked to stuttering.

- Stuttering may have its etiology in congenital factors for some stutterers. These may include physical trauma at birth or *in utero*, cerebral palsy, retardation, and emotionally stressful situations.
- Slightly more boys begin to stutter than girls, but girls are more likely to recover, so by school age and beyond, there are many more boys who stutter than girls.
- Early childhood stuttering may be either transitory, in which the child recovers naturally within 18 months, with no or minimal treatment, or persistent, in which the child, if not treated, stutters 3 years or more.
- Persistent and transitory stuttering appear to be the result of a common genetic factor (either a single gene or several), but the persistent form of stuttering may have additional genetic factors that impede recovery.
- Natural recovery from stuttering seems to be associated with the following factors: (1) good scores on tests of phonology, language, and nonverbal skills; (2) either no family history of stuttering or family members who had natural recovery from stuttering; (3) early age of onset of stuttering; and (4) being a girl.
- Brain imaging studies of adults who stutter have shown various anomalies during speaking and especially during stuttering. One anomaly is overactivation in right-brain areas homologous to left-hemisphere speech and language structures typically used by nonstutterers. Another anomaly is deactivation in the left auditory cortex.
- Neuroanatomical differences seen via brain imaging include (1) anomalies in the planum temporale (related to auditory processing) and in gyri (raised areas on the brain's surface) in speech and language areas and (2) less dense and less myelinated white matter fiber tracts connecting speech perception, planning, and execution areas.
- Recent theoretical views based on neuroanatomical evidence have suggested that stuttering may be the result of dysfunction of the neural "loop" that sends signals from the planning area of the cortex to the basal ganglia and then to the thalamus and back to the motor area cortex. This dysfunction is thought to perturb the timing signals that control the initiation, continuation, or termination of motor programs for speech.
- Inducement of short-term or long-term fluency in stutterers is accompanied by decreases in right-hemisphere activations and increases in activation of left-hemisphere speech, language, and auditory areas.

STUDY QUESTIONS

1. How does each of the areas—family studies, twin studies, and adoption studies—provide evidence that stuttering is inherited?
2. A couple comes to you for advice. They tell you they are thinking of having children but are worried because each has a relative who stutters. What more information would you like to get from them? What would you tell them about the likelihood that they would have a child who stutters and whether they should be concerned?
3. How do studies provide evidence that stuttering is a product of both heredity and environment?
4. How would you summarize the major findings about brain differences in stutterers to someone who is not a professional in our field?
5. Why is it important to study the brains of children who stutter as well as adults who stutter?
6. Researchers have found many differences between groups of stutterers and nonstutterers. Why can't we always say that these differences cause stuttering?
7. What research finding in this chapter do you think has the most relevance for the treatment of stuttering? Defend your answer.

SUGGESTED PROJECTS

1. Talk to someone who stutters and plot out their family tree, noting relatives who stutter (and whether they recovered or not) and relatives who have other speech, language, or learning problems.
2. Make a family tree of your own relatives indicating which, if any, currently have or in the past have had speech, language, hearing, or learning disabilities. Describe how you got the information and what the disabilities are.
3. On which side of your brain do you process speech and language? Find out how you could ascertain this information by asking speech-language pathology researchers or audiologists you know if they have tests you could take to find out. If this doesn't lead to a test for this kind of laterality, search the internet for self-administered tests, which tell you whether you are more "left-brained" or more "right-brained." Does the answer make sense to you? (I came out more right-brained).

SUGGESTED READINGS

Bloodstein, O., Ratner, N. B., & Brundage, S. (2021). *A handbook on stuttering* (7th ed.). Plural Publishing.

This is a totally revised, new edition of the classic reference book containing reviews of the latest research and theoretical perspectives on stuttering. The book provides many excellent tutorials that give reader-friendly overviews of complex topics. It is also filled with many new illustrations that make complicated concepts clearer. The new Handbook gives extensive coverage not only about the nature and development of stuttering but also about assessment and treatment strategies.

Chang, S. E., & Guenther, F. H. (2020). Involvement of the cortico-basal ganglia-thalamocortical loop in developmental stuttering. *Frontiers in Psychology, 10*, 1–9. doi:10.3389/fpsyg.2019.03088

Although this important publication focuses extensively on the basal ganglia's role (in concert with other midbrain structures and the cortex) in the etiology of stuttering, it also provides a review of neuroimaging studies that support the authors' theoretical perspective.

Doidge, N. (2007). *The brain that changes itself*. Penguin Books.

This is an inspiring book by a psychiatrist interested in neuroplasticity. It describes research suggesting that the brain is more changeable that previously believed.

Doidge, N. (2016). *The brain's way of healing*. Penguin Books.

A follow-up to Doidge's 2007 book. This one has many stories of individuals who overcame serious brain injuries and diseases by helping their brains change and thereby modify their disorders.

Etchell, A., Civier, O., Ballard, K., & Sowman, P. (2017). A systematic literature review of neuroimaging research on developmental stuttering between 1995 and 2016. *Journal of Fluency Disorders, 55*, 6–45. doi:10.1016/j.jfludis.2017.03.007

This is a review of both brain structure and function differences in people who stutter—at least those found up to 2016.

Guenther, F. (2016). *Neural control of speech*. The MIT Press.

This is a comprehensive account of how the brain controls speech. The author, a computational and cognitive neuroscientist, emphasizes how the cortex, in conjunction with subcortical structures, functions to produce typical speech. He also presents his theoretical views about the brain dysfunctions that account for stuttering, dysarthria, apraxia of speech, and other neurological disorders of speech.

Ingham, R., Ingham, J., Euler, H., & Neumann, K. (2018). Stuttering treatment and brain research in adults: A still unfolding relationship. *Journal of Fluency Disorders, 55*, 106–119. doi:10.1016/j.jfludis.2017.02.003

A good review of the effects of treatment on the brain and explorations of potential new approaches to treatment.

Neumann, K., & Euler, H. (2010). Neuroimaging and stuttering. In B. Guitar, & R. McCauley (Eds.), *Stuttering treatment: Established and emerging approaches* (pp. 355–377). Lippincott Williams & Wilkins.

This chapter begins with a history of brain imaging and stuttering and then describes the most important findings (up to that point) in structural and functional brain imaging related to stuttering. This is followed by a section on neuroimaging findings before and after treatment, a specialty of the authors.

Smith, A., & Weber, C. (2017). How stuttering develops: The multifactorial dynamic pathways theory. *Journal of Speech, Language, and Hearing Research, 60*, 2483–2505. doi.org/10.1044/2017_JSLHR-S-16-0343

Although this publication will again be recommended at the end of Chapter 6 on Theories of Stuttering, I mention it here because the authors review research relevant to this chapter: genetics and neuroimaging, as well as speech motor control via the brain.

3

Sensorimotor, Language, and Emotional Factors in Stuttering

Chapter Outline

Chapter Objectives

After studying this chapter, readers should be able to:

- Describe differences in these areas found between groups of individuals who stutter and groups of individuals who don't: (1) central auditory processing, (2) sensory processing other than auditory, (3) reaction time, (4) fluent speech, (5) nonspeech motor control
- Suggest why differences in each of these areas could be related to stuttering
- Describe how language development and performance in individuals who stutter have been found to differ from individuals who don't
- Describe the ways in which stuttering and emotion may be related

Key Terms

Proprioception: Sensory information from the body that conveys position of structures and movement of structures

Sensorimotor control: The way all movement is carried out with sensory

information used before, during, and after to improve the precision of movement
Sensory processing: Activity of the brain as it interprets information coming from the senses, such as sounds arriving via the ears and auditory nerves
Temperament: Aspects of an individual's personality, such as sensitive versus thick skinned, that are thought to be innate rather than learned

In the previous chapter, I discussed the role of genetics and brain anomalies in stuttering. Now I will explore how those factors may result in sensory and motor deficits that can give rise to stuttering. Following that, I will describe two other factors that may trigger the onset of stuttering and affect its development and possible persistence: language and emotion. Figure 3.1 depicts examples of these deficits that appear to be associated with stuttering in some individuals. There are many interactions among these factors and exactly how the factors and their interactions work to produce stuttering in any individual is not always clear. It is possible, of course, that some or all of the deficits do not cause stuttering, even indirectly. They may be simply a side effect of the many anomalies in brain function and structure that we described in Chapter 2.

SENSORIMOTOR FACTORS

As we have just noted, sensory and motor deficits may be key factors in stuttering. Sensory and motor functions usually work together, as "sensorimotor" functions. However, some of the research on sensory ability is often done by testing perception and processing of sound or touch without involving motor activity at the same time. Thus, the first topics of this sensorimotor section will be just sensory. Then research on motor abilities will be discussed under the heading of "**sensorimotor control**."

As you read this section, you may be puzzled about how some of these findings relate to the actual behaviors of stuttering. Why would stutterers have abnormal electrical activity in their brains in response to various auditory or visual stimuli? Researchers often have theories about the underlying causes of stuttering and need to test their theories by assessing stutterers' sensory or sensorimotor abilities. As an example of why someone would assess stutterers' perceptions, let me tell you about an experiment in my lab. Based on some previous research, one of my students thought stuttering may be caused by a person's inability to regulate the timing of speech movements. He thought that stutterers have a basic inability to judge time intervals of all sorts. So, he tested groups of stutterers and nonstutterers on their ability to judge the durations of short auditory tones and the intervals between them. He found that individuals who stutter were significantly poorer at judging the length of the tones and intervals. But he also unexpectedly found that by dividing the *nonstutterers* into more fluent and less fluent individuals, the accuracy of temporal judgments separated these two groups of normal speakers (Barasch et al., 2000). Thus, he not only provided support for the timing dysfunction hypothesis but also discovered an unexpected link between stuttering and normal disfluency. Note that by assessing sensory processing, the student was able to look into the brain structures and functions that provide timing information, presumably for speaking as well as for judging durations of sensory stimuli.

Sensory Processing

There are at least two arguments to support the position that fluency may be affected by sensory processes. First, patients with various injuries and diseases have taught us that normal speech depends on intact auditory as well as proprioceptive (feeling of position and movement) and tactile (feeling of touch) feedback. For example, previously normal speech can be disrupted by loss of hearing and by the reduction of feeling that you experience when the dentist numbs your mouth. Therefore, researchers have been curious to determine whether, in people who stutter, abnormal speech might be the result of some disturbance of sensory feedback. Second, experiments that have *altered* **sensory processing**, such as delayed auditory feedback (DAF) (Barrett & Howell, 2021; Black, 1951; Lee, 1951), have created repetitions, prolongations, and blocks in normal speakers, prompting scientists to ask whether this disturbance of feedback might be the cause of stuttering.

Central Auditory Processing

As you probably know, auditory processing begins in the external, middle, and inner ear. Sound information passing through these stages of the peripheral auditory system is then transmitted, via the cochlear nerve, to the auditory cortex, located in the temporal lobe of the brain. Then central auditory processing takes place, analyzing the sounds and making meaning of them. In typical speakers, central auditory processing largely takes place in the left hemisphere, but in stutterers, this may not be the case—both hemispheres may be involved.

As I suggested in Chapter 2, functional problems may be explained by structural anomalies. The brain imaging studies reviewed in that chapter suggested weaker white matter connections many areas, including the auditory system (Chang et al., 2015). These structural deficits may underlie central processing problems, such as underactive left and

Sensorimotor factor: Deficit in Auditory Perception

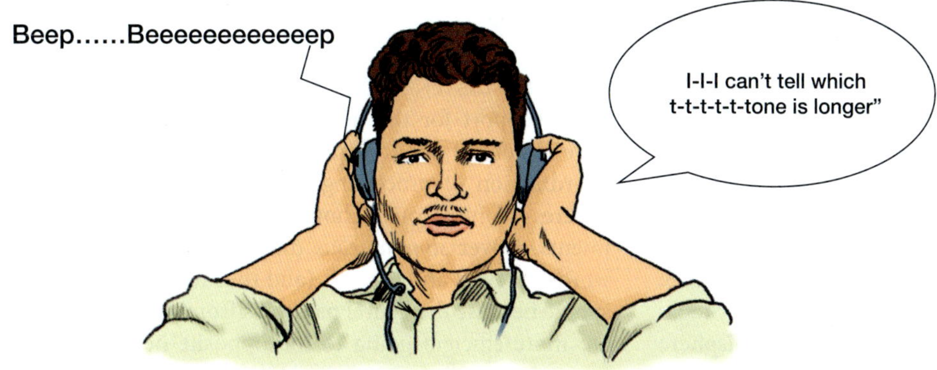

Beep......Beeeeeeeeeeeep
I-I-I can't tell which
t-t-t-t-t-tone is longer"

An example of the effect of language demands on stuttering

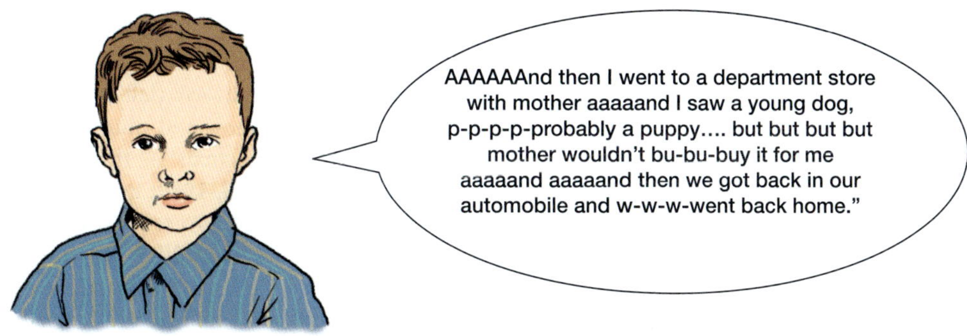

An example of the effect of emotion on stuttering

Bad boy! You broke it!"
Bu-bu-but I-I-I
didn't' mean to
bu-bu-break it."

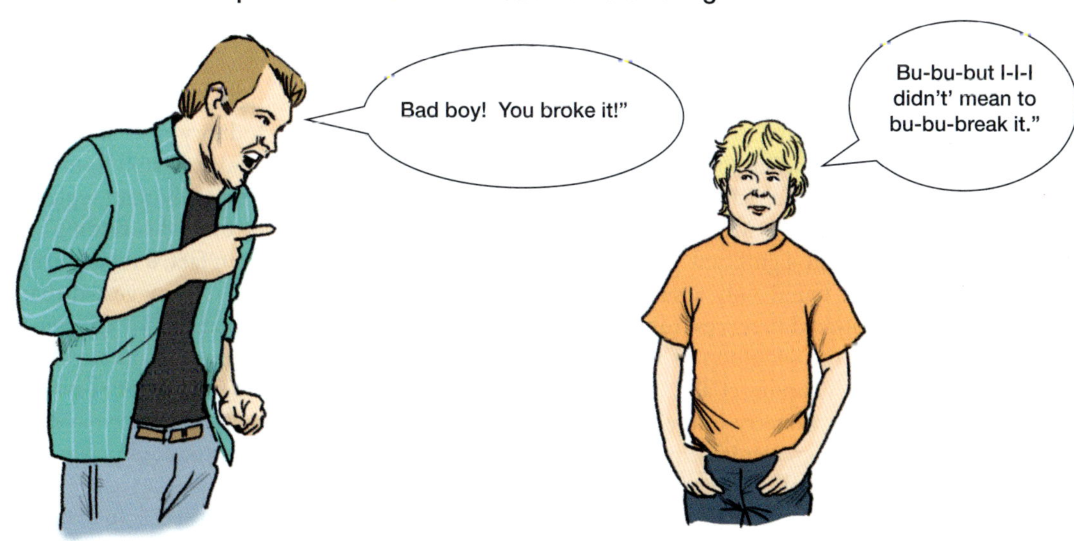

Figure 3.1 Sensorimotor, language, and emotional factors in stuttering.

right auditory cortices when individuals are stuttering (Beal et al., 2007; Brown et al., 2005, Budde et al., 2014; Kikuchi et al., 2017). That is, those areas may not be as fully engaged in the process as is required for fluent speech. Even mutations in certain genes associated with stuttering have been shown to affect auditory-motor integration for speech (Benito-Aragon et al., 2020). It would not be surprising, then, if these brain anomalies affect the fluency of speech.

Speech and Sound Perception

Researchers have demonstrated that individuals who stutter (compared to individuals who don't) have deficits in perceiving speech and other sounds under conditions that stress auditory perceptual processing (Bakhtiar et al., 2019; Hall & Jerger, 1978; Herndon, 1967; Kramer et al., 1987; Liebetrau & Daly, 1981; Molt & Guilford, 1979; Toscher & Rupp, 1978).

Interestingly, one study, which did not find these differences, used individuals who stuttered who became more fluent after they received treatment (Hannley & Dorman, 1982). This finding may be explained if by evidence that treatment for stuttering repairs deficits in auditory processing—an idea supported by several studies (De Nil et al., 2003; Ingham, 2003; Kell et al., 2009; Neumann et al., 2003; Stager et al., 2003). Perhaps treatment increases left-hemisphere participation in both speech production and speech perception, activating more effective auditory perception centers.

Another unexpected finding about speech and sound perception (described earlier in this chapter) is that when more fluent and less fluent *nonstuttering* speakers are compared on tests of auditory perception, the more fluent speakers perform significantly better than the less fluent speakers—even when they are not speakers who stutter (Barasch et al., 2000; Wynne & Boehmler, 1982). This might reflect some commonality in the neurophysiological functioning between people who stutter and typical speakers who are highly disfluent. It suggests that intact central auditory processing is required for high levels of fluency.

Brain Electrical Potentials Reflecting Auditory Processing

Studies of electrical brain activity in response to auditory stimuli have provided further evidence that auditory processing is often abnormal in individuals who stutter. A variety of publications have shown that some or all groups of individuals who stutter have abnormalities in neural electrical activity when responding to a variety of auditory stimuli (Daliri & Max, 2018; Dietrich et al., 1995; Hampton & Weber-Fox, 2008; Hood, 1987; Molt, 1997; Toyomura et al., 2020). While most found significant group differences, Hampton and Weber-Fox found only a subgroup of individuals who stuttered showed differences from controls. This finding is reminiscent of the subgroup of individuals who stuttered described in the Foundas et al. (2004) study with an anomalous rightward asymmetry in the planum temporale. This subgroup showed a greater improvement in fluency while speaking under DAF than did those individuals who stuttered with more typical planum temporale asymmetry. In other words, not all individuals who stutter may have auditory processing anomalies. Only a subgroup may have both structural and functional deviations from the norm, and this subgroup may benefit from therapeutic approaches that help them compensate for these deviations. Perhaps a subgroup that becomes fluent under DAF would benefit from treatment that uses DAF to induce fluency and then weans them from DAF to speak fluently without it. Ideas like this suggest that understanding auditory processing can help us understand not just what is going wrong during stuttering but also how to fix it.

Dichotic Listening Tests

More support for the notion that individuals who stutter have abnormal auditory processing—in this case involving coordination of processing involving both cerebral hemispheres—comes from dichotic listening studies. These experiments deliver *simultaneous* different auditory stimuli (eg, words) to right and left ears (and thus to the opposite hemisphere because the neural pathways from the ear to the brain are more efficient going to the opposite hemisphere). The researchers are interested in whether the subjects more often report hearing the words delivered to right ear (called a right ear advantage) than the left ear. Typical speakers report hearing more of the words delivered to the right ear, indicating that they process language best in the left hemisphere. Most (but not all) of these studies indicate that individuals who stutter do not show the right-ear (left hemisphere) advantage that typical speakers show and thus may be processing language-related auditory signals in the right hemisphere (Blood, 1985; Blood & Blood, 1989; Brady & Berson, 1975; Curry & Gregory, 1969; Davenport, 1977; Liebetrau & Daly, 1981; Quinn, 1972; Robb et al., 2013; Rosenfield & Goodglass, 1980; Sommers et al., 1975; Strong, 1977). Because the right hemisphere is neither structurally nor functionally designed to process language and speech, stutterers' processing may be impaired.

Sensory Processing Other Than Auditory

The few studies that have been conducted of other sensory systems besides auditory also show some deficits, but the results are mixed. Baker (1967) found that people who stutter performed more poorly than typical speakers on tests of oral sensation. However, this finding was not replicated by Jensen et al. (1975). In fact, a review article by Namasivayam and van Lieshout (2011) suggested that the literature does not support the hypothesis of deficits in orosensory function in stuttering. However, on a test that required subjects to match spatially ordered visual patterns with temporally ordered auditory patterns, Cohen and Hanson (1975) found that individuals who stuttered performed more poorly than those who didn't. Chuang et al. (1980) evaluated abilities of individuals who stuttered to make the smallest movements possible with their jaws and tongues. The stuttering group had significantly larger "difference limens" (smallest detectable difference) with or without the assistance of visual feedback for such movements. This means that they did not have the degree of fine sensorimotor control of the jaw and tongue that the nonstuttering group did. De Nil and Abbs (1991) followed up this study and demonstrated that individuals who stuttered had less sensorimotor control for minimal movements with their jaws, lips, and tongues (but not finger movements) compared to individuals who did not stutter, when using only kinesthetic (awareness of position or movement of parts of the body) feedback. There were no differences between the groups when using visual feedback.

The review by Namasivayam and van Lieshout (2011), mentioned previously, did suggest that individuals who stuttered appeared to benefit from increased kinesthetic feedback by using larger articulatory movements or by using a slower speech rate. This temporary increase in fluency via increased kinesthetic feedback is advocated as a therapeutic strategy called "**proprioception**" that is described in the chapters on treatment of school-age children and treatment of adults. Proprioception is a key element in the treatment for stuttering developed by Van Riper (1973a). In an experiment involving vibrotactile feedback—perhaps comparable to the increased kinesthetic feedback just cited—Cheadle et al. (2018) found that this sort of feedback increased fluency in stutterers without slowing their speech rate. These authors then suggested that the development of a portable vibrotactile (awareness of vibration through sense of touch) feedback device might be a useful and discrete therapy tool that stutterers could use to increase fluency without affecting the naturalness of their speech.

Summary of Findings on Sensory Processing

Together with the findings about the auditory system, these studies of other sensory modalities may indicate that as a group, individuals who stutter have some difficulty using auditory, tactile, and proprioceptive (position and movement) information to control speech. But Namasivayam et al. (2009) provided evidence that individuals who stutter are as capable as those who don't in using sensory feedback to stabilize speech motor control in the face of experimental perturbations (masking noise and tendon vibration). If they are as good as individuals who don't stutter at using sensory feedback to nullify the effects of external interference with speech movements, individuals who stutter may be using sensory feedback to also nullify the effects of internal interference with speech (ie, their innately poorer speech motor skills). In other words, when individuals who stutter are fluent, as they naturally are some of the time, they may be achieving this fluency by making extra use of sensory feedback (van Lieshout et al., 2004). In summary, this literature is full of conflicting findings, and it is not clear whether all individuals who stutter have deficits in sensory feedback or only a subgroup. It is possible that deficits in sensory processing may be quite widespread in individuals who stutter, but that it varies in people tested in these experiments depending on the task and on the day. After all, stuttering itself varies from day to day in each of us who have the disorder. Table 3.1 summarizes sensory processing factors in stuttering.

Sensorimotor Control

There are three major areas of research that I will discuss in this section: Reaction Time, Fluent Speech, and Nonspeech Motor Control. Research in these areas examines how sensory information is used to influence motor action. Interestingly, studies in all three areas show anomalies in timing that are characteristic of stuttering subjects, as a group. Aspects of speech sounds or movements are shown to be slower for stutterers than for fluent speakers or the sequence of movements is somehow mistimed. These findings have been cited or predicted by numerous authors in the past. For example, in his last publication, "Final Thoughts on Stuttering," Charles Van Riper suggested that "....stuttering is essentially a neuromuscular disorder whose core consists of tiny lags and disruptions in the timing of the complicated movements required for speech." (Van Riper, 1990).

Reaction Time

Reaction time studies are used to examine sensorimotor control in speech production because in stuttering, it is thought that timing may be particularly compromised. Figure 3.2 depicts an example of a reaction time experiment. The participant is told to watch the computer screen for a picture of an object and to say the name of the object the instant it appears. The time between the appearance of the object on the screen and the first sound made by the participant is her reaction time. As indicated, reaction time involves sensory analysis, response planning, and response execution. It is, therefore, a potentially useful measure in stuttering research if it is thought that the core deficit is a delay in some aspect of sensory processing, planning, or motor execution.

Among the early experiments demonstrating sensorimotor control difficulties related to stuttering were those that found that people who stutter were slower than nonstutterers in initiating and terminating a vowel sound in response to a buzzer (Adams & Hayden, 1976; Starkweather et al., 1976). This research and the research that followed tended to support the hypothesis that reaction times of stutterers as a group were usually slower than that of fluent speakers, probably reflecting generally slow central nervous system processing making it difficult for them to speak at a typical speech rate and remain fluent. Later experiments showed that people who stutter were slower than people who don't in reacting to auditory and visual stimuli with respiratory (exhalation) and articulatory movements (lip closing) (McFarlane & Prins, 1978; Watson & Alfonso, 1987). They were also slower in producing movements involving parts of the body used in speech whether they were responding to auditory or visual signals (eg, Cross & Cooke, 1979). Children who stutter were also found to have slower reaction times in similar studies by Bakhtiar and Zhang (2019), Cross and Luper (1979, 1983), Cullinan and Springer (1980), Maske-Cash and Curlee (1995), and Till et al. (1983).

TABLE 3.1 Sensory Processing Factors in Stuttering

Important Findings	Major Implications
Individuals who stutter show the following differences from their fluent peers: Poorer central auditory processing, especially of temporal information (eg, Budde et al., 2014; Kikuchi et al., 2017). Poorer perception of speech and nonspeech sounds, under difficult listening conditions (eg, Bakhtiar et al., 2019). Longer brain wave latencies and lower amplitudes in people who stutter compared to people who don't when listening to linguistically complex stimuli—or at least for a subgroup of individuals who stutter (eg, Daliri & Max, 2018; Toyomura et al., 2020). Smaller right-ear/left-hemisphere advantage in dichotic listening studies in people who stutter, especially in more severe stutterers and more likely when stimuli are linguistically complex (eg, Robb et al., 2013). Poorer processing of tactile, kinesthetic, and visual information among people who stutter, although found in only a small number of studies (eg, Namasivayam & van Lieshout, 2011). Decreases in the frequency and severity of stuttering when self-monitoring of speech is altered using masking or other means of changing the way they hear themselves (eg, Namasivayam et al., 2009).	Dysfunction of auditory system and perhaps other sensory systems is implicated as a contributing factor in the etiology of stuttering. More disfluent typical speakers may also show some of these deficits, suggesting a link between these two groups. Treatment may improve deficits in sensory processing. Temporary fluency can be obtained by masking or distorting auditory feedback. Possible use in treatment.

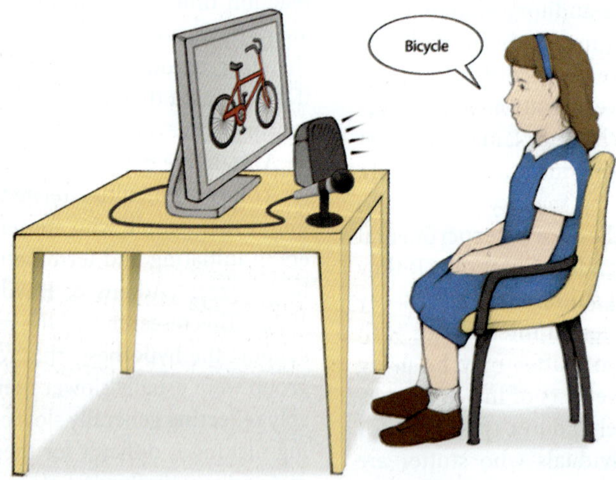

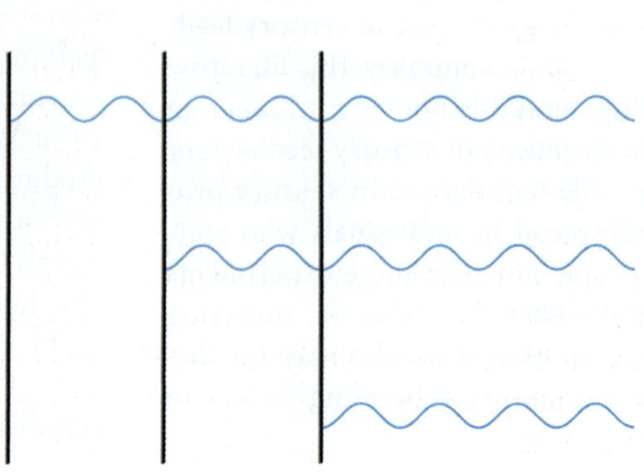

Figure 3.2 Processing stages in a reaction time task.

Although not all studies showed clear-cut significant group differences, De Nil (1995) pointed out that about 75% of the 44 voice reaction time studies that he reviewed found that people who stutter were significantly slower than people who don't stutter and that most of the other studies showed trends in that direction. He further noted that when investigators used linguistically meaningful stimuli (that they had to react to, as fast as they could) to test reaction times, 80% of the studies found significant differences between people who stutter and people who don't. These findings are likely to be related to the evidence from brain imaging studies indicating that individuals who stutter have anomalies in areas used for **sensorimotor processing** of speech and language. Not surprisingly, these anomalies may affect sensorimotor reaction times on nonspeech tasks but are most evident in tasks requiring linguistic processing.

Studies of Fluent Speech

The fluent speech of individuals who stutter has been a focus of numerous studies because clues to the nature of stuttered speech may be hidden in these individuals' fluent utterances. That is, the deficits that create moments of perceptible stuttering—differences in coordination and timing—may sometimes be present, but so subtle that stuttering itself does not appear. However, fine-grained analysis of this apparently fluent speech may show tiny differences in coordination and timing. Here are some findings related to that idea: Acoustic studies have demonstrated that, on average, people who stutter (compared with people who don't stutter) have longer vowel durations, slower transitions between consonants and vowels, and delayed onsets of voicing after voiceless consonants even when speaking fluently (Colcord & Adams, 1979; DiSimoni, 1974; Hillman & Gilbert, 1977; Starkweather & Myers, 1979). Consider how each of these differences at a certain magnitude might be associated with the phenomena we see in stuttering. The results of these acoustic studies have been supported by "kinematic" research, which has measured the movements of speakers' speech structures (eg, Alfonso et al., 1987; Zimmerman, 1980). As a group, people who stutter tend to move their lips and jaws more slowly, even during fluent speech, than do people who don't stutter (eg, Zimmerman, 1980). Kinematic research has also shown that some individuals who stutter demonstrate abnormal sequencing of articulator movement onsets and velocities (Caruso et al., 1988). Walsh et al. (2015) demonstrated that boys who stutter showed less stability (more variability) in motor speech control, compared to girls who stutter and less stability compared to fluent children. Other kinematic studies, however, have not found group differences or have found them only in individuals who stutter and who had recently undergone therapy (eg, McClean et al., 1990), which may have taught them to speak more slowly. Smith and Weber (2017) provide an excellent review of many studies from their research group at Purdue University that have shown that both children and adults who stutter have less stable articulatory coordination than their peers.

Three different explanations have been put forth by researchers for why many individuals who stutter speak more slowly or use different sequences of articulatory movements than nonstuttering speakers even when they are fluent. First, some researchers think that these findings reflect delays or other dysfunctions in processing incoming and outgoing signals. Individuals who stutter may be unable to process neural signals fast enough to make the rapid, precise movements of normal conversational speech, especially when they are under the stress of planning a complex sentence or competing with other talkers. Their delays in voicing onset, slower transitions, and abnormal sequencing during fluent speech may just reflect a slower mechanism working at its limited rate (eg, Etchell et al. 2014; 2015). Second, other researchers, perhaps more skeptical ones, have suggested that such differences simply reflect the way individuals who stutter have learned to talk to avoid stuttering, either on their own or as a result of therapy, and this way of speaking keeps them fluent even with an inefficient speech motor system. An example of this view can be found in a review of the evidence supporting a "speech motor skills" approach to stuttering by Namasivayam and van Lieshout (2011). They suggested that a slower speech rate in the fluent speech of individuals who stutter is a compensatory strategy that gives the speaker more time to use sensory feedback to guide articulator movement. This increased sensory feedback is thought to stabilize the speech motor system and prevent stuttering.

Yet a third interpretation of slower movements on the part of people who stutter in fluent speech is that these slow movements are the result of heightened tension in muscles having antagonistic functions for speech production (Starkweather, 1987). For example, increased tension in both muscles that move a structure forward (agonists) as well as muscles that hold it back (antagonists) would make movement of that structure considerably slower. Imagine two people pulling a rope in opposite directions. Even if one were stronger, that person would make slow progress in their direction because the other, weaker person would create a drag. These slowed movements of speech structures in those who stutter would account for not only slower reaction times but also the longer movement durations in their fluent speech.

Findings from a number of studies support this third view that muscle tension may be responsible for slower speech and contribute to stuttering. They have shown that people who stutter co-contract agonist and antagonist muscles of both the laryngeal (Freeman & Ushijima, 1975; Shapiro, 1980) and articulatory (Guitar et al., 1988) muscle groups during stuttering. These studies, like Starkweather's (1987) review, have noted that such co-contraction of agonist and antagonist muscles appears even in some apparently fluent speech of stutterers. This finding has led many researchers to posit that stuttering is not an "all-or-nothing" event (Adams & Runyan, 1981; Bloodstein, 1987; Smith & Kelly, 1997). Sometimes, people who stutter may speak freely, without a trace of excess tension. At other times, they may have excess tension that isn't heard by listeners as stuttering. At still other times, muscle tension may be great enough that both listeners and the person who stutters are acutely aware of stuttering. This continuum of fluency reflects the subjective impression of many individuals who stutter, including me.

Of course, not all researchers believe that excess muscle tension is an important component of stuttering. Walsh and Smith (2013), for example, did not find evidence of perioral (around the mouth) muscle tension in preschoolers who stutter. As you will see, in Chapters 5 and 6, I make the argument that tension is a response to stuttering that may appear as children experience excessive disfluencies that feel "out of control." Perhaps the preschoolers that Walsh and Smith studied were not reacting to their disfluencies with tension (their stuttering was not threatening to them yet) or perhaps the researchers' measurements, which were limited to perioral muscles, did not reflect tension in other musculature.

Nonspeech Motor Control

Researchers have been curious about whether stuttering is the result of a general motor timing/coordination problem rather than a problem limited to speech production. In a study of both sequential finger movements and sequential counting aloud fluently, Borden (1983) found that individuals who stuttered severely, but not those who stuttered mildly, were slower than their fluent peers in executing both finger movement and speech tasks. Thus, severely stuttering individuals may have substantial deficits in certain sensorimotor tasks that require coordination of sensory and motor processing in addition to stuttering, but those who stutter mildly may only have slight deficits that would require more sensitive tasks to uncover.

Webster (1993a) developed a finger movement task—10 years after Borden's study—in which participants tapped four numbered keys in a predetermined sequence. To make the task somewhat like speech, participants were assigned a novel sequence of keys at the beginning of each trial (3-2-4-1 or 4-1-2-3, etc.). In both timed and untimed tests, subjects who stuttered made more errors sequencing and were slower initiating the task but were comparable to their fluent peers in execution time (once the movement was started). Unlike Borden's study, no effort was made to analyze the results by subjects' stuttering severity. Webster thought that these results suggested that individuals who stutter may have difficulty in "response planning, organization, and initiation" (Webster, 1993b, p. 84) of novel sequences of movements.

To answer the question of why this difficulty may be present only intermittently in individuals who stutter (after all, they have a great deal of fluent speech), Webster (1993b) postulated what others (Cross et al., 1985; Curlee, 1993; Peters & Guitar, 1991) have also considered that at times—especially under emotional stress—there is interference with speech motor control, or "cross talk." Specifically, the idea is that activity in the right cerebral hemisphere, which plays an important in processing negative emotions such as fear, interferes with sequential movement control in the left hemisphere. It's as if signals from the right hemisphere compete with signals for sequential movement in the left hemisphere, making the transmissions slow down.

To test this, Webster (1993b) used a task in which participants performed sequential finger tapping with the right hand while turning a knob with the left hand, in response to an auditory signal. If his hypothesis were true, the stuttering group's left hemisphere—controlled finger tapping would be vulnerable to interference by the right hemisphere—controlled knob turning. Indeed, the stuttering group's performance was significantly poorer than that of the nonstuttering group on both the sequential finger tapping task and turning a knob.

Later, in 1997, Webster wondered whether interference of left-hemisphere sequential movement control mechanisms might be the result of an inability to focus attention on the left-hemisphere task and ignore interference from a competing source, whether from the right or left hemisphere. To test this, Webster used a procedure developed to investigate attention focus in right- and left-handed people. Participants were required to tap twice with one hand for every tap they made with the other hand. They were tested with the right-hand double tapping and the left-hand single tapping, as well as vice versa. The individuals who didn't stutter were able to perform the task significantly better when they tapped twice with the right hand and once with the left; however, people who stuttered and nonstuttering left handers performed the task equally well with either hand doing the double tapping. Webster interpreted this outcome as suggesting that individuals who stutter and left-handed individuals who didn't stutter did not have the ability to focus predominantly on the left hemisphere but had equal focus on both, making their left hemispheres vulnerable to interference from other activities. Webster's model of stuttering, derived from these experiments, postulates that individuals who stutter are unable to protect the integrity of speech production centers from interference or "cross talk" from right-hemisphere emotions. So why, then, don't all of those left handers who are right-hemisphere dominant for speech stutter? I would presume that this model proposes that individuals who stutter have both a deficit in the sequencing of processing underlying speech production (unlike fluent left handers) as well as an inability to focus on the left hemisphere.

Following up on Webster's studies, Subramanian and Yairi (2006) experimented with a version of the finger-tapping task, using not only individuals who stuttered and controls but a third group of "high-risk" participants. The high-risk individuals were parents or siblings of the subjects who stuttered—of special interest because they were thought to be carriers of genetic material that could create stuttering except for the absence of some critical factor that would presumably cause them to stutter, too. All participants were right handed. They all tapped in several conditions, including tapping at a comfortable rate and at a fast rate. Among the findings of this study was evidence that in the comfortable rate condition, the stuttering group and the high-risk group were slower than the control groups. However, in the fast rate condition, the stuttering group tapped faster but at a more variable rate than either of the other groups, both with their right hand and with their left hand. In contrast, the high-risk group had slower tapping rates than either the stuttering group or the control group but had relatively low variability. The authors speculated that these findings may reflect that those in the stuttering and high-risk groups have motor systems that operate best at slow rates. Under pressure to operate at a faster rate, the high-risk group was able to control their rate and maintain stability (low variability), whereas the stuttering group tapped very rapidly but stably because they had pushed their motor systems beyond their optimal operating speed.

It is probably not too great a leap to imagine that individuals who stutter speak more rapidly than is optimal for their speech planning and execution systems, thus becoming disfluent. However, it may also be the case that close relatives of individuals who stutter and, therefore, may have inherited a predisposition for stuttering don't develop stuttering because they are able to speak at slower speech rates, more appropriate for the limitations of the speech motor production system. When I read this finding, I was reminded of meeting a young man at a social gathering who said that he had a first cousin who stuttered, but he himself didn't. As I talked with the young man, I realized that he talked quite slowly (but fluently). This seemed to confirm the hypothesis that some relatives of individuals who stutter may have some genetic material for stuttering but are able to control their speech rates and thereby remain fluent. But several weeks afterward, I realized this was an example of "confirmatory bias"—confirming your hypotheses on the bases of selected observations. I was ignoring the many fluent and fast-talking relatives of people who stuttered whom I had met over many years.

But back to the idea that those who stutter may be talking more rapidly than their speech production systems allow: This perspective was supported by research of Kloth et al. (1995, 1998) who found that in a high-risk-for-stuttering population (one or more parents stuttered) of 93 children studied prior to onset of stuttering, the 26 children who did develop stuttering spoke more rapidly than the 67 children who didn't. However, both groups' speech rates were within the normal range.

Prepare yourself: The following paragraph may seem rather complicated, but the essential message is that stutterers may be using both the right and left hemispheres when speaking and, therefore, may be vulnerable to interference from one hemisphere on the other. Fluent speakers, on the other hand, can focus entirely on the left hemisphere when speaking and are thus protected from right hemispheric interference.

Subramanian and Yairi (2006) found evidence that could support Webster's (1997) hypothesis that individuals who stutter suffer from an inability to focus entirely on the left hemisphere when performing motor tasks. Instead, people who stutter may activate both hemispheres for speech, as brain imaging studies have shown (eg, Brown et al., 2005; Budde et al., 2014). Specifically, Subramanian and Yairi's (2006) data showed that when participants were asked to tap simultaneously with both hands, but tap twice as fast with one hand as with the other, the stuttering and high-risk participants (parents and siblings of the subjects who stuttered) performed equally well with either the right or left hand tapping twice as fast. The control group participants (fluent speakers not related to anyone who stuttered) were better when they tapped twice as fast with their dominant (right) hand as with their left hand. This finding supports the hypothesis that the stuttering and high-risk groups did not suppress the right hemisphere and focus entirely on the left hemisphere.

Subramanian and Yairi's (2006) finding, described earlier, that adults who stutter manifest greater *variability* in a nonspeech motor task (rapid finger tapping) was also found in children who stutter. Olander et al. (2010) studied 17 children who stuttered and controls, ages 4 to 6, using a task that required children to clap their hands in time to a metronome and then continue to clap at that rate after the metronome was turned off. Their results indicated that although 40% of the children performed like the control group, 60% showed variability outside the range of the controls. They speculated that nonspeech motor variability may be related to speech motor control deficits and that these deficits might be predictive of recovery or persistence of stuttering. However, Hilger et al. (2016) found in a larger study (70 children who stuttered) that there were no differences—between children who stuttered and those who didn't—in the timing of hand clapping in preschool children. The authors suggest that the use of a large sample is vital to assessment of differences between those who stutter and those who don't.

The last studies of nonspeech motor control I will review concern the use of auditory input to control nonspeech motor output. A common paradigm in these studies is to have participants track or follow the changing frequency (pitch) of a target sound with a second sound, called a "cursor." A computer controls the pitch changes in the target's sound, and participants follow these changes by using their hand or their jaw to move a lever that changes the pitch of the cursor. Using this paradigm, Sussman and MacNeilage (1975) found that normal speakers made fewer errors tracking the target sound when the cursor tone was presented to the right ear and the target tone to the left ear. Those who stuttered, on the other hand, made equal numbers of errors whether the cursor tone was in the right ear and the target tone in the left or vice versa, suggesting that they did not have a left-hemisphere advantage for integrating auditory information with motor output as the nonstutterers did. These effects were seen when the jaw was used to control the cursor, but not the hand, suggesting the laterality findings are related to speech movements.

Researchers in Australia replicated and extended this work on tracking (Neilson, 1980; Neilson & Neilson, 1987, 1988) using both visual and auditory targets and cursors. They demonstrated that participants who stuttered were significantly poorer using auditory targets and cursors than when using visual ones to guide their movements. They also showed that when both stuttering and nonstuttering participants practiced the tasks beforehand, the differences between the groups were even larger than when they had not practiced. The Neilsons proposed that those who stuttered were slow in developing a mental auditory-motor model of the relationship between their movement of the cursor control and the resulting sound change. They further hypothesized that the basic deficit in stuttering is difficulty in forming or accessing auditory-motor models of what speech movements are needed to produce the sounds they want to make. The Neilsons' perspective on stuttering is given in detail in Chapter 6. I suspect that the Neilsons would agree that individuals who stutter can use their auditory-motor models better in situations where the demands on their neural resources are low but have more trouble when the demands are high.

Brain imaging studies have provided evidence of possible neural substrates (brain structures or functions) underlying the difficulty that individuals may have in accessing auditory-motor models of speech sounds. Chang et al. (2015) reported that the biggest differences in white matter tracts, between individuals who stutter and those who don't, are in "areas supporting auditory-motor and somatosensorimotor integration for speech motor production" (p. 706). These areas are apparently crucial for using stored auditory-motor models of sounds to plan and execute the articulatory gestures needed for speech.

As the Neilsons were working on their experiments in Australia, researchers at Baylor University College of Medicine in Texas were also studying the auditory-motor tracking abilities of individuals who stutter. In a series of publications (Nudelman et al., 1987, 1989, 1992), these researchers described experiments that required participants to hum along with a tone that suddenly changed pitch. The pitch of the target tones was sometimes changed rapidly, sometimes slowly, while researchers measured how quickly participants could change their humming to match the changing pitch of the auditory target tone. The researchers found that the subjects who stuttered were significantly slower than those who didn't in responding to changes in the target's frequency, suggesting that subjects who stutter need more time to process auditory signals and make motor responses.

In a motor skill task with adults who stuttered and adults who did not, Bauerly and DeNil (2015) found that adults who stuttered were poorer than control subjects at a monosyllable nonsense word repetition task, suggesting that stuttering may be related to a deficit in speech motor sequencing. Interestingly, the stuttering group consisted of a number of individuals who performed well and others who performed quite poorly. This supports a hypothesis that there is heterogeneity among people who stutter. Some may have a speech motor deficit and others may have a different disability that contributes to their stuttering.

A different motor task was developed for children who stuttered by another research group. Tendera et al. (2020) gave a series of multifinger sequence learning tasks to children who stuttered, children who had recovered from stuttering, and children who never stuttered. Their results suggested that in the early part of the experiment, children who stuttered did more poorly than either the children who recovered or the children who never stuttered. They improved later in the experiment, suggesting that given enough time and practice the stuttering children could perform adequately. However, the children who stuttered also showed less ability to have well-timed motor responses. The authors suggested that their findings support a view of stuttering being a problem of overall motor performance.

Once again, we find that research has produced evidence that, as a group, people who stutter have difficulty performing sensorimotor tasks. This may be related to the findings of Chang (2010), Chang et al. (2015), Cykowski et al. (2010), and Sommer et al. (2002) that brain areas used for sensorimotor integration are not efficiently connected to motor planning/motor execution areas. Chang et al. (2011) found this lack of connectivity between programming and premotor areas for nonspeech as well as speech movements in adults. This inefficiency in sensory-motor integration may be a basic problem for some who stutter. As you may remember from Chapter 2, Benito-Aragon et al. (2020) found that mutation of the gene GNPTG that is associated with stuttering is also associated with inefficiencies in the neural networks that support auditory-motor integration.

Table 3.2 summarizes sensorimotor control factors in stuttering.

Summary of Findings on Sensorimotor Control

Most, but not all, studies of reaction times show that both children and adults who stutter demonstrate slower reaction times than controls, particularly if linguistic processing is required in the task. Studies of the apparently fluent speech of individuals who stutter show anomalies when detailed analyses of acoustic and kinematic (movement) signals are carried out. Overall, the results suggest that individuals who stutter have slower articulatory movement, sequencing errors, and excess variability compared with controls.

Researchers have also examined nonspeech motor control in stutterers to explore whether deficits are only found

TABLE 3.2 Sensorimotor Control Factors in Stuttering

Important Findings	Major Implications
Compared to nonstutterers, individuals who stutter appear to have these differences:	Training in auditory speech motor control could possibly improve fluency.
Slower reaction times in people who stutter, especially when linguistically meaningful stimuli are used (De Nil, 1995).	Slower performances on a variety of tasks suggest that using slower speech rate may facilitate fluency.
Slower fluent speech, with longer vowels, slower transitions, and delayed onset of voicing in individuals who stutter than in their fluent peers. Also slower completion and more errors on nonspeech tasks of sequencing particularly for more severely stuttering individuals (eg, Namasivayam & van Lieshout, 2011).	If people who stutter try to speak at fast rates, they may be more likely to stutter because of unstable speech motor control.
Although individuals who stutter are slower tapping with their hand at a comfortable rate, they are faster than controls during fast-tapping conditions but more variable. Close relatives of stutterers have slower tapping rates than stutterers and controls but less variability.	It is possible that some close relatives of people who stutter may be predisposed to stutter but may prevent stuttering by speaking more slowly. Modeling slow speech by parents of young children at risk may prevent stuttering by inducing a slower speech rate in children.
Results of hand-tapping task experiment suggested that individuals who stutter are not as able to focus on left-hemisphere motor control and may be vulnerable to interference from the right hemisphere or other areas of the left hemisphere (eg, Subramanian & Yairi, 2006).	Results of hand-tapping task experiment suggested that individuals who stutter are not as able to focus on left-hemisphere motor control and may be vulnerable to interference from the right hemisphere or other areas of the left hemisphere.
Individuals who stutter are poorer at auditory-motor tracking; they may not have left-hemisphere advantage for auditory-motor tracking, and they may be slower at developing a mental model of auditory-motor relationships (eg, Neilson, 1980; Neilson & Neilson, 1987, 1988).	Brain imaging studies support findings of poorer auditory-motor control in people who stutter because of anomalies in auditory-motor areas of the brain.

when the speech mechanism is engaged. Finger movement and sequencing tasks have revealed that both children and adults who stutter have difficulty in accurate sequencing of finger movements and more variability than control subjects. Some studies have required subjects to track auditory tones by moving a cursor with their hand or jaw and have found poorer performance in those who stutter compared to those who do not. Some of these researchers have suggested that these results indicate that individuals who stutter may have deficits in sensorimotor integration. Remember from Chapter 2 that brain imaging studies have suggested that similar anomalies appear when connections among brain areas are examined (eg, Chang et al., 2008; Cykowski et al., 2010; Watkins et al., 2008).

LANGUAGE FACTORS

Language and speech are intimately connected. What you say influences how you say it. How you say it may also influence what you say. We will first focus on how language acquisition in children affects the onset and development of stuttering, then how the language structures used by stutterers affect their stuttering.

Language Effects on Children Who Stutter

The very onset of stuttering itself—which occurs in most children between the ages of 2 and 5 years—has been linked to rapid pace of language acquisition at this same time (Bloodstein et al., 2021; Smith & Weber, 2017; Yairi & Ambrose, 2005). You can imagine that if a child has a vulnerable speech production system in the first place and, therefore, needs extra neural resources to maintain fluency, the demands of emerging language may overpower fluency. Even after early language is mastered as the child gets to be 5 and then 6 years old, the stress of producing long and complex sentences at rapid rates will cause fluency breakdowns. After all, even adults who can be said to have mature language system and do not stutter continue to have disfluencies, although rarely of the kind we refer to as stuttering.

The relationship between language development and stuttering has long been a focus of research. Studies by Berry (1938), Andrews and Harris (1964), Accordi et al. (1983), and Bernstein Ratner and Silverman (2000) have shown that children who stutter frequently have delays in language development. More recent studies have confirmed these delays and some have found that children who stutter are more likely to have language deficits or "dissociations" among language components (one language area like syntax being more advanced than another, like vocabulary) than their fluent peers (eg, Anderson & Conture, 2000; Anderson et al., 2005; Bloodstein et al., 2021; Luckman et al., 2020; Ntourou et al., 2011; Zackheim & Conture, 2003). Several studies have even used event-related potentials (electroencephalography) to assess neural correlates of language processing in children who stutter. They have shown that young children who stutter have anomalies in brain activity related to language processing (eg, Mohan & Weber, 2015; Usler & Weber-Fox, 2015). Some of these studies have also shown that a few of these brain activity deviations predict whether the children will recover from stuttering or not (eg, Leech et al., 2019). In addition, there is evidence that delays in phonological development predict which children will recover from their stuttering.

A meta-analysis of 11 studies of stuttering persistence versus recovery has shown that poorer accuracy in speech sound production and lower scores in expressive and receptive language predict persistence of stuttering (Singer et al., 2020). Moreover, a relatively large longitudinal study of preschool children that included a multitude of factors found that among the best predictors of persistence in stuttering were poorer performance on a test of articulation/phonology and lower accuracy on a nonword repetition task. These studies (which are reviewed in more detail in Chapter 1) and others consistently find that language factors assessed in preschoolers predict persistence of stuttering.

Recently, researchers have begun to demonstrate that delays in language, especially the sound structure of the language, or phonology, can help predict which children who stutter may fail to stop as they grow older. In their review of many studies of stuttering children compared to their peers, Smith and Weber (2017) remind us that (1) there are many individual differences in language ability and performance in children who stutter, with some children having above-average abilities and others below; (2) complex interactions among language skills and between language and speech skills will be different for different children; and (3) these interactions involve many subsystems that are developing rapidly during childhood. Thus, stuttering in individual children will emerge at different times from different combinations of factors, including some that related to speech and language.

Language Effects on Adults Who Stutter

Research on the effect of language on stuttering may be somewhat easier to conduct in adults than in children because adults can be trained to do complex tasks that challenge their speech and language processing. The trick is to develop these complex tasks. One example of such research is the work of Bosshardt (1999, 2002, 2006), who found that in many cases, adults who stutter are poorer at tasks requiring linguistic processing while engaging in other cognitive activities at the same time. Specifically, he used a mental addition task for the cognitive activity to be performed at the same time subjects were repeating three-syllable words or generating and producing sentences. In interpretation of his results (eg, stutterers produced less complex sentences), Bosshardt hypothesized that individuals who stutter have speech production systems that are less protected (compared to typical speakers) from the heavy demand of complex language, where complexity includes unrelated multisyllable words and generating and producing sentences.

Another approach to examining language processing in adults who stutter was developed by Anne Smith's research group at Purdue University. Rather than adding on cognitive processing tasks, as Bosshardt did, Kleinow and Smith (2000) studied the stability of articulator coordination (using a measure of stability called "spatiotemporal index" that reflect variability in articulatory movements) during fluent speech as their subjects were asked to produce more linguistically complex utterances. A baseline phrase, "Buy Bobby a puppy" was compared with longer and more complex phrases such as "You buy Bobby a puppy now if he wants one." The underlying assumption was that adults who stutter have vulnerable speech production systems that would show "breakdown" in articulatory coordination even before any stuttering appeared. Kleinow and Smith demonstrated that longer and more syntactically complex sentences produced significantly more instability in the speech production of individuals who stutter, compared to their production of simpler and shorter sentences. The same was not true for individuals who don't stutter; rather, this group showed more consistent/stable articulatory movement patterns for both simple and complex utterances. As you might expect, Kleinow and Smith interpreted these findings as suggesting that in individuals who stutter, speech production systems are more vulnerable to breakdown when language complexity is great. Ten years later, Smith et al. (2010) found increasing interarticulatory coordination breakdown (variability in upper and lower lip movements across repetitions of the utterance) as phonological complexity increased for adults who stutter but not control subjects who didn't stutter. Similarly, findings about syntactic complexity have been reported by Smith et al. (2012) and by MacPherson and Smith (2013). Table 3.3 summarizes language factors in stuttering.

A more detailed summary of both older and more recent research on language factors in stuttering can be found in Chapter 10: "Cognitive and Linguistic Abilities" in Bloodstein et al. (2021). Note that the chapter also summarizes research on cognitive abilities of individuals who stutter.

Summary of Findings on Language Factors in Stuttering

The demand on neural resources as preschoolers develop language at a break-neck pace may trigger the onset of stuttering in a child whose speech production system is weak. Research

TABLE 3.3 Language Factors in Stuttering

Important Findings	Major Implications
Association of stuttering with preschool language development (Bloodstein et al., 2021). Slightly less robust language processing abilities in children who stutter compared to their fluent peers (eg, Luckman et al., 2020). Increased stuttering in more complex sentences; stuttering is influenced by linguistic factors such as lexical class of word, length, and location in a sentence (Smith & Weber, 2017). Poor performances by adults/children who stutter on many speaking tasks when more linguistically complex stimuli are used (eg, Bosshardt, 1999, 2002, 2006).	Findings of deficits in language processing and more stuttering under greater linguistic demands support a model of stuttering wherein a vulnerable speech production mechanism breaks down under the demands of language learning and using more complex language. To help develop an idea of possible causal roots when evaluating a child who has recently begun to stutter, it is important to determine if the child is/was in a period of intense language development when stuttering started. A complete evaluation of a child who stutters should include assessment of receptive and expressive language as well as subcomponents of language. Decreasing linguistic load on children who are beginning to stutter may reduce their stuttering. In addition, the use of pauses and slower speech rate in older children and adults who stutter may increase fluency by decreasing linguistic demands on the speech production system.

since the 1930s has confirmed that many children who stutter have slower language development than their typically speaking peers. Studies have also suggested that children who stutter may have imbalances among subsystems of language—such as more advanced receptive versus expressive language or more advance syntax than vocabulary.

Even adults who stutter have been shown to have vulnerable speech production systems that may break down under the demands of complex language. Even in fluent utterances, they may show instability (more variability) in their articulatory coordination when saying long and grammatical complicated sentences.

Table 3.3 summarizes language factors in stuttering as well as their clinical implications.

EMOTIONAL FACTORS

Emotions have many components—physiological arousal (which we will also call emotional arousal), associated behaviors, and conscious experience. I will touch upon all of these as I review the research on stuttering and emotions and add my interpretation of the findings.

Stuttering as a Result of Emotional Arousal

Relatively few studies have investigated whether momentary increases in emotional arousal are associated with occurrences of stuttering. A direct connection between emotional arousal and stuttering-like behavior in people who didn't stutter was suggested by an important, but almost forgotten, study conducted many years ago by Hill (1954). Subjects were trained to produce a sentence describing a picture in response to a red light flashing on. After several trials, when the red light came on, they were then given a mild electric shock while speaking the sentence. Subsequently, no shock was given during sentence production, but the red light was assumed to be associated with electric shock. When speaking under the anticipation of shock when the red light flashed on, subjects produced "compulsive and preservative" repetitions, prolongations, and blocks. Hill reported that many responses appeared to be "indistinguishable from what is generally termed stuttering. [Moreover, the responses of several subjects] would have been classed as severe [stuttering] in any speech clinic" (p. 302). Electromyographic sensors that had been placed on the sternocleidomastoid muscle of the neck—because it is easily accessible and indicative of generalized tension—detected increased muscle tension during these stutterlike responses. Thus, it appears that even individuals who don't stutter will show stuttering-like behaviors under threat of penalty, and some people who don't stutter show severe instances of this. This study demonstrates that emotion (probably negative arousal, in this case) can result in stutterlike disfluencies, as well as increase muscle tension in anticipation of stuttering. Many of the studies of emotional arousal and stuttering focus on negative arousal because stutterers themselves report that negative arousal (eg, fear) triggers stuttering. However, in later sections, we will discuss studies that demonstrate that positive emotional arousal can also elicit stuttering.

Several researchers have examined how stuttering frequency and severity, in people who stutter, are affected by emotional arousal. Three studies in the 1990s found that when people who stutter are more emotionally aroused—assessed by various physiological measures like heart rate, skin conductance, and level of cortisol—they stutter more (Caruso et al., 1995; Miller, 1993; Weber & Smith, 1990). The study by Weber and Smith examined the period just preceding moments of stuttering as well as during stuttering and found that for both conditions, higher levels of physiological arousal (skin conductance, peripheral blood volume, and heart rate) were associated with instances of stuttering. Additionally, severity of moments of stuttering was associated with higher levels of arousal.

Other studies have used a more indirect approach, using emotionally laden words to examine the effect of emotional arousal (low vs high arousal) on the speech production system. Hennessey et al. (2014) found that people who stutter had longer speech reaction times (ie, took longer to begin to say the word) in response to emotionally loaded words (eg, inferior, inept, foolish) compared to neutral words. These longer reaction times correlated significantly with the amount of stuttering that the subjects showed in conversational speech recorded in the same session. This suggests that the speech production system of those who stutter is vulnerable to emotion and more so for those who stutter more frequently. Similar results were found by van Lieshout et al. (2014) who showed that aspects of the speech production system of people who stutter were affected by saying emotionally loaded words. While words weren't stuttered, reaction time to begin to speak and articulator movement coordination were affected by threatening words (eg, "rape" and "loser"). These five studies (the three studies in the 1990s and the two studies in 2014—all cited above) are indirect support for the hypothesis that emotional arousal has an effect on the speech of those who stutter more than those who do not.

Anxiety and Sensitive Temperament in People Who Stutter

This section reviews research on whether people who stutter are more anxious than people who don't. Do they carry around more worry and dread about events in the future? Also, do they have a **temperament** that is more easily emotionally aroused?

Anxiety

Just to make sure that we're on the same page about anxiety, I'm not referring to the immediate effect of encountering something threatening, like a coiled snake or a strange creature under your bed. That immediate emotion we usually call fear. Anxiety, on the other hand, is a more ongoing emotion that usually involves worries about something bad that might happen in the future. Like many questions about stuttering, questions about anxiety and stuttering wrestle with the issue of cause and effect. Does anxiety cause stuttering or does stuttering result in anxiety—or do effects occur in both directions?

An early study of anxiety and stuttering is of interest because of what it might tell us about emotion, speech physiology, and stuttering. Horovitz et al. (1978) looked at a phenomenon called the stapedial reflex, which had been previously shown to increase during anxiety in typical speakers. The stapedial reflex is muscle contraction in the middle ear, triggered by activation of the internal branch of the superior laryngeal nerve just prior to speaking, decreasing the loudness with which a speaker hears their own voice. The researchers found that individuals who stutter demonstrated an increased stapedial reflex when they became more anxious (as measured by a physiological assessment of anxiety—the amount of sweat on the subject's palm), compared to a low-anxiety condition. A group of matched fluent speakers showed no increase in stapedial reflex when their anxiety increased, despite earlier studies showing increased stapedial reflex in typical speakers during anxiety. Participants in both groups increased their anxiety (sweated more) by imagining themselves in stressful speaking situations. Although the results of this study are hard to interpret, it appears to show that an increase in anxiety in stutterers may result in changes in speech-related physiology even when only imagining some difficulty speaking. It may be relevant that the increase in stapedial reflex may have been brought about by an increase in laryngeal nerve activity (McCall & Rabuzzi, 1973). This connection between autonomic arousal and heightened laryngeal muscle activity may reflect a conditioned response that becomes part of the learning that many believe maintains stuttering in some individuals. I will revisit this connection between laryngeal tension and autonomic arousal when I discuss temperament and stuttering in Chapter 6.

Researchers have asked whether people who stutter are generally more anxious than people who don't. Some of the authors I cited earlier, who showed that physiological evidence of greater anxiety was associated with more stuttering (Caruso et al., 1994; Miller, 1993; Peters & Hulstijn, 1984; Weber & Smith, 1990), also compared anxiety (autonomic arousal) between a group of people who stuttered and a control group in a situation that involved speaking. They found no differences between the groups.

Because anxiety and stuttering have long been a controversial topic, Ashley Craig edited a special issue of *Journal of Fluency Disorders* (volume 40, 2014) devoted to this subject. Nine studies—some of them analyzing the literature and others presenting new experimental results—comprised the special issue. I recommend reading this issue of the journal to get an in-depth view of stuttering and anxiety. My "take" on the findings is that the authors generally agreed that the anxiety relevant to stuttering is the anxiety that derives from a speaker's repeated experiences stuttering in social situations. This doesn't mean, to me, that all people who stutter have social anxiety disorder; they may just feel anxious about stuttering in social situation. Sometimes, the anxiety develops because listeners' reaction to the stuttering is sometimes clearly negative; at other times, the speaker interprets a relatively neutral reaction as negative. Both experiences create a general dread of speaking and expectations of negative listener reactions, but this varies greatly among individuals. Anxiety, of this type, contributes to the problem of stuttering in several ways. It causes people who stutter to develop avoidance behaviors related to the moment of stuttering as well as to speaking situations. The anxiety is also part of the suffering experienced by people who stutter, making it imperative that, to the extent a specific client does have anxiety, this part of the problem is treated along with the speech itself.

Sensitive Temperament

Many of us who work with children who stutter have often heard parents describe their children as particularly sensitive. Upon questioning, these parents frequently say that even before stuttering began, the child was more easily upset by changes in routine or was shyer with strangers than their siblings. These emotional and behavioral characteristics may be a part of the child's inherited temperament. The idea of different people having different temperaments goes back at least as far as the ancient Greek physician Hippocrates who suggested that personalities could be categorized as sanguine, choleric, melancholic, or phlegmatic. These different temperaments were thought to be determined by different bodily fluids or "humors." Today, we think of temperament as determined by genes and epigenetics, interacting with the environment.

Jerome Kagan's (eg, Kagan, 1994b; Kagan et al., 1987) work on temperament has influenced my thinking about the relationship between temperament and stuttering. His view of temperament places children on a continuum from cautious and shy (inhibited) to fearless and outgoing (uninhibited). Much of his research has studied children on the extreme ends of this continuum, using behavioral observation and acoustic/physiological measurements to compare the two groups. Among his many observations, he and his colleagues have found that more inhibited children (children who are typically fluent; he has never studied children who stutter) show an increase in laryngeal muscle tension under more stressful conditions (Kagan et al., 1987). This finding may be related to changes in the topography of stuttering as it progresses, as I suggest in Chapter 5.

Rothbart (2011) has also done extensive research on temperament in typical children. She and her coworkers conceptualize temperament as based in the child's biology and observed as differences in children's reactivity and self-regulation. Reactivity, a term also introduced by Kagan, refers to how arousable the child's motor, cognitive, and emotional systems are to various stimuli. Self-regulation refers to how the child deals with those stimuli, for example, avoiding negatively arousing situations. A number of studies have used Rothbart's model of temperament to compare children who stutter and those who don't, using the Children's Behavior Questionnaire (Rothbart et al., 2001). In the next section, I will summarize these results and other relevant studies after a brief historical account of how various authors have speculated that temperament may play an important part in the development of stuttering.

Theoretical Considerations About Stuttering and Sensitive Temperament

An important early conceptualization of stuttering, temperament, and anxiety can be found in Brutten and Shoemaker's (1967) landmark book *The Modification of Stuttering*. Rather than using the term "temperament," they referred to "individual differences in conditionability and autonomic reactivity." They suggested that some individuals have predispositions to stutter because they are constitutionally more likely to have an anxiety-based speech breakdown under stressful conditions. Moreover, these individuals are also thought to be more conditionable because of their autonomic reactivity, making it more likely that initial breakdowns under stress will develop into well-learned stuttering behaviors.

Following Brutten and Shoemaker (1967), a number of authors have speculated about the possible importance of considering this kind of reactive temperament in gaining a better understanding of the nature of stuttering (eg, Bloodstein, 1987, 1995; Bloodstein et al., 2021; Conture, 1990; Guitar, 1997, 1998, 2000; Peters & Guitar, 1991; Walden et al., 2012). Many of us have suspected that a reactive temperament, for example, might trigger increased struggle, physical tension, and avoidance in children when they are initially disfluent and thus create a learned cycle of mild stuttering begetting more severe stuttering, leading to chronic stuttering. On the other hand, a placid temperament in equally disfluent children might allow them to stay relaxed, ignore the disfluencies, and thereby outgrow early stuttering. Questionnaire studies have found indications that both adults and children who stutter are more sensitive than nonstutterers. This has been corroborated by studies of physiological measures of sensitivity, which I will discuss later in this section (Anderson et al., 2003; Karrass et al., 2006; Zengin-Bolatkale, 2016).

With this evidence in hand that at least some individuals who stutter have more sensitive temperaments, we need to ask how this may shed light on the disruption of fluency by emotion. Psychologists who study temperament have looked carefully at the regulation and expression of emotion in persons with sensitive temperaments. Studies of both normal and brain-damaged patients provide good evidence that the regulation of emotion is a lateralized function (Kinsbourne, 1989; Kinsbourne & Bemporad, 1984). These authors suggest that some emotion-based behaviors are more regulated by one cerebral hemisphere than the other. Emotions regulated by the left hemisphere seem to motivate such behaviors as approaching new situations or new stimuli, exploration, and action, whereas emotions regulated by the right hemisphere motivate behaviors such as avoidance, withdrawal, and the arrest of action. Studies of electrical activity in the brain indicate that individuals with sensitive temperaments are right hemisphere dominant for emotionally based behaviors (Ahern & Schwartz, 1985; Calkins & Fox, 1994). This means that if individuals who stutter are temperamentally reactive as a group, they may have an inborn proclivity toward behaviors motivated by right-hemisphere emotions—avoidance, withdrawal, and the arrest of action.

How this association of emotions and hemispheres may affect speech is not yet clear, but Webster (1993b) speculates that when individuals who stutter are emotionally aroused, then right-hemisphere proclivities, such as avoidance and withdrawal, could affect their left-hemisphere supplementary motor areas, interfering with planning and initiation of speech. My own speculation about the relationship between emotion and stuttering is that one important aspect of right hemisphere—dominant, emotionally based behaviors—is the arrest of ongoing behavior. This phenomenon is especially well described by Gray (1987), a psychologist who has studied the central nervous system's response to stress. He proposes that when an individual experiences fear or frustration, a behavioral inhibition system in the brain increases three distinct forms of behavior: (1) freezing, which involves widespread muscular contractions that produce tense and silent immobility; (2) flight; or (3) avoidance. It is possible that such behaviors may be manifested in stuttered speech by both core behaviors (repetitions, prolongations, and blocks) and secondary behaviors (escape and avoidance).

Gray's hypothesis of an individual's increasing tension under stress is supported by a study by Coster (1986) (cited in Kagan et al., 1987). Coster, studying children who had no stuttering or any other speech disorder, found that more sensitive children manifest their reactivity by generating higher levels of physical tension, particularly in laryngeal muscles, when they are speaking in unfamiliar or threatening situations. It is particularly relevant to stuttering that Coster found increased tension in laryngeal muscles in typical speaking children. This is because some sensitive children who stutter and are embarrassed by may respond to these disfluencies by increasing physical tension, especially in laryngeal muscles. As Van Riper (1971) has observed, "When the child becomes aware of his basic stuttering behaviors as frustrating or unacceptable to others, tension appears in the speech musculatures involved in the repetitions and fixations [silent blocks]" (p. 123). This physical tightening of muscles may further interfere with speech, producing the abruptly terminated repetitions, as well as prolongations, pitch rises, and blocks that develop in many children when stuttering persists. Other children who are highly sensitive and predisposed to stutter may show tense prolongations and blocks in response to emotionally difficult situations at the onset of their stuttering. The heterogeneity of individuals who stutter and their unique patterns of stuttering will be discussed further in upcoming chapters on developmental factors and on learning.

More speculation about the effect of emotion on stuttering is prompted by brain imaging studies that have shown extensive activity during stuttering in an area called the right insula, shown in Figure 2.5 in the last chapter (Fox, 2003), and the anterior cingulate cortex (Braun et al., 1997a, 1997b; De Nil et al., 2000). Both of these areas have strong connections with the amygdala (Allman et al., 2001; Habib et al., 1995), a major structure in fear conditioning (LeDoux, 2002, 2015). A number of studies have found that right-hemisphere activity is heightened during stuttering and reduced during induced fluency (Braun et al., 1997a, 1997b; De Nil et al., 2000; Forester & Webster, 2001; Fox et al., 1996, 2000; Neef et al., 2018; Weber-Fox et al., 2013), findings that may reflect negative emotional arousal. My reasoning is as follows. First, many of the studies reviewed in the previous chapter suggest that in individuals who stutter, speech planning and production are localized in right-hemisphere regions homologous to Broca's, Wernicke's, and interconnecting areas in the left hemisphere. Second, emotions lateralized to the right hemisphere in the human brain are those associated with fear—avoidance, escape, and arrest of ongoing behavior (Gray, 1987; Kinsbourne, 1989). Third, because strong emotions tend to dominate the neural processes in surrounding areas (LeDoux, 2002), these emotions may disrupt ongoing speech processing in ways analogous to how they affect all behavior, including avoidance behaviors, escape behaviors, and blocks.

The section you have just read—on emotions and stuttering—suggests that emotions play a major role in the development of stuttering. In some cases, emotions may trigger the onset of stuttering. An interesting theoretical perspective on stuttering and emotions has been proposed by Conture and Walden (2012) and Walden et al. (2012). Although their view ("dual diathesis-stressor model of stuttering") incorporates both emotional variables and speech-language variables, I will only describe what they hypothesize about emotions. They suggest that children who stutter may have constitutional predispositions (diatheses) that make them highly emotionally reactive to novel stimuli. This predisposition will be greater or lesser in different children. For the predisposition to be "activated," the child must encounter some environmental stress. Thus, the child may stutter more or less in any given situation, depending on the stress they experience and the degree of predisposition they have. The stimulus the child is reacting to in this case is the experience of having some difficulty speaking (disfluencies or other speech disturbances). The child's emotional reaction to the difficulty will increase the difficulty in a cyclical fashion, with early emotional reactions to milder disfluencies causing them to become more severe, which in turn would cause stronger emotional reactions, resulting in even more struggle and avoidance behaviors. Of course, any given child will have other predispositions, such as language or speech deficits that will interact with the emotional diathesis.

Complete theoretical models of stuttering must, of course, incorporate all of the constitutional factors described in this and the previous chapter—genetics, epigenetics, brain structure and function, sensory processing, sensorimotor control, language, and emotion (see Smith & Weber, 2017). In addition, developmental and environmental factors must be included as well. An unexpected connection between genetics, emotion, and stuttering comes from a study mentioned earlier, by Kang et al. (2010). This work has identified a gene associated with stuttering (GNPTG) that is associated with both motor control and emotional regulation. Exploration of how individuals with this gene respond to treatment and how treatment may be adjusted to modify the effect of this gene promises be a vital step forward.

Empirical Evidence About Stuttering and Sensitive Temperament

Greater sensitivity in children who stutter has been reported by several studies. Fowlie and Cooper (1978) reported that mothers of children who stutter viewed them as more sensitive than did mothers describing children who do not stutter. In a questionnaire study, Oyler (1992) found that adults who stutter were more emotionally sensitive than were adults who don't stutter; however, this hypersensitivity could be the result of many years of stuttering. Oyler and Ramig (1995) found that parents of children who stutter rated them as more sensitive than did control parents rated nonstuttering children. A follow-up study of behavioral inhibition in children who stuttered was conducted by Ntourou et al. (2020). This study developed a scale to assess behavioral inhibition (similar to hypersensitivity) in children and establish its reliability and validity. Using 225 children who stutter and 243 children who did not stutter, the Short Behavioral Inhibition Scale, as it is called, was shown to be reliable and valid as a tool for differentiating children with a high degree of behavioral inhibition from those who not so behaviorally inhibited, and to be assessing a single, homogeneous construct. Results also indicated that children who stutter had a significantly higher level of behavioral inhibition and higher levels were associated with greater frequency and severity of stuttering.

The connection between temperament and stuttering severity was made convincingly by Kraft et al. (2014) and replicated 5 years later with an impressively large (*n* = 98) cohort of children (ages 2 to 12 years) who stuttered (Kraft et al., 2019). These authors looked at a component of temperament called "effortful control," the ability to regulate attention so that activation or inhibition can be used to control behavior, which is influenced by both heredity and environment, making it possibly amenable to therapeutic change (Eisenberg & Sulik, 2012). The researchers were able to show that effortful control was a strong predictor of stuttering severity as rated by both parents and clinicians. Of particular interest was the evidence that when additional measures of the child's home environment and history of life events (possible stressors) were included in the study, only effortful control was significantly predictive of stuttering severity. Kraft et al. (2014, 2019) strongly suggest that those children who score low on effortful control can benefit from treatment that includes a combination of appropriate clinical management of stuttering and training in self-regulation. Such training may help a child use effortful control to limit overreacting to events that might otherwise trigger stuttering.

Using the concept of "difficult" temperament, which includes some aspects of sensitivity as well as restlessness and impulsiveness, both Wakaba (1998) and Embrechts and Ebben (1999) found that parents of children who stuttered rated their children as having this type of temperament to a greater degree than did parents of nonstuttering children. LaSalle (1999) presented a paper indicating that, in contrast to parents of young children who don't stutter, parents of young children who do stutter rated their children as having high frustration reactions and lack of persistence. Both of these traits have been associated with sensitive temperament (Thomas & Chess, 1977). Anderson et al. (2003), using the Behavioral Style Questionnaire (McDevitt & Carey, 1978), found that parents of children who stutter rated their children as slower to adapt to novelty compared with how parents of nonstuttering children rated their children. They related this to Kagan's (1989, 1994b) description of this personality trait as also being shyer and more fearful when encountering unfamiliar events and people. More evidence of children who stutter having a more reactive temperament comes from an important study by Karrass et al. (2006). Their findings, using a scale of children's reactions to everyday stressful situations completed by parents, suggested that when compared to nonstuttering children, children who stutter are more emotionally reactive and are less able to regulate their emotional responses. The authors speculated that these traits may make it more likely that children who stutter will react emotionally to their disfluencies, producing more disfluencies in a cycle of reactivity and increased stuttering, which the authors call "reverberant interaction."

Kurt Eggers conducted several studies on children who stuttered compared with those who did not. His initial study (Eggers, 2012) included 69 children who stuttered and 149 children who did not; all children were between 3 and 8 years old. Using the Children's Behavior Questionnaire (Rothbart et al., 2001), Eggers found that children who stuttered scored higher in negative reactivity (Kagan's category of "inhibited") and lower in self-regulation. Relating this to Rothbart's interpretation of these factors, this study suggests that children who stutter tend to have greater motor, cognitive, and emotional responses to stimuli. They also may show more inhibition and avoidance (see Fig. 1.1 in Eggers, 2012).

Compared to the research on temperament in children who stutter, only a small amount of research has been done on adults. Some researchers (eg, Kagan, 1994a, 1994b) have advocated for physiological or behavioral studies, rather than parent rating of children's temperament. In this spirit, using a physiological measure of sensitivity, Guitar (2003) found that the acoustic startle responses of adults who stutter were significantly greater than those of adults who do not. The startle paradigm, which measures the magnitude of the eye blink in response to a burst of white noise, is believed to differentiate individuals whose nervous systems have low thresholds of arousal from those whose nervous systems require larger stimuli to react (Vrana et al., 1988). Moreover, that paradigm has been used to demonstrate differences between children who have been categorized as temperamentally inhibited and those categorized as temperamentally uninhibited (Snidman & Kagan, 1994). Guitar (2003) also found substantial correlations between startle responses and scores on the nervous subscale of the Taylor-Johnson Temperament Analysis (Taylor & Morrison, 1996). That subscale assesses the individual's tendency to be tense and excitable.

Importantly, two later studies, Alm and Risberg (2007) and Ellis et al. (2008), failed to replicate Guitar's (2003) findings. This suggests that a sensitive temperament may not be a characteristic of all adults who stutter, and it is certainly not a trait limited to those who stutter. To the extent it is a component of stuttering for many individuals, it probably interacts with a basic predisposition for difficulty with speech motor control.

Some studies of sensitive temperament in children who stutter have used electrophysiological measures of brain activity as well as parent questionnaires to compare children who stutter with those who don't. Zengin-Bolatkale (2016, 2017) used late positive potential—a measure of electroencephalography activity in response to stimuli—to assess both groups' response to pleasant and unpleasant pictures. Higher levels of late positive potential are thought to reflect emotional reactivity, and this study was able to show that children who stutter had significantly more emotional reactivity to unpleasant pictures, and this reactivity was significantly correlated with parent report of the child's sensitive temperament. Zengin-Bolakale (personal communication, November 27, 2017) also showed that this emotional reactivity was significantly and positively correlated with the children's severity of stuttering.

The findings that children who stutter are more temperamentally reactive are important because they may explain why some children who have vulnerable speech production systems may begin to stutter under relatively normal stress. They also help us understand why some of these children are susceptible to conditioning that can turn mild intermittent stuttering into more severe and persistent stuttering. This line of thought will be explored more fully in Chapter 5, on learning. Table 3.4 summarizes emotional factors in stuttering.

Summary of Findings on Emotional Factors in Stuttering

Several studies have shown that emotional arousal is associated with stuttering behaviors. One study found that even in nonstuttering speakers, negative emotional arousal was associated with stuttering-like behaviors (Hill, 1954). In stuttering speakers, more emotional arousal was associated with more frequent and severe stuttering. This emotional factor—arousal—is a time-limited, situational response, whereas another emotional factor—anxiety—is more long term.

It has been shown that increases in anxiety in stutterers (but not nonstutterers) are correlated with increased muscle tension in muscles associated with speaking. Most experts agree that the anxiety associated with stuttering is social anxiety that results from repeated negative experiences when stuttering and experiencing (or anticipating) rejecting listener responses. Thus, the anxiety related to social situations makes it more likely they will stutter in these situations and avoid them if they can. An important part of therapy involves reducing this anxiety by making stutterers more comfortable

TABLE 3.4 Emotional Factors in Stuttering

Area of Interest	Important Findings	Major Clinical Implications
Anxiety	Many, but not all, studies find that individuals who stutter are not more anxious than individuals who don't stutter, but a few do indicate they are more anxious.	For many individuals with persistent stuttering, their treatment programs may benefit from components that facilitate the unlearning of fear-based stuttering behaviors.
Autonomic arousal	Anxiety or autonomic arousal in individuals who stutter is associated with stuttering. Emotion caused by threat of electric shock can cause disfluencies even in individuals who don't stutter.	Treatment should consider addressing anxiety and fear in clients who manifest them.
Temperament	There is some evidence that children and adults who stutter tend to have a more sensitive or inhibited temperament; there is speculation that this may be related to right-hemisphere activity associated with stuttering. Sensitivity may influence physical tension.	There may be a subgroup of particularly reactive/sensitive individuals who need more focus on emotions during treatment.

with their stuttering when talking in public or in social gatherings.

In regard to temperament, this is an underlying personality trait rather than anything situational, and it is probably, in part, genetic. There are several theoretical views that incorporate a child's sensitive temperament into models of how stuttering develops from mild repetitions and prolongations into tenser and more severe stutters—especially blocks. In terms of data on temperament and stuttering, multiple studies have indicated that individuals who stutter are more likely to have more sensitive temperaments (sometimes described as more behaviorally inhibited) than nonstuttering individuals. The more sensitive the child is, the more frequent and more severe the stuttering tends to be.

SUMMARY

- Strong evidence indicates that individuals who stutter have deficits in sensory processing, such as auditory perception, cortical speech processing, dichotic listening, and control of movement using kinesthetic feedback. These deficits may signal some weakness in use of sensory information to make movements used in speech production.
- Many studies have found that sensorimotor responses, like reaction times, in individuals who stutter are slower than in typical speakers. Movements in fluent speech are also slower, reflected by acoustic and kinematic measures.
- Individuals who stutter appear to have deficits not only in speech motor control but also in nonspeech motor tasks, such as sequential finger tapping and using auditory input to control motor output.
- A number of studies, some using brain imaging and others focused on genetics, have suggested that individuals who stutter have difficulty with sensorimotor integration (using sensory information in planning and making movements) to produce fluent speech.
- Many researchers have theorized that stuttering occurs because some individuals—through heredity or cerebral injury—have a vulnerable speech production system that may break down under stress of various kinds.
- One type of stress that may produce stuttering in such a vulnerable system is from demands of language. It is hypothesized that the demands of language learning during, especially between ages 2 and 5, may overwhelm the speech system and result in the onset of stuttering. In adults, it has been shown that those who stutter show problems in motor speech coordination as the components of language (eg, syntax or phonology) become more complex.
- Another stress that may cause breakdown in a vulnerable speech motor system may come from emotional arousal. Heightened emotion has been shown to affect those who stutter more than those who don't. In addition, there is evidence that a sensitive temperament may characterize both adults and children who stutter, making them more prone to emotional reactivity and less ability to regulate responses to emotion. Emotion may interfere with smooth motor coordination, lead to more muscle tension, and make classical conditioning (learned emotion-based responses) more likely.

STUDY QUESTIONS

1. Why do researchers study sensory processing in stutterers when stuttering is clearly a movement disorder?
2. What are some reasons why individuals who stutter might be slower in their reaction times and in speech movements during fluent speech?
3. Why would people who stutter have problems with motor movements that have nothing to do with speech, like finger tapping?
4. Explain how language demands might cause the onset of stuttering between ages 2 and 5.
5. Given that adults have already learned their languages, why would adults who stutter have more stuttering with utterances that are more complex?
6. Do you think stuttering causes people to be more sensitive or do you think more sensitive people tend to stutter?
7. Why would an easily emotionally reactive person be more likely to be affected by classical conditioning? (You may need to find out more about classical conditioning to answer this. See Chapter 5.)
8. Researchers have found many differences between groups of people who stutter and their fluent peers. Why can't we say that these differences cause stuttering?
9. What research finding in this chapter do you think has the most relevance for the treatment of stuttering? Defend your answer.

SUGGESTED PROJECTS

1. Assess your own reaction time under different conditions. Use a stopwatch (how fast can you turn it on and off?) or similar instrument to determine your reaction time. Try this under many different conditions, such as at several times during the day and when sick or tired versus when feeling alert. Determine what variables affect your reaction times, and determine whether it is true for other people. Using this information, suggest why different studies of reaction times in individuals who stutter get different outcomes.
2. Find a temperament test (many are available online at no cost), and take it yourself. Do you think the results accurately describe you? Here's one to start with: www.TemperamentQuiz.com/.
3. Record yourself saying a brief sentence and then a long, complex sentence. Time each sentence and then count the number syllables in each and calculate the rate at which you said each sentence (in syllables per second). If you said the long, complex sentence at a slower rate, can you say it faster? Do you have more disfluencies when you said it faster than when you said it slower? If so, do you think people who stutter ought to be urged to talk more slowly? Do you think parents of young children who are starting to stutter should talk more slowly to their child? If you do think that, how could that help?

SUGGESTED READINGS AND OTHER RESOURCES

Bloodstein, O., Bernstein Ratner, N., & Brundage, S. (2021). *A handbook on stuttering.* (7th ed.). Plural Publishing, Inc.

This is the most recent edition of a classic reference book on stuttering. It provides a thorough update of "the most important research in stuttering." Moreover, it is really enjoyable to read. Chapters 7, 8, 9, and 10 cover the areas discussed in this chapter—Sensorimotor, Emotional, and Language Factors in stuttering.

Craig, A. (Ed.). (2014). Anxiety and stuttering [Special issue]. *Journal of Fluency Disorders*, 40, 1–140.

This issue of the journal contains review articles as well as empirical research on the relationship between anxiety and stuttering. It gives a good overview of this topic as of 2014.

Smith, A., & Weber, C. (2017). How stuttering develops: The multifactorial dynamic pathways theory. *Journal of Speech, Language, and Hearing Research*, 60, 2483–2505.

This article is an excellent review of research—much of it from Smith and Weber's own research group—supporting a view that motor, linguistic, and emotional factors combine and interact to precipitate and maintain childhood stuttering.

StutterTalk: Changing how you think about stuttering…one podcast at a time. www.stuttertalk.com

This website is a gold mine of information about stuttering research and treatment. Founder Peter Reitzes and other hosts interview scientists, clinicians, and people who stutter about stuttering—its nature and treatment. At present, there are more than 700 recorded interviews you can listen to on your computer or mobile device. Episodes 558, 561, 564, 568, and 571 are interviews on topics covered in this chapter on constitutional factors in stuttering.

Van Riper, C. (1982). *The nature of stuttering* (2nd ed.). Prentice-Hall.

Although somewhat dated, this book reviews an impressive amount of world literature on stuttering, from as long ago as the 20th century BC. *In a synthesis of the research, Van Riper presents his venerable hypothesis that stuttering is a disorder of timing.*

Yairi, E. & Ambrose, N. G. (2005). *Early childhood stuttering.* Pro-Ed.

The authors give an in-depth description of the results of 14 years of research on the development of stuttering conducted at the University of Illinois-Urbana/Champaign. Chapters are devoted to the onset and development of stuttering, characteristics of children's disfluency, genetics, and cognitive, psychosocial, and motor factors in stuttering. Elaine Paden and Ruth Watkins contributed chapters on phonological and language abilities of children who stutter, respectively. Like Wendell Johnson's magnum opus The Onset of Stuttering, *this book reflects a monumental effort focused on childhood stuttering.*

4

Developmental and Environmental Factors in Stuttering

Chapter Outline

Chapter Objectives

After studying this chapter, readers should be able to:

- Explain how factors related to physical development can interfere with fluent speech
- Explain how factors related to speech and language development can interfere with fluent speech
- Explain how, in some cases, increasing language development may decrease disfluencies

- Explain how factors related to cognitive development can interfere with fluent speech
- Explain how factors related to social-emotional development can interfere with fluent speech
- Describe the evidence for the role of parents, the speech-language environment, and life events in the onset and development of stuttering

Key Terms

Competition for neural resources: This is the concept that the brain has a limited amount of resources that can be applied to tasks such as learning to speak and learning to walk. If some task requires a great deal of attention or involves extensive neural activity, other tasks performed at the same time will have fewer resources and may thus be less well performed

Language complexity: This refers to gradually more adultlike language acquired by children as they develop. When children use more advanced phonology, morphology, and syntax (eg, passive vs active voice), their fluency may suffer. Parents are encouraged to use only the level of language complexity their child uses when they speak with them

Life events: These are typically stressful events or circumstances in a child's life, such as moving to a new home, the birth of a sibling, or a death of a parent. Very sensitive children may find some typical events (such as a visit to relatives' homes) stressful—so much so that this event may cause the onset of stuttering or worsening of existing stuttering.

Speech and language environment: The communication style that characterizes people in a child's environment—usually his or her home. For example, some parents, siblings, and other relatives of a child may speak very rapidly, use advanced forms of language, or interrupt the child frequently. These aspects of the speech and language environment are thought to stress the child.

The two preceding chapters described the constitutional factors (eg, less dense and less myelinated white matter fiber tracts connecting speech perception, planning, and execution areas) that put a child at risk for stuttering. These factors usually lie dormant until the child's language reaches the two-word stage or even later, while motor and cognitive abilities are also developing rapidly. Further, it is not uncommon for the child's environment at this point to consist of a busy household with competing demands and distractions. These are the conditions under which stuttering first appears, then disappears, continues, or grows worse.

Although developmental and environmental influences can be pressures that bring on stuttering, but they can also ameliorate or protect. For example, a child's rapidly developing language abilities may enable them to keep up with a desire to produce long and complex sentences, thus bridging a gap that might otherwise have resulted in stuttering. Alternatively, if parents are able to change a child's environment, so that demands from a garrulous, fast-talking family can be tempered by quieter one-on-one time when a parent talks slowly with a child and lets them speak when they want to on a topic of their choosing, while the parent listens, this can sometimes reverse the development of stuttering.

Figure 4.1 depicts the influence of developmental and environmental factors on the onset and development of stuttering.

The developmental and environmental factors that interact with constitutional factors to give rise to stuttering often work quietly. The ordinariness of the child's life when stuttering first appears is reflected in this observation by Van Riper (1973a, p. 81):

> *In the great majority of children we have carefully studied soon after onset, we were unable to state with any certainty ... what precipitated the stuttering. In most instances there simply were no apparent conflicts, no illnesses, no opportunity to imitate, no shocks or frightening experiences. Stuttering seemed to begin under quite normal conditions of living and communicating.*

Children's lives often seem to be on an even keel when stuttering first emerges, an observation consistent with the results of careful research examining critical developmental and environmental factors affecting its onset and progression proving inconclusive. Thus, defining immediate or local causes of stuttering onset is a domain of educated guesses and tentative hypotheses. Evidence for developmental factors is inferred from the fact that almost all onsets of stuttering occur when children are developing most rapidly during their preschool years (Andrews et al., 1983; Bloodstein et al., 2021; Wingate, 1983; Yairi & Ambrose, 2005, 2013).

Evidence of environmental influences comes in part from clinical reports of associations between the onset of stuttering in the presence of some environmental stresses and its remission as these stresses are lessened (eg, Jones et al., 2014; Van Riper, 1973a, 1982a). Environmental factors are also

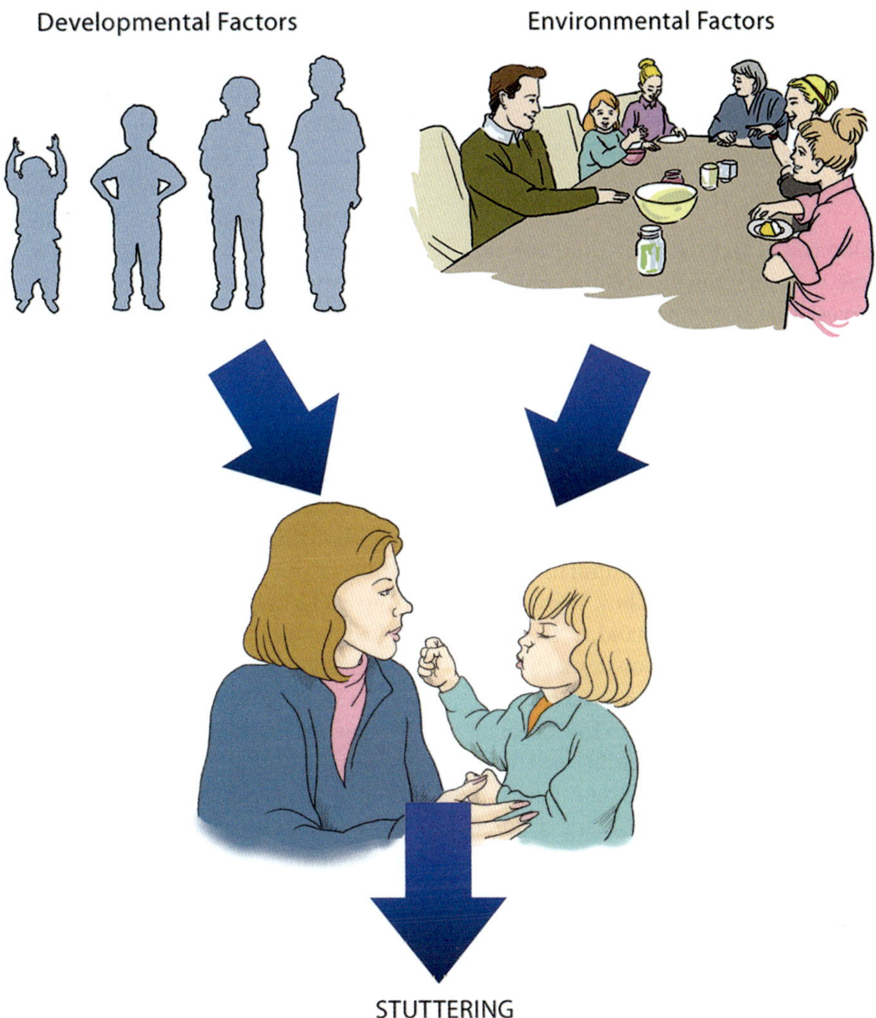

Figure 4.1 Developmental and environmental factors can interact with constitutional factors to precipitate or worsen stuttering.

implicated by higher incidences of stuttering in those cultures that appear to be more competitive, with high standards and less tolerance of differences, like the United States and Japan (Van Riper, 1982a). A high incidence of stuttering has also been found in certain West African countries like Cameroon and Nigeria (Bloodstein et al., 2021). This is partly attributed to stress placed on children by their parents for high achievement and low tolerance of differences like stuttering, such as in the Ibo culture (Bloodstein et al., 2021). By contrast, some communities around the world have been reported as having no stuttering and no term to label stuttering. Morgenstern (1956), Johnson and Moeller (1967), Bloodstein et al. (2021) discussed these reports and suggested that certain societies such as in New Guinea, among Polar Eskimos, and in the aborigines of Australia may have little or no stuttering because parents raise their children permissively and these cultures are very accepting of individual differences. Evidence of cultures with little stuttering, presumably because of easy-going child rearing practices, provided support for the theory that stuttering is caused by parents' overreaction to typical disfluencies (this was termed the "diagnosogenic" theory). More recent evidence of the importance of genetic factors and findings that most parents are usually accepting of the mild disfluencies seen at the onset of the disorder have discredited the diagnosogenic theory.

Finally, some sources of evidence for genetic factors in stuttering are also evidence for environmental factors—in other words, genetic factors do not account for all stuttering. Genetic studies—described in Chapter 2—show that genes alone do not explain stuttering in all children, but rather some other factors—probably environmental—must also play a part (eg, Andrews et al., 1991; Fagnani et al., 2011; Felsenfeld et al., 2000; Ooki, 2005; Van Beijsterveldt et al., 2010). However, this research has not been able to identify with certainty which environmental factors might be involved.

In this chapter, I have divided developmental and environmental factors into separate sections, although they do not operate independently. For example, if a child is in the early stages of speech and language learning, it may be hard for them to keep up with a chattering, interrupting, and raucous household. Excess disfluencies and then perhaps stuttering may appear because of this interaction pattern. Every child and every family are different, of course. Thus, an evaluation needs to explore recent changes in each child's developmental level and the challenges of their environment.

DEVELOPMENTAL FACTORS

My view of how developmental factors affect children's fluency assumes that there is in the growing child **a competition for neural resources**. That is, the brain must divvy up its resources in coping with the "great blooming, buzzing confusion" (James, 1890) of the sounds, sights, and feelings of childhood. Like a computer, the brain can work on several things at once—but as the brain nears its maximum capacity, the more tasks it performs simultaneously, the more slowly and less efficiently it does each one—or at least does some of them. For humans, there are ways in which multiple things can be done simultaneously. If the tasks are dissimilar, such as driving a car and talking about cool stuff to buy, there is less interference between them. On the other hand, if the tasks are similar, such as using one hand to rub your stomach while using the other to pat your head, there is more interference between them (Kinsbourne & Hicks, 1978). The problem of shared resources is more acute in children because their immature nervous systems have less processing capacity to draw on (Hiscock & Kinsbourne, 1977, 1980). Some children are especially at risk for straining their developing resources. For example, their speech and language skills may be delayed, yet they have to compete in a highly verbal environment. Or, their language development may surge ahead of their speech motor control skills, giving them much to say, but limited capacity to say it rapidly and fluently. It is as though they were trying to herd a dozen cats through a small door, in a hurry, resulting in a catastrophe. Children with some uneven development across different skills may become excessively disfluent as other developmental demands—for example, language growth may compete with their ability to coordinate the complex movements of rapid, articulate speech. As you'll see later in this chapter, research has been carried out to quantify the extent to which differential maturation of components related to speech and language production is characteristic of children who stutter.

Here is an example of the competition between burgeoning language and slower motor development. Several years ago, I evaluated a 4-year-old girl whose uncle and grandmother stuttered. Her parents were concerned because she had been repeating words and sounds excessively for a year and a half, sometimes up to 20 times per instance. However, her language development was well above average; she began to talk with single words at 9 months and to produce sentences intelligibly at 12 months. In contrast, her motor development was somewhat slower; she had not walked until 18 months. I think it is possible that her disfluencies emerged as a result of a high proportion of her cerebral and other neural resources being used to formulate and express language while her capacities for motor activities, including fluent speech, were less mature. In other words, a disparity between language facility and motor speech ability may have been an important contributor to the emergence of stuttering for this child.

To appreciate how many skills and abilities the child is developing at the same time, look carefully at Figure 4.2. This chart covers only social, motor, and language domains, but it is clear that children have to master many different abilities simultaneously. If a child's development is slower in one or more areas (ie, dyssynchronous), their road to maturity may be steep at times.

The question of dyssynchronous development is an important one, because if it involves domains relevant to producing fluent speech, dyssynchrony may be a contributing factor in stuttering. To understand dyssynchrony, imagine trying to prepare a huge dinner, but having trouble getting all the parts of the meal ready at the same time. The string beans may be done, but the roast beef may be only half cooked. Another example is a tricycle factory (Fig. 4.3) that sometimes malfunctions because some parts of the tricycle are ready to be assembled when other parts are delayed. If the team preparing the wheels is much slower than the team making the frames, delays will result. Extra resources will be suddenly needed by the wheel team to resolve the problem, taking away resources from other teams, making the factory go into momentary disarray (ie, stuttering).

So, let us look at some of the domains of development and how they might contribute to the onset of stuttering.

Physical and Motor Development

In my clinical experience, children at risk for stuttering may sometimes show an increase in disfluencies or the onset of stuttering when great strides in physical growth are made. Motor development, specifically speech motor control, may be delayed in children who stutter, particularly in children who persist in stuttering (eg, Spencer & Weber-Fox, 2014).

Demands of Physical and Motor Development

The mother of a 3-year-old child who recently began to stutter told me "Whenever he has a spurt of physical growth, his stuttering seems to increase." Why would this be? Between ages 1 and 6 years, children grow by leaps and bounds. Their bodies get bigger. Their nervous systems form new pathways and new connections. Their perceptual and motor skills improve with maturation and practice. This intensive period of growth is a two-edged sword for children predisposed to stuttering. Neurological maturation may provide more neuronal resources that support fluency, but it also spurs development of other motor behaviors that may compete with fluency. An example of such competition is the common observation that children usually learn to walk first or

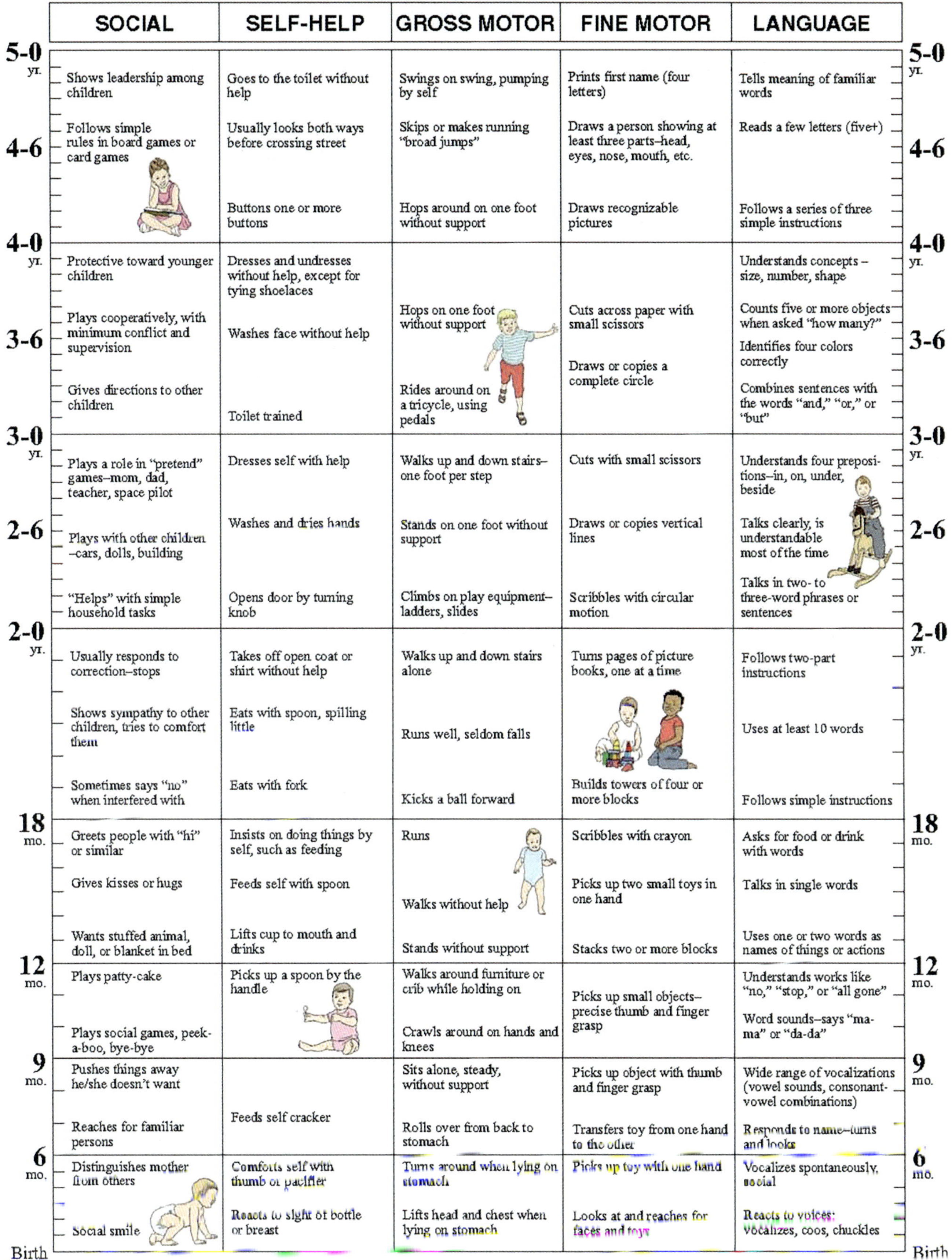

Age	SOCIAL	SELF-HELP	GROSS MOTOR	FINE MOTOR	LANGUAGE
4-0 to 5-0 yr. (4-6)	Shows leadership among children Follows simple rules in board games or card games	Goes to the toilet without help Usually looks both ways before crossing street Buttons one or more buttons	Swings on swing, pumping by self Skips or makes running "broad jumps" Hops around on one foot without support	Prints first name (four letters) Draws a person showing at least three parts–head, eyes, nose, mouth, etc. Draws recognizable pictures	Tells meaning of familiar words Reads a few letters (five+) Follows a series of three simple instructions
3-0 to 4-0 yr. (3-6)	Protective toward younger children Plays cooperatively, with minimum conflict and supervision Gives directions to other children	Dresses and undresses without help, except for tying shoelaces Washes face without help Toilet trained	Hops on one foot without support Rides around on a tricycle, using pedals	Cuts across paper with small scissors Draws or copies a complete circle	Understands concepts – size, number, shape Counts five or more objects when asked "how many?" Identifies four colors correctly Combines sentences with the words "and," "or," or "but"
2-0 to 3-0 yr. (2-6)	Plays a role in "pretend" games–mom, dad, teacher, space pilot Plays with other children –cars, dolls, building "Helps" with simple household tasks	Dresses self with help Washes and dries hands Opens door by turning knob	Walks up and down stairs– one foot per step Stands on one foot without support Climbs on play equipment– ladders, slides	Cuts with small scissors Draws or copies vertical lines Scribbles with circular motion	Understands four prepositions–in, on, under, beside Talks clearly, is understandable most of the time Talks in two- to three-word phrases or sentences
18 mo. to 2-0 yr.	Usually responds to correction–stops Shows sympathy to other children, tries to comfort them Sometimes says "no" when interfered with	Takes off open coat or shirt without help Eats with spoon, spilling little Eats with fork	Walks up and down stairs alone Runs well, seldom falls Kicks a ball forward	Turns pages of picture books, one at a time Builds towers of four or more blocks	Follows two-part instructions Uses at least 10 words Follows simple instructions
12 mo. to 18 mo.	Greets people with "hi" or similar Gives kisses or hugs Wants stuffed animal, doll, or blanket in bed	Insists on doing things by self, such as feeding Feeds self with spoon Lifts cup to mouth and drinks	Runs Walks without help Stands without support	Scribbles with crayon Picks up two small toys in one hand Stacks two or more blocks	Asks for food or drink with words Talks in single words Uses one or two words as names of things or actions
9 mo. to 12 mo.	Plays patty-cake Plays social games, peek-a-boo, bye-bye	Picks up a spoon by the handle	Walks around furniture or crib while holding on Crawls around on hands and knees	Picks up small objects– precise thumb and finger grasp	Understands works like "no," "stop," or "all gone" Word sounds–says "ma-ma" or "da-da"
6 mo. to 9 mo.	Pushes things away he/she doesn't want Reaches for familiar persons	Feeds self cracker	Sits alone, steady, without support Rolls over from back to stomach	Picks up object with thumb and finger grasp Transfers toy from one hand to the other	Wide range of vocalizations (vowel sounds, consonant-vowel combinations) Responds to name–turns and looks
Birth to 6 mo.	Distinguishes mother from others Social smile	Comforts self with thumb or pacifier Reacts to sight of bottle or breast	Turns around when lying on stomach Lifts head and chest when lying on stomach	Picks up toy with one hand Looks at and reaches for faces and toys	Vocalizes spontaneously, social Reacts to voices; vocalizes, coos, chuckles

Figure 4.2 Child development in the first 5 years. (Courtesy of Harold Ireton, Ph.D.)

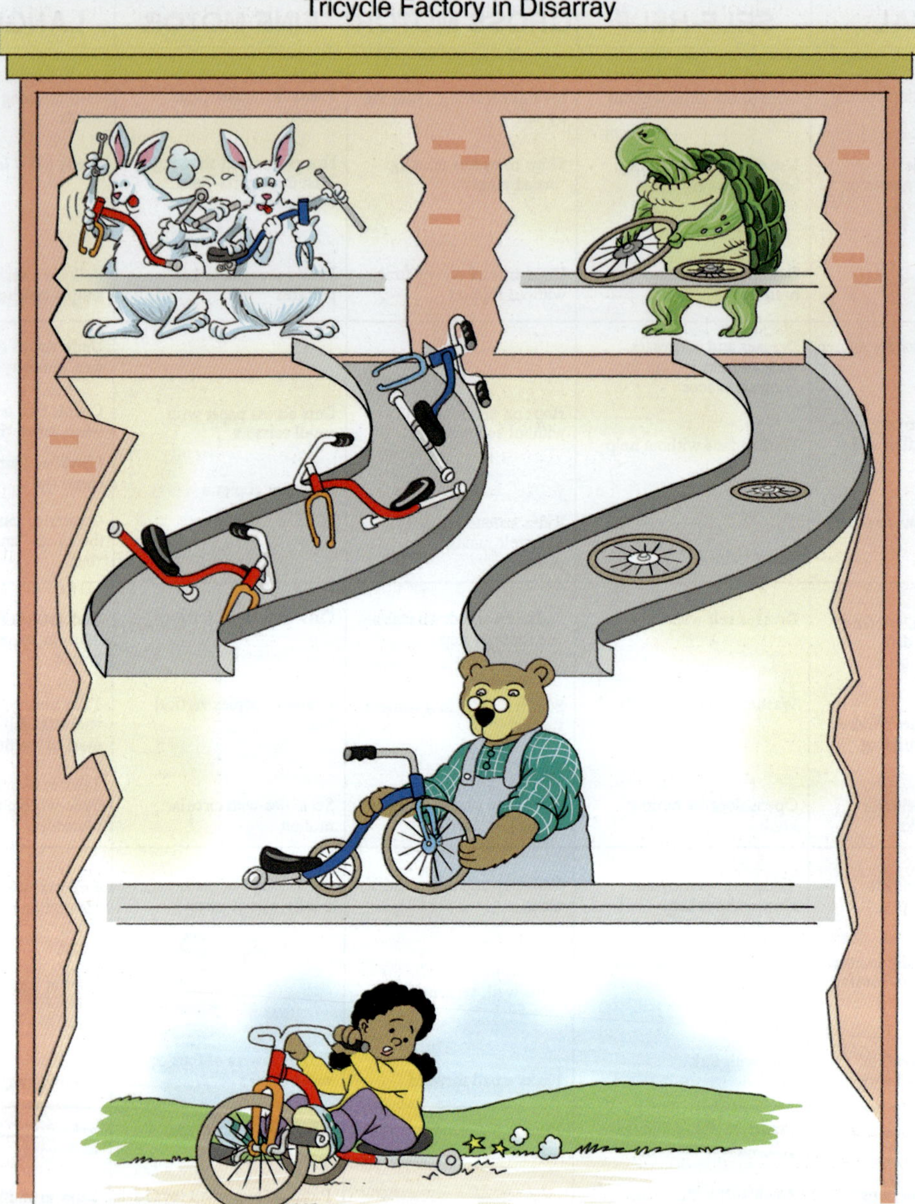

Figure 4.3 A tricycle factory in disarray and using extra resources.

talk first, but not both at the same time. For example, Netsell (1981, p. 25) said of this trade-off, "The practice of walking or talking seems sufficient to 'tie up' all the available sensorimotor circuitry because the toddler seldom, if ever, undertakes both activities at once." Likewise, Berk (1991, p. 194), in his text on child development, suggested "when infants forge ahead in spoken language, they seem to temporarily postpone mastery of new motor skills or vice versa." Other possible evidence for competition between cognition and motor control (Beurskens et al., 2014) also suggests that if one domain is heavily engaged, the other domain may suffer deficits. This argues for the possibility that rapid physical and motor development may interfere with the cognitive resources needed for fluency. In the chapter on theoretical perspectives on stuttering, I will introduce the "capacities and demands" view of stuttering, which may be a useful framework for understanding the competition for resources that I have been discussing.

Research is never simple. In some cases, it can be downright confusing. A very different perspective from the one described in the preceding paragraph has been presented by Walle and Campos (2014), who found that in 44 infants between ages 10 month to 13.5 months (assessed every 2 weeks), *learning to walk* was associated with a significant *increase in receptive and expressive language*. Thus, the supposed "competition for neural resources" that suggests learning to walk interferes with learning to talk may not be as simple as once thought. Perhaps learning to walk stimulates cognitive aspects of language development, such as growth of vocabulary, but competes with motor aspects of talking, such as fluency.

Another possible challenge to speech motor control posed by physical development in children is rapid change in the vocal tract between ages 2 and 5 years. During this time, structures in a child's head, neck, and torso undergo their most accelerated growth; moreover, different structures grow at different rates (Kent & Vorperian, 1995, 2007). As children's speaking mechanisms change, the shape, size, and biomechanical properties of muscles and bones are different one day to the next. Despite that, children continue to produce intelligible speech. Callan et al. (2000) hypothesized that children maintain a stable speech output in the face of daily changes in their speech structures by using feedback to continuously update the motor commands they send to their muscles to produce specific sounds. What their brains told their muscles to do yesterday must be adapted to the new size, shape, and biomechanical properties of the vocal tract today. Auditory feedback, integrated with proprioceptive and other muscle feedback, helps children discover errors in their motor commands and adjust the commands to the new dimensions of the vocal structures.

You can see from these demands of speech motor development just described that the preschool child's brain is occupied with a multitude of tasks to keep up with their developing speech mechanism. No wonder that children with a fragile speech motor system—children predisposed to stutter—will develop repetitions and prolongations as they juggle the demands of growing, changing sensorimotor mechanisms, the need to speak ever faster, and the ability to employ increasingly more complex language.

Delays in Motor Development

As I have just suggested, the many competing demands of normal development stress typical children, but children who begin to stutter may be extra stressed because the inherent weaknesses of their speech production systems. As you will remember from Chapter 2, there is much evidence for motor delays in children who stutter. Brain imaging studies (eg, Chang et al., 2015; Choo et al., 2016; Çykowski et al., 2010; Sommer et al., 2002) suggest that, in children who stutter, the neurological structures, pathways, and networks used to produce sounds and words may be inefficient (less well myelinated, where myelin provides a form of insulation that carries signals more efficiently). Moreover, these neural pathways and networks are crucial in helping the child speak accurately as their system changes in development. When children with compromised neural pathways are ready to speak and need quick access to the stored plans for production, this access may be slow in coming, and stuttering may result.

Problems in neural networks related to speech production have been detected using various measures of motor coordination or movement stability. A good review of studies of motor coordination in people who stutter can be found in Chapters 6 and 7 (devoted to central neurological findings and to motor, sensory, and metabolic function) of Bloodstein et al. (2021). Whereas earlier studies were inconclusive in their search for deficits in speech motor control, more recent studies, many of which have been conducted at Purdue University, have provided stronger evidence that children who stutter have a delay in development of motor control. As mentioned in the section on nonspeech motor control in the Chapter 3, Olander et al. (2010) at Purdue demonstrated a deficit in motor timing during a rhythmic clapping task in a large subgroup of preschool children who stutter. When tested on nonsense words produced fluently in a later study (Smith et al., 2012), preschool children who stuttered showed greater variability (similar to that of younger children) in articulator movement than did the control children. Thus their mechanisms are less stable.

Also at Purdue, MacPherson and Smith (2013) assessed speech motor variability when children who stutter speak fluently. They found that many, but not all, of the stuttering children had greater variability (less stability) than their nonstuttering peers in articulator movements even during fluent speech. The Purdue group then followed these children to see if there were differences in measures of speech-motor abilities over the time span in which some of them recovered and some didn't. For example, Spencer and Weber-Fox (2014) found that tests of accuracy of phonological production and nonword production showed a greater deficit in those children who persisted in stuttering than those who did not. A year later, similar conclusions about persistent stuttering were published by researchers at the University of Illinois (Ambrose et al., 2015). They followed a large cohort of 58 children who stuttered. They observed the children from near the onset of their stuttering to several years later when many had recovered. Their findings in motor development supported the conclusions of Spencer and Weber-Fox described above. Specifically, they demonstrated that, when motor performance was measured acoustically, children who persisted in stuttering tended to show more immature speech motor development for their age compared to both the children who recovered and those who had never stuttered.

Immature speech motor development may be related to poorer speech auditory-motor learning. This possibility was suggested by the finding by Kim et al. (2020) who found that children who stutter have deficits in both auditory-motor and visuomotor learning compared to peers, especially in younger children compared to older children who stuttered. Such a deficit in auditory-motor learning would make it difficult for these children to develop accurate internal models for speech production and adapt them as their speech mechanisms grow over time. In the domain of nonspeech motor ability, Tendera et al. (2020) found that motor sequencing of finger movement was poorer in children who stuttered compared to children who recovered from stuttering and children who never stuttered. Finger movement motor sequencing probably depends on the same motor resources used to sequence the rapid speech gestures required for fluent speech, suggesting once again that stuttering may be related to an overall motor problem rather than one confined to speech motor ability.

Absolute delays in development may not be as important in stuttering as differences in the rate of development among components. Building on previous research (Anderson et al., 2005) that compared the relative maturation of different components of the speech-motor-language system, Choo et al. (2016) compared children who stuttered with children who didn't on many aspects of performance. At the same time, they also compared white matter tract density of the two groups using diffusion tensor imaging (a type of magnetic resonance imaging—to detail tissue structure using random motion of water molecules). These researchers found more dissociations (uneven abilities) in the development of motor performance in children who stuttered compared to typical children. In fact, they found delays and uneven development in speech and language areas as well as motor performance. This was more pronounced in boys and all left-handed children who stuttered. These delays and dissociations in motor development were also reflected in their brain imaging data suggesting less dense white matter tracts (in the children who stuttered compared with those who didn't) in areas supporting speech motor and auditory-motor development.

Summary of the Effects of Physical and Motor Development on Fluency

The demands of motor development on neural resources affect even children who are developing typically. They may have to postpone learning complex levels of phonology, morphology, syntax, and semantics as they master walking, climbing, hopping, and kicking a ball. Children with compromised speech motor development (including children who stutter) may be affected even more. This possibility is important to note because recent accumulations of evidence suggest that children who stutter demonstrate motor delays and that these delays appear to be greater in children who persist in stuttering rather than those who recover. Additionally, research suggests greater dissociations (unevenness of abilities) in the relative development of motor abilities and language abilities in children who stutter compared to those who don't. Such dissociations may contribute to the onset or persistence of stuttering because of the strain this may put on neural resources (Anderson et al., 2005; Coulter et al., 2009).

Speech and Language Development

Language Learning and the Onset of Stuttering

In Chapter 3, I made the point that language growth may affect fluency because individuals who stutter may have a fragile speech production system that would be stressed by the increasing demands of producing more and more complex language as the child grows. I also suggested that typically developing children may also have increasing disfluencies because of the heavy load that language learning puts on neural resources. However, the relationship between language development and fluency is not always simple and linear (Bloodstein et al., 2021). In this section, I want to expand on this idea that early language learning can be a stress frequently associated with the onset of stuttering.

A quick review of some of the facts of typical language development from single words, which are usually produced about age one, through the preschool years may be helpful, given that this is the time period in which stuttering typically starts. Between ages 1 and 2, children typically move from predominantly one-word to two-word utterances and develop a vocabulary of about 50 words. Between the ages of 2 and 3, a child's vocabulary often jumps from about 50 to well over 500 words; in fact, toward the end of this year, five to seven new words may be learned each day (Studdert-Kennedy, 1987). As the child's utterances increase in length and complexity, intonation becomes more adultlike (Branigan, 1979; Veneziano, 2013). Thus, across this time period, the child's speech graduates from a simple "syllable-timed" prosody for single words to complex prosodic rhythms that span multiple words and begin to reflect "stress-timing," in which stressed syllables, rather than individual syllables appear at regular intervals (Allen & Hawkins, 1980; Peppé & Wells, 2014).

As children are implementing these changes in their speech, they are also upgrading their language storage system. At first, you can think of their "shelves" as stocked with whole words in the form of articulatory routines or gestural patterns. Then, as the number of words increase, children change strategies and begin to stock, not whole words, but segments that can be combined in various ways to form a multitude of words (Kent, 1985; Nittrouer et al., 1989; Sternberger, 1982; Tilsen, 2016). During these same preschool years, children also progressively learn active, negative, and passive constructions as well as present, future, and past tenses. Further, they increase the length and linguistic complexity of their sentences, along with the rate at which they are spoken, to match the rates and rhythms of their families', with whom they have a growing urge to communicate (Prelock & Hutchins, 2019; Velleman, 2015).

This huge array of language and speech production tasks is a challenge even to the fluency of nonstuttering children. Normal disfluencies of children also increase from ages 2 to 4, peaking when they tackle the task of producing long, complex sentences (Ito, 1986). It is not surprising, then, that children begin stuttering during this same period.

Many clinician-researchers have speculated on the connection between language learning and stuttering. Dalton and Hardcastle (1977) commented that "it is tempting to see the ever-increasing demands on linguistic competence and articulatory proficiency as major factors in the onset of some disfluency" (p. 69). Sheehan (1975) said, "The age of onset of stuttering is consistently related to certain stages in the developmental sequence. Most notably, the 'period of resonance,' or high readiness in language learning...is also the period during which stuttering develops and flourishes" (p. 142). Andrews et al. (1983) pointed to the demands placed on speech by rapidly developing language, noting that "stuttering [has] a maximal frequency of onset at a time when an explosive growth in language ability outstrips a still-immature speech-motor apparatus" (p. 239).

Several studies have examined difficulties in language acquisition in conjunction with other variables such as vulnerable temperament to show that children who stutter are more likely to have problems in both areas (Conture & Walden, 2012; Singer et al., 2019). Kefalionos et al. (2017), however, found that children who successfully acquired strong language skills were more likely to recover from stuttering, but that there was no relationship between recovery and vulnerable temperament. In another study of language development and stuttering, Choo et al. (2016) tested 66 children who stuttered and 53 who did not, examining multiple variables in the children between ages 3 and 10 and found many "dissociations" of cognitive, language, and motor development (unequal development in some areas compared to others) to be associated with white matter neuroanatomical deficits. These studies gave support to the hypothesis that problems with language acquisition are associated with the onset or persistence of stuttering.

Many, but not all, studies of children have found that greater length and complexity of language are associated with more stuttering. This is a developmental factor because stuttering may first appear when children use longer and more complex utterances as they mature. For example, research on natural conversational speech of children who stutter has shown that more complex utterances contain more stuttering (Brundage & Bernstein Ratner, 1989; Gaines et al., 1991; Logan & Conture, 1995; Yaruss, 1999). However, Hollister et al. (2017) found that as children who stutter increased their linguistic abilities, they did *not* have more disfluencies in longer and more complex utterances compared to shorter and simpler utterance. This finding may have been the result of the children having fairly advanced linguistic abilities by the time that disfluencies in longer and more complex were assessed. These children at this point may not have had their neural resources stressed by the increased linguistic demands.

Some research suggests that utterance length may have a greater effect on stuttering than does complexity (Hollister et al., 2017; Logan & Conture, 1995; Wilkenfeld & Curlee, 1997; Yaruss, 1999). Experimental studies, in which children were asked to produce both more and less complex utterances, show that both children who stutter (Bernstein Ratner & Sih, 1987; Stocker & Usprich, 1976) and fluent children (Gordon et al., 1986; Haynes & Hood, 1978; Pearl & Bernthal, 1980; Yaruss et al., 1999) increase their disfluencies (stuttering and typical disfluencies) as **language complexity** is increased. On a similar topic, a study of articulatory coordination variability in both typically developing children and children who stuttered indicated that both groups demonstrated more variability—thus, more tendency toward discoordination—for longer sentences (MacPherson & Smith, 2013). This suggests that as both typically developing and stuttering children use longer utterance as their language matures, articulatory coordination may become less stable, giving rise to increased normal disfluency as well as stuttering. Unfortunately, there is little longitudinal research that bears directly on the question of how and when emerging language is associated with stuttering. Some research, however, has looked longitudinally at the issue of typical disfluencies and language development (Colburn & Mysak, 1982a, 1982b; Wejnen, 1990).

One of the few studies of the appearance of disfluencies in individual children over time was Norma Colburn's analysis of the disfluencies of four nonstuttering children using data originally gathered by Bloom (1970) for her work on normal language development. Publications of Colburn's analysis (Colburn & Mysak, 1982a, 1982b) suggested that these children's normal disfluencies did not emerge when they first learned a new language construction but appeared as they began to master a new construction and started using it regularly. Explanations suggested for this result include the possibility that a child who has learned, but not completely automatized, the use of a new construction allocates fewer resources than are necessary for its production (Kent & Perkins, 1984) or the possibility that as a child masters the new construction they produce it at an increased rate, thereby straining capacity (Starkweather, 1987).

A single-case study by Wijnen (1990) explored the relationship between syntax acquisition and normal disfluencies. Weekly speech samples were obtained from a boy from age 2 years, 4 months to 2 years, and 11 months. The number of repetitions, revisions, and incomplete phrases was assessed in relation to the length and complexity of utterances. It was reported that disfluencies were randomly distributed initially but eventually clustered on function words and sentence-initial words and then declined. Wijnen concluded that the eventual decline in the child's disfluencies was associated with his mastery of a routine type of sentence (pronoun + verb + some other word) and that the early stages of learning this routine involved so much of his processing capacity that speech production was short-changed and disfluencies resulted. This preliminary study needs to be followed up with many more cases to test the hypothesis that the process of making sentence productions more automatic through routinization of several sentence types is at least initially is associated to increases in typical disfluency.

What is happening in the brain to precipitate stuttering during this speech and language growth spurt? You will remember from Chapter 2 that brain imaging studies of children who stutter have shown some anomalous patterns of activity during speech. For example, there are abnormally high levels of activity in some regions of the right hemisphere and abnormally low levels in some areas of the left—the hemisphere typically used for speech and language. In addition, recent findings with children who stutter suggest that white matter tracts connecting areas of the brain used for integration of articulator planning, sensory feedback, and motor execution are compromised (eg, Chang & Guenther, 2020; Chang et al., 2008, 2015). Thus, planning and production of speech and language may have to rely on less robust neural pathways and compromised gray matter areas that may be slow or inefficient. However, despite these inadequacies, the demands are growing ever greater as a child attempts longer, faster, and more complex sentences. Tasks using different neural networks for segment selection, grammatical formulation, and prosodic planning must be orchestrated precisely so that each element is in place at the proper time for utterances to be produced and produced fluently. If some components are ready but others are delayed, initial sounds or syllables may be repeated, prolonged, or even blocked, waiting for all the elements of each sentence to be put together in the brain.

Before we leave the topic of language development and the onset of stuttering, I would like to bring up the view that language development may, in some cases, decrease stuttering. A longitudinal study by Hollister et al. (2017) examined the language development and disfluencies of three groups of children: typically developing children, stuttering children who would recover, and stuttering children who would persist in stuttering. Their findings indicated that of the three groups, only the children who would recover had fewer disfluencies as their mastery of grammar and syntax increased (independent of age). This suggests that as the recovering children were more easily able to manage the demands of producing longer sentences, their speech production systems were not as frequently overloaded to the point of disfluency.

Delayed and Deviant Language Development

For an example of a child whose language was delayed and then developed stuttering, watch the video of David Wilkins' mother in which she describes the onset of her son's stuttering. Go to *Lippincott Connect* and watch "A Mother's Experience with Her Child's Stuttering."

Because available evidence suggests that stuttering frequently arises from constitutional differences (eg, inheritance or congenital injury), it is natural to wonder whether the brain anomalies that give rise to stuttering also delay overall language development as well. It's possible that delays in language development could co-occur with stuttering, but not cause it. On the other hand, language delays could cause children to become frustrated with their difficulty expressing themselves, thereby instigating fears about speaking, which could lead to stuttering. For a description of this perspective, see the Communicative Failure and Anticipatory Struggle Theory in Chapter 6—Theories About Stuttering. For a more detailed explanation of this theory, read the chapter on "Theories and Models of Stuttering" in *A Handbook on Stuttering* (Bloodstein & Ratner, 2021). In support of this theory is a study many years ago indicated that language-delayed children have a significant amount stuttering-like disfluencies when they are given language therapy—significantly more stuttering-like disfluencies than matched language-delayed children not in therapy and more than matched typically developing children (Merits-Patterson & Reed, 1981). This suggests that the combination of language delay and pressure to produce language and ensuing frustration may generate signs of stuttering.

What is the evidence for language delays in children who stutter? Some published studies have found that language delays or difficulties are more common among children who stutter than those who don't, but the findings are neither simple nor clear-cut, and their implications are unclear. Unfortunately, this is often the nature of research, but persistence in trying to answer this question will eventually pay off. After surveying many studies of language abilities in children who stutter, Nippold (2012, 2019) concluded that there are no consistently demonstrated differences in language capability in children who stutter compared to those who don't and that language deficits are not associated with stuttering onset, nor its persistence. Supporting this position, Watts et al. (2014) examined language abilities in a large community sample of children ages 2 to 5 (181 children stuttered; 1,438 did not). They found that the children who stuttered scored higher on all the language measures. It should be noted that many of the younger children who stuttered may have later grown out of stuttering, so the sample is probably a mix of recovered and persistent children who stuttered. In contrast to these and Nippold's findings, research groups in Illinois and Wisconsin (Ambrose et al., 2015) over a period of several years compared 58 children who stuttered (ages 2-4) with 40 who did not over a period of several years. By the end of the study, the children who stuttered at the first visit could be classified as Persistent ($n = 19$) or Recovered ($n = 39$). Analysis of standardized language testing indicated that the Persistent group's performance was significantly poorer than those of either the Recovered or the Control group on the first tests of language, although it was within the normal range. The Recovered group's performance was similar to that of the Controls on all language tests. In summary, as a single group, children who stutter appear to have similar language skills compared to fluent children. However, when the stuttering children were subdivided into those who persisted in stuttering and those who recovered, the persistent stuttering children scored slightly below those who recovered in measures of language. This finding could be affected by the possibility that the persistent stuttering children could have been more severe at the first assessment making them more reluctant to speak or not as experienced in speaking and thus appear to make them have slightly less developed language.

A number of researchers have approached the language question in a slightly different way—examining the relative advancement of different subcomponents (Anderson et al., 2005; Choo et al., 2016). A possible reason for the conflicting findings about language delay in children who stutter may be due to considerable variability in the overall levels and patterns of language skills in children who stutter. Some may have above-average ability in one area of language but average in another. Some may have below-average ability in one area but average in another. Such variable patterns could result in group averages that are within the typical range but with many individual cases in which there is a disparity in the child's abilities in subcomponents of language, as it is usually assessed. In fact, research has suggested that this very phenomenon—unequal rates of maturation of different abilities required speech and language production—may be an important contributor to stuttering. Neuropsychologists studying neurological patients developed a statistical procedure to identify when "dissociations" (unequal abilities in subcomponents) were truly occurring at rates that seem unlikely to be due to chance (Bates et al., 2003). Anderson et al. (2005) used this statistical procedure to test for dissociations among speech and language skills in 45 children who stuttered and 45 who did not. They found that the group of children who stuttered had generally poorer speech and language skills but were still within the normal range. However, three times as many children who stuttered had dissociations among speech and language skills than those who did not stutter. The authors hypothesized that these dissociations may lead to stuttering because neural resources may be suddenly taken away from fluent speech production to resolve the mismatch between the readiness of some components compared to others, to be produced.

The work of Choo et al. (2016), mentioned earlier in regard to motor development, revealed more dissociations among language areas in children who stuttered compared to typically developing children and less white matter coherence in "left dorsal language pathways" that support these language areas. This disparity in dissociations was particularly pronounced among boys who stuttered compared to girls and in left- compared to right-handed children who stuttered.

Summary of the Effect of Speech and Language Development on Fluency

The onset of stuttering, commonly between ages 2 and 5, is the period when children are most intensively learning to understand and produce language. It has been suggested that the heavy and fluctuating load placed on neural resources during language learning puts an extra and unpredictable strain on the child's speech production system so that stuttering may come and go during this period—particularly if the child's speech production system is less robust, or even fragile, compared to those of children who do not stutter.

Research studies are conflicted about whether children who stutter have language delays compared to children who do not. There may be a subgroup of children whose language, while within the normal range, is somewhat delayed. These children may be those whose stuttering persists.

Some components of speech and language may be developing more slowly than other components in some children who stutter. This dyssynchrony in development may put an extra strain on the speech production system and result in stuttering. In these children, the white matter nerve tracts supporting language also appear to be developing more slowly or abnormally.

Cognitive Development

I use the phrase "cognitive development" to refer to the growth of executive function, perception, attention, and working memory that play roles in spoken language. These abilities can be considered separate from spoken language because they are also involved in many other kinds of learning and problem-solving but necessarily intertwined with language as well, given the importance of these variables in speaking and listening. Even though I will be discussing changes in cognition as the child matures, I will begin with a brief summary of cognitive deficits that have been identified in individuals who stutter. After all, whether it's plants or people, deficits at birth will affect development. Premature babies will not reach developmental milestones at the same time as a full-term baby. Similarly, children who stutter and who have problems in cognition can be expected to experience more stress as their language surges forward.

An excellent review of cognition in stuttering is provided in Chapter 10 ("Cognitive and Linguistic Abilities") in Bloodstein et al. (2021). Those authors conclude that although there are many conflicts among research findings about the cognitive abilities of children and adults who stutter, overall the evidence suggests that, as a group, individuals who stutter show weaknesses in such cognitive areas as overall executive function (eg, Anderson & Ofoe, 2019; Doneva, 2019, Ntourou et al., 2018), including attention and inhibition, working memory, and cognitive flexibility. These skills contribute to an individual's abilities to process language and regulate emotion—abilities that may undermine speech production.

Cognitive development may affect stuttering in two ways. First, growth spurts in some but not all aspects of cognitive development may trigger the onset of stuttering or may exacerbate it. In this view, competition for neural resources as the child tries to compensate for areas of deficit may deprive the child of resources needed for fluent speech. Second, as a child who stutters develops more advanced cognitive abilities, they are more likely to become aware of and even self-conscious about their stuttering. This embarrassment could then be exacerbated by the child's being unable to ignore fearful stimuli and inhibit emotions that result, or both, thereby triggering threat- or fear-based behaviors that interfere with fluency.

Cognitive Development Related to the Onset and Fluctuation of Stuttering

Parents frequently report that the onset of their child's stuttering occurred under the most commonplace circumstances, when there are no unusual stresses in the household and no apparent increases in the child's anxiety. The same commonplace circumstances are also frequently present when there are sudden changes in the ongoing stuttering of a preschool child. Suddenly, the child's stuttering is worse, and just as suddenly, it's better. One factor that may not be obvious to the parent but nonetheless may be an influence on stuttering is the child's cognitive growth. Earlier in this chapter, I suggested that aspects of physical development may affect stuttering; for example, learning to walk may make great demands on sensorimotor abilities, making fewer resources available for fluency. Now, I am proposing that learning to think, remember, problem-solve, and plan may make great demands on neural resources, leaving fewer resources available for rapidly producing fluently spoken language.

This argument has been made before. Lindsay (1989) pointed out that during Jean Piaget's "preoperational period" of childhood development from 2 to 6 years, a child goes through a series of transitions in which new cognitive learning must be assimilated and consolidated with existing knowledge. These transitions are times when a child's linguistic and cognitive systems are temporarily unstable before new concepts are mastered. As a consequence, children's speech and language production during this period of adjustment may be vulnerable to disfluencies.

Even in children with stable, age-appropriate cognitive function, high cognitive demands in their communicative environments may make stuttering temporarily worse (Starkweather, 1987). Consider, for example, how "on the spot" a 4-year-old child feels when asked to play "telephone" with a group of people. In this parlor game, participants sit in a circle, and one person starts by whispering a complex message to the person next to them. The last person to receive the message has to say aloud what they heard. The fun comes from the fact that the whispered message gets hilariously distorted in its journey around the circle. The agony comes from the fact a child who stutters has to remember what they heard, consider whether to alter it, then either say it to the next person or, sometimes, if they are the last person, say it aloud to the whole circle. Even decades later, this experience still haunts me.

A number of studies suggest that the incidence of stuttering is unusually high in individuals who have cognitive impairments, such as those with a developmental disability, especially Down syndrome (Kent & Vorperian, 2013; Van Borsel et al., 2006; Van Riper, 1982a). An explanation has been suggested by Starkweather (1987) based on the observation that developmentally delayed individuals are generally slower in their overall acquisition of speech and language. Their extended period of acquisition may make them more vulnerable to speech breakdown because competition between language acquisition and motor speech production for limited neurological resources occurs over a relatively long period of time. Motor speech production itself may be stressed because there is evidence that individuals with Down syndrome often have deficits in motor speech skills (Kent & Vorperian, 2013).

Individuals who have had traumatic brain injury, which usually affects cognitive functions such as memory and attention, also have an increased risk for fluency disorders (Jokel et al., 2007; Strasberg et al., 2016; Theys et al., 2008). This may be because typically rapid and complex speech and language production depend on fully functioning perception, attention, working memory, and executive functions. When these processes are compromised, breakdowns in spoken language are likely to result. As an example, consider the effect of a faulty working memory on rapid retrieval of vocabulary or syntax. If some components of language are mistimed in relation to others, repetitions of words or syllables may result, just as an engine with an unsteady fuel supply will stop and start, stutteringly.

Yet another link between cognition and stuttering was found in a study by Yairi, Ambrose, Paden, et al. (1996) that indicated that poorer cognitive skills are associated with lack of ability to recover from stuttering. Of the study's 32 children who began to stutter, 12 continued to stutter for 36 months and perhaps longer. The two groups of stutterers—those who recovered and those who did not—were compared with a control group of nonstuttering children on an intelligence test—the Arthur Adaptation of the Leiter International Performance Test (Arthur, 1952). The group of children who continued to stutter scored significantly lower than the nonstuttering control group, although their mean score was not below the norm for the test. However, the children in the recovered group performed just like the control group. Thus, some abilities associated with cognition may be related to a neural resilience allowing recovery from stuttering. In other words, children with slightly higher cognitive functioning may have the extra resources needed to reorganize their speech and language processing, allowing them to develop a work-around for the problem that caused them to stutter.

The research by Choo et al. (2016) that I cited earlier in my discussion of disassociation among language areas assessed cognitive functioning in the group of children who stuttered and the group who did not. As with speech, language, and motor measures, the children who stuttered scored below the nonstuttering children on cognitive measures and exhibited dissociations among these areas. They also showed less dense white matter tracts in areas underlying all these skills and abilities.

Cognitive Development and Reactions to Stuttering

In the preceding section, I have suggested that children's cognitive development may influence the onset of stuttering—or momentary increases in stuttering—through competition for resources in the child's brain. Now, I would like to suggest that the role of cognitive development is also important in explaining how and when a child begins to form negative attitudes and beliefs about themselves and their speech. Between ages 3 and 4, children's cognitions mature enough so that they internalize the standards of behavior of those around them, including peers (Fagan, 2002). It is only at this point, according to Lewis (2000), that children can evaluate how they are performing in comparison to others and will experience the "self-conscious" emotions of embarrassment, shame, and guilt.

In regard to stuttering, once children who stutter compare their speech with others, they are likely to conclude that they are not doing as well and perhaps that they are doing something wrong. Some of the conclusions that children who stutter draw about their speech may come from other children's reactions to their speech. A study by Ezrati-Vinacour et al. (2001) is relevant here. These researchers looked at awareness of stuttering in typically developing children and found that some children were aware of stuttering in puppets at age 3, but most were not aware until age 5. Notably, most children at age 4 showed a preference for fluent speech, suggesting a negative evaluation of disfluent speech. Thus, peers of children who stutter may respond negatively to the speech of stuttering children at this age. In many children who stutter—particularly those who are more sensitive—this response from peers and others will cause them to feel embarrassed, ashamed, and will lead to avoidance and escape behaviors.

In two studies of preschoolers' attitudes toward other preschoolers who stuttered, Weidner, St. Louis, Burgess, and LeMasters (2015) and Weidner, St. Louis, Nakisci, and Ozdemir (2017) found that fluent preschoolers had negative attitudes about stuttering in their peers, but their regard for their peers who stuttered was positive. One of these studies was conducted in the United States and the other in Turkey, suggesting that negative attitudes toward stuttering itself is widespread. The authors suggest that education programs be developed to ensure that preschoolers understand how to appropriately respond to their peers' stuttering. Thus, it is probable that young children who stutter do experience negative responses to their stuttering, wherever they live.

A study by Boey et al. (2009) found that children as young as 2 years old appear to have some awareness of their own stuttering, although it is not clear that they are comparing their speech to other children. The signs of awareness of the youngest of these children were more in terms of being frustrated or angry, and it was not until they were older that they were showing some sadness about their speech, which may reflect comparison with other children.

The authors of a meta-analysis of 18 studies on the attitudes of children who stutter (Guttormsen et al., 2015) concluded that negative communication attitudes increase with age, in both preschoolers and in school-age children. It was suggested that this increase in negative attitudes may arise from more negative experiences with speech, including bullying, as children get older. This meta-analysis is a rich source of information for readers who want to delve deeper into communication attitudes, as well as emotional and behavioral reactions to stuttering.

Emotions such as embarrassment and shame that arise from the increasing cognitive maturity of children who stutter and their peers may play an important role in the discomfort children feel when they stutter, and thus, it may affect the persistence of the stuttering. The emotions that some children feel about their stuttering may be important factors that give rise to increases in tension, escape, and avoidance responses that may make stuttering a self-sustaining disorder and increasingly difficult to overcome. In my experience, most children who recover completely from stuttering with or without treatment are younger than 5, perhaps a significant age, given the evidence cited above about self- and peer awareness of stuttering.

Summary of the Effect of Cognitive Development on Fluency

The stresses of ongoing cognitive development may deplete the extra neural resources some children need to compensate for a vulnerable speech motor system. Stuttering may appear or worsen during this stress. Children who have cognitive limitations (or even slightly lower than typical cognitive abilities in some areas) may be more stressed during cognitive development as they try to compensate for these limitations. This also may precipitate or worsen stuttering. As children who stutter advance in cognitive development, they become more likely to be aware of their stuttering and may develop negative attitudes toward communication as a result.

Social and Emotional Development

In this section, I will discuss how children's development in the preschool years may be disrupted by social challenges and emotional stresses that may trigger or worsen stuttering. Evidence that children who stutter have more social and emotional problems than their nonstuttering peers comes from a cross-sectional study of children that used a large community sample (McAllister, 2016). The 18,818 children in McAllister's study who were tested with the Strengths and Difficulties Questionnaire (Goodman, 1997) with samples taken at 3, 5, and 11 years of age. All parents were asked if their child stuttered. A total of 537 children were identified as stuttering: 173 children at age 3, 194 at age 5, and 170 at age 11. Statistical analysis of the Strengths and Difficulties Questionnaire results indicated that at each of these ages, the children who stuttered showed more emotional and social problems than their nonstuttering peers. It is not clear if the problems result from stuttering or if the problems cause stuttering, or if it goes both ways. The following sections suggest how emotional and social problems may affect fluency.

Interference of Speech by Emotion

At some time in your life, you have probably experienced the effects of strong emotion on your speech. If you've been nervous when talking in front of an audience, your voice may have quavered or you may have been talking faster than you meant to but couldn't help it. When you get really worked up, like when you have to make a phone call in an emergency, rapid breathing and tension in your larynx can make it difficult to talk. The same sort of interference by emotion may be even more prevalent in early childhood, because a child's speech neural networks are immature, are not fully myelinated, and, therefore, may not be buffered from "crosstalk," or interference by the limbic (emotional) system structures and pathways involved in the regulation and expression of emotion (eg, Dolcos & McCarthy, 2006). Such interference may be even more likely among many children predisposed to stutter. Their slower maturing speech production system may not be optimally localized or adequately insulated from interference because of poorer myelinization of white matter tracts (Chang et al., 2015, 2017).

Moreover, their neural networks for speech may be closer to centers of emotion in the right hemisphere, a hypothesis I discussed in Chapter 3 in the section on emotion. Thus, when such children are emotionally aroused, fluency may suffer because neural signals for properly timed and sequenced muscle contractions may be interrupted or degraded from the excess activity resulting from emotion. I see evidence of this when I ask parents when their child first began to stutter. They frequently tell me that they noticed stuttering for the first time when their child was highly excited about something.

Excitement is commonly mentioned in the literature as a stimulus that elicits disfluency. Starkweather (1987) noted "all children speak more disfluently during periods of excitement." Davis (1940), who conducted one of the first studies of normal disfluency, reported that of the 10 situations in which children showed repetitions in their speech, "excitement over own activity," was when they most frequently repeated sounds and words. In a later study, Johnson et al. (1959) asked parents of children identified as stuttering to describe the situation in which they first observed their child's stuttering. They most often reported that the first appearance of stuttering occurred when the child was in a hurry to tell something or was in an excited state. Thus, both stuttering and normal disfluency seem to occur most often or noticeably during states of transitory emotional arousal.

More recent evidence of the relationship between heightened emotion and stuttering comes from a study by Ntourou et al. (2013) that examined emotional reactivity and emotional regulation in children who stutter. Among other things, they found that children who stuttered showed more negative emotion in an experimental task designed to disappoint them than children who didn't. There was also a tendency for children who stutter to show more stuttering while speaking when they were trying to regulate their negative emotions. In discussing their results, the authors concluded that "...present findings support the notion that emotional processes are associated with childhood stuttering and may possibly contribute to the difficulties that at least some CWS have establishing normally fluent speech" (p. 271). As to how emotions exert that influence, they suggest that "...children's emotional arousal may divert limited attentional resources from an already, for some CWS, vulnerable speech-language planning and production system (eg, Ntourou et al., 2011) and in turn contribute to disruptions in their speech fluency" (p. 270).

Having explored the connection between emotions and the occurrence of stuttering, let us now turn to children's progress through stages of social-emotional development and their influences on fluency.

Stages of Social and Emotional Development

As children grow, they pass through several stages of social and emotional development, some of which may provoke more stress than others. Rothbart (2011) describes the development of many personality features during childhood that result from the interaction between the child's inborn attributes such as temperament and the child's environment, including parents and peers. For example, the attachment between infants and their mothers can be a critical foundation for growing children's sense of security and their ability to learn to cope with stress and to regulate their own emotions. If the child experiences a mother who is able to meet the child's needs, to soothe the child when distressed, the child develops better coping skills and can more easily attach to others. If attachment to the mother is not secure, stresses will have a greater negative effect on the child. All this, of course, is greatly affected by the child's biological inheritance, including temperament. These interactions are described in detail by Rothbart (2011). Note that Rutter (1981) has shown that significant maternal attachment can be replaced by strong attachments to others both inside and outside the family. Thus, when a child's attachment to their mother is not effective, efforts should be made to establish attachment with another adult in the child's life.

Emotional Security

As a young child grows older, other members of the family besides the child's primary caregiver, usually the child's mother, play a role in social and emotional changes. Although a child's father and siblings comprise a wider support system, a child's resentment at having to share his mother's attention may elicit feelings of anger, aggression, and guilt. It seems possible that if such feelings are punished or ignored, transient disfluency or more severe stuttering may result in some children.

One of the more common provocations for feeling resentment is the birth of a sibling. I discuss the effect of a sibling's birth on fluency later in the section on environmental factors, but it warrants mentioning here, too, because a child's strong emotions may often reflect his developmental level as well as the environmental event that triggered the emotions. Theodore Lidz (1968, p. 246), a developmental psychiatrist with interests in speech and language, provided this example:

> *Psychoanalytically oriented play therapy with children also indicates that many of their forbidden wishes and ideas have relatively simple access to consciousness. A 6-year-old boy who started to stammer severely after a baby sister was born was watched playing with a family of dolls. He placed a baby doll in a crib next to the parent dolls' bed and then had a boy doll come and throw the baby to the floor, beat it, and throw it into a corner. He then put the boy doll into the crib. In a subsequent session, he had the father doll pummel the mother doll's abdomen, saying, "No, no!" At this point of childhood, even though certain unacceptable ideas cannot be talked about, they are still not definitely repressed.*

This vignette may seem out of date, but with many individuals who stutter the threat that triggers stuttering may be nonconscious, and psychological counseling or play therapy may help to reduce the threat and improve fluency. Many threats to feelings of security can create emotional stress that may disrupt the speech of children who are predisposed to stutter. As we will see in the section on treatment, we have found that therapy strategies that increase a child's sense of security and help them learn to speak more fluently will suffice for many children who begin stuttering under these emotional stresses.

Development of Self-Consciousness and Sensitivity

As we noted earlier in the section on cognitive development, the emergence of self-consciousness, which begins during the child's second year and gradually increases, may be another source of social and emotional stress. This reflects the child's growing awareness of how they are performing relative to adult expectations. Although this process is not thoroughly understood, Kagan (1981) presents an interesting description of it in his book, *The Second Year*. In a relevant example, Kagan proposes that the self-corrections a child makes in his speech are evidence of this self-awareness. Taking this further, we can surmise that increased self-awareness in a child who is excessively disfluent might lead to self-corrections and stoppages that only worsen the problem.

In Chapter 3, in a section on temperament, I discussed the hypothesis that people who stutter, as a group, may have unusually sensitive temperaments. Research on temperament in nonstuttering children, especially the longitudinal studies of Calkins and Fox (1994) and Kagan and Snidman (1991), indicates that the social-emotional traits of fearfulness and withdrawal that accompany more sensitive temperaments can change over the course of a child's preschool years. Some children become better able to regulate their temperamental tendencies, but others remain hostage to their temperaments. Such individual adaptations may be crucial in determining which children who begin to stutter will continue to do so and which will stop. In addition, it has been reported (Singer et al., 2019) that children who stutter who have more sensitive temperaments are slower in their development of receptive vocabulary. This interference by temperament with the development of language may be yet another drain on neural resources that contributes to stuttering.

Reports on sensitive temperament have included the positive as well as negative aspects of this personality type. In an overview article, Ellis and Boyce (2008) suggest that a reactive temperament in a child may produce very different outcomes, depending on whether a child encounters a stressful environment or a nurturing one. For example, Boyce et al. (1995) found that, compared to relatively unreactive children, sensitive children in stressful environments had more respiratory illnesses than typical children, whereas sensitive children in nurturing environments had fewer than typical children. In other words, a sensitive temperament can give a child protection against illness if the environment is favorable. What are the implications for stuttering? We will revisit this in Chapter 6, "Theories About Stuttering," but it is pretty clear that a nurturing environment could help a sensitive child predisposed to stuttering be less reactive to his disfluencies.

I previously cited several studies that support the hypothesis that many children who stutter are born with a sensitive temperament. However, a strong case has been made for the opposite view—that children who stutter, as a group, do not have an inherently sensitive temperament, but that developmental and environmental factors have given rise to the anxiety and sensitivity often seen in children who stutter. Smith et al. (2014) reviewed many studies related to anxiety and sensitive temperament in stuttering and concluded that there is no clear evidence for an inherited anxiety or hypersensitivity. They suggest that repeated negative social consequences of stuttering, in later childhood and adolescence (and beyond), give rise to increased anxiety in many people who stutter. Others disagree (eg, researchers at Vanderbilt University, including Jones et al., 2014; Ntourou et al., 2013; Walden et al., 2012). A strong and data-based answer to this question has been made by Eggers (2012). He found that children who stutter have higher "negative reactivity" and lower "self-regulation" than children who do not stutter. My impression of his findings and those of the researchers at Vanderbilt is that they strongly suggest that these temperamental differences are inherent, rather than a consequence of stuttering.

Summary of the Effect of Social and Emotional Development on Fluency

Many of the normal social and emotional stresses that children experience as they grow up may result in disfluent speech, although the evidence is mostly anecdotal.

Children who are neurophysiologically predisposed to stutter may be especially prone to disfluency when social conflicts and emotions create extra "noise" in their neural circuitry for speech. This would be particularly true for those children who are both predisposed to stuttering and who have emotionally reactive temperaments. This combination of constitutional traits could be associated with the onset and development of stuttering. These same traits may also be related to the persistence of stuttering in some children.

Some researchers believe that emotional reactivity and anxiety are not one of the causes of stuttering but the result of social encounters in which negative listener reactions create the anxiety and sensitivity. Others think that emotional reactivity or sensitivity is innate.

Important findings, key speculations, and clinical implications about developmental factors are summarized in Table 4.1.

TABLE 4.1 Developmental Factors in Stuttering

Area of Interest	Important Findings and Key Speculations	Clinical Implications
Development in general	Competition for neural resources may diminish resources available for speech-motor control.	When a child is going through a period of intense developmental growth in any domain, stuttering may increase.
Physical and speech motor skill development	Physical growth can compete with neural resources for speech. Developmental changes in the speech motor system require neural resources to continually update sensorimotor "maps" for fluent speech. Evidence that children who stutter—especially those who persist—have less mature speech motor control than typical children. Some studies suggest that uneven development of speech motor abilities in children who stutter may be as detrimental to fluency as delayed development.	Possibility that adult modeling of slower speech rate could promote fluency. Predicting which children will persist in stuttering rather than recover may be possible using measures of speech motor control.
Speech and language development	Evidence that as children learn to use longer and more complex sentences, both typical disfluencies and stuttering increase. Studies conflict about whether children who stutter are more delayed than those who don't. However, several studies found that children with persistent stuttering are more delayed (than typical children or those who recover) in language when tested when they first begin to stutter. Even this research, however, found that children who stutter have language within the normal range. Some researchers have found among stuttering children "dissociation" or uneven development of subcomponents of language, even though overall language scores of children who stutter are not different from those of typical children. As with uneven development of motor abilities (see above), these disparities in development of language subcomponents may drain neural resources as stuttering children try to cope with them.	Adult models of shorter and less complex sentences may promote fluency in children beginning to stutter.

TABLE 4.1 Developmental Factors in Stuttering (*Continued*)

Area of Interest	Important Findings and Key Speculations	Clinical Implications
Cognitive development	In the preschool years, children pass through several stages of cognitive development. At each new stage, neural resources may be taxed, stressing the fragile speech motor system of children at risk for stuttering. This competition for resources may precipitate or worsen stuttering. Individuals with cognitive limitations—such as those with Down syndrome—appear to be at greater risk for stuttering (or excess disfluencies) because of competition for neural resources during development (and thereafter). Some evidence shows that children who stutter have slightly lower scores on cognitive assessments. There is also evidence that children who persist in stuttering may have slightly lower (but in normal range) scores on cognitive assessments. Although a few younger children who stutter may be unaware of their stuttering, most children do develop awareness and negative attitudes toward their stuttering. These negative attitudes increase with age—perhaps because of more negative experiences—and may contribute to the persistence of stuttering.	Information about fluctuations of stuttering with cognitive development may help parents understand why stuttering can be better at some times and more severe at others. They may be reassured they aren't causing the changes. Parents with children who have cognitive limitations may find this information helpful to understand their child's speech. Evidence of slightly lower than average cognitive scores may predict persistence and warrant immediate treatment. Treatment of stuttering should take into consideration negative communication attitudes in children who stutter. Children with little awareness of their stuttering may benefit from indirect treatment. Children who are negatively aware of their stuttering may need treatment components that change attitudes as well as behaviors.
Social and Emotional Development	Increases in emotion tend to be associated with increases in stuttering. As children grow, they pass through various stages of social and emotional development, some of which may be stressful and precipitate more stuttering. Threats to a child's sense of security, for example, may increase stuttering. The development of self-consciousness, especially in sensitive children, may cause them to feel more negatively about their stuttering.	Heightened emotion—whether positive or negative—may temporarily increase stuttering. This may explain otherwise puzzling changes in stuttering. Increasing a child's sense of security may help increase fluency. Children who are negatively aware of their stuttering may be helped by treatment procedures that decrease this negative emotion, such as pretending to stutter in a variety of ways, especially if you and the child can invent funny ways to stutter (if the child seems OK with that).

ENVIRONMENTAL FACTORS

Environmental factors that influence the onset and progression of stuttering are stresses and pressures in the child's home, playground, and daycare or school. One example is a conversational style in the child's home that is characterized by lots of interruptions and rapid, complex speech that is beyond the child's level. As you can imagine, there are many things in a child's environment—some subtle and some not so subtle—that can add enough stress to a child with a predisposition to stutter to trigger the onset and promote the development of stuttering. Environmental stresses interact with genetic factors as well as developmental pressures to have their effect on the child. Table 4.2 summarizes environmental factors that may influence children's stuttering.

I begin the discussion of environmental factors by reviewing research on the most important factor in family environments—the parents.

Parents

In the 1930s and 1940s at the University of Iowa, Wendell Johnson developed the "diagnosogenic" theory of stuttering (Johnson et al., 1942). This theory proposed that a child's

TABLE 4.2 Environmental Factors in Stuttering

Area of Interest	Important Findings and Key Speculations	Clinical Implications
Parents	Theory that parents caused stuttering by misdiagnosing normal disfluencies has been disproven. Some evidence shows that parents of children who stutter may be a little more anxious and demanding than parents of typical children, but other research refutes this idea. Parents may be more hypervigilant about disfluencies if they have family members who stutter, but there are no data confirming this.	Families should be reassured that there is no evidence that parents or families cause stuttering. In a diagnostic evaluation, parent-child interactions should be evaluated to assess whether there may be demands on the child that could be reduced to see if this improves fluency. Parents will benefit from learning what aspects of their child's speech are typical disfluencies, compared to actual stutters.
Speech and language environment	There is evidence that some parents of children who stutter speak to their children with a higher speech rate, interrupt more, ask more questions, and use more complex language, compared to parents of children who are developing typically. But because there are conflicting data, it is probably best to assume that parents of children who stutter may be using speech and language at nearly normal levels but their children would benefit from less conversational pressure.	For younger children, treatment may focus on helping parents and families use slower speech rates, allowing their children plenty of time to talk without interruptions, asking fewer questions (but using comments instead), and using language at the child's level.
Life events	Stuttering may first appear or worsen after stressful life events, such as emotional trauma. This cause of stuttering may be more likely in cases where there is no family history of stuttering.	If onset or worsening of stuttering is associated with an emotional life event, child should receive psychological counseling as well as stuttering therapy. When the clinician is qualified, these may be carried out by the same individual.

parents were the cause of stuttering because they misdiagnosed normal disfluencies as stuttering. Parents' reactions to the "stuttering" then caused the child to try to avoid these normal disfluencies and, in avoiding them, the child hesitated and struggled in a way that eventually became real stuttering. Johnson's diagnosogenic theory generated a great deal of research on parents of stutterers. Were they different from the parents of nonstutterers? Were they unusually critical? Did they have unreasonably high standards of speech?

Early studies by Johnson and his colleagues conducted to answer these questions suggested that parents of children who stuttered appeared to be more critical and perfectionistic and had higher standards of behavior than parents of children who did not. These findings, as well as details about the types of disfluencies reported by parents, were collected and published in a book titled *The Onset of Stuttering: Research Findings and Implications* (Johnson et al., 1959). Johnson interpreted these data as showing a great deal of similarity between the disfluencies of stuttering and nonstuttering children. He suggested that the same disfluency types that parents of nonstuttering children considered normal were reported by parents of stuttering children as the earliest signs of stuttering. Johnson used this as evidence to support the diagnosogenic hypothesis that the problem was parents' interpretation of their child's disfluencies, or as some often put it, "the problem was not in the child's mouth but in the parent's ear."

Later researchers disagreed. McDearmon (1968), for example, argued that Johnson's findings actually showed that the disfluencies of normal children were notably different from those in the stuttering children. Syllable repetitions, sound prolongations, and complete blocks were reported to have occurred much more frequently in the stuttering children, whereas phrase repetitions, pauses, and interjections were reported more frequently in the nonstuttering control group. This reinterpretation of Johnson's data and new findings about genetic and constitutional factors in stuttering have caused the diagnosogenic view of stuttering to be largely abandoned.

Somewhat more recent studies of parents of children who stutter and parents of typically speaking children focused on parent characteristics rather than disfluency types. In a summary of these studies, Yairi (1997b) found mixed results. Some indicated that parents of stutterers were more anxious or more rejecting, while others found no differences. On balance, Yairi suggests, it seems likely that some children who stutter grew up with parents who were a little more demanding or anxious than average, and this may have made a difference. Assuming they already had a constitutional predisposition to stutter, these children's early speech may have been peppered with disfluencies, which would have alarmed their parents. The children then, picking up on their parents' dismay, may have become self-conscious about their minor disfluencies and thus have unwittingly added tension and struggle, which blossomed into more noticeable stuttering. However, Yairi's strong conclusion is that parents do not cause their children to stutter, although they may have passed along genes that increased the risk for stuttering.

A recent study has shown that parents of children who stutter are indeed more perfectionist and control oriented. For example, in a study of 427 parents of children who were in an Australian preschool treatment program, Park et al. (2021) found that half of the parents failed a screener for identifying "Anankastic Personality Disorder" when they completed the International Personality Disorders Examination Questionnaire prior to their child's treatment. This disorder is classified as a type of obsessive-compulsive personality by the *International Classification of Diseases* 11th edition (Fineberg et al., 2014). Such a personality in a parent of a child who stutters may stress the child when the parent expresses—overtly or covertly—anxiety or disapproval about the stuttering. This may, in turn, cause the child to try to stop stuttering by increasing tension in an effort to hold the stutter inside.

It is interesting to speculate that in some cases, a child's hypersensitivity to parents' concern and the child's increased tension as a response to his disfluencies are a component of an overall vulnerable temperament found in some children who stutter (Anderson et al., 2003; Choi et al., 2016; Eggers, 2012; Karrass et al., 2006; Oyler & Ramig, 1995; Walden et al., 2012), and which may be inherited. The parents, the genetic source of these temperaments, may be the anxious, overprotective mothers or fathers that have been described in the literature on parents of stutterers. Such children are, therefore, in double jeopardy for persistent stuttering because of the children's own temperaments and because one or both parents, having a sensitive temperament themselves, may be overly concerned about their children's stuttering. On the other hand, some parents may have a beneficial and calming effect on their child's vulnerable temperament, making it possible for a child who begins to stutter and who is emotionally reactive to recover from stuttering. In a discussion of environmental influences on biological predispositions of children who do not stutter, Calkins and Fox (1994) said that "the child's interactions with a parent provide the context for learning skills and strategies for managing emotional reactivity" (p. 209).

Once again, we see that influences on stuttering are numerous and complex, coming from both the child and the environment. Some of these influences may precipitate stuttering, others may interact to make remission difficult, and still others may provide the kinds of support that make remission possible.

Summary of the Effect of Parents on Fluency

The "diagnosogenic" theory of stuttering onset—that parents cause stuttering because they misdiagnose normal disfluencies as stuttering—has been largely refuted.

Nonetheless, some research suggests that parents of children who stutter may be a little more demanding or perfectionistic than parents of typical children. The results, however, are mixed and some studies find no differences between these two groups of parents.

Any stress that comes from parents may be the result of the fact that stuttering is often inherited and parents may have relatives who stutter, making them hypervigilant about stuttering in their children. Or, these parents may have a hypersensitive temperament (which they may have passed on to their children), making them (and their children) more anxious and reactive to an excess of disfluencies.

Of course, the home environment for the child includes not only parents but other family members as well—siblings, grandparents, cousins—whoever lives in the household or comprises the extended family. Figure 4.4 is a photograph of a family at a formal dinner. The young child is stuttering and the child's mother (on the child's immediate left) is showing possibly negative emotion in her facial expression. This environment may be stressful to the child, not only because of

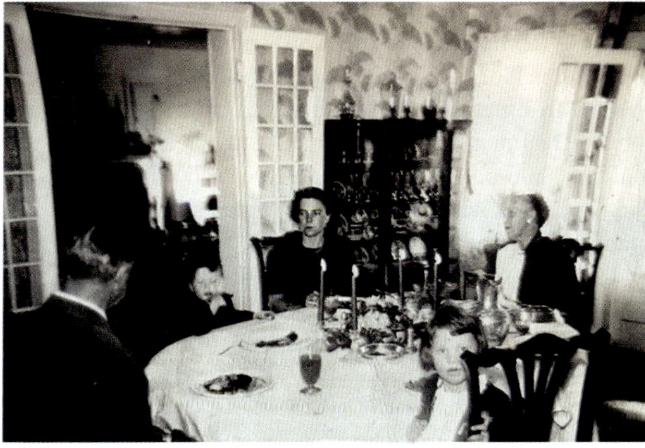

Figure 4.4 A young child stuttering when he is questioned in a formal family gathering.

demands for speech but also because of some family members' responses to his stuttering.

Speech and Language Environment

Because every preschool-age child is tuned into the speech and language around him, especially that of his parents, the communication style in their home may be an important influence on the child who stutters. Van Riper (1973a) expressed the situation this way: "Stuttering usually begins at the very time that great advances in sentence construction occur, and it seems tenable that, when the speech models provided by the parents or siblings of the child are too difficult for him to follow, some faltering will ensue" (p. 381).

Many other clinical researchers have also speculated that **speech and language environments** are a potential source of stress for children who stutter (eg, Gottwald, 2010; Richels & Conture, 2007; Shapiro, 1999; Starkweather et al., 1990; Zebrowski & Kelly, 2002).

Treatment approaches focused on the child's speech and language environment have shown some success. A colleague and I conducted an experimental treatment of a stressful speech and language environment using an ABAB design[1] with a 5-year-old during dinner table conversations (Winslow & Guitar, 1994). This child had a strong family history of stuttering and had himself developed quite severe stuttering at age 3. By the time he reached age 5, his stuttering was not as severe, but it continued, especially when he was competing with his older brother for his parents' attention—for example, at the dinner table. In this situation, everyone talked at the same time, making it hard for the child to be heard. Treatment focused on conversational turn-taking and the two children were supplied with wooden blocks they had to raise up in the air to be recognized for their turn to speak. Even the parents carefully took their turns speaking. The children were rewarded with praise for limiting their talking to when they raised their block and praised when they held back from talking as they waited their turn. Over 15 sessions, alternating between no treatment (the boys were allowed to talk simultaneously, competing for attention) and treatment (each boy held up his block to ask for speaking time), it became clear that the treatment sessions reduced the child's stuttering and the no treatment sessions saw stuttering return. Soon, the children (and parents) learned to give each other an opportunity to speak without being interrupted and the 5-year-old gradually became typically fluent.

In addition to treatments that take into account speech and language stresses, theoretical models have emerged to explain how the speech and language environment influences children's stuttering. Crystal (1987) proposed an "interactive" view of many speech and language disorders, which suggested that demands at one level of language production (eg, syntax) may deplete resources for other levels (eg, prosody or phonology) and result in breakdown. His supporting data nicely illustrate how stuttering may be exacerbated by a child's use of advanced language. He presented evidence that the more complex the syntax and semantics that a child used, the more they stuttered. Starkweather (1987), describing a demands-and-capacities view of stuttering, commented "the production of speech and the formulation of language place a simultaneous demand on the young person. If the demands in either of these two dimensions are excessive, performance in the other dimension may be reduced." These two views imply that stuttering may increase when an individual uses longer words, less frequently occurring words, more information-bearing words, and longer sentences. Stuttering may also increase when the individual is uttering a more linguistically complex sentence. By implication, the child's speech and language environment—usually conversation by adults talking to the child—may be responsible for influencing a child to use more advanced language.

What do we know about the speech and language of parents of children who stutter and its influence on stuttering? Research has concentrated on four major characteristics of parent speech: (1) rate of speech, (2) interruptions of children's speaking, (3) frequency of questions that parents ask children, and (4) the linguistic complexity of parent speech. I'll summarize the research in each area.

Rate of Speech

Meyers and Freeman (1985a, 1985b) compared the speech of mothers of stuttering children with that of mothers of nonstutterers. They found that mothers of children who stuttered spoke more rapidly than did the mothers of nonstutterers. This may be critical, since a mother's high speech rate may encourage a child to try to speak faster than his optimal speed (eg, Jaffe & Anderson, 1979). The possibility that rapid speech rates may lead to stuttering is consistent with Johnson and Rosen's (1937) finding that adults who stutter were more likely to stutter when they spoke more rapidly than their habitual rates. Children who stutter may be even more vulnerable to fluency breakdowns during rapid speech than adults who stutter by virtue of the fact that children's natural rates of speech are slower and their temporal coordination less skillful than those of adults (eg, Kent, 1981).

However, Kelly and Conture (1992) found no differences in the speaking rates of mothers of these two groups of children. In a subsequent study, Kelly (1994) found no differences in the rates of fathers of the two groups. Using another method to compare rates, Yaruss and Conture (1995) found no differences in the articulatory rates (the rate at which each individual phrase is spoken, in contrast to "speaking rate," which includes pauses between phrases) between mothers of stuttering children and mothers of nonstuttering children. However, the latter researchers did find a significant correlation

[1]An ABAB design is a single-subject experiment in which a baseline of the behavior in question is established (A) and then a treatment (B) is introduced and the behavior is again measured. Then the baseline of the behavior is done when treatment is not present (the second A) and this is followed by a second introduction of treatment (B) in which the effect of the treatment on behavior is again measured.

between children's severity of stuttering and parent-child differences in speaking rate; greater differences in parent-child speech rates were associated with more severe stuttering in the children. These results could have been obtained if more severely stuttering children talk more slowly than other children and their parents have speech rates similar to other parents in the study. It is also possible that greater parent-child differences in rate make a child who already stutters stutter more severe.

A study by Dehqan et al. (2008) found results that appear to confirm the findings of Yaruss and Conture (1995). They assessed mothers' speaking rates, their children's rates, and the severity of their children's stuttering and found that faster rates by mothers were associated with more severe stuttering in their child. As expected, the more severe the child's stuttering, the slower was his speaking rate. This study suggests many follow-up questions: (1) Did these mothers' speech rates increase from the time of their child's stuttering onset to when it was measured? (2) If the mothers were taught to slow their speech rates, would the frequency of their children's stuttering decrease? (3) If the parents were taught to use a response-contingent intervention such as Lidcombe Program, would the mothers' speech rates decrease as their children's stuttering severity decreased?

Interruptions

Another suspected stress, in addition to rapid speech rates, is the frequency with which parents (or other listeners) interrupt their children. One of Meyers and Freeman's (1985a) reports presented some unexpected evidence about interruptions. The mothers of both stuttering and nonstuttering children interrupted most frequently when a child was disfluent. It seems possible that such parental interruptions, some of which may have been elicited by the child's disfluencies, may in turn elicit changes in the child's speech. Some children might increase tension and rate, thereby developing the struggled behaviors of stuttering. Others might suppress disfluencies to avoid interruptions and eventually be "taught" by parents not to be disfluent.

In a later study, Kelly and Conture (1992) found no significant differences in the interruptions of mothers of stuttering children and those of mothers of nonstuttering children. However, a closer inspection of their data revealed a correlation between the duration of "simultalk" (one person talking at the same time another is talking) of the mothers of children who stutter and the severity of their stuttering. Thus, mothers of more severe stutterers did more simultalk when their children were talking than did mothers whose children stuttered less severely. In a later study of fathers, Kelly (1994) found no differences in the interruptions of fathers of children who stutter and those of fathers whose children don't stutter. Moreover, the correlation between these fathers' simultalk and severity of stuttering was not significant.

In an unusual study, Livingston et al. (2000) deliberately interrupted the speech of several children who stuttered (ages 5-6) and found that stuttering did not increase very much. They were reluctant to emphasize reducing parental interruptions of children who stutter, especially for this age group.

Asking Questions

Another variable of children's speech and language environments that has been studied is the extent to which parents ask questions. Meyers and Freeman (1985a) found no significant difference in the number of questions asked by mothers of children who stutter compared to mothers of children who do not. In contrast, Langlois et al. (1986) found significant differences when making a similar comparison. Langlois and Long (1988) then conducted an experimental treatment of a 4-year-old who stuttered, in which the mother was taught to reduce the number of questions she asked, among other changes. After 16 treatment sessions in which the mother had markedly reduced her number of questions and given her child more speaking turns, the child no longer stuttered. This finding is especially interesting because it is tempting to assume that asking questions results in more stuttering. However, subsequent studies tested this assumption and failed to support it. In a study of eight stuttering children in conversations with their parents, Weiss and Zebrowski (1992) found that the children stuttered less when they answered questions than when they made assertions. This appeared to be related to the fact that questions were often answered with brief responses, but assertions by children were often longer utterances. A more direct test of the effect of parents asking questions was carried out by Wilkenfeld and Curlee (1997), who used a single-subject ABAB design to vary an adult's verbal behavior (questions vs comments) in conversations with a child who stuttered. Their results with three children who stuttered demonstrated that stuttering did not appear to be related to whether the adult asked questions or commented but was more likely to occur in either condition when the child's utterances were longer.

Complexity of Language

Most studies of parents' speech have focused on comparing parents of children who stutter with parents of children who do not. Kloth et al. (1999) took a different approach, with a longitudinal study of speech and language of parents whose children were at risk for stuttering (ie, one or both parents stuttered). They assessed the complexity of the mothers' language, measured in terms of mean length of utterances (MLU) in words in conversations with their child, both before and immediately after the onset of stuttering. They found that the language of the mothers of children who persisted in stuttering was significantly more complex than that of the mothers of children who recovered, when measured both before their children began to stutter and again after stuttering began. In a later study of persistent and recovered stutterers, Rommel et al. (2000) assessed the complexity of the language of 71 mothers soon after their children had begun to stutter, rather than before stuttering began. They followed these children for 3 years and found that one of the more powerful predictors of whether or not a child would recover was "the linguistic demands to which the child is exposed" (p. 181). More specifically, these researchers found that the more complex the mother's syntax (MLU)[2] and the greater number of different words she used in talking to her child, the more likely that her child would not recover over the following 3 years. The language abilities of the children themselves had no predictive value (Rommel et al., 2000).

Using a more traditional approach rather than looking at persistence and recovery, Miles and Ratner (2001) assessed the complexity of the language of parents of children who stuttered, gathering samples of conversations from 12 mother-child pairs involving stuttering children and 12 involving fluent children. All children were between 27 and 48 months of age, and the stuttering children were within 3 months of the onset of their stuttering. Mothers' utterances were assessed for syntactic complexity, lexical diversity and rarity of words, and mean number of utterances per turn. No significant differences between the mothers of the stuttering children and the mothers of the fluent children were found. These studies suggest that parents of children who stutter may not use more complex language than parents of typically speaking children, but for at-risk or stuttering children, less complex language is associated with better likelihood of recovery.

TABLE 4.3 Possible Speech and Language Stressors

Stressful Adult Speech Models	
Rapid speech rate	Complex syntax
Polysyllabic vocabulary	Use of two languages in home
Stressful Speaking Situations for Children	
Competition for speaking	Hurried when speaking
Frequent interruptions	Frequent questions
Demand for display speech (eg, "Tell Mrs. Tiggiewinkle what you did today")	Excited when speaking
Loss of listener attention	Many things to say

[2]MLU is a measure of mean length of utterance. This reflects the level of syntax with higher MLU indicating more advanced syntax.

[3]The acronym SLP stands for Speech Language Pathologist, the title of workers in the field of Communication Sciences and Disorders.

Summary of the Effects of Speech and Language Environment on Fluency

Speech models by parents, siblings, and others may precipitate or worsen stuttering if they are too far above the child's level. This may occur because of the demand on already stressed or somewhat inadequate neural resources. Table 4.3 lists a variety of sources of possible stress from the speech and language environment.

Life Events

Certain **life events** can deliver a blow to a child's stability and security. When this happens, stuttering may suddenly appear out of nowhere, or previously easy repetitions may be transformed into hard, struggled blocks. To move to a new home, to be hospitalized for an operation, or to have parents divorce is difficult even for adults, but it is especially difficult for children. Although there are not many published studies supporting this idea, Van Riper (1982a) discusses reports of emotional stress triggering the onset of stuttering but is cautious about accepting all the clinical anecdotes in the literature. In my own case, a move from Connecticut to South Carolina was associated with a worsening of my stuttering, and the move back to Connecticut a few years later was associated with it becoming noticeably more severe. In an odd coincidence, as I was writing this section, I received an e-mail from an SLP[3] asking advice about a child who had experienced just such a life event. This child was from a family of migrant workers and had begun to stutter after he and his family became homeless for several months. I am hoping that after some help with the emotional trauma, accompanied by therapy for his stuttering, he will improve his fluency and become a mostly fluent boy again. As you might imagine, many children go through stressful experiences and adapt to them without apparent major problems. But children who are more sensitive often show the effects of such events in their speech. Kagan (1994a) noted that some children who begin life with relaxed temperaments might even become shy and fearful under the onslaught of stressful events. This may well set the stage for stuttering if other constitutional factors predispose the child for it. You may wonder what the mechanism is by which stress can precipitate or worsen stuttering. I don't know the answer, but it seems likely that if a child's brain pathways for speech and language are compromised, extra resources are needed to maintain fluency. When stress increases negative emotions such as anxiety, it seems possible that the negative emotions would consume the extra resources. It is also possible that crosstalk between emotion centers in the brain and neural networks for speech may affect fluency in these children, as I suggested in the earlier section "Interference of Speech by Emotion."

There is little hard research on the relationship between stressful life events and stuttering, but many authors have observed the connection. Starkweather (1987), for example, wrote, "All children speak more disfluently during periods of tension—when moving or changing schools, when their parents divorce, or after the death of a family member" (pp. 146–147). These increases in disfluency could easily result in the onset of stuttering or in increased stuttering in children who are vulnerable to such stresses. Johnson et al. (1959) noted that the following events were among the 16 situations in which parents first noticed their child's stuttering: (1) child's physical environment changed (eg, moving to a new house); (2) child became ill; (3) child realized his mother was pregnant; and (4) a new baby arrived. In discussing the onset of stuttering, Van Riper (1982a) acknowledged that various studies have found no differences in the amount of emotional conflict in the homes of children who developed stuttering versus those who didn't. However, he went on to note, "Nevertheless, we have studied individual cases in which stuttering did seem [to be] triggered by such conflicts, and it is difficult for us to ignore these experiences" (p. 79).

My own clinical experience is similar. In the past many years, for example, during which I've evaluated many children who stutter, I've encountered four children in four different families who began to stutter when their parents were in the early stages of divorce. However, this turmoil was not the only factor in their stuttering. Three of the children had relatives who stuttered, and the father of the fourth child stuttered himself. Moreover, all four were preschoolers and were probably experiencing various growth and development pressures. Nonetheless, for all four of these children, their parents' divorce appeared to be a factor that pushed them from normal speech to stuttering.

In another case of a life event precipitating stuttering, I evaluated a 9-year-old girl who began to stutter when her classroom teacher had an emotional breakdown that became very apparent in the classroom. The teacher's outbursts of anger and crying, interspersed with high demands for rapid performance on frequent examinations, were apparently extremely stressful for this student. Under this stress, she developed tight blocks, with physical tension at the level of the larynx and abdomen. Even though I was convinced through extensive interviews with the family that the child had no prior stuttering, I noted several predisposing factors for stuttering. First, her younger sister had significant learning disabilities, including auditory processing problems. Second, her mother described herself and her daughter who stuttered as shy and emotionally reactive. These two factors—a family history of learning disability and a vulnerable temperament—may have provided a fertile matrix for the sudden germination of stuttering when a stressful life event occurred. Happily, after a year of treatment, this child became fluent. This child, now a young woman, discusses this stressful time with her mother in the video "Onset of Stuttering Related to a Stressful Life Event" on *Lippincott Connect*.

Another client whose stuttering began after a traumatic life event was a young woman in her thirties who came to our clinic with noticeable blocks characterized by facial grimaces and complete stoppage of speech for several seconds. Her stuttering had begun at age 5 when her mother unexpectedly gave birth to a sibling at home. Our client told us that she had witnessed a difficult birthing process with her mother experiencing severe pain and profuse bleeding. She began to stutter immediately afterward. Because when she arrived at our clinic, she was well adjusted and not upset by her stuttering, we treated her with a fluency-shaping program based on using delayed auditory feedback to slow her speech rate to a fluent drawl. After two intensive days of treatment, during which she was gradually speeded up to a normal rate, the client declared that she was fluent and needed no more treatment. We followed her for several weeks, sometimes using clinic visits and, once, a phone call disguised as a survey about gas prices in her neighborhood (which we revealed as a ruse, at the end of the call), and found her to be entirely fluent. Thirty years after the initial treatment, we again interviewed her and were impressed by her continuing fluency. Her successful life adjustment had somehow enabled her to use a slowed speech rate in our clinic to become fluent and then to use a normal rate to continue to speak fluently for years afterward.

An unusual life event—an earthquake—precipitated stuttering in three children (one girl age 4 and a girl and boy age 5) at the same time (Jafari et al., 2019). A 6.6 magnitude quake struck near their homes in Kerman, Iran and they began to stutter with repetitions of sounds, syllables, and words. They showed excessive fear, urinary incontinence, and a brief period of not talking, before the stuttering started. None of the children had stuttered previously nor had any relatives who stuttered. After several months, the children still continued to stutter and their families brought them to a speech-language pathologist for treatment.

More ordinary life events can also be associated with the onset of stuttering in children who appear to have no genetic predisposition to stuttering. As cited in Chapter 2 on constitutional factors, Poulos and Webster (1991) examined 57 clients with no family history of stuttering and found that 37% reported childhood events or illnesses that were associated with stuttering onset. For example, three individuals reported experiencing intense fear associated with the onset of stuttering. These fears arose from being attacked by an animal, being bombed during a war, or being alone in a thunderstorm. When this sort of life event triggers stuttering, a predisposition for stuttering may or may not have existed prior to the event, rather than a genetic inheritance specifically of stuttering. Other neurologically predisposing conditions such as ADHD (Alm & Risberg, 2007; Briley et al., 2021) or sensitive temperament (Karass et al., 2006) may have existed in these children. Other life events, such as head injury or diseases of the nervous system, may precipitate stuttering without a predisposing condition because the event may damage the speech motor control system.

Table 4.4 lists some of the life events that I have found to be detrimental to children's fluency.

TABLE 4.4 Stressful Life Events That May Increase a Child's Disfluency

The child's family moves to a new house, a new neighborhood, or a new city.
The child's parents separate or divorce.
A family member dies.
A family member is hospitalized.
The child is hospitalized.
A parent loses their job.
A baby is born, or a child is adopted.
An additional person comes to live in the house.
One or both parents go away frequently or for a long period of time.
Holidays or visits occur, which cause a change in routine, excitement, or anxiety.
There is a discipline problem involving the child.

Summary of the Effects of Life Events on Fluency

Many clinicians have suggested that stressful life events may precipitate stuttering or increase its severity. Some research suggests that among individuals who stutter without family history of stuttering, there is more evidence of emotional trauma, sickness, or injury associated with the onset of stuttering than in those with family history of stuttering. This suggests that in some cases, stressful life events, rather than a genetic inheritance of stuttering, can cause stuttering.

In the preceding section, I described the environmental factors that can interact with developmental factors and with a child's constitutional predisposition to produce and worsen stuttering. Fortunately, some of these environmental factors can be modified or compensated for to improve fluency.

SUMMARY

- Physical and motor development uses a great deal of neuronal resources in the brain, perhaps leaving fewer resources available for speech fluency. This may be potentially crucial in children with compromised or delayed neural systems for speech production.
- Children's learning of phonology, morphology, syntax, and semantics may strain resources for the establishment of fluent speech. In addition, *differences in the rate of development* of different components of speech and language may result in more disfluency.
- The demands of cognitive development (memory, attention, executive function) may stress the development of fluency, resulting in the onset of stuttering or increase in it.
- Normal social and emotional conflicts in children predisposed to stutter may trigger onset or worsening of stuttering.
- Communication stress in the home (rapid speech rates, frequent interruptions, questions, and complex language) may precipitate or worsen stuttering.
- Traumatic or stressful life events may trigger or worsen stuttering in children who have a family history of stuttering and/or have a vulnerable temperament.

STUDY QUESTIONS

1. The effect of a child's development on fluency has been likened to the effect of too many users on a website. Explain this analogy or suggest another analogy that depicts some sort of "overload" that could be like the many demands placed on a child as they develop.
2. It has been said (though not by everyone) that children usually do not learn to walk and talk at the same time. If this is true, what does this suggest about how motor development might affect fluency?
3. There is a high incidence of stuttering among individuals with cognitive impairment. What might this suggest about the relationship between cognition and fluency?
4. What aspects of social and emotional development might threaten fluency?
5. What evidence is there that emotional arousal might increase disfluency?
6. What is the possible connection between atypical hemispheric localization and the effects of emotion on fluency?
7. Why would children's speech and language development be likely to put greater pressure on fluency than would their physical or cognitive development?
8. What aspects of parents' behavior might put pressure on a child who is disfluent?
9. Is there anything in Figure 4.4 that might suggest some family members may have "Anankastic Personality Disorder"?
10. Identify several characteristics of parents' speech that may create difficult models for a disfluent child to emulate.

11. Name several life events that have been suggested to increase a child's disfluency.
12. The communicative failure and anticipatory struggle view proposes that experiencing a communication failure may cause a child to anticipate difficulty speaking and begin to stutter as a result. What characteristic of the child may be another important factor?
13. Johnson et al.'s (1959) revised view of stuttering suggested that it results from an interaction among the following three factors: (1) the extent of the child's disfluency, (2) the listener's sensitivity to that disfluency, and (3) the child's sensitivity to his own disfluency and to the listener's reaction. Relate these factors to constitutional, developmental, and environmental factors in stuttering.

SUGGESTED PROJECTS

1. Record a natural speech sample from someone who stutters, and analyze the relationship between the occurrences of stuttering and the linguistic level of the utterances in which they occur.
2. Develop an experimental protocol to assess the relationship between linguistic variables and stuttering. For example, compare the variables of length of utterance, syntactic level of utterance, and phonological complexity of utterance to the likelihood of the utterance being stuttered.
3. Interview several people with typical speech and ask them if they had major life events in their childhood that impacted their lives. Compare these events with the life events mentioned in this chapter that may affect stuttering.
4. Study the effect of your speech rate on other people by designing and carrying out an experiment in which you vary the speed at which you talk. Record conversations in which you talk slowly for several minutes and then talk rapidly for several minutes. Measure the effect on your conversational partner's speed of talking. You will need to practice varying your rate beforehand.
5. In the section called Speech and Language Development, research on language abilities of children who stutter is reviewed. Some studies found that children who stutter have poorer language abilities, and other studies did not. Review these studies and suggest what might be causing this disagreement in the literature.

SUGGESTED READINGS

Andrews, G., & Harris, M. (1964). *The syndrome of stuttering*. W. Heinemann Medical Books.

These authors present data from longitudinal studies of 1,000 families in Newcastle, England. The interpretation of results presents evidence that both genetic and environmental influences are at work to create stuttering. This book gives an early version of the "capacities and demands" view that stuttering is due to a lack of capacity for some aspect of speech and language processing. This book is a classic but may be hard to find.

Bernstein Ratner, N. (1997). Stuttering: A psycholinguistic perspective. In R. Curlee & G. Siegel (Eds.), *Nature and treatment of stuttering: New directions* (2nd ed., pp. 99–127). Allyn & Bacon.

This is an insightful review of the many connections between language and stuttering. The author's background in language acquisition and development allows her to use linguistic theories and evidence from child language studies to discuss how language influences the loci of stuttering in speech, how parent-child interactions may affect stuttering, how language development may be important in stuttering onset, and the role of feedback on speech, language, and stuttering development.

Bloodstein, O., Ratner, N., & Brundage, S. (2021). *Chapter 10: Cognitive and linguistic abilities.*

This chapter provides a good view of how cognitive and language abilities may interfere with fluency. It is clearly written and filled with recent research.

Choo, A., Burnham, E., Hicks, K., & Chang, S. E. (2016). Dissociations among linguistic, cognitive, and auditory-motor neuroanatomical domains in children who stutter. *Journal of Communication Disorders*, 61, 29–47.

This article examines dissociated (uneven) development across speech, language, cognitive, and motor domains and relates those findings to density of white matter nerve tracts. Important implications for persistent versus recovered stuttering are provided.

Crystal, D. (1987). Towards a "bucket" theory of language disability: Taking account of interaction between linguistic levels. *Clinical Linguistics and Phonetics*, 1, 7–22.

This is a theoretical discussion of interaction among levels of speech and language, with an illustrative case of a child whose stuttering increases when language demands are greater. The article makes a clear argument for the influence of speech and language development on stuttering.

Guttormsen, L., Kefalianos, E., & Naess, K. A. (2015). Communication attitudes in children who stutter: A meta-analytic review. *Journal of Fluency Disorders*, 46, 1–14.

This is an excellent overview of the many studies that have been conducted on the attitudes of children who stutter. Their findings include evidence that children who stutter have much more negative attitudes about speaking than their fluent peers and that these negative attitude increase with age. The authors discuss the bidirectional nature of these attitudes: more negative attitudes can create more severe stuttering and more severe stuttering can result in experiences that make attitudes more negative.

Hollister, J., Van Horne, A., & Zebrowski, P. (2017). The relationship between grammatical development and disfluencies in preschool children who stutter and those who recover. *American Journal of Speech-Language Pathology*, 26(1), 1–13.

In its introductory review of the literature, this article presents a good description of how language demands may interact with language abilities to produce disfluencies. One important finding discussed is that for children who recover, as their mastery of syntax and grammar increases, their disfluencies decrease. Relationships between frequency of disfluencies and sentence length and sentence complexity were also explored.

Johnson, W. & Associates (1959). *The onset of stuttering.* University of Minnesota Press.

This book presents extensive data on parents' perceptions of the onset of their child's stuttering, compared with other parents' perceptions of their child's normal disfluency. Johnson eloquently lays out his view of stuttering as the product of an interaction between the child's disfluency, their sensitivity, and the listener's reactions. A classic, but perhaps hard to find.

Paden, E. P. (2005). Development of phonological ability. In E. Yairi & N. Ambrose (Eds.), *Early childhood stuttering* (pp. 197–234). Pro-Ed.

This chapter focuses on the phonological development of children who stutter with particular emphasis on comparisons between children who recover without intervention and those who persist in stuttering. The author brings to light several aspects of her research that are intriguing puzzles for future researchers to solve.

Watkins, R. V. (2005). Language abilities of young children who stutter. In E. Yairi & N. Ambrose (Eds.), *Early childhood stuttering* (pp. 235–251). Pro-Ed.

Although evidence reviewed in this chapter suggests that language abilities of children who stutter and those who don't are similar, language factors appear to play an important role in stuttering. The author discusses several interesting relationships between language and stuttering, including the role of language factors in the occurrence of stuttering in an utterance and the finding that early onset of stuttering is often associated with advanced language skills.

5

Learning and Unlearning

Chapter Outline

Chapter Objectives

After studying this chapter, readers should be able to:

- Explain classical conditioning, operant conditioning, and avoidance conditioning
- Describe how each of these types of conditioning plays a role in the development of stuttering
- Describe what the tension response is, what it is a response to, and how it affects the development of stuttering
- Describe the role of learning new behaviors and unlearning old ones in the treatment of stuttering

Key Terms

Classical conditioning: Learning caused by the association of a neutral stimulus with a stimulus that strongly provokes a response, usually through a physiological or psychological process that occurs without awareness. The conditioning process will cause a formerly neutral stimulus to eventually provoke a response. As an example, imagine that you have encountered an aggressive goat that one of your neighbors has just acquired as a pet; they keep it outside, on a rope that reaches the sidewalk. Despite the goat's cute looks, it has a bad habit of butting you in the backside you when you walk by the neighbor's house. You naturally develop a fear of getting butted whenever you have to walk by the house. Before the goat arrived, the neighbor's house was an *unconditioned stimulus* (UCS). But now it is a *conditioned stimulus* (CS) because it elicits threat and fear. Your fear in response to getting butted was an *unconditioned response* (UCR) because it was a natural, protective reaction. But now that the fear is elicited just by seeing the house it has become a *conditioned response* (CR) because the house is now associated in your mind with getting butted

Operant conditioning: Learning caused when a behavior is immediately followed by a reward or punishment or the relief from punishment. Imagine that, in the butty goat situation, your neighbor comes out of his house and shows you how to hold out your hand and sing out, "Oh what a good goat you are!" and give it a clump of grass. You try it, and then the goat rubs its head gently against you. Now you want to try it the next time the goat comes out to greet you. It works, and you feel immense relief. That feeling of relief is the reward that makes you want to repeat the whole experience of walking by the neighbor's house and feeding the goat. That is operant conditioning

Avoidance conditioning: Learning that teaches an individual to engage in behavior that *prevents* an unpleasant consequence. It is thought to combine classical and operant conditioning in the following way. If, as in the goat example, you start avoiding that neighbor's house and walk on the other side of the street, you would find it rewarding that you don't experience the conditioned fear because you no longer go right near the house. The association of the house with the fear caused by the butting goat is classical conditioning. The reward you experience by avoiding the house is operant conditioning. Together, they make up an example of avoidance conditioning

Here are four examples of how learning can affect stuttering after it begins. See if you can identify the type(s) of learning that each describes.

- Children who stutter often begin with repetitions of the first sound of words, like "Ca-ca-can I have some milk?" If stuttering is progressing, children will start to have longer repetitions (more iterations) with tense articulators and laryngeal muscles, as a result of the threat that stuttering creates for them. They will also speed up their repetitions. Imagine that you can hear a slight rise in pitch and less time between each iteration as a child says, "Co-co-co-co-co-cookie."
- If children have been stuttering for several months, they may begin to have more prolongations, like, "Mmmmm-mmmmmy name is Joe." If a prolongation lasts for several seconds, you may hear pitch rises as the prolongation continues. The laryngeal tension causing pitch rise may be a result of the threat and fear that stuttering creates.
- Children's repetitions and prolongations may turn into blocks as their muscles tense even more. As their tension increases and the stutters feel really stuck, children may insert extra sounds, such as, "uh," or nod their head to get out of the stutter and finish the word. It is rewarding to get out of a frustrating stutter.
- As children feel more frustrated, embarrassed, and even ashamed by their stuttering, they may begin to not use words they think they may stutter on and not go into situations that they associate with stuttering. They feel relieved when they have not had to say a feared word or go into a feared situation.

In the next sections, I will discuss learning concepts and terminology and explore them with you in many ways. See if you can apply them to four examples just presented. Learning can be complex, so I will try to present concepts and terminology in several ways, in hopes that the underlying ideas will become second nature to you. Ideally, then, you can use them to create effective evaluation and therapy strategies.

LEARNING

In this section, you will find out how learning works in the development of stuttering, so that you will understand your clients' stuttering behaviors and be able to help them change. Specific types of learning are often referred to as different kinds of conditioning. These include **classical conditioning, operant conditioning, and avoidance conditioning**. As I describe the ways in which stuttering behaviors are learned,

I will be drawing on many sources, but two books have been particularly helpful: *Learning and Behavior: A Contemporary Synthesis* by Bouton (2016) and *Anxious: Using the Brain to Understand and Treat Fear and Anxiety* by LeDoux (2015). For more details, see the Suggested Readings at the end of the chapter.

Classical Conditioning

Classical conditioning was first described by the Russian physiologist Ivan Pavlov. As with many discoveries, it came as a complete surprise. Pavlov and his colleagues had been studying how dogs digest their food, which the scientists assessed by measuring the dogs' saliva when they were fed. One morning when Pavlov first walked into his laboratory in his white coat and bushy beard, he noticed that the dogs salivated just in response to seeing him, even though he hadn't fed them. Pavlov realized that the dogs associated his appearance with their food. Just his walking into the lab triggered their salivation. Experimenting with different cues, he tried ringing a bell just before they were fed. After many pairings (the conditioning), he saw results—the bell alone elicited salivation without the food.

Note that the bell is the stimulus used in the rarefied atmosphere of a laboratory. Everyday classical conditioning happens in a more complex context. For example, your phone ringing at night may be a neutral stimulus at first, simply arousing your curiosity about who is calling. However, if your special person starts calling you at night to tell you how much they love you, the phone ringing may become a conditioned stimulus (CS) arousing your excitement and desire. You may even salivate. The phone is your Pavlov's bell.

Pavlov's observation provided the first scientific understanding of classical conditioning. Since then, classical conditioning has been studied extensively, and scientists have been able to describe how it takes place. Figure 5.1 depicts the "paradigm" (a model or diagram of how a process takes place) for classical conditioning.

For classical conditioning to take place, several things must occur:

- A stimulus that reliably elicits a response must be present (like food elicits salivation). This new stimulus is called the unconditioned stimulus (UCS). The response it elicits—often a reflexive or hardwired response—is called an unconditioned response (UCR).
- For humans, encountering a snake when walking in the woods is often a UCS for a threat response such as freezing in your tracks.
- Then, a neutral stimulus that doesn't elicit any particular response is paired with the UCS. The neutral stimulus is called the CS because it alone elicits a response. In the example of the snake, a neutral stimulus might be a pile of rocks where snakes could hang out if you saw the previous snake near a pile of rocks.
- After repeated pairing of the CS (the pile of rocks) with the UCS (the snake, which reliably elicits the UCR of freezing), the CS is then presented without the UCS, and voila! The CS elicits the freezing (which then becomes a CR). If you have encountered snakes around a pile of rocks many times, the next time you suddenly stumble upon a pile of rocks while hiking, you will momentarily freeze in your tracks (and probably look around for snakes).

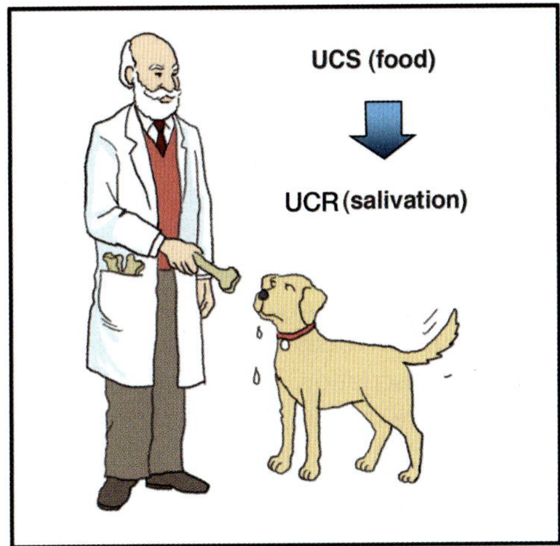

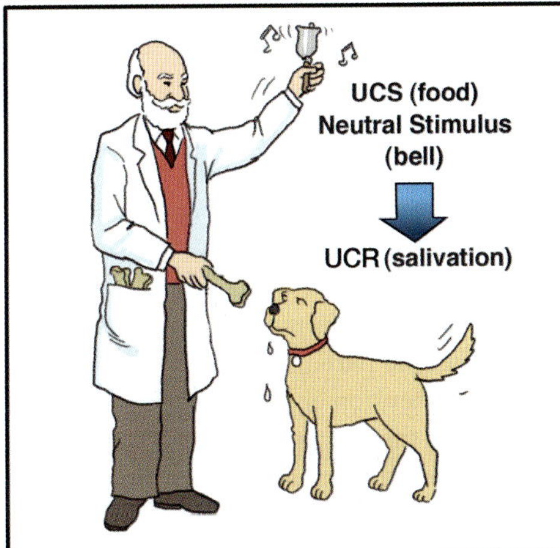

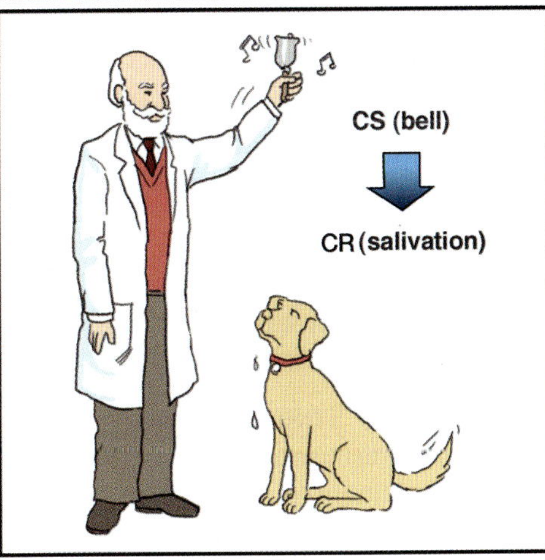

Figure 5.1 Classical conditioning paradigm. Dog salivates naturally when given food. Food is paired frequently with sound of bell. Bell without food eventually elicits salivation without the food. CR, conditioned response; CS, conditioned stimulus; UCR, unconditioned response; UCS, unconditioned stimulus.

Classical Conditioning and Stuttering

An excellent theoretical account of classical conditioning and stuttering was provided by Eugene Brutten, a speech-language pathologist, and Donald Shoemaker, a psychologist, who worked together at the University of Southern Illinois (Brutten & Shoemaker, 1967). They hypothesized that the earliest stuttering symptoms (often repetitions) result from the cognitive and motor disorganization that occurs when a child's anxiety or negative emotion is associated with speech.

Although the description of classical conditioning and stuttering I give here owes much to Brutten and Shoemaker's pioneering work, I believe classical conditioning is seldom responsible for the earliest signs of stuttering. Instead, I believe, along with Van Riper (1982a), that "the real contribution of classical conditioning theory as it is applied to stuttering lies in its ability to explain the *development* [emphasis added] of the disorder." (p. 294) I also agree with a similar assessment by Starkweather (1987, p. 372) that "it seems likely that neurophysiological sources play more of a role in stuttering onset, whereas conditioning processes play more of a role in stuttering development."

If you follow the arc of most children's stuttering development, you will see that in most cases, the earliest signs of stuttering are multiple part- and single-syllable whole-word repetitions without tension or hurry (see Fig. 5.2A). The child often doesn't notice them at first. These appear to be the result of dyssynchronies in the child's speech production system caused by delays or deficits in the development of some neural circuits and systems. Many researchers believe that some components of the word or phrase to be produced are ready to be articulated while others are not. The part that is ready for production is spoken, but it is repeated, awaiting the next part. In the following section, I describe how those relatively simple disfluencies become transformed into more complex stuttering.

Classically Conditioned Components of Stuttering

Initial Conditioned Stimulus

The initial stuttering disfluencies, as just described, are most often excessive repetitions of syllables or words. At first, the child may have no reaction to these repetitions. This is depicted in Figure 5.2A. Gradually, as the repetitions go on and on, they may elicit negative reactions from listeners or make the child feel that their mouth is running away from them doing something they don't want it to do. At that point, the child may understandably experience these repetitions on a nonconscious level as threatening (Fig. 5.2B). The threat or alarm caused by these out-of-control repetitions could then trigger an UCR to the UCS of repetitions or other disfluencies. In my opinion, the UCR is increased physical tension of the muscles of speech and perhaps other muscles as well. This is a reflexive, nonconscious co-contraction of agonist-antagonist muscle pairs that increase the stiffness of muscle groups. Stiffening of muscle groups such as this appears to be a type of "freezing" response that animals and humans may show when threatened (Gray, 1987; Hagenaars et al., 2014; LeDoux, 2015). Such freezing would often stop the repetitions in their tracks (cf., Guitar et al., 1988). Such a hard-wired, nonconscious response to threat may be understood by appreciating that children probably experience distress by their runaway mouth and by their listener's negative response to their stuttering (Fig. 5.2B and C). The conscious experience that we know as fear occurs when neural processes bring the presence of the threat into conscious awareness. When this response occurs again and again, the disfluencies become the CS that elicits the tension response, now the conditioned response (CR).

Like other threat responses, the tension response to the feeling of being out of control in stuttering is probably processed through the amygdala. It is nonconscious and may be the specific area controlling increased muscular tension[1] described by Bloodstein in his theory of stuttering (Bloodstein, 1975). This view of stuttering is also reflected in several studies of adults' perception of what stuttering is like to them (Bloodstein & Shogun, 1972; Tichenor & Yaruss, 2019). The study by Tichenor and Yaruss surveyed 430 adults who stuttered, asking them to describe what stuttering was like for them. The authors summarized respondents answers this way: "Common experiences include physical tension, struggle, or bodily movements. Many speakers discussed these aspects as deeply ingrained experiences that occur with the sensation of being stuck or losing control." (p. 4361). Tichenor and Yaruss also suggested that a common sentiment was that "...the primary impairment in stuttering can be described not as the overt behaviors that listeners may observe but rather as an internal sensation of being stuck or losing control." (p. 4363). The findings of this survey strongly support the view that loss of control along with physical tension are common phenomena. One has the impression that the physical tension is not something the speakers decide to initiate but rather something that happens to them, in the way that a nonconscious, reflexive response would be experienced.

This perspective is reinforced by Bloodstein et al.'s (2021) summary of the Bloodstein and Shogun (1972) and the Tichenor and Yaruss (2119) studies just mentioned: "the two essential features of real stuttering referred to repeatedly [in these studies] were its tension and its involuntary quality...." (p. 11). These qualities, it seems to me, are the essence of the threat (involuntary or out-of-control) and the reflexive response to the threat.

---

[1]Many others have suggested that increased tension is a common reaction to the feeling that one is unable to control one's actions. For example, Oliver Bloodstein has suggested that "Whenever we are faced with the threat of failure in the performance of a complex activity demanding accuracy or skill, we are likely to make use of abnormal muscular tension" (Bloodstein & Ratner, 2008a, p. 46). Reacting to walking on a slippery surface illustrates this nicely.

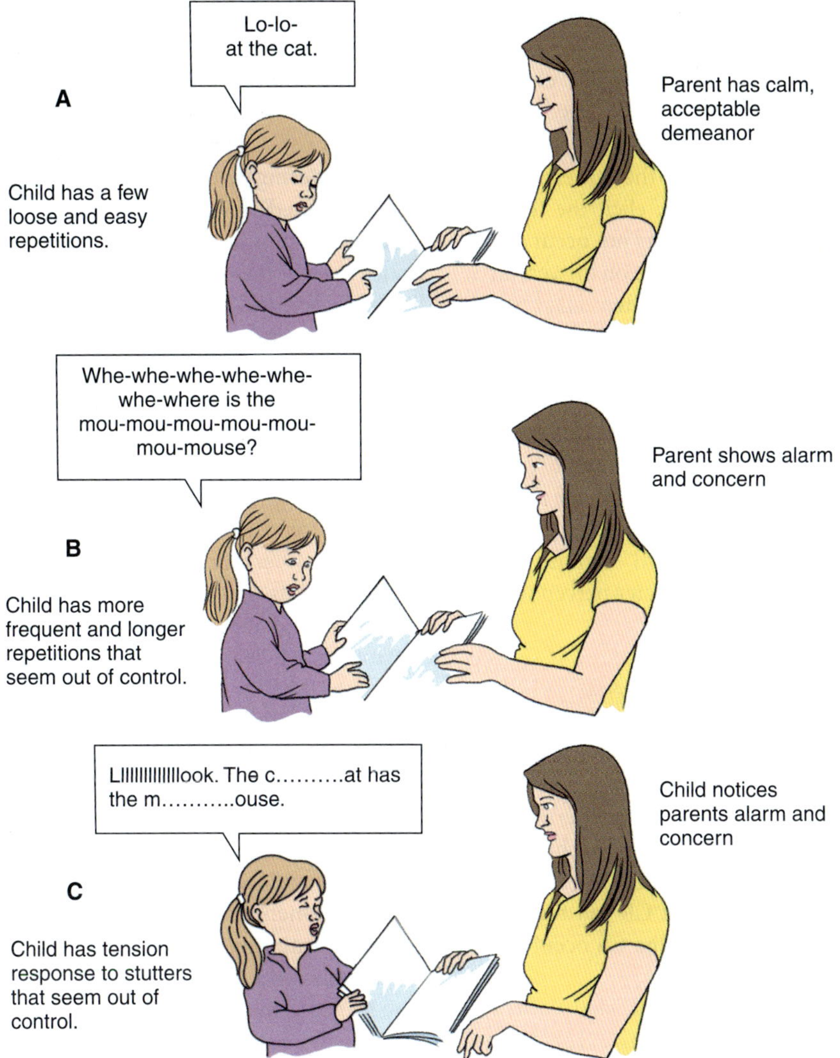

Figure 5.2 Changes in child's speech and parent's response as stuttering becomes more severe. Frame **A** depicts a child's earliest signs of stuttering and parent's calm response. Frame **B** depicts stuttering becoming more serious as more and longer repetitions occur and parent shows concern in her facial expression. Frame **C** depicts a child's more severe stuttering with tense prolongations and blocks. Parent shows alarm and child notices parent's worried facial expression.

Spread of Conditioning

Classical conditioning is an active and continuing process, and it spreads from the initial setting to many, many more situations. When children are disfluent and experience the tension response, a host of stimuli are present in that context. When they stutter, they are talking to someone, uttering a particular word or sound, speaking in a particular room, and talking about a particular topic. Because of the power of classical conditioning, the pairing of these other stimuli with the CS (in this case, the out-of-control repetitions) gives the other stimuli (specific listeners, activities the speaker is involved in, etc.) the potency to elicit the tension response when children are disfluent but also even before any disfluencies occur. The particular sound on which the children stutter, for example, may become conditioned to elicit the tension response, so in the future the children are more likely to produce that sound with tension. As conditioning takes place again and again, the stimulus becomes a complex of many things, as mentioned, including words and sounds, listeners, and physical surroundings or situations. This chaining of stimuli is called "higher-order conditioning" or "second-order conditioning." Gradually, past experiences of the threat stored in the medial temporal lobe memory systems (LeDoux, 2015) create conscious fear in children whenever the memories resurface, and this adds to the dynamics of the spread of conditioning.

The spread of conditioning to other conditioned stimuli results in changes in stuttering as well. Initially, children might emit several repetitive disfluencies or a long prolongation before the tension response occurs. Soon, however, muscle tension occurs earlier and earlier in the stutters. When other conditioned stimuli, such as words, elicit the tension response, the easy repetitive disfluencies may not occur at all. Instead, children may increase muscle tension on the very first sound they try to utter, resulting in what are often called "fixed articulatory postures" that are a sign of advancing stuttering.

As children's stuttering frequency increases as a result of the spread of conditioning to more and more stimuli, the duration of their stuttering may also increase. This can be explained by the fact that the tension response soon becomes a stimulus that itself elicits more tension. After all, the tension response (co-contracted muscles) makes it harder to utter a word, and the experience of "squeezing hard" without being able to speak for a second or two elicits greater perception of threat, leading to a longer tension response.

Extinction of the Conditioned Response

For maintenance of the effects of the out-of-control repetitions or other disfluencies causing the tension response, negative emotion must occur periodically. If negative emotion doesn't occur when there is some mild stuttering, the CR (tension) may stop occurring. That is, in psychological terms, it may be "extinguished." Bouton (2016, pp. 166–171) provides an excellent discussion of how a CR can be extinguished. The heart of the process is that the CS occurs and the CR is prevented.

How does extinction relate to stuttering? Imagine a treatment for stuttering that involves desensitizing clients to the threat of stuttering (eg, Guitar, 2019; Sisskin, 2018; Van Riper, 1973a). The aim of this approach is to present the stimulus repeatedly without arousing negative emotion and thus without the CR. One stage in such treatment might involve having clients repeatedly stutter but in contexts designed to engender a milder emotional response, perhaps even a positive emotion (if, eg, the clinician and a group of colleagues cheer and clap whenever the client stuttered). With enough of this treatment, the expectation of stuttering may no longer elicit the tension response and the client's stuttering may become like a normal disfluency or even fluency. This extinction of the conditioned tension response will usually be done in a specific context: a clinic setting and the presence of a clinician. Several factors—well understood in rat psychology—will influence the durability of the extinction of the CR. Consider ways we can change them as you read about them in the following paragraph.

The simple passing of time after the extinction may cause the CR to reappear. This is the relapse seen so often after stuttering treatment. Not only the passage of time but also change in context can cause relapse. When the client leaves the clinical setting (the treatment situation and the clinician), the tense stuttering (the CR) will often return. Bouton (2016) makes the point that this reappearance affirms the claim that extinction does not destroy the original CR. It stays in the memory of the client, basically forever, especially if the CR (tense stuttering) is learned in childhood and continues to be "reconditioned" for several years. This may happen as stuttering continues to be experienced as a threat and thus continues to elicit the tension response. It seems likely to me that listener responses of alarm or dismay may contribute to the threatening nature of the runaway repetitions or other disfluencies that feel out of the child's ability to cope with them. In children who are cognitively advanced enough, the nonconscious perception of threat is gradually conceptualized by the child as fear. Another thing that may happen is that the individual begins to imagine that the listener has a negative response even though the listener response may be actually neutral. In other words, as children develop cognitively, they develop beliefs that their stuttering is bad and listeners will always be impatient with them when they stutter.

How do we deal with the continuing experience of threat associated with stuttering and the reappearance of stuttering (relapse) after treatment? A key strategy is to begin treatment early, when children can be bathed in positive responses to their speaking, and reactions to their stuttering can be empathetic and accepting. This can extinguish the CR because the stuttering is associated with much less negative emotion. On the other hand, when clients have been stuttering for many years, treatment can involve more extensive disconnection between stuttering and negative emotion, as suggested in the desensitization procedure mentioned earlier. In addition, new learning may be used to teach clients a way to stutter more easily, that feels comfortable and doesn't elicit negative listener responses. To diminish the likelihood of relapse, careful modifying of the therapeutic context should take place. The clinician should work with clients in many situations outside the clinic and should help clients take over the role of being their own clinicians: planning assignments, evaluating the outcomes, and devising improvements. Visits with the clinician can be faded from every week to every other week, to monthly, and gradually less and less frequently. If stuttering reappears in force, frequent visits can be reinstated, until the tension response is extinguished again. Because the memory of the initial conditioning may be permanent, work can also be done via counseling and support group meetings to change the way clients feel about their stuttering—both in the hopes of reducing its occurrence, but even more in hopes of reducing its impact on their feelings of self-worth: an effective communicator and intact individual. Thus, the benefit of Stuttering Pride and the view that Stuttering is OK can both be conceived of within a learning paradigm as well as in other paradigms.

Individual Differences in Conditioning

Before we leave our discussion of classical conditioning, I would like to touch on the topic of individual differences and conditioning. The rapid learning and widespread generalization that is apparent in most stuttering may parallel the "prepared classical conditioning" of some animals that are rapidly and deeply conditioned to naturally dangerous stimuli as snakes (Mineka, 1985). Preparedness in animals—humans included—refers to sensitivity to various objects that could have caused harm to our ancestors (eg, snakes, spiders, hostile strangers). Evolution favored humans, and other animals who were more sensitized to harmful stimuli would have had a greater chance for survival. Thousands of years later, rapid conditioning can occur in individuals with temperaments that are more alert to threatening stimuli. For example, individuals with an anxious temperament are more prone to acquire fears and phobias (Biederman et al., 1995; Mineka & Oehlberg, 2008) and animals that have been exposed to stressful situations—especially those that are unpredictable and uncontrollable—are more easily classically conditioned (Mineka & Oehlberg, 2008; Shors et al., 1992). Thus, it seems likely that those children who stutter and who are especially sensitive may rapidly condition to such threatening stimuli as being unable to say a word, a critical listener response, or a peer who makes fun of their stuttering. This conditioning may be most etched into memory if that word, listener, or peer is particularly important to the child, as might be the case if the word were the child's name, the listener was their parent, or the peer was a close friend or sibling. Brutten and Shoemaker (1969) and Brutten (1986) have made a similar point: that individual differences in emotional reactivity and conditionability are important factors in the developmental patterns of stuttering. A small study by Arenas and Zebrowski (2013) confirmed that individuals who stuttered, compared to a group of nonstutterers, were more autonomically reactive and were more easily classically conditioned. These differences in conditionability, when they occur in children who stutter, may relate to stuttering persistence versus recovery.

Illustration of Classical Conditioning and Stuttering

Let me give you a description of how classical conditioning might actually work in the development of childhood stuttering. I would like to present a girl named Ashley (Fig. 5.3) as an example because, with her kind permission, I have been able to provide a video clip of her early stuttering. You can find the video clip on *Lippincott Connect* under Chapter 1. video "A Young Preschool Child: Borderline Stuttering."

Let's assume that Ashley was born with a predisposition to stutter in the form of a vulnerable speech production system. When Ashley was just 2-and-a-half years old and her

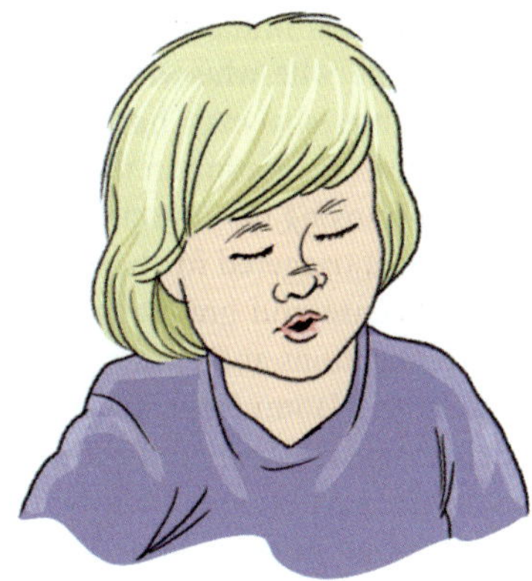

Figure 5.3 Ashley: a young preschool child with borderline stuttering. (see Chapter 1 video "A Young Preschool Child" on Lippincott Connect.)

language development was galloping along, she began to have easy whole- and part-word repetitions in her speech, like "I-I-I" and "whe-whe-whe-when." She didn't even notice them at first.

But, as Ashley's repetitions occurred more and more often, she began (I believe nonconsciously) to react to them as a threat and her response was to "freeze"—a typical response that a person or animal has to threat. Her paired muscles (agonists and antagonists) related to speaking co-contracted simultaneously and her runaway repetitions were stopped in their tracks, so to speak. Ashley's squeezing of her speech muscles were akin to the way your body would tense up if your car started sliding around on an icy road and headed for a tree. This is a reflexive, nonconscious response.

Let's go back to how classical conditioning worked in Ashely's case. Her repetitions were typically most frequent (and she tensed up to stop them) when her mother asked her questions about a picture book they had read together. This context eventually became a CS for Ashley's tension response.

Ashley's tension response was at first a UCR: automatic and nonconscious. However, after many days, the context of her mother asking questions and the repetitions that followed elicited the tension response. Then, the context of her mother asking questions elicited the tension response whenever Ashley tried to answer. That is, because Ashley had often experienced repetitions in answering her mother's questions about the picture book, and she had responded with increased tension, the context of her mother asking questions (previously a neutral stimulus) became a CS for the tension response (previously a UCR) and that became a CR.

Although Ashley's increasing tension in response to her repetitions first occurred with her mother asking her questions, it began to spread or generalize to more and more situations. After many repeated pairings, Ashley began to stutter and do so more tensely to other people and in other places. Several things were responsible for this development of her stuttering. First, the stimulus or cue of her mother became associated with other listeners who asked questions, and then to when Ashley herself initiated the conversation, such as when she asked "Whe-whe-whe-whe-when are we going home?" Then, over time, she may have been consciously aware of "proprioceptive" (sensation in the articulators) cues signaling that she was tensing her muscles before even starting to talk. This, in turn, triggered further tension that made her repetitions more tense and gradually changed some of the stutters into prolongations and blocks.

One of my students, Naomi Rogers, carried out a study that found that children who stuttered showed significantly more pitch rises in their repetitions than typically speaking (control) children showed in their natural repetitions. Pitch rise in repetitions as well as prolongations can be a useful diagnostic sign, indicating that the child is beginning to react to their stuttering and may need treatment.

Operant Conditioning

Here, I will describe another aspect of learning that is key in the development of stuttering: operant conditioning. It differs from classical conditioning in that classical conditioning focuses on the pairing of two stimuli (food and a bell), whereas **operant conditioning** deals with a behavior and its consequences (a rat pushing a lever and receiving a food pellet). These two types of learning have also been contrasted by noting that classical conditioning builds upon an involuntary physiological reaction (eg, salivation; tension as a result of threat) and operant conditioning builds upon a voluntary action. Here's how operant conditioning was first scientifically studied: In the 1930s and 1940s, a psychologist named B.F. Skinner conducted a series of experiments that involved putting a rat in a box that had a lever mechanism for delivering a food pellet. Whenever the rat accidentally hit the lever in the box, a food pellet would roll out of a chute, and, of course, the rat would gobble it up. The rat soon learned to hit the lever deliberately rather than accidentally to receive a food pellet reward. This approach to learning is called operant conditioning, and it happens when an animal (or person) is free to make a response whenever it wants and the response is followed by some consequence. For example, you are free to push an elevator button whenever you feel like it to get the elevator to stop on your floor. You quickly learn to push the button when you want the elevator (your positive reinforcement). You've probably learned it so well that you push the button multiple times if the elevator doesn't come quickly enough.

Operant conditioning is simply the occurrence of a consequence after a behavior is performed that changes the frequency of the behavior. Consequences can be one of three things:

- A positive reinforcer (such as a food pellet), which increases the behavior that preceded it (lever pressing).
- A negative reinforcer (such as experiencing an electric shock and then having it stop). This may be a little harder to grasp, but it works because it is a reinforcer that terminates an unpleasant experience. If a rat is placed on an electric grid and given a continuous shock, the rat will make random movements. One of the random movements may include jumping off the electric grid onto the floor of the cage. This jump will stop the animal from feeling the shock and will increase (reinforce) the behavior (jumping off an electrified grid).
- A punishment (eg, a traffic ticket) during a behavior, which decreases the behavior (speeding in a school zone).

Operant Conditioning and Stuttering

Many clinicians and researchers have suggested that the complicated stuttering behaviors we see in most adults who stutter result from a combination of classical and operant learning (Bloodstein et al., 2021; Brutten & Shoemaker, 1967; Van Riper, 1971a, 1982a). They suggest that whereas classical conditioning is probably responsible for the child's learning to respond to certain stimuli with excess muscle tension suffusing repetitions, prolongations, and blocks, operant conditioning teaches the child to use a variety of secondary behaviors *in response* to the unpleasantness of being stuck. A common secondary behavior is using the articulators to push out a word that is stuck because of the tension that is meant to stop the stutters. If simple pushing doesn't work, then the individual may add a sudden movement of the face or eyes or even of the arms or legs to escape from feeling "jammed up" by having muscle groups that are so tense that movement is impossible. A typical facial movement to release a word is squeezing the eyes shut. The first time this occurs, it might be the result of random struggle behavior. When the squeezing is followed by release of the word, this relieves the emotional pain of being stuck in a stutter and feeling frustrated and embarrassed. The negative reinforcement—escaping a painful experience—makes it more likely the speaker will use the same eye squeezing when stuttering happens again. This is the beginning of an individual's own personalized pattern of stuttering. However, the squeezing of the eyes may not always work to release the stutter, and when it doesn't, the speaker needs to add something else like making a sound such as "uh." Then, the several "escape behaviors"—pushing with the articulators, squeezing the eyes shut, and saying "uh," one right after the other—become part of the speaker's habitual way of responding to being stuck in a stutter. Sometimes one is used and not the others, but in most cases, the child develops a repertoire of escape behaviors.

Illustrations of Operant Conditioning and Stuttering

Ashley, the child we described earlier as being classically conditioned to respond to various speaking-related cues with tension, soon began to show escape behaviors as part of her pattern of stuttering. For example, when she was stuck in a repetitive stutter, she would often just stop trying to say the word and continue talking, omitting the stuttered word. This was an escape behavior that was negatively reinforced; specifically it occurred during the uncomfortable feeling of "stuckness" and was rewarded by relief from that feeling. The video of Ashley on Lippincott Connect (Chapter 1 video "A Young Preschool Child: Borderline Stuttering") shows that escape behavior.

Another child, Katherine, who was a year older than Ashley, developed much tenser blocks than Ashley. After a few months of increasingly tense repetitions and prolongations, Katherine's stuttering had become complete blocks. These blocks created even greater negative emotion, which elicited even greater tension, in a worsening spiral. In fact, occasionally, Katherine's escape behaviors included not just a panicky flailing of her arms when she was jammed up but swinging her arm to hit her mother until the block was released. See Chapter 1 video "An Older Preschool Child: Beginning Stuttering" for an example of this.

Avoidance Conditioning

Avoidance conditioning has been something of a puzzle to learning theorists because it could be considered a type of operant conditioning, but psychologists have been hard-pressed to identify what the reinforcement is (Bouton, 2016). That is, if a child who has previously enjoyed going to his friend's house suddenly starts avoiding his friend's house, why is that rewarding? Probably the best explanation of the dynamics of avoidance learning was given by the psychologist O.H. Mowrer in his "two-factor theory" (Mowrer, 1939; Mowrer & Lamoreaux, 1942). Bouton (2016) suggests that Mowrer's description of avoidance learning is generally accepted today by psychological scientists. Mowrer suggested that the first factor in avoidance learning is Pavlovian or classical conditioning, in which the organism (typically a rat in Mowrer's lab) was given a warning signal such as a buzzer that was followed by an electric shock. In this way, the buzzer became a CS for threat that was aroused because of the impending shock. The rat then learned that if it leapt to another part of its "shuttle box" when the buzzer sounded and the shock was given, the shock stopped. Soon, the rat learned to jump to another part of the box whenever the buzzer sounded, but before the shock was given. The rat could thus avoid the shock by jumping to the safe part of the box when the buzzer sounded. Mowrer postulated that the buzzer elicited fear. This was a key element in the classical conditioning component. But then the avoidance was reinforced by the reduction of fear (threat). This reinforcement was the operant conditioning component. This explanation was confirmed in many later experiments by a legion of psychologists (eg, Brown & Jacobs, 1949; Miller, 1948). According to Bouton (2016), Mower's two-factor theory has been the basis for the analysis and treatment of many human behaviors such as "agoraphobic" avoidance that often accompanies panic disorder and compulsive hand washing in obsessive-compulsive disorder. In agoraphobia, individuals stay home and avoid public places because of a learned fear of crowds that might result in a panic attack. In compulsive hand washing, people wash their hands frequently because of a learned fear of germs. Treatment often consists of systematically extinguishing the fear by helping patients accept the fear and gradually become calm in a threatening situation, with the help of the therapist. LeDoux (2015) supports Mowrer's model as a basis for treatment but suggests that it is not fear (the word Mowrer used) that is extinguished but the nonconscious defensive state that is triggered by the CS (threat). If components of the defensive state in stuttering are nonconscious, extinguishing it in people who stutter will require real creativity.

In the example I gave earlier, in which a child suddenly starts avoiding his friend's house, we would probably find that classical conditioning has caused the friend's house to trigger a defensive state (nonconscious threat) in the child. This could happen if the friend had a birthday party in his house and his parents had invited a clown to perform at the party. The child who developed the avoidance behavior may have been terrified by the clown, and thus the friend's house became a CS associated with the defensive state triggered by the terrifying clown. Once that association has been made, the child's avoidance of his friend's house is rewarded by easing the defensive state ("fear," if it is conscious) when they meet somewhere else—not the friend's house, but the child's own house.

Avoidance Conditioning and Stuttering

The history of stuttering theory and speculation is brimming with ideas about the cause of stuttering itself being avoidance behavior. Many figures in the "Stuttering Hall of Fame" have formulated a view of stuttering as essentially an avoidance reaction to being punished for normal nonfluency. Here are examples: "stuttering is an anticipatory, apprehensive, hypertonic avoidance reaction" (Johnson, 1938); "the stutterer has originally established an avoidance reaction" (Wischner, 1950); stuttering is a result of "anticipatory struggle" (Bloodstein, 1958). I, personally, think it's more accurate to put avoidance behaviors among the secondary symptoms that appear after stuttering has started and learning has taken place, rather than an explanation of its onset. As you now know, stuttering's onset is probably the result of a vulnerable speech production system breaking down under stress. However, I think avoidance is a key concept in the development of stuttering and, therefore, an important aspect of treatment. Avoidance behaviors in stuttering are probably triggered both by nonconscious and conscious cues. These are cues signaling that the person is about to be trapped in a stutter. The avoidance behaviors—such as putting in extra sounds before starting a feared word usually stuttered on, substituting easy words for ones that may be stuttered, or not volunteering in a class discussion—are learned because they reduce the threat and fear and are thus negatively reinforced. They become part of the individual's stuttering pattern, they maintain the emotional response to stuttering, and they may need to be identified and confronted in treatment.

Illustration of Avoidance Conditioning and Stuttering

David began stuttering when he was 3 years old; the onset of his stuttering occurred after his parents were away for a weekend and he and his sister were taken care of by a babysitter. David's mother recalled that she first noticed David's stuttering right after that weekend, while driving him somewhere in the family car with David in a car seat behind her. He started to say something and he got stuck in a tense repetitive stutter, something like "I-I-I-I-I-I" and immediately put his hand over his mouth. In the months following, when he got stuck in a stutter, he would roll his eyes and tense his jaw. It wasn't long before he began to use avoidance behaviors such as putting in extra sounds before saying a feared word and changing how he pronounced words (see how he says "amount" in the video described below) to keep from stuttering on them.

Some examples of David's avoidance behaviors are in the video clip of him on Lippincott Connect, Chapter 1 video "A School-Age Child: Intermediate Stuttering." In Segment 1, notice how he puts in extra words like "and then" and extra sounds like "um" to reduce the fear he feels as he tries to say what he wants to say but can't. In Segment 2, he uses "and then" and another sound like "um" to postpone his attempt on "whoever." In Segment 3, talking to the clinician, he again uses repetitions of "he" to reduce fear as he gets up his courage to say "automatically"—on which he blocks and pushes back in his chair to escape from the block and finish the word. David's avoidance behaviors were very well established by the time he started treatment at age 6. For the first year of therapy, he would only let me indirectly address his stuttering, resisting my attempts to talk with him about it or to show him how to change it. Our initial work together was mostly through play therapy during which I laced my speech with examples of an easier form of stuttering. Then, gradually, with the use of tangible rewards (Jolly Rancher™ candies), I was gradually able to get David to put easier stuttering into his own speech.

SUMMARY

The development of stuttering is a complex process. As you've seen, it involves the accumulation of classical (increasingly tense stuttering), operant (increasing escape behaviors), and avoidance (increasing avoidances) conditioning. As a child stutters more and more over months and years, a host of cognitive and emotional characteristics become wrapped around the stuttering. The question I will be addressing at great length in this book is: How do we unwind this complicated, attitudinally knotted, and emotionally twisted ball of human behavior?

UNLEARNING

In this section, I will describe the unlearning of the three types of learned behavior discussed earlier—classical, operant, and the form that includes both classical and operant conditioning—avoidance. After I describe the general unlearning process for each type of conditioning, I'll briefly depict how the procedure can be applied to stuttering. Note that with stuttering, the unlearning of classical conditioning must be approached differently at different ages because very young individuals will probably not have been conditioned to the same extent that older individuals have. Moreover, the techniques used with adults will be inappropriate for children, given their differences in linguistic and cognitive skills.

Unlearning Classical Conditioning

People with fears and anxieties about spiders, snakes, large crowds, or clowns can be taught to let go of their fears and live without constant worry about these apparent "threats." Imagine a child who developed a fear of a nearby zoo because, once when visiting the zoo with his parents, a large monkey jumped at the bars in front of the child and shrieked. In this case, the zoo started out as an UCS. The child's sudden experience of threat in response to the monkey jumping and shrieking would be nonconscious and natural and is an UCR. Because of the pairing of UCR (threat) and the environment where it happened, the zoo becomes a conditioned stimulus (CR), causing it to elicit the threat and soon after conscious fear. This is like a child's stuttering at first being neutral but if a listener responds badly, chastising the child for stuttering, or if the stuttering begins to feel scary and out of control to the child, it can be experienced as a threat and fear can soon follow.

Back to the child's zoo fear, this fear can be unlearned if the parents soothe the child and give them pieces of their favorite candy when they are near but outside the zoo. Gradually, the child can be taken into the zoo, away from the monkey's cage, given candy and helped to feel calm. Little by little, the child can be brought to the monkey's cage, soothed and given candy. As with clients who stutter, this process is most effective if the relationship between child and parents is strong and supportive. For the child, the initial threat may still be present, but dormant, because it was processed by the amygdala and stored in implicit memory. It can be kept inactive if enough "deconditioning" (undoing the conditioning) takes place to keep the link between the CS and CR uncoupled.

A good example of this approach when working with anxiety disorders comes from the work of Michelle Craske and her team at UCLA (Craske et al., 2014). Treating a young woman (whom she called Julia) who had developed posttraumatic stress disorder as a result of a sexual assault that occurred at a party, the therapist was able to help her deal with recurrent traumatic memories and handicapping avoidance behaviors. Craske and her team used exposure therapy that decoupled the CS-UCS link (the connection between stimuli associated with the sexual assault and the experience of threat triggered by the amygdala). A warm and supportive clinician was able to help Julia explore the imagined bad outcomes from leaving her house, attending parties, and dating. Subsequently, the clinician was able to support Julia in participating in more and more of those activities. Julia discovered that when she didn't avoid these opportunities, bad outcomes didn't occur. Gradually, this treatment reduced Julia's threat-based physiological and emotional experiences substantially, and she was able to resume her normal life. In my opinion, the supportive relationship established by the clinician is as powerful in this treatment as the exposure therapy. In my own experience, my therapist—Charles Van Riper—provided the ideal of a supportive relationship that made all the difference in my ability to turn my stuttering, first, into a minor problem and, eventually, into a source of pride. He appeared to see deep into my soul, and still accept me with all the foibles, faults, and failings he must have seen. He became a partner with me as I battled my years of stuttering fear and shame.

Unlearning Classical Conditioning and Stuttering

With stuttering, as with other classically conditioned behaviors, the aim in treatment is to decouple the link—etched into the amygdala and other areas of the brain—between the CS and the CR. In stuttering, this is the link between the stuttering (and anticipated stuttering) and the defensive tension response (a type of freezing) and eventually negative emotion (which triggers increased muscle tension—the CR). This decoupling can be done in different ways, depending on the client's age. For example, we work with very young children (ages 2-4) to prevent the CS of multiple repetitions from eliciting negative emotion and the resulting tense muscle cocontractions. Changes in the family environment are made to boost the child's natural fluency and prevent or reverse the child's bad feelings about his early stuttering. It is essential for the family to respond to the child's stuttering with acceptance as part of an overall strengthening of the caregiver-child bond. Open acknowledgment of the child's stuttering accompanied by comments that let the child know that stuttering is OK will help (eg, Bloodstein et al., 2021). At the same time, the family is using strategies—like a slow speech rate with many pauses—to facilitate the child's growing fluency.

When children are slightly older (ages 4-6), but still in their preschool years, we also use a combination of increasing natural fluency by having parents and clinician use a slow but natural speech rate and pauses, as well as preventing negative emotion from being associated with speaking. This is done through much more structured practice and the use of rewards and very gentle requests for the child to say the word again, followed by praise when they repeat it fluently. For us, we may carry out this unlearning by using the Lidcombe Program, but other effective approaches are available. de Sonnerville-Koedoot et al. (2015) found that an approach that reduced demands on the child and enhanced the child's capacities was as effective as the Lidcombe Program when children were reassessed 18 months after treatment. All approaches require extensive warm support and guidance by a speech-language pathologist with expertise in stuttering.

Once the child reaches school age (ages 6-12), treatment can be targeted to elicit the CS (the CS of stuttering) and make sure it is followed not by the CR (the UCS of a defensive reaction or negative emotion) but instead by neutral or even positive emotion. For example, the exercises in Danra Kazenski's "Silly Stuttering" program described in Chapter 14 (see the figure depicting Danra and her client) are designed to reduce the defensive reaction and negative emotion associated with stuttering. In most effective treatments for school age children, treatment is done in a very supportive context in which the child engages in games and activities to decouple the links with defensive reactions and negative emotions. Treatment provides children repeated activities in which they experience the stuttering as being under their control and thus nonthreatening. This leads to reduced negative anticipation of stuttering, which promotes fluency. As with all ages, undoing the conscious and nonconscious beliefs about negative listener responses is critical. The clinician should form a warm and accepting relationship with the client. This can be the basis of a "re-transcription" of the individual's conscious and nonconscious memory of listener rejection. In other words, a strong relationship with a caring clinician can help the clients relearn that listeners will—for the most part—accept the stuttering and even more so if the client accepts it themselves.

In adults and adolescents, the decoupling of the CS (CS of stuttering) with the CR (CR of defensive reaction and negative emotion) is done more directly, by educating the client about the likelihood that his stuttering is "kept hot" by negative feelings associated with the anticipation and experience of stuttering, as well as by his avoidance and escape behaviors. When they are ready, these individuals are shown how to go directly into the stutter (without avoidances) and experience it as tolerable, draining away the negative emotion, via coaching and praise by a clinician who has forged a strong relationship with the client (Fig. 5.4).

This therapy is done by gradual desensitization (reducing the threat and fear) of clients to their stuttering, starting in the safe environment of the clinic and moving to more and more challenging real-world situations while keeping up the clinician's support and praise. In our clinic, we often take clients out on the sidewalk or to a nearby store, where we stop passers-by and practice open and easy stuttering as we pile on the admiration of the clients' work. As clients stop fighting

Unlearning Classically Conditioned Tense Stuttering

Before Treatment

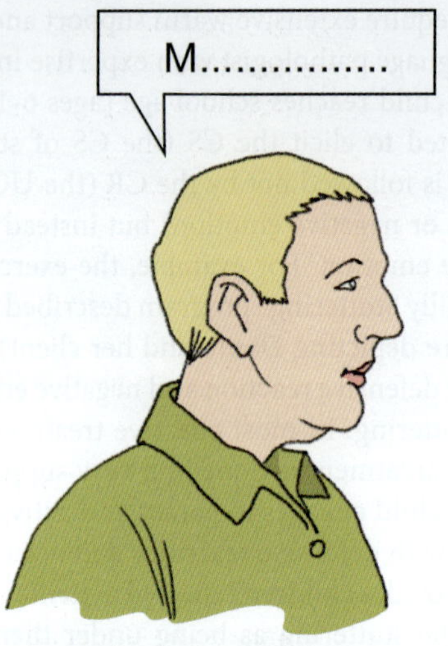

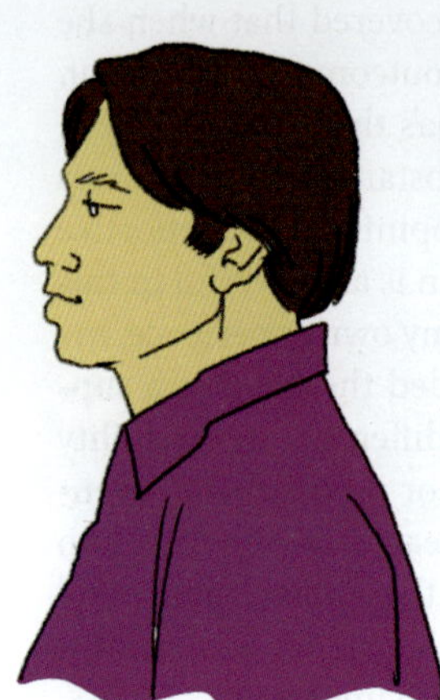

During Treatment

CS
Being in stutter
CR
Relaxed stuttering
M....MMMMM
Just stay in the stutter. Good job! Nice!

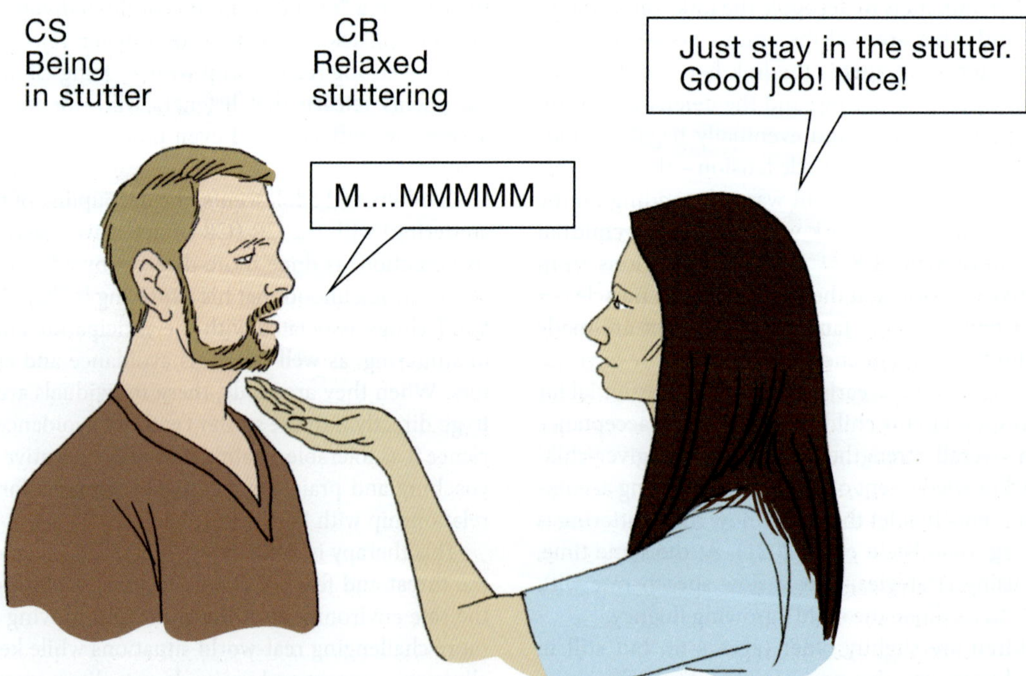

Figure 5.4 Unlearning classically conditioned tense stuttering. CR, conditioned response; CS, conditioned stimulus.

the stutter and are able to reduce the feeling of threat and fear that the stuttering has typically elicited, they discover that the physical tension in their muscles reduces and they are able to release the word more easily. Through repeatedly being able to release the stutter without struggle, the individuals stop being threatened by and being afraid of their stuttering and are able to stop using avoidance and escape behaviors. This sounds simple enough, but most individuals require extensive support and coaching before they can accomplish this. As I described earlier in this chapter in the section on extinction of the CR and possible subsequent relapse, it is important that the decoupling of the CS and the CR continue to take place—both with the clinician's support and by clients on their own—in a host of real-world contexts.

Unlearning Operant Conditioning

An example of the unlearning of operantly conditioned behaviors is the treatment for drug addiction. Drug users become drug users in part because of operant conditioning. Heroin and methamphetamine, for example, provide a reward so strong and so immediate that an addict is willing to forgo food, friends, and family just to get a fix. Some addicts can unlearn their addictive behaviors if operant condition is used to reward healthy behaviors and punishment immediately follows bad behaviors. A partner can provide love and attention to an addicted person who comes home after work "clean." The same partner could also withdraw love and attention by going to their room and locking the door if the addicted person comes home high. Treatment for addiction is notoriously difficult, but the principles of immediately rewarding drug-free behavior with a truly valued activity and strongly punishing addictive behavior can be successful for some addicts in a highly controlled program (Horvath et al., 2016).

Unlearning Operant Conditioning and Stuttering

Most theorists and clinicians do not believe that the core behaviors of stuttering—repetitions, prolongations, and blocks—are caused by operant conditioning (eg, Bloodstein et al., 2021). However, there is agreement that much of the abnormality of stuttering—escape behaviors such as facial contortions, eye blinks, head nods, and finger snapping—are maintained by operant conditioning (eg, Van Riper, 1982a). With children, treatment often produces fluency without the need for specific undoing of the escape behaviors. Children learn to speak more fluently, are relieved of the bad feelings tied to stuttering, and stop using the escape behaviors, all as happy side effects of learning to talk with easier stuttering.

The same side effects may occur when older children, adolescents, and adults are taught to stop fighting the moment of stuttering, accept the stuttering, and release the word easily. However, on the way to this goal, the clinician may need to educate the client about why the slow, easy release of a stuttered word is critical: because it stops the tension, struggle, and escape behaviors from being operantly reinforced by the reward and relief of getting the word out.

Unlearning Avoidance Conditioning

In my earlier example of unlearning classical conditioning, I described the treatment of Julia, a young lady who avoided parties, dates, and going out to visit friends and family because she had been sexually assaulted at a party. Thanks to treatment, Julia was able to uncouple the association between the CS (conditioned stimuli that now reminded her of the terrible incident—such as being at a party) and the UCS (the experience of threat and terror). As the therapist helped her gradually feel more and more comfortable leaving the house, she was able to stop avoiding parties and dates and resume her active life.

Unlearning Avoidance Conditioning and Stuttering

I will start this section with a clinical warning about working with older children and adults who stutter: Don't take away avoidance behaviors before you've helped the individual to deal with the stuttering. I learned this lesson the hard way. Once, I suggested to a client on our waiting list that he didn't need to use the "uh" that he was using as an avoidance behavior (a starter) before saying a feared word. He was not scheduled to start treatment for another month. When he did come in for therapy, he had dropped the "uh" but replaced it with "mmm...well, well, well...that is" followed by a mighty head snap that accompanied his attempt to say a word. I had made his stuttering worse because I had taken away his avoidance behavior without helping him first manage his stuttering.

After your clients learn how to handle anticipated stuttering and the threat and fear that often accompany anticipated stuttering, they may spontaneously drop their avoidance behaviors. In my treatment of older children, adolescents, and adults, after I establish a strong supportive relationship, I teach them first to go right into the sound they fear and stay in it while I help them reduce the negative emotion. A crucial aspect of this is to provide an environment in which stuttering is accepted and clients' staying in the moment of stuttering is rewarded. As the negative emotion subsides, they find that the physical tension diminishes and they are able to finish the word more easily and slowly. You can see this in several of the videos on Lippincott Connect. For example, in the Chapter 11 video called *CM Trial Therapy* (02:50 to 04:45), you'll see a young boy holding onto stutters and loosening them. After he has had a little therapy, the same boy is able to demonstrate this in *Cam's Popcorn Video* (Chapter 15). Watch a few minutes of the video, beginning at 02:44. As my clients gradually master this technique, they can drop the avoidances they have built up over the years and go right into the word they plan to say and feel better about facing down the fear that was the driving force behind their avoidances. For many individuals, this isn't easy. It will take some time before they reduce their fears and learn that actively seeking out difficult situations and using feared words gives them increased fluency and confidence in saying whatever they want to say wherever they want to say it.

In the treatment sections of the book, I will describe other approaches designed to achieve the same outcome.

SUMMARY

- The onset of stuttering in children is typically the result of neurophysiological differences manifesting as multiple part-word and single-syllable whole-word repetitions. These signs of stuttering often appear when developmental and/or environmental stresses are strong.
- The development of stuttering—from repetitions to prolongations and blocks with concomitant escape and avoidance behaviors and with attitudinal and emotional overlays—is driven by learning factors.
- Because of classical conditioning, milder stuttering is linked to a nonconscious defensive state that triggers increased tension (a form of "freezing"). As stutters become increasingly tense, they are transformed from repetitions into prolongations and blocks.
- As stuttering continues to be experienced as an unpleasant threat, the child will use escape behaviors to terminate the unpleasant experience. An example of an escape behavior is a child being caught in a series of tight repetitions and then squeezing their eyes shut to get the word out. Because of operant conditioning, this behavior will occur more frequently; the escape from the unpleasant threat rewards the squeezing.
- Children who stutter also learn to avoid stuttering as well as escape from it. If children have learned to associate particular words or situations with the unpleasant, threatening experience of being caught in a stutter, they will also learn to change words or stay away from certain situations, so that they will not encounter that threatening experience. Both classical and operant conditioning play a role in this avoidance learning.
- As suggested in the previous paragraph, the conditioning process gradually spreads to more and more cues, like sounds, words, people, and situations.
- Important individual differences affect the learning process. More rapid conditioning occurs with people who have more anxious temperaments and are, therefore, more alert to threatening stimuli.
- The conditioning that has caused stuttering to develop can be unlearned or even prevented: (1) In young children who have not experienced their stuttering as threatening, parents can do much to keep this from happening. (2) In slightly older preschool children whose stuttering does create the experience of threat and fear, increased fluency can be learned, and the conditioned negative experiences of stuttering can be undone through positive experiences. (3) In older children, adolescents, and adults who experience much threat and fear and many escape and avoidances, new learning can gradually extinguish the tension response and the secondary behaviors and attitudes.

STUDY QUESTIONS

1. Some stuttering experts in the past have suggested that the onset of stuttering is caused by operant conditioning. What ideas could you come up with to support the idea that the onset of stuttering is the result of operant conditioning?
2. How would you explain to a parent, in simple language, that classical conditioning has caused their child's stuttering to change from easy, loose repetitions to tightly squeezed blocks? Can you think of analogous experience that the parent might have had?
3. Describe how someone might develop a fear of spiders. Use the classical conditioning paradigm, indicating what are the unconditioned and conditioned stimuli and responses.
4. Add to the above example the concepts of "preparedness" and "anxious temperament."
5. Design a strategy ("treatment") for someone who has developed a fear of public speaking.
6. Explain the separate roles of classical conditioning and operant conditioning in avoidance conditioning.
7. If a child learns to decrease their conditioned tension response (and thus learns to stutter easily and loosely) only in a therapy room, what might happen when the child stutters in their classroom?
8. Go back to the four examples of how learning can affect stuttering after it begins that were given in the Introduction section of this chapter. Identify the type of learning that takes place in each example. Then describe the therapy you would apply to undo the learning in each example.

SUGGESTED READINGS

Bouton, M. (2016). *Learning and behavior: A contemporary synthesis* (2nd ed.). Sinauer Associates, Inc.

This is a clear and lively description of the principles of learning, as well as how these principles can be applied to treatments. Bouton has been called "the leading expert in the study of extinction [of behaviors] in animals" (LeDoux, 2015) and presents the latest research and thinking about learning.

Brutten, E. J., & Shoemaker, D. J. (1967). *The modification of stuttering*. Prentice-Hall, Inc.

This is a classic book in the field of stuttering. It describes a theory of stuttering that ascribes the initial symptoms of childhood stuttering to the effect of anxiety on fluency and ascribes the later symptoms to learning. The authors go on to suggest therapeutic approaches that derive from their model.

LeDoux, J. (2015). *Anxious: Using the brain to understand and treat fear and anxiety*. Viking.

LeDoux has written other landmark books, such as The Emotional Brain, Synaptic Self, and The Deep History of Ourselves: The Four-Billion-Year Story of How We Got Conscious Brains.

However, the book titled Anxious is the most relevant to stuttering. It advances LeDoux's views on fear and anxiety and their treatment. From his perspective, fear is not a basic response to threat, but a cognitively synthesized emotion. Fear and anxiety derive from nonconscious responses to threat. These low-level defensive automatic responses include hypertonic behaviors such as freezing. I think our understanding of stuttering may be improved if we take these into consideration.

6

Theories About Stuttering

Chapter Outline

Chapter Objectives

After studying this chapter, readers should be able to:

- Explain what a theory is and what hypotheses are
- Identify trends in/approaches to theories of stuttering
- Describe the author's integrated two-factor view of stuttering

Key Terms

Anomalous neural organization: Brain structure and function that differ from the typical. This sometimes refers to delayed development in myelination of white matter that interferes with connections between different areas of the brain. In some cases, the developing brain substitutes other structures or uses other, sometimes longer and, therefore, less efficient pathways to try to resolve the problem

Autonomic reactivity: The tendency of the autonomic nervous system to respond quickly and strongly to particular stimuli. The sympathetic part of the autonomic nervous system is responsible for the flight-or-fight response and causes the heart, respiratory system, and other organs to be ready for action

Behavioral inhibition system: A view developed by psychologist Gray (1987) that humans are endowed with a hard-wired protective response to a threat; the body's response in this situation is freezing, flight, or avoidance. Freezing has been described as a response to threat that involves immobility created by increased muscle tonus (Hagenaars et al., 2014). Flight occurs if the threatening object (eg, a predator) is encountered. Avoidance takes place quickly and often even before conscious awareness if the individual can detect or predict the threatening object before it is encountered. Actions can then be taken so that the threatening object is not encountered

Capacities and demands: A view of stuttering (often called the demands and capacities model) that suggests that stuttering results when the demands (eg, pressure to talk rapidly) put on a child's speech are greater than the child's capacity for fluency (eg, capacity to manage the complex components of spoken language production while speaking rapidly)

Communicative failure and anticipatory struggle: A view of stuttering that supposes that stuttering begins when a child experiences problems with communication (eg, having many repetitions or being told they must try harder to say sounds correctly). The child may develop a fear of having difficulty, which then causes tension and fragmentation of speech

Corticobasal ganglia thalamocortical loop: A neural circuit that processes signals from the cerebral cortex going to several basal ganglia structures and back to the cortex for execution. This circuit is responsible for timing and sequencing of speech segments to ensure the smooth, rapid flow of articulation. Several authors have proposed ways in which various components of the circuit may be dysfunctional in stuttering

"Covert repair" hypothesis: An explanation of stuttering suggesting that stuttering occurs as the result of the brain's stopping production of speech when it detects an error in the plan that the brain has made to produce a word

Diagnosogenic theory: The idea that stuttering is caused by the misdiagnosis of typical disfluencies as stuttering, usually by parents. This misdiagnosis causes parents to respond to typical disfluencies with disapproval and anxiety, thus causing children to try not to be disfluent, making their disfluencies tenser, with more struggle, escape, and avoidance behaviors

Hemispheric dominance: In general, the phenomenon that one hemisphere of the brain (left or right) takes the lead or is stronger for a particular function. In the context of this chapter, hemispheric dominance refers to the fact that the left side of the brain is usually more specialized for speech and language than the right side

Hypothesis: A specific and testable proposition derived from a theory. For example, in a theory that proposes that stuttering is caused by lack of hemispheric dominance for speech, a hypothesis might be that, using brain imaging, all individuals who stutter will show equal activity in right and left sides of the brain rather than the expected greater activity in the left side of the brain consistent with hemispheric dominance

Inverse internal models of the speech production system: A concept about how your brain functions when you learn to talk as a child and as you are talking as an adult. The basic idea is that as a child hears speech in his environment, they store auditory and kinesthetic images of the sounds and words. During babbling, they learn how to send motor commands to their muscles to make those sounds and words. These connections create the internal model for speech production. They are called inverse because they start out as the auditory and kinesthetic images or targets but get "inverted" to become the motor commands needed to hit those auditory targets

Multifactorial dynamic disorder: Stuttering may be seen as multifactorial because many factors (eg, genetic, emotional, cognitive, social, environmental) interact to create it. It is also dynamic because the overt signs of stuttering are seen as surface manifestations of an ever-changing neurophysiological process underlying the disorder

Myelination: The development of an insulating sheath around nerve fibers, increasing the speed and integrity of neural transmission. Myelination occurs primarily before age 5, although it continues until early adulthood and is achieved in left-hemisphere frontotemporal tracts before the right-hemisphere tracts

Primary stuttering: Early stuttering, near the onset of the disorder, that is usually characterized by loose, easy repetitions. For those children who begin stuttering in this fashion, it is assumed that initially they are unaware of their stuttering and do not react to it

Secondary stuttering: Stuttering characterized by tension and struggle and sometimes by escape behaviors and avoidances. In some views, this type of stuttering is thought to be a reaction to primary stuttering, as the child becomes self-conscious and frustrated by their difficulty with speaking

Sensorimotor modeling: The process of building "maps" that code the motor commands to hit the auditory (and kinesthetic and proprioceptive) targets that the speaker intends; a bidirectional process in which maps that code the motor commands are adjusted if errors are detected in the auditory and kinesthetic signal

Sensory targets: These are essentially the auditory targets mentioned in the last definition, but actually the targets contain not only auditory information but also information about the movements of the articulators (kinesthetic and proprioceptive information)

Theory: A comprehensive explanation of a phenomenon. Regarding stuttering, a theory might explain why some people stutter and others don't. Theories are expected to be quite formal, so I use the term "theoretical perspective" to indicate the rudimentary explanations available thus far to help us understand stuttering

What are theories, and what can we learn from them? A **theory** puts together findings in a systematic way so that past phenomena are explained and future ones are predicted. For example, a theory about tsunamis explains that they are caused by earthquakes on the ocean floor, explains the processes by which they are caused, and predicts that when a large undersea earthquake occurs again, another tsunami will occur. A theory about stuttering would take the many facts, findings, and observations that you have been reading about in the first five chapters and put them together to explain why one person stutters and another does not, and why one child recovers from stuttering without treatment and another does not. A complete theory would also explain why a person stutters on some words and not others or in some situations and not others and why people who stutter do the things they do when they stutter. When a theory can explain these things well, we believe it can lead to more effective treatments. When we know much more about what causes stuttering, we hope to have a better chance of being able to modify the conditions leading to it and thereby even prevent it.

Scientists often use the word "theory" to mean a formal set of hypotheses that explain the important causal relationships in a phenomenon. These hypotheses are then tested, and the theory may be thrown out, improved, or partially confirmed as a result. The field of stuttering research and treatment hasn't developed far enough to have a formal theory of stuttering, although there are a number of informal theories that might be called "theoretical perspectives" or theoretical models.

In this chapter, I present several theoretical perspectives on stuttering as well as my own attempt to integrate research and clinical findings into a two-factor theoretical perspective. I have organized existing perspectives according to how they approach the descriptive task but will also connect these with the constitutional, developmental, and environmental factors, and learning processes they entail. Theoretical models in stuttering change every few years as more data are gathered on stuttering and new information is generated in related areas. Without a doubt, the explanations of stuttering I summarize in this chapter, including my own, will be superseded by others in a few years. I have chosen several contemporary views of constitutional factors to discuss in the following sections. Although the views differ, they are not mutually exclusive. If linked together, they provide us with some interesting notions about what factors might be inherited or acquired and how that might result in stuttering.

THEORETICAL PERSPECTIVES ABOUT CONSTITUTIONAL FACTORS IN STUTTERING

Stuttering as a Disorder of Brain Organization

Many studies of both normal speakers and brain-damaged patients have demonstrated that the left hemisphere is dominant for language in most people. This means that areas in the left hemisphere are specialized for processing language and that the right hemisphere is subservient to the left, playing a less important, but still significant role in the production and comprehension of language.

One early theory of stuttering suggested that it is caused by lack of **hemispheric dominance** (the Orton-Travis theory of stuttering referred to in Chapter 2). The theory came about in the following way: In an atmosphere of intense scientific curiosity and collaboration among researchers at the University of Iowa in the 1920s, Samuel Orton, a neurologist, and Lee Edward Travis, a psychologist and speech pathologist, observed that many stutterers seemed to have been left handers whose parents changed them into being right handed (Travis, 1931). Because the therapy that derived from the theory depended on switching stutterers back to being left handed turned out to be unsuccessful, the original cerebral dominance theory of stuttering languished for many years.

In the 60s and 70s, evidence began to mount that stutterers may not, after all, have normal left-hemisphere dominance for language. Then, in 1985, a new version of the cerebral dominance theory of stuttering was proposed. Two neurologists, Norman Geschwind and Albert Galaburda, suggested that many disorders, including stuttering, dyslexia, and autism, resulted from delays in left-hemisphere growth during fetal development that led subsequently to right-hemisphere dominance for speech and language (Geschwind & Galaburda, 1985). The delay in left-hemisphere growth accompanied by timely development of the right hemisphere that resulted in what appeared to be predominantly male disorders was thought to be caused by a male-related factor. Geschwind and Galaburda hypothesized that these delays might result from fetal exposure to excess testosterone during embryonic development. So far, however, no evidence has been found to support their **hypothesis** about testosterone. In fact, Neilson et al. (1987) provided some evidence against this hypothesis, but the idea of a delay in left-hemisphere development continues to be of great interest.

In Geschwind and Galaburda's hypothesis, underdevelopment of the left hemisphere as the central nervous system matures causes specialized nerve cells for speech and language to migrate to the more well-developed right hemisphere instead. These specialized cells then organize themselves as "networks" of neural activity in the right hemisphere for processing of speech and language. However, because the right hemisphere is not designed by its architecture and interconnections for this function, speech and language operate inefficiently there. Figure 6.1 shows the result of the inappropriate location of speech networks in the right hemisphere combined with inefficient speech networks in the left hemisphere: poorly timed speech with disruptions.

William Webster proposed another version of the view that stuttering results from a different problem with brain organization—one in which a dysfunctional left hemisphere

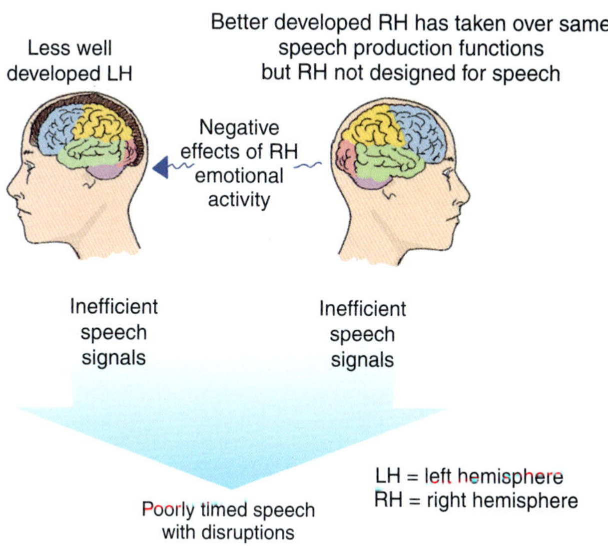

Figure 6.1 Stuttering as a disorder of brain organization.

continues to be the main location for activity involved in speech and language production. Webster hypothesizes that the supplementary motor area (SMA), typically involved in the motor speech production, is vulnerable to disruption by activity in other areas of the brain. In particular, he suspected that individuals who stutter often may have overactive right hemispheres and speculated that overflow of right-hemisphere activation, especially from right hemisphere–regulated emotions (eg, threat, fear, excitement), could disrupt SMA functions in planning, initiating, and sequencing speech motor output being generated by the left hemisphere.

Stuttering as a Disorder of Timing

Several authors believe that the known facts about stuttering point to the value of conceiving it as a disorder of timing (Fig. 6.2). For example, Van Riper (1982a, p. 415) stated that "when a person stutters on a word, there is a temporal disruption of the simultaneous and successive programming of muscular movements required to produce one of the word's integrated sounds..." Building on Van Riper's view, Kent (1984) marshaled several lines of evidence to support a hypothesis that stuttering arises from a deficit in temporal programming. He speculated that this deficit reflects the inappropriate localization of speech and language functions to the right hemisphere. Like a conductor of a symphony orchestra who determines when each section plays, as well as its speed or tempo, mechanisms in the brain control the rate at which we speak and the order of movements for producing sequential sounds. Just as the conductor integrates the timing of an orchestra's several sections, the brain must coordinate complex timing relationships for phonemes, syllables, and phrases of speech, as well as prosody.

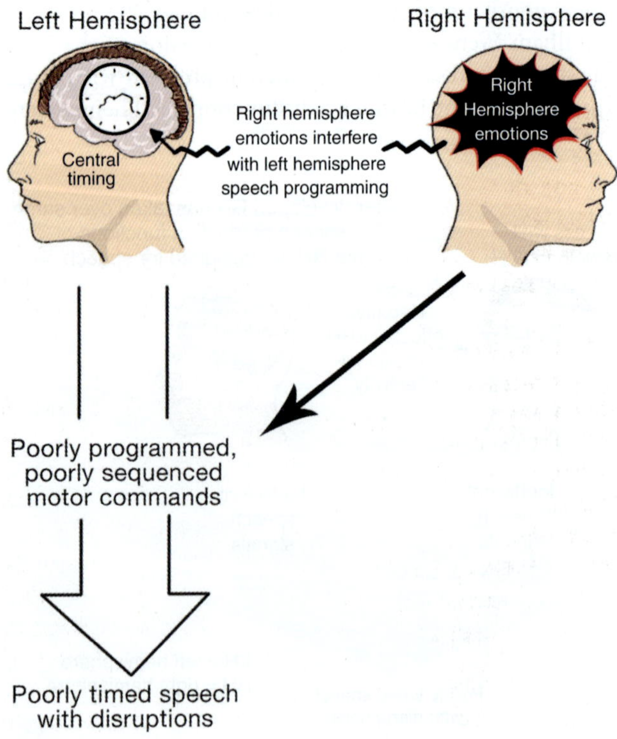

Figure 6.2 Stuttering as a disorder of timing.

Kent (1984) suggested that the inability to perform precise timing functions consistently may stem from the problem that the left hemisphere of a person who stutters may be less well developed than the right hemisphere (cf., Geschwind & Galaburda, 1985) and may be vulnerable to interference from right hemisphere negative emotions. Because the left hemisphere is specialized for processing brief, rapidly changing events such as those needed for fine motor control of verbal output, a person who stutters may be disadvantaged when trying to process at the rapid speed required for normal speech. This central timing function, Kent points out, not only must regulate left-hemisphere aspects of speech production but also must integrate the production of rapid, left hemisphere–generated speech segments with the slower prosodic elements of speech that are generally functions of the right hemisphere.

Kent also noted that emotion may play an important role in disrupting the timing of the speech of someone who stutters. As I indicated earlier, the right hemisphere is believed to be heavily involved in the regulation of certain negative emotions. The deficit of a person who stutters, then, may be that his timing functions for speech are arranged so that they are (1) less efficient than those of nonstutterers and (2) vulnerable to interference by right-hemisphere activity during increased emotion. How exactly this deficit causes the repetitions, prolongations, and blocks we hear in stutterers' speech is not explained in this theory.

Another view of stuttering as a disorder of timing was proposed by Alm (2004). As explained in the next section, he attributed much of the problem to malfunctions in the basal ganglia.

Stuttering as a Problem in the Corticobasal Ganglia-Thalamocortical Loop

As you may remember from Chapter 2: "Primary Etiological Factors in Stuttering," the basal ganglia are a group of interconnected subcortical structures at the top of the brainstem. Working together, these structures regulate body movement, facilitating and inhibiting motor programs. In typical speech production, it is the left hemisphere corticobasal ganglia-thalamocortical loop (hereinafter referred to as the "BG loop") that is active and where the deficits for stuttering are thought, in this view, to be located. The first stage of activity of the BG loop for speech production is that the cortical networks in cognitive, sensory, and motor areas of the language-dominant hemisphere send information about movement plans and intended execution down to the *striatum*. This is a part of the basal ganglia composed of the *caudate nucleus* and the *putamen*. Other parts of the basal ganglia include the *globus pallidus*, the *substantia nigra*, and *subthalamic nucleus*. Control of movement by these structures is almost like highway flaggers using their signs to facilitate traffic flow (voluntary movement) by stopping some traffic, but allowing other traffic to flow. In the corticobasal ganglia-corticothalamic loop, motor programs for syllable production can be instantly initiated or terminated so that speech flows rapidly from one syllable to the next. The signals from the cortex controlling motor movement can follow two different pathways. In the "Direct Pathway," which initiates movement, signals go through the striatum (caudate nucleus and putamen) and to the globus pallidus *internus* to prevent that structure from inhibiting the signals from the thalamus. This disinhibition allows the thalamus to send excitatory signals back up to the motor cortex, which then releases the next appropriate motor program for the desired syllable. The "Indirect Pathway" does the opposite. It stops inappropriate movement, causing the just-completed syllable to cease, and it also stops competing (similar-but-wrong) motor programs from being executed. The indirect pathway consists of the signal from the cortex going through the striatum to the globus pallidus *externus*. This then sends signals to the subthalamic nucleus, which, in turn, sends signals to the globus pallidus internus to cause it to inhibit the thalamus from sending "go" signals to the motor cortex.

In our metaphor of flaggers controlling traffic flow on a highway under construction, in order to speed up traffic flow, flaggers nowadays use two-way radios to communicate quickly with each other when to start and when to stop traffic flow. Similarly, the basal ganglia use *dopamine*—a neurotransmitter—to ramp up the speed of exciting or inhibiting the production of syllables via the motor cortex. Dopamine is released by the substantia nigra and goes to the striatum where it acts on both the direct and indirect pathways. Dopamine's action on the direct pathway increases activation of movement via the first dopamine receptor (D1) in the striatum. When the D1 receptor is stimulated by dopamine, a signal goes out to the globus pallidus internus to cause the thalamus to send a particularly strong activation signal to the cortex to stimulate movement. In contrast, dopamine's action via the D2 receptor in the striatum is to send inhibitory signals to the globus pallidus externus, which would typically be involved in inhibition of movement, but because D2's role in disinhibition of the globus pallidus externus, the end result is that the thalamus is enabled to activate inappropriate movements via the cortex. Thus, a very careful balance of dopamine flow is critical for maintaining the activation and inhibition patterns that allow for (1) rapid initiation of appropriate motor programs at the right time and (2) inhibition of "finished" motor programs at the right time, as well as (3) inhibition of inappropriate competing motor programs.

How does this go wrong in stuttering? One of the earlier perspectives on the role of the basal ganglia in stuttering was suggested by Alm (2004). As a person who stutters, Alm was very aware of the ameliorative effect on stuttering of imposed timing cues, for example, through singing, choral reading, and speaking in time to a metronome. His personal commitment inspired him to write his Ph.D. thesis on how the basal ganglia and its interconnections with the cerebral cortex may be critical in providing internal timing cues to control speech production and how this may go wrong (Alm, 2005). Before he finished his thesis, he published a detailed account of how the basal ganglia and its interconnections may be involved in stuttering (Alm, 2004). He suggested that parts of the basal ganglia loop are malfunctioning. As I said earlier, the BG loop begins with signals from the cortex to the striatum (putamen and caudate) and ends with the signal from the thalamus back to the cortex, activating appropriate movement via the SMA. In this case, when the BG loop malfunctions, there are no appropriate *internal* timing cues for initiation of movement and appropriate stoppage of movement, coming through the BG loop. Fluency can only be sustained by *external* timing cues (metronome, etc.) coming through the lateral premotor cortex.

Alm (2004) speculated that one cause of the BG loop's breakdown may be excessive activity in D2 receptors and greater D2 density compared to D1 density. The excess activity in D2 receptors causes the release of inappropriate motor activity, which is usually (but not in this case) inhibited through the thalamus. The breakdown may also come from excess release of dopamine overall and, possibly, deficits elsewhere in the BG loop. It is interesting that Turk et al. (2021) hypothesized that excess dopamine in the basal ganglia may disrupt laryngeal coordination in stuttering. One piece of evidence supporting the excess D2 hypothesis is the effectiveness of the dopaminergic drugs (antipsychotic medications) such as haloperidol (a D2 blocker) in reducing stuttering severity (Gattuso & Leocata, 1962). However, other studies have found that a dopamine stimulant drug—amphetamine, that has the opposite effect of haloperidol (a tranquilizer)—is effective with a different group of stutterers than those helped by haloperidol (Fish and Bowling, 1962, 1965). This evidence led Alm to endorse the idea that stuttering is a heterogeneous disorder with multiple subtypes.

Another hypothesis about the role of the BG loop in stuttering was proposed by Smits-Bandstra and De Nil (2007). These authors reviewed four research studies they had conducted demonstrating that subjects who stuttered were poorer than control subjects at learning sequences. The first task involved reading sequences of nonsense syllables; the second tested subjects' abilities to finger tap in a certain sequence; the third task involved reading nonsense syllables and remembering them at the same time they were involved in another task; the fourth task involved finger tapping while also engaging in another activity at the same time. In each study, findings indicated that the individuals who stuttered were poorer at sequence skill learning and automatization of this skill. These researchers then made the case that the BG loop (the basal ganglia and their connections with the cerebral cortex) must be dysfunctional in stuttering. Smits-Bandstra and De Nil presented research from many other scientists over many years to support the argument that the BG loop is critical in sequence skill learning and automatization. They also make strong arguments about why this hypothesis explains the period of onset of stuttering and the sex ratio and recovery patterns of stuttering. Unfortunately, it appears that many reviews of work on the BG loop appears to overlook Smit-Bandstra and De Nil's several published studies on this topic.

In a more recent publication, Chang and Guenther (2020) presented a model influenced by Alm's (2004) hypothesis that the dysfunctions in the corticobasal ganglia-corticothalamic loop may be the basis for many cases of stuttering. Using the GODIVA, their computer-based simulation of how the brain produces speech, the authors developed a digital representation of the corticobasal ganglia loop and proposed three possible problems in the BG loop that could cause stuttering. Figure 6.3, from Chang and Guenther (2020), depicts these three areas of dysfunction.

Before describing these dysfunctions, I'll briefly retrace the activities of the BG loop. Syllable production begins with planning of the desired syllable in the desired context, taking into account where the articulators are and what is needed to enact the appropriate motor program. This information is transmitted from the cerebral cortex to the striatum (putamen and caudate nucleus). From there, with involvement of dopamine receptors (D1 and D2), signals progress to the globus pallidus and the substantia nigra. Using messages of activation and inhibition, the signal goes on to the thalamus and then to the motor cortex (SMA). In this way, the BG loop initiates the syllable, terminates it at the appropriate time, starts the next one, and inhibits competing motor programs from interfering. The *first* dysfunction, Chang and Guenther suggested, is within the basal ganglia itself and results from either excess dopamine or paucity of dopamine. Excess dopamine, as Alm (2004) hypothesized, would allow activation of competing motor programs, interfering with the execution of the desired program. On the other hand, paucity of dopamine would lead to a poorly activated appropriate motor program, preventing initiation of the syllable. The *second* impairment of the corticobasal ganglia loop is hypothesized to be inadequate signal strength in cortex-to-striatum projection. This would interfere with information about the cognitive-sensory-motor context that is sent to the basal ganglia. Thus, proper initiation and termination of the next syllable would not take place. Chang and Guenther cite a number of studies that support such a dysfunction in

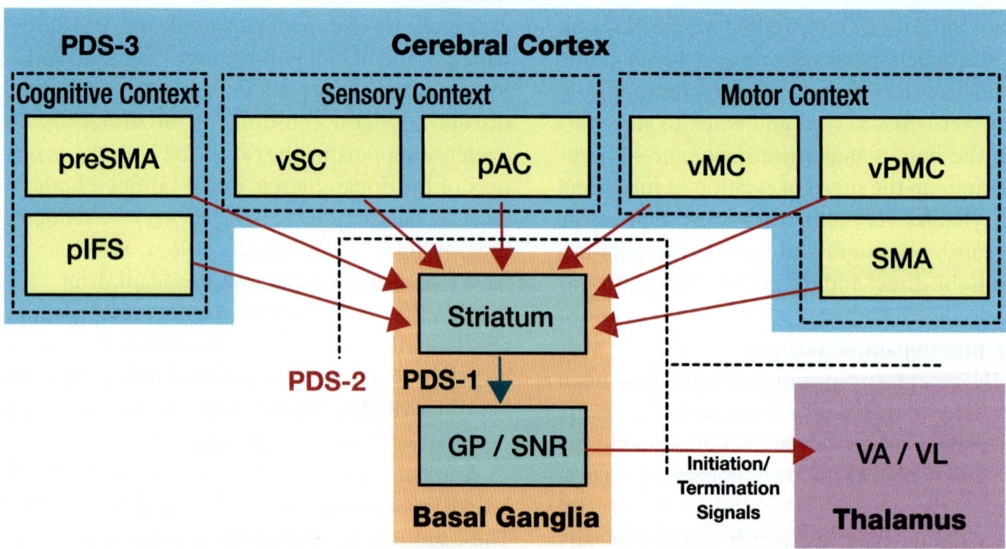

Figure 6.3 Potential impairments of the basal ganglia loop that may contribute to stuttering.

the corticostriatum connection. One example is research by Chang and Zhu (2013) that showed impaired connectivity between the left putamen and left hemisphere cortical areas that are key in speech production. The *third* possible problem with the BG loop is in the cortical regions that provide to the basal ganglia information about cognitive context, sensory context, and motor context. To support this hypothesis, the authors cite research by Chang et al. (2011) and Beal et al. (2013) that found, in children and adults who stuttered compared to those who did not, structural anomalies in prefrontal and/or premotor cortical areas of the left hemisphere. Chang and Guenther provide many other examples of deficits in left hemisphere cortical areas in individuals who stuttered.

Both Alm (2004) and Chang and Guenther (2019) emphasized that the different and separate impairments in the BG loop suggested distinct and separate etiologies for subgroups of individuals who stutter. They also concluded that the specific anomalies that they described may be only part of multifactorial combinations of difficulties that cause stuttering—some of which will be considered in the section on Stuttering As a Multifactor Dynamic Disorder.

Stuttering as Reduced Capacity for Internal Modeling

Another view of constitutional factors in stuttering was advanced by Megan and Peter Neilson, whose research on stutterers' tracking abilities was reviewed in Chapter 3. The Neilsons proposed that the repetitions of beginning stutterers are the result of a deficit in their ability to create and use "**inverse internal models of the speech production system**" (Neilson & Neilson, 1987). This rather complicated sounding model can be easily understood if we go back to an assumption about how children learn to speak.

During the first year of life, infants store up perceptions of the speech sounds they hear around them and begin to play with speech sounds, trying to imitate what they hear. Gradually, as they grow older, children learn how to make these sounds accurately. Some scientists, like the Neilsons, believe that too much of the brain's neural resources would be required if children had to remember each of the movements needed to produce each sound of their language in every possible phonetic context. Instead, children are thought to develop a mental "model" of the relationship between their speech movements and sounds they hear. Just as someone beginning to play a trombone must learn the relationship between the movements of the trombone slide (the arm that changes the tones as the trombonist moves it) and the sounds that result, experienced trombonists have established mental models of the relationship of their arm movements to the sounds produced and are able to move the slide to produce a desired sound without having to think about it in any deliberate way.

A child, then, develops a mental model of the relationship between speech sounds and motor commands. The mental model in the brain might be called a **sensorimotor model** for speech, which the Neilsons call an "inverse internal model" of how speech is produced. It is an "inverse" model because it transforms or inverts **sensory targets** (ie, heard speech sounds) into the motor commands needed to produce them. As infants learn to produce the sounds they hear, they constantly use and refine their sensorimotor model for speech. They plan a word or sentence in terms of what it should sound like (the target) and then rely on their sensorimotor model to generate the motor movement commands that will produce the speech targets they are trying to hit.

The process of learning to speak is something like learning to drive a car. At first, keeping the car on the road requires constant vigilance. But as we learn the relationships between turning the wheel, stepping on the accelerator, and going where we want, the linkage becomes automatic, even when driving a stick-shift vehicle in stop-and-go traffic. Moreover, the linkage is refined as we encounter different driving conditions and different cars (eg, cars with loose steering wheels and sticky accelerators). Just as drivers establish sensorimotor models for driving, children develop sensorimotor models for speaking.

Figure 6.4 is a schematic depiction of how the brain may transform desired sensory (perceptual) targets into motor commands for speech. In the figure, the desired output (the word or phrase, eg, that a child intends a listener to hear) is fed into the internal inverse model of the speech production system. Here, the desired output is entered as sensory code of its expected auditory and kinesthetic results, which is "inverted" by the model to generate its output as movement codes or motor commands. Experience, practice, and vocal play help the child to acquire these inversions or transformations. Moreover, this internal model is continually updated as a child's speech and language skills mature and the speech production system changes with age. The internal model's motor commands are sent to the muscles of the speech production system, whose coordinated contractions produce the acoustic output that result in a planned utterance. Concurrently, ongoing planning and feedback of this process are fed into the modeling circuitry.

Let us retrace our steps for a moment. When motor commands are sent to muscles, a copy of these commands, which is called the "efference copy" by motor physiologists, is also sent to the modeling circuitry. Here, the efference copy is transformed into its hypothetical output, which is a model, or template, of the output that should be produced based on the motor commands. This hypothetical output is continuously compared with feedback on the current positions and movements of the speech mechanism so that the inverse internal model can update its ongoing motor commands, if necessary, to produce the desired output more accurately. These components of the speech production process are assumed to involve the corticocerebellar structures and pathways that are commonly described in neural models of speech output (eg, Neilson & Neilson, 1987, 2005a, 2005b; Neilson et al., 1992).

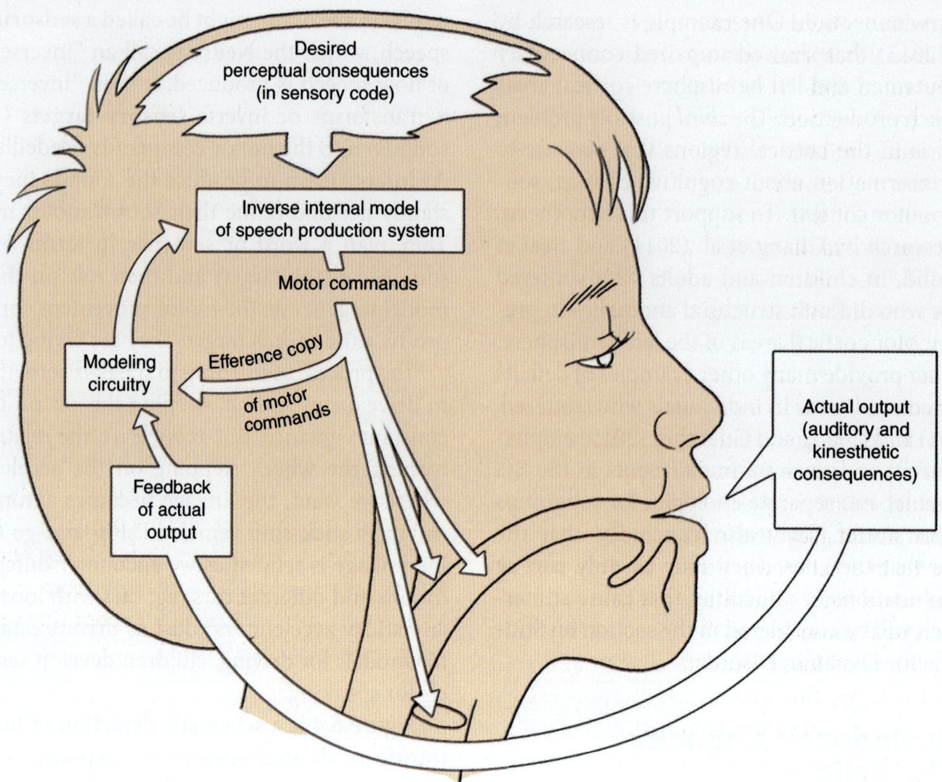

Figure 6.4 Schematic of the inverse internal model theory of speech production.

The Neilsons and their coworkers have used the inverse internal model of the speech production system to understand the performance of stutterers in experiments that tested their ability to track an auditory tone whose pitch changed unpredictably (Neilson et al., 1976). The subjects heard an unpredictably changing "target" tone in one ear and a "cursor" tone, which they could control with a handheld device, in the other ear. Their task was to track the pitch of the target tone with the cursor tone as accurately as possible. The Neilsons' experiments found that people who stutter were poorer than people who don't stutter in tracking auditory tones that went up and down in pitch. People who stutter were still poorer than people who don't stutter even after practicing the task. These findings suggested to the Neilsons that if stutterers had difficulty learning the relationships between the sounds they want to say and the movements required to produce them as young children, they would also, therefore, have difficulty making the sensory-to-motor and motor-to-sensory transformations required by the tracking tasks.

However, they hypothesized, this difficulty would not always result in stuttering. When circumstances don't call for much of the brain's functional capacities in speech and language areas, people who stutter should be able to compensate for their slight weaknesses. On the other hand, when large portions of the brain's functional capacity are allocated for language tasks, such as choosing new or unfamiliar words or constructing complex sentences, the diminished neural capacity cannot be accommodated, and more repetitions would result. As these researchers put it, "whether one will become a stutterer depends on one's neurological capacity for these sensory-to-motor and motor-to-sensory transformations and the demands posed by the speech act" (Andrews et al., 1983, p. 239).

How do these intermittent deficits in available functional neural capacity result in the symptoms of stuttering? This theory attempts to account only for the core behaviors of early stuttering, that is, repetitions and prolongations. According to the theory, repetitions and prolongations result from inadequate transformations of sensory targets, transformations that should generate the motor commands for speech. A speaker with reduced functional neural capacity may begin to speak but be unable to plan and carry out the rest of his utterance without disruption. Repetitions or prolongations may occur if a speaker is attempting to push ahead with speech while his brain is still planning the syllables that follow and how to link them with the initial sound.

Other researchers have also used the concept of inverse internal models to explain the behaviors of stuttering. The Neilsons' view was echoed in the perspective described in Guenther (1994), and their model was later adapted by Max et al. (2004) to propose a theoretical model of stuttering based on unstable or insufficiently activated internal models. One of their hypotheses parallels the Neilsons' proposition that some children are predisposed to stutter because of the difficulty learning the relationships between their motor commands and the desired acoustic output. This difficulty would result in an inaccurate inverse internal model of the speech production system (Fig. 6.4), which would generate output that would not match the desired perceptual consequences. The speech production system would then "reset" itself to try again, producing repetitions (one for each mismatch). This resetting process would continue until the child's error-correction process could update the model sufficiently to make the output match the consequences. If this could be done quickly, only one or two repetitions would occur; if not, then many repetitions would occur. The Max team's proposal has other hypotheses and an extensive review of the literature to support them.

The proposal by Max et al. (2004) is particularly effective in relating various stuttering phenomena to aspects of the model. For example, the findings that articulatory movements of a person who stutters movements are slower during fluent speech (see Chapter 3) and the evidence that slow speech can induce fluency are both explained by the possibility that a slower rate of speech production would allow the individual more time for feedback to update the internal model. With a properly updated internal model, the actual speech acoustic output would match the intended perceptual consequence. Therefore, the system would not produce the repetitions that are thought to be a result of inaccurate speech output that doesn't match the intended perceptual consequences. In other words, slower speech makes corrections possible while a syllable is being produced rather than after it is completed. Note that if this hypothesis is accurate, errors would be found in the unsuccessful repetitions of a person who stutters. Can you devise a study that would investigate this?

Research by Cykowski et al. (2010) has supported this perspective on stuttering as a deficit in using inverse internal models for speech. Their work suggests that specific pathways in the brain used for sensorimotor integration—within the superior longitudinal fasciculus (SLF III)—are less efficient in adults who stutter compared to adults who do not. This is also shown by Chow and Chang's (2017) study of children who stuttered (those who would recover and those who would become persistent) compared to control children. They found that the children who stuttered who would become persistent had significantly less density (and less growth of density over time) in white matter tracts compared to control children. The most problematic areas appeared to be those that would be critical in an inverse internal model for speech production: white matter tracts responsible for sending motor commands and creating expectations of their auditory and somatosensory consequences, so that the motor commands could be adjusted when errors are detected.

To apply these views to the first signs of stuttering, children's repetitions may be the result of motor commands creating a first syllable of an utterance, but this output may be flawed (or detected as flawed). Repetitions would then occur as corrections are attempted. It is also possible that the first syllable is adequate but the system is not functioning well enough to plan and carry out the following syllables. Hence, the first syllable is uttered again and again while the system awaits the plans and commands for the next.

Treatment aimed at making a slower speech rate natural for these children would be appropriate.

Stuttering as a Language Production Deficit

Many researchers have been intrigued by the influence of linguistic factors on stuttering. For example, stuttering often begins when a child enters a period of intense language development (eg, Bloodstein et al., 2021; Yairi & Ambrose, 2005). Similarly, stuttering is most frequent when the load on language functions is heaviest (eg, in longer utterances, at the beginnings of sentences, and on longer, less familiar words) (Bloodstein et al., 2021). These factors have prompted several theorists to propose that stuttering reflects an impairment in some aspect of spoken language. I use the term "spoken language" because these theorists believe the major problem is not in the motor execution of speech but rather in the planning and assembly of language units, such as phonemes, that occur before speech is actually produced.

Kolk and Postma (1997) developed the **"covert repair" hypothesis** to explain stuttering from a language production point of view. Typically, speech flows smoothly, like the bicycle factory in Figure 6.5.

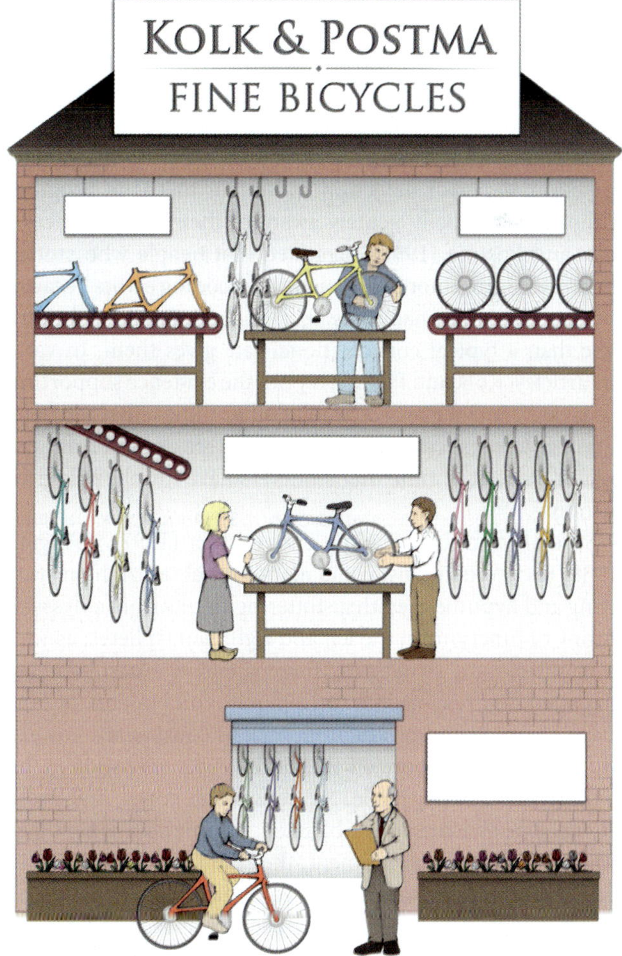

Figure 6.5 Quality control in a bicycle factory as an analogy for part of the language production system in the brain.

However, In Kolk and Postma's model, when internal monitoring during speech production detects an error in the phonetic plan (eg, using the speaker's perception of their own speech), speech production is interrupted and repair is needed before production can continue. Thus, the halting of production and the repair process is thought to cause the disfluencies of both normal speakers and individuals who stutter. In stuttering, however, there are both the time pressure to produce speech at a normal rate and the concern felt by the speaker when the repair process takes time.

To Kolk and Postma (1997), the most common stuttering disfluencies (repetitions, prolongations, and blocks) are the result of correcting or "repairing" the phonological (rather than semantic, syntactic, or lexical) errors detected in the phonetic plan before they are spoken. In the case of part-word repetitions, if a speaker detects an error in the final part of a syllable (eg, the /p/ in "cup"), he restarts the phonological encoding process ("cu-cu-") and keeps going until the phoneme is encoded correctly and the entire syllable can be produced. In contrast, prolongations are thought to occur when the phoneme of a word or syllable preceding the error is a continuant (eg, the /l/ in the word "lip" when the error involves the vowel). In this case, the continuant, /l/, is prolonged until the speaker successfully encodes the vowel, /i/, following /l/.

Blocks are thought to result from errors in the initial sounds of words or syllables. When an error is detected, speech production is halted for repairs, but the speaker may try to plunge ahead, building up muscle tension, unaware of the automatic error detection and repair that is in progress (although potentially acutely aware of their consequences). Kolk and Postma (1997) suggested that people who stutter are prone to have more phonological encoding errors because they are constitutionally slower in encoding and need more time than a typical conversational rate gives them. In various articles, Kolk and Postma lay out the evidence supporting their views and suggested, among other things, that the benefits of a slower speech rate on stuttering are derived from the greater amount of time that stutterers have for phonological encoding.

Several years before Kolk and Postma (1997), Wingate (1988) reviewed linguistic and neurological research on stuttering and hypothesized that stuttering results from a dyssynchrony of functions in the left and right hemispheres, as well as in subcortical structures. These different areas, Wingate suggested, are responsible for different components of language planning and production, such as consonants, vowels, and prosody. He theorized that when speakers produce the initial portion of a syllable, the consonant, vowel, and prosody must be synchronously blended. If some component lags behind at this critical moment, the result is a disruption in speech production that we observe as stuttering, although he does not explain how this halt appears in speech as a repetition, prolongation, or block.

Perkins et al. (1991) proposed another theory of stuttering as a deficit in language production. These authors suggested that stuttering results from a dyssynchrony between two components of language production. The "paralinguistic" component is a right hemisphere–controlled social-emotional process that is responsible for vocal tone and prosodic functions. The other component is linguistic and involves a left hemisphere segmental system that is responsible for the content and structure of language (semantics, syntax, and phonology). The two components must be integrated before spoken language is produced. If one lags behind the other for whatever reason, the resulting dyssynchrony produces disfluency.

Perkins et al. (1991) added two elements to this dyssynchrony that must also be present if the resulting disfluency is stuttering, rather than just a normal disfluency. First, the speaker must experience time pressure from either an outside source or an inner feeling, so that they continue trying to speak even though the dyssynchrony in paralinguistic or linguistic processes has resulted in an incomplete or anomalous speech motor program. Second, the speaker must experience a feeling of "loss of control," which arises from being unaware of why they cannot say the word. These elements appear in the bicycle factory metaphor in Figure 6.6.

Packman et al. (2007) and Packman and Attanasio (2010) have suggested another perspective on the language production dyssynchrony model. They believed that the challenge of producing variable linguistic stress from syllable to syllable triggers moments of stuttering. The problem, according to these authors, first appears in children's speech as they move from the simple production of single words to the more complex production of phrases. Phrases demand stress contrasts that tax the child's unstable speech production system. Having said the first syllable, the child is unable to move on because they cannot program the needed stress contrast between the first and second syllable. They hypothesized that the difficulty in children have in starting utterances is located in the SMA—6 region of the brain involved in initiation of speech. Children are unable to move forward beyond the first syllable because of this problem and, according to Packman and Attanasio, they revert to a babbling-like repetition of the first syllable until brain resources allow the speech production system to move ahead to the following syllables.

Stuttering as a Multifactorial Dynamic Disorder

For almost 25 years, Anne Smith and her colleagues carried out a systematic program of research on stuttering, developing a theory that at the core of stuttering is a motor speech disorder, the appearance and severity of which are influenced by a multitude of cognitive, linguistic, and psychosocial

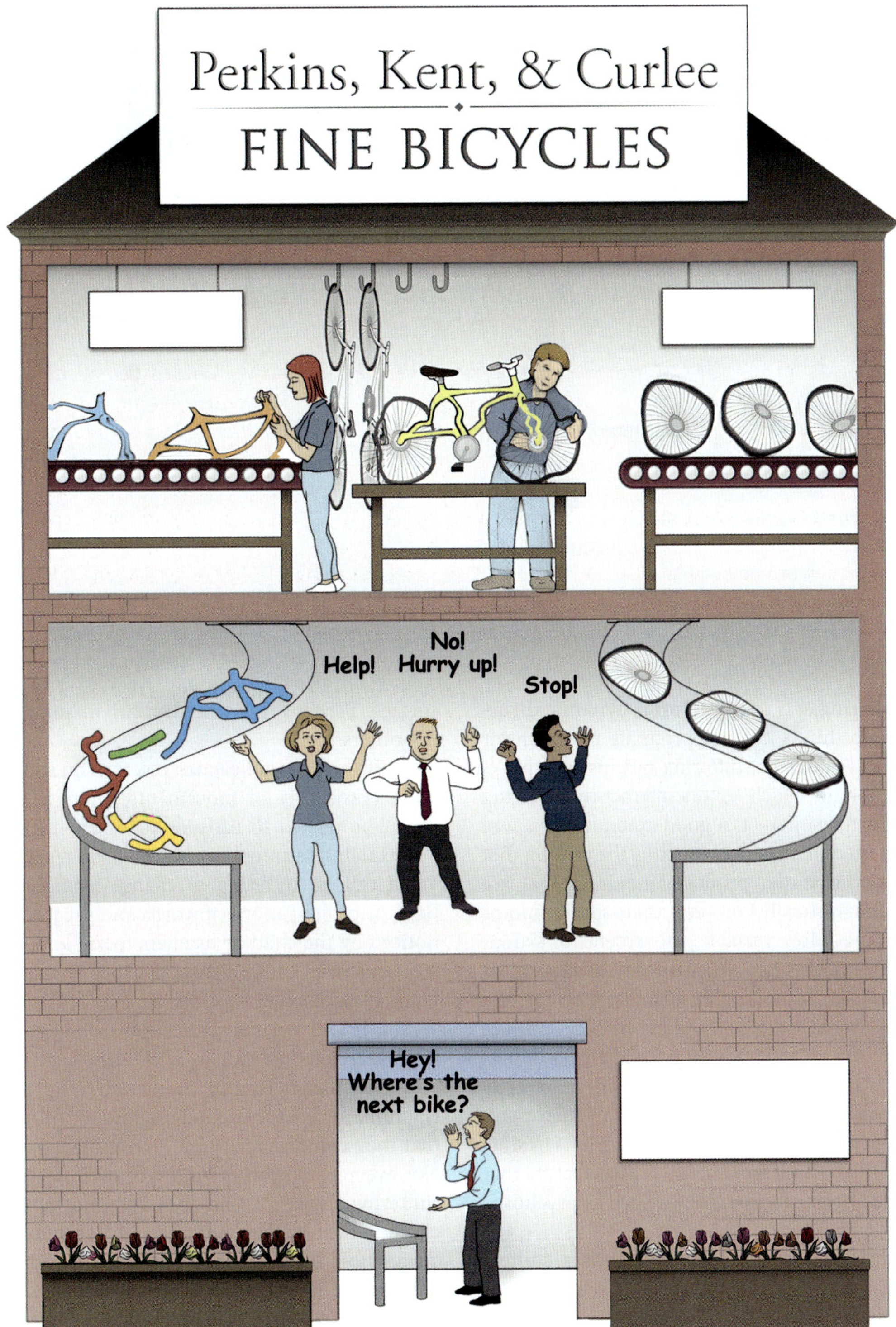

Figure 6.6 Disarray in bicycle factory when breakdown occurs and workers feel loss of control and time pressure. Like language production breakdown and resultant stuttering.

factors (eg, Smith, 1999; Smith & Goffman, 2004; Smith & Kelly, 1997; Smith & Weber, 2017; Zimmerman et al., 1981). In arguing for the multifactorial nature of stuttering, Smith quotes Van Riper (1982a), who makes the point that not only are there multiple factors acting in concert that determine if individuals stutter but that different individuals will have unique combinations of factors—different amounts of various factors—that determine their own stuttering fate.

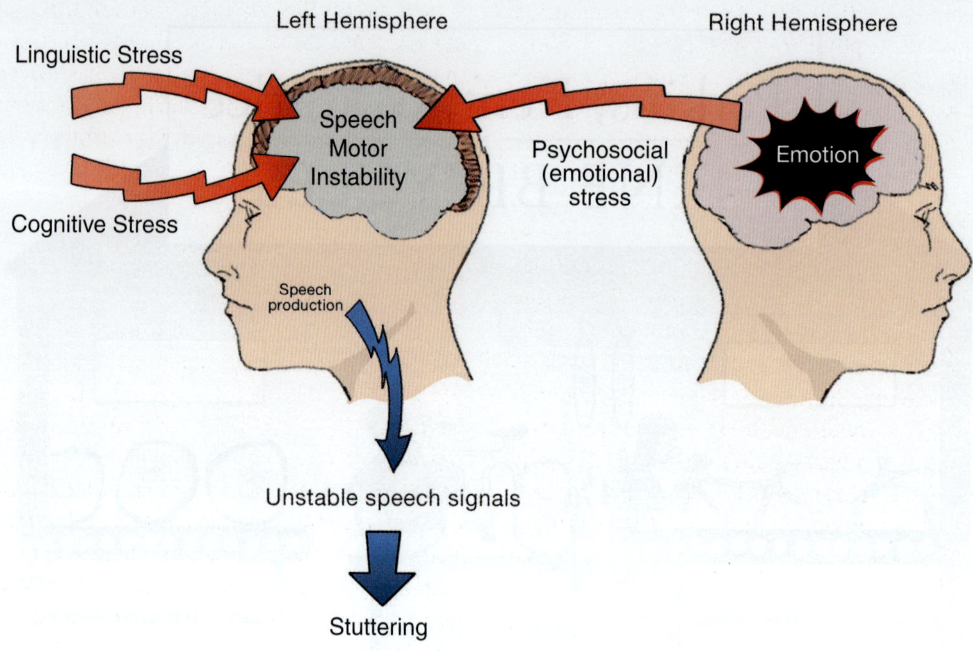

Figure 6.7 Stuttering as a multifactorial dynamic disorder.

Portraying stuttering as a **multifactorial dynamic disorder** (Fig. 6.7), Smith thinks it is inappropriate to search for a single underlying "cause" of stuttering but instead thinks it's important to look for which factors interact in stuttering and determine how they interact. A good example of the way this view is manifested in Smith's research is the finding that when individuals who stutter produce utterances that are longer and more linguistically complex, their speech motor coordination becomes more variable (movements of articulators appear less regular when standard deviations—measures of variability—are computed for many repetitions of a phrase), compared to individuals who don't stutter (Smith et al., 2010). Despite the greater variability in their coordination, the individuals in the stuttering group did not overtly stutter as they produced the utterances in this experiment. Exactly how this greater variability sometimes results in stuttering will probably await further study of other factors that can be manipulated in these experiments, such as psychosocial stress.

The multifactorial, dynamic view characterizes stuttering as a "dynamic" disorder because the "stuttering events" of repetitions, prolongations, and blocks are seen as only the outward manifestation of an underlying, ever-changing process resulting in these events erupting to the surface from time to time. So, in the experiment described above involving longer and more complex sentences, there may be increasing speech motor instability as linguistic load increases, and if psychosocial stress were increased (as part of the underlying, ever-changing process), some stuttering events might surface. Perhaps this would occur in some individuals but not others.

Smith and her colleagues' research on speech motor instability (variability of movements) hints at a substrate that might be related to early or **primary stuttering**, but what can explain the secondary reactions of tension and struggle? What causes stuttering to change from brief, easy repetitions or prolongations of words and syllables that are hardly noticed by the child or listeners to the long, tense blockages that frustrate, embarrass, and upset both the speaker and, often, his audience?

Smith and her colleagues have done some research on this aspect of stuttering as well. They have found that some moments of stuttering are characterized by rapid (5 to 12 Hz), rhythmic, oscillatory neural input to the muscles of speech so that they contract in a rapid, tremorlike way (Smith, 1989). Not every person who stutters shows these tremors during stuttering, however, and they may not appear in younger children who stutter but are only detected in older children whose stuttering has persisted for some time and may have developed maladaptive reactions. As Kelly et al. (1995) pointed out, it is also possible that these tremors are evoked or magnified by autonomic arousal or the emotion that arises in response to the expectation or occurrence of speech difficulties.

Several writers have linked emotional stress with stuttering and suggested that the tiny tremors that appear in everyone's speech muscles may be amplified by emotion to a level that interferes with talking (Fibiger, 1971, 1972; Van

Riper, 1982a; Weber & Smith, 1990). The effects of emotion on tremor may provide a physiological explanation of how the mild disfluencies of young children become the more severe blockages we see as beginning stuttering evolves into advanced stuttering. Even mild disfluencies may trigger emotional responses in some children that result in increased tremors that block speech. Emotional responses may also explain the unusual cases of severe blocks at the onset of stuttering, especially when stuttering begins during conditions of stress and strong emotion. The interaction of very strong emotion with a child's vulnerable speech motor system may create sudden severe stuttering because it amplifies tremors in the speech musculature. Such tremors may be analogous to the quivering lip of a toddler who is about to burst into tears when frightened by a barking dog or by a yelling parent. Just how magnified tremors block or slow the forward movement of speech is not known, but Van Riper's (1982a, p. 126) description of tension and tremor may give us some clues. He suggested:

> *What usually seems to happen is that tremors begin when the stutterer creates a fixed closure, invests its antagonistic musculatures with tension, and then suddenly produces an increase of air pressure behind or below the closure. At the moment this increase occurs, the antagonistic musculatures become suffused with a sudden burst of further tension and the stuttering tremor comes into being. Then it persists...*

Why a person who stutters would create fixed closures is a mystery. Perhaps it is one of the body's responses to threat that Gray (1987) described as a behavioral inhibition system, which I discuss later in the section on secondary stuttering and temperament.

THEORETICAL PERSPECTIVES ON DEVELOPMENTAL AND ENVIRONMENTAL FACTORS

Serious academic interest in identifying factors causing and explaining stuttering did not occur until well into the 20th century. Among the earliest theories was one that placed the entire burden of the disorder on parental reactions to disfluencies occurring in their children's speech. Specifically, in the 1930s, Wendell Johnson and other researchers at the University of Iowa, noting similarities in the disfluencies of both children who were viewed to be stuttering and those who were not, developed the **"diagnosogenic" theory**. In that theory, the parents' reactions to their child's speech as abnormal—that is, their diagnostic reactions—led to the development of increasingly less typical disfluencies—actual stuttering, in these children. Although this theory had many immediately negative consequences, including vilification of parents of children who stuttered, it nonetheless prompted lively reactions among the research community.

With regard to theories that are more active in affecting current research and clinical practice, however, two theories deserve special attention because they explore a myriad of internal and external factors that may help us understand stuttering and may promote key therapeutic approaches.

Communicative Failure and Anticipatory Struggle

The theoretical view of **Communicative Failure and Anticipatory Struggle**, developed by Bloodstein (1987, 1997; Bloodstein et al., 2021), proposes that stuttering emerges from a child's experiences of frustration and failure when trying to talk. The child's original difficulty in talking may be the typical disfluencies of childhood, but other frustrations might also make the child feel that talking is difficult. Many types of communication failure may lead the child to anticipate future problems with speech and thus increase tension. It is common, Bloodstein noted, to find delays in the development of articulation and language, cluttering, and other speech problems in the histories of children who begin to stutter. Table 6.1 lists some of the circumstances that Bloodstein suggested might cause some children to believe that speaking is difficult. If a child cannot make himself understood or is penalized for the way they talk, they may begin to tense their speech muscles and fragment their speech—reactions that become the core behaviors of the child's stuttering. And these behaviors in turn result in more frustration and failure in communication, which the child anticipates with dread. A video of my interview with Oliver Bloodstein about this theory can be found on Lippincott Connect. It is titled "Communicative Failure and Anticipatory Struggle."

Other aspects of the child's "internal" and "external" environments and his development also play important parts. The child's personality may be hypersensitive,

TABLE 6.1 Experiences That May Make Some Children Believe Speaking Is Difficult

1. Normal disfluencies criticized by significant listeners
2. Delay in speech or language development
3. Speech or language disorders, including articulation problems, word finding difficulty, cerebral palsy, and voice problems
4. Difficult or traumatic experience reading aloud in school
5. Cluttering, especially if listeners frequently say, "Slow down" or "What?"
6. Emotionally traumatic events during which child tries to speak

perfectionistic, or they may harbor the need to live up to parental expectations. The child's family may have high standards for speech, find any speech abnormality unacceptable, or otherwise pressure the child to conform to standards beyond their reach. The presence or absence of these sorts of developmental and environmental pressures may cause some children to interpret an articulation difficulty, language problem, or disfluency as a failure, whereas other children only shrug it off.

This perspective on stuttering accounts for the wide variability of disfluency among children. Most typical children experience temporary frustration when learning to talk as they produce the mild fragmentations of speech we associate with typical disfluency. Children who stutter for just a few weeks may encounter unusual difficulty when first learning to talk but soon master the fundamentals and feel successful. Children who develop persistent stuttering may be those who repeatedly experience communication failure, have a sensitive temperament, and/or grow up in an environment fraught with communicative pressure.

Here is a case—a client of mine—whose experiences illustrate some of the environmental pressures that some children who begin to stutter may experience. Susan grew up in the oil fields of Oklahoma, where her parents set themselves apart from the rest of the community by their aloof manner and precise speech. They raised their children to feel that they were more cultured than their neighbors; in fact, Susan's father would often say, "We speak better than other people." Unfortunately, Susan's speech development was delayed. When she did begin talking in sentences at about age 3, she began to stutter with mild repetitions. When she started school, she worried that her father was embarrassed by her speech. Then she tried to speak better and began to push out the words instead of repeating the first parts of them. She soon developed severe secondary stuttering.

Although we have no way of knowing for sure, Susan's critical father may have been a major factor in the onset of her stuttering. However, many children who grow up in families that are critical of speech don't develop stuttering. Perhaps both a constitutional deficit, which led to her delayed speech development, and family pressure for perfect speech were necessary to produce Susan's stuttering. Neither may have been sufficient by itself to create stuttering, but together they may have been enough to tip the balance.

Treatment implications for the Anticipatory Struggle view of stuttering are many. Children's families can radiate acceptance by their nonverbal communications such as showing interest in what their children are saying, and also verbally, by saying, "It's OK when you have a little trouble saying a word; lots of kids do." More formal stuttering therapy can help older children and adults become desensitized to the moment of stuttering. As the desensitization continues, they can learn how to get into a word with a looser and easier approach that helps them feel in control even if the word feels slightly stuck.

Capacities and Demands

Another view of stuttering that considers many factors interacting is proposed by the **Capacities and Demands** theory. Others have called this a "demands and capacities" view, but I prefer to put capacities first, because they exist in children before demands are placed on them. This view suggests that disfluencies as well as real stuttering emerge when a child's capacities for fluency are not equal to speech performance demands. Earlier in this chapter, I briefly discussed a narrow version of this view in describing the reduced capacity for internal modeling theory of stuttering. Andrews et al. (1983) stated that "whether one will become a stutterer depends on one's neurological capacity…and the demand posed by the speech act" (p. 239). These authors indicated that some demands come from the rapid development of language between ages 3 and 7 years. Other demands may come from fast-talking parents, whose speech rates may be hard for a child to keep up with. Demands for speech performance sometimes come from within the child, sometimes from outside stimuli, and sometimes from both.

Sheehan (1970, 1975) expressed an early variation of the capacities and demands view when he wrote that "a child who has begun to stutter is probably a child who has had too many demands placed on him while receiving too little support" (Sheehan, 1975, p. 175). The demands that Sheehan pinpointed were primarily those of parents who have high standards and high expectations for their child's behavior. The support he refers to appears to be the environment's capacity to provide love, care, and encouragement. In addition, he believed that "there are persisting reasons for retaining the possibility that some kind of physiological predisposition for stuttering exists" (Sheehan, 1975, p. 144). Thus, Sheehan, who is best known for a theory that stuttering is learned, professed the view that stuttering is precipitated by the demands of the environment interacting with a predisposition to stutter.

Starkweather (1987) added considerable detail to the concept of capacities and demands as an explanation of stuttering onset and development. He called his theoretical perspective "Demands and Capacities." A typical child's capacities, he pointed out, include the potential for rapid movement of speech structures in well-planned sequences that are coordinated with the rhythms of his language. Demands on children include those of their internal environment, such as their increasingly complex thoughts to be expressed, which require more sophisticated phonology, syntax, semantics, and pragmatic skills. The external environment often places demands on children's fluency through parents' interactions. Parents may ask questions rapidly, interrupt frequently, and use complex sentences choked with big words. They may show impatience about the children's typical disfluencies and may make children feel that they meet their expectations only when they perform at high levels. These kinds of interactions can stress any child but are likely to push a slowly developing child to try to speak beyond their capacity for fluency.

Because a child's capacities develop in spurts and environmental demands fluctuate, stuttering may wax and wane in cycles. Children may be highly fluent for a day or a week when they have mastered new speech and language skills and when external demands are low. But their stuttering may suddenly flare up if their capacities become strained by their efforts to use more advanced syntax or if the demands of the external environment suddenly increase when their fast-talking, interrupting, big-city cousins arrive for the Fourth of July holiday weekend.

The capacities and demands view provides a way to account not only for the day-to-day variability of stuttering within an individual but also for the great differences between one individual who stutters and another. As Adams (1990) pointed out, some children may grow up in an environment with typical levels of demand but have limited speech production capacities. Others may have normal capacities for speech production but grow up with excessive demands for rapid, fluent speech.

Treatment based on this model would begin with a careful evaluation of the child's capacities and the demands they experience. Therapy would be designed to enhance capacities, decrease demands, and provide support for the child and their family while these changes are taking place. Starkweather, his colleagues, and other clinical researchers have used this approach to formulate a sensible and effective program of stuttering prevention (de Sonnerville-Koedoot, Stolk, et al., 2015; Gottwald, 2010; Gottwald & Starkweather, 1984, 1985; Starkweather & Gottwald, 1990; Starkweather et al., 1990). Figure 6.8 depicts the ratios of capacities and demands in a child predisposed to stutter. In one view, the demands are greater than the child's capacities and stuttering occurs. In the second, the demands are lessened, and although capacities stay the same, stuttering is diminished.

Consequentially, I would opine that hereafter-
Look here, don't you "opine" me, and furthermore, I'm going on that business trip! - Suzie stop that!
Ca-ca-can I-I go to Anne's?
Capacity
Demands
Suzie, when you finish playing with Daddy, would you like to take a walk over to Anne's with me?
Capacity
Demands

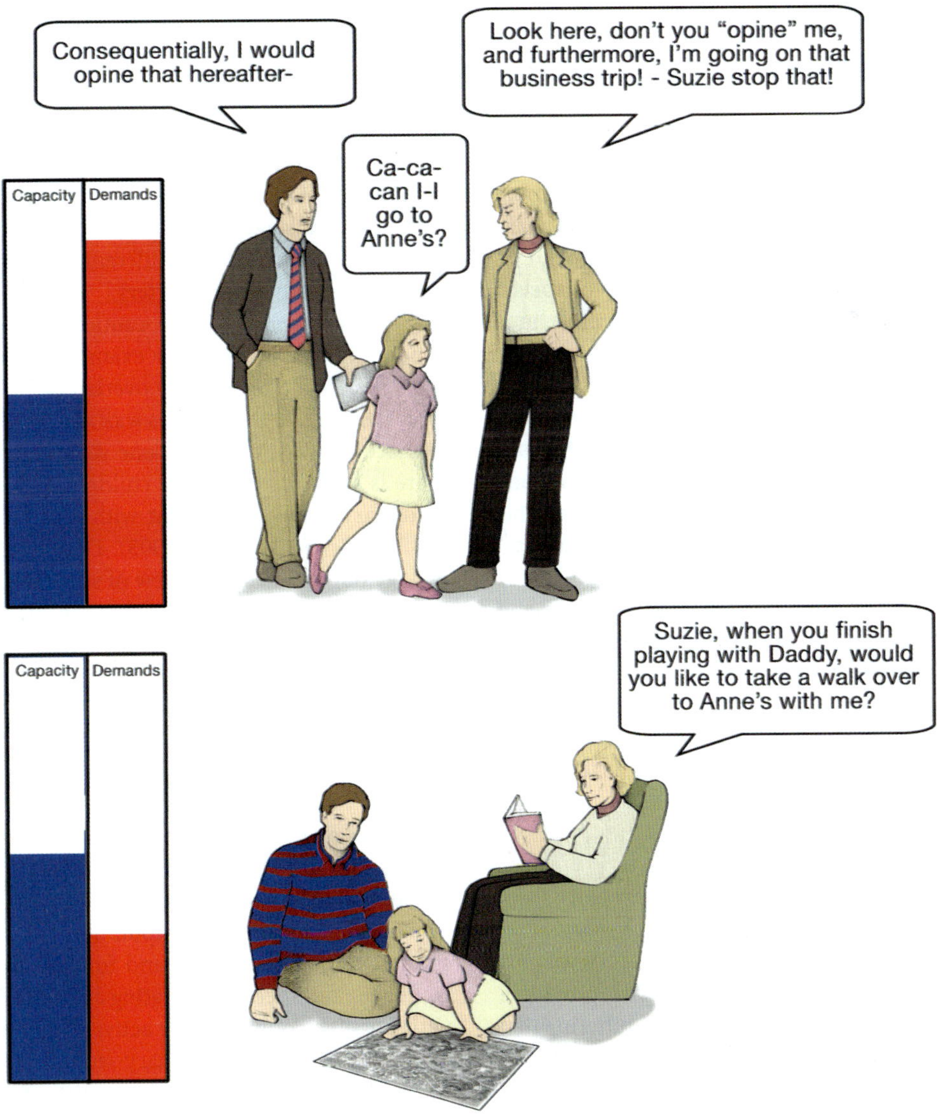

Figure 6.8 Two different ratios of capacities and demands and their hypothesized effects on fluency.

To illustrate the capacities and demands view more fully, the following case is from my own experience. Gina was a bright, happy 7-year-old. Her mother had been a severe stutterer as a child, but through treatment and her own perseverance, she had largely recovered. When Gina began the second grade, she had no history of stuttering or any problem with school. Sometime before Christmas that year, however, when her class was learning to read, Gina began to dislike school, and her mother soon discovered that she was having problems academically. After testing, it was discovered that she had a learning disability that had not been apparent before; however, once reading was required, it became obvious. As Gina struggled to cope with her reading problem throughout the rest of the second grade, she began to stutter. Over the course of the next 2 years, she stuttered noticeably but did not receive therapy. She was, however, given extra help for her reading disability. By the fourth grade, Gina was making headway with reading, and her stuttering had diminished to an inconsequential level without treatment.

Although there are various ways to account for the onset of Gina's stuttering and recovery, a capacities and demands view would see it this way: Gina was predisposed to stutter, but it lay dormant until she was faced with the challenge of reading. Reading, at least when first learned, involves a highly conscious use of linguistic processes, in contrast to the more automatic linguistic processing used in listening and speaking. Consequently, learning to read puts a heavy demand on the pool of available resources that are also used for speech and language processing. Such demands may result in a reduced capacity (ie, fewer available resources) for speech production, which may result in disfluency for a vulnerable child. In this case, Gina did not seem to develop a persistent fear of speaking as a result of her stuttering. Thus, when she overcame her initial reading difficulty and reading became more automatic (ie, demanded fewer resources), her available capacity for speech processes increased, and she "outgrew" her stuttering.

Once again, the reader is reminded that the capacities and demands view is a model for describing relationships that appear again and again but are not well understood. As such, its major function is to help students and clinicians organize the complex interrelationships of variables associated with stuttering into a set of principles that may guide its treatment and suggest hypotheses for research.

INTEGRATION OF PERSPECTIVES ON STUTTERING

In this section, I draw upon the theoretical views just described coupled with my own speculations to provide a description of the etiology and development of stuttering that can guide your assessment and treatment. Figure 6.9 depicts the major components of this perspective. A special component of this integrated approach is its attempt to explain the development of stuttering to include not only the easy repetitions often first seen at onset but also the tense repetitions, prolongations, and blocks as well—the pattern seen in most people who have stuttered for a time.

A Two-Stage Model of Stuttering

Many years ago, a child psychiatrist who stuttered, Charles Bluemel, observed that stuttering begins in most children as repetitions, of which they are hardly aware and to which they don't react. He thought that over time, many of these children become aware of their disfluencies and react to them by increasing the tension and tempo of their repetitions. These repetitions then become fast, irregular, and halting as children are bothered by them and do what they can to stop them. As they tense further, the repetitions become blocks and sometimes prolongations. This can happen overnight in some children and over a period of months for others. Bluemel (1932) called the beginning behaviors "primary" stuttering and the later reactions "secondary" stuttering. Brutten and Shoemaker (1967) also described stuttering as deriving from two factors or having two stages of development, as I mentioned in Chapter 5 on Learning and Unlearning. This view of stuttering as having two separate stages or components seems useful to me also and suggests the possibility that each component may have a different etiology. Understanding the nature of each stage may help us choose the most appropriate treatment—which may be different for each stage—as well as for each individual who stutters.

There are reasons to be cautious about embracing this apparently simple view. For example, primary and secondary stages of stuttering may overlap in children because the forces that create these stages wax and wane and make it hard to place children clearly in one stage or another. Moreover, there is evidence that some children begin stuttering in the secondary stage—or at least with tense blocks (Van Riper, 1982a; Yairi & Ambrose, 2005). Despite these exceptions, I will lay out an integrated view of stuttering on the presumption that there are, for most children, two stages of stuttering, and I describe how the exceptions themselves can be explained in this view.

A Perspective on Primary Stuttering

In Chapters 2 and 3, I reviewed studies of genetics, brain structures and functions, and sensorimotor function. These studies support the view that individuals who stutter have differences in the way their brains process sensory information and produce motor output. Many of the brain imaging studies point to structural and functional anomalies in the language- and speech-generating areas of the left hemisphere with possible compensatory activity in homologous areas of the right. In addition, primary stuttering can appear when children who have the above-mentioned deficits also experience stress on their speech production abilities from their language development and stresses from their environments,

INTERNAL AND EXTERNAL FACTORS
RESULTING BEHAVIORS
Left Hemisphere Differences
• Dysfunction in neural networks essential for speech production, especially sensorimotor processing
• Less well-myelinated neural circuits that are thus Vulnerable to disruption from activity in other areas of left- and right-hemispheres
Right Hemisphere Differences
• Relocation of some aspects speech production to less efficient areas
Stresses from Language Development and Environment Pressures
Frequent repetitions of single-syllable words and part-words
Less-likely: prolongations and blocks
A
INTERNAL AND EXTERNAL FACTORS
Left Hemisphere Differences
• Dysfunction in neural networks essential for speech production, especially sensorimotor processing
• Less well-myelinated neural circuits that are thus Vulnerable to disruption from activity in other areas of left- and right-hemispheres
Right Hemisphere Differences
• Relocation of some aspects speech production to less efficient areas
Stresses from Language Development and Environment Pressures
Sensitive temperament/ emotional reactivity
TENSION
RESULTING BEHAVIORS
Tense repetitions & prolongations
Tense, struggled blocks

Escape behaviors
Avoidance behaviors
Reactions to these disfluencies
Frequent repetitions of single-syllable words and part-words
Less-likely: prolongations and blocks
B

Figure 6.9 A two-factor view of stuttering: primary stuttering **(A)** and secondary stuttering **(B)**.

such as rapid, competitive speaking situations and psychological pressures in their families.

The source of these internal differences in the central nervous systems in people who stutter appears to be the result of genetic inheritance or early brain injuries or other trauma. Either of these factors would affect how the brain grows during embryonic development or how the brain responds to injury. Let's look more closely at this process.

The development of speech and language networks in the brain begins—soon after conception—with the proliferation, migration, and differentiation of neural cells, a process guided by genetic predisposition and affected by external events, such as experience, injury, and disease (Chase, 1996; Edelman, 1992; Lagercrantz, 2016). As neural cells continue to proliferate and differentiate, millions of synapses are formed, and pathways of communication emerge when clusters of cells send information back and forth in response to stimulation. Cells that communicate readily among themselves become self-organizing, functional neural circuits that perform various tasks. For example, after birth as an infant interacts with the outside world, groups of circuits and systems in the infant's brain bind together to form "maps" or representations of the outside world to help the infant process incoming sensory information and produce appropriate motor responses (Edelman, 1992). A related phenomenon is the development of networks that are anatomically and functionally connected to achieve various tasks, such as speech and language production. Using a variety of neuroimaging tools, researchers have identified anomalies in networks vital to speech production, particularly in the left hemisphere, such as in the frontal aslant tract (FAT) (Neef et al., 2018) and the Default Mode Network (DMN) (Chang et al., 2018).

When there are anomalies in speech and language areas of the left hemisphere due to inheritance or injury, the developing brain can deal with them in a number of different ways. The most common way is by extensive anatomical reorganization, including growth of new fibers, new synapses, and entire new cortical tracts (Hadders-Algra & Forssberg, 2002). This reorganization would attempt to establish the functional circuits necessary for the development of spoken language in whatever structures are available. If reorganization involves relocation of these circuits to areas that have not naturally evolved to serve these circuits, or if reorganization entails neuronal groups being placed at an unusual distance from each other, these circuits will be both inefficient and vulnerable to disruption by other brain activities occurring in nearby areas. Vulnerability to disruption may occur if new circuits or even the original ones are insufficiently myelinated (insulated by a protective sheath), an outcome that would result in less-efficient transmission of neural signals. In fact, several researchers (Chang et al., 2015; Chow & Chang, 2017; Cykowski et al., 2010; Karlin, 1947) have suggested that inadequate **myelination** itself may be the reason why neural circuits for speech and language are inefficient or vulnerable to disruption in the brains of those who stutter.

Which neural circuits underlying spoken language may be inefficient or vulnerable to disruption? One of the functions that often seems to be atypical in stuttering is sensorimotor processing, particularly auditory-motor processing. Because auditory processing plays a major role in infants' use of the sounds of adult speech and the sounds of their own babbling, a dysfunction in this area would obviously have an influence on the development of interacting neuronal circuits for speech and language production. The sounds of adult speech give infants auditory targets to aim for when they are learning to speak. The sensorimotor activity in babbling helps a child develop internal models that specify what articulatory gestures are needed to produce desired auditory targets (Guenther et al., 2006; Hickok et al., 2011; Hickok & Poeppel, 2007; Neilson & Neilson, 1987, 2005a, 2005b). Moreover, the auditory information from babbling allows the child to adapt his internal auditory-articulatory model to his rapidly growing speech production mechanism (Callan et al., 2000). Because these circuits are self-organizing, they may develop a variety of solutions to the auditory processing problem. Some individuals may use homologous right-hemisphere structures for auditory processing, others may continue to use inefficient areas of the left hemisphere, and still others may use both.

Many of the brain imaging studies described in Chapter 2 suggested that there are problems in the very pathways that would be expected to support sensorimotor modeling for speech. The findings of Sommer et al. (2002), Chow and Chang (2017), Chang et al. (2008), Watkins et al. (2008), Cykowski et al. (2010) and Jossinger et al. (2022) suggested that individuals who stutter have less dense bidirectional fiber tracts connecting sensory and motor areas. If these fiber tracts are less dense, they are probably less efficient for rapid transmission of signals.

Rapid information flow between sensory and motor areas is critical for accurate and fluent speech. If there is a delay in the information needed to generate the motor plans and execute them, repetitions may occur. This often happens after the speaker produces the first sound. This sound can be produced because it can be based on already obtained sensory information about the resting state of the speech system structures. But new information is needed to go forward—information required for production of the next sound, syllable, or word. However, that information is often delayed because it depends on rapid updating of information about the new state of the speech system (sensory analysis) and the rapid analysis of the sound just produced (comparison of efference copy of motor commands and feedback of actual output). Return to Figure 6.4 for a visual description of the process.

This description of dyssynchrony in the assembly of components of speech and language production is intended only as a possible explanation of primary stuttering, which is a stage of stuttering usually characterized by relatively relaxed repetitions and occasional prolongations that typically occur, as Bloodstein et al. (2021) have suggested, at the beginnings of phrases or sentences. As indicated in the paragraph above, the first sound or syllable may be fluent but the second is often a repeat of the first, li-like this. Most children who begin to stutter outgrow their disfluencies as their speech and language systems mature or as they develop effective ways to work around the problem. The work of Chow and Chang (2017) suggested that at least some of the children who do not outgrow their stuttering but persist in it have a slower growth rate in the myelination of white matter tracts interconnecting speech motor areas. This, they suggested, continues to interfere with the feedforward (the preview of what is about to be produced) and feedback needed for fluent speech production in the inverse internal model of speech production described earlier.

Another factor that may be operating to make some children persist in stuttering as well as become more severe is the child's reactions to their primary stuttering. Why do some children react to their primary stuttering by increasing the tension and speed of their disfluencies? Why do they go on to develop the characteristics of secondary stuttering: blocks, escape behaviors, and avoidance reactions? The answer, in part, can be found in the temperament of these children, interacting with the processes of learning.

A Perspective on Secondary Stuttering

In earlier sections, I mentioned that several authors (eg, Brutten & Shoemaker, 1967; Van Riper, 1982a) have suggested that the tensing, speeding up, escape, and avoidance behaviors of **secondary stuttering** are a reaction to the simple repetitions and sometimes prolongations of sounds and syllables that often characterize stuttering when it first begins. I now want to make the case that the child's general temperament and his in-the-moment emotional responses interacting with learning can explain the behaviors of secondary stuttering.

Temperament

This section focuses on the personality or temperament of children and uses both "sensitive" and "reactive" to refer to the same thing: a behavioral and emotional style characterized by being easily aroused by novel stimuli, as well as a tendency to withdraw when confronted by unfamiliar people or situations. Others use "inhibited" to describe the same traits (eg, Kagan, 1994a, 1994b; Kagan et al., 1987). There is evidence, which was discussed in Chapter 3, that individuals (even adults) who stutter tend to have more sensitive or reactive temperaments (Anderson et al., 2001; Eggers, 2012; Eggers et al., 2021; Embrechts & Ebben, 1999; Fowlie & Cooper, 1978; Guitar, 2003; LaSalle, 1999; Ntourou et al., 2013, 2020; Onslow & Kelly, 2020; Oyler & Ramig, 1995; Wakaba, 1998). If so, such reactivity may explain why some children who stutter eventually respond to their disfluencies by tightening their muscles, a reaction indicative of a response to a perceived threat, as I described in Chapter 5. Research on even nonstuttering children who are typically developing and have sensitive temperaments suggested that they respond to novel, threatening, or unfamiliar events by increasing their physical tension in the larynx—as measured acoustically in terms of decreased fluctuations in pitch (Coster, 1986; Kagan et al., 1987). The same has been shown with adults who stutter. Long ago, Lee Edward Travis assessed the effects of emotion on laryngeal tension in individuals who stutter (Travis, 1925). Using 19 subjects who stuttered and 18 who did not, Travis measured pitch fluctuations under two emotional conditions. First, he had subjects prolong an "ah" while relaxed. Then Travis induced emotional upset by questions and suggestions, followed by his firing a gun (!), after which he administered an electric shock. In the nonstuttering subjects, the emotional upset produced fluctuations in pitch, but in the subjects who stuttered, pitch changes over the few seconds of "ah" were markedly reduced during the emotional condition, suggesting to Travis that this was caused by "muscular fixation" in the larynx. We have seen similar results in our lab, but without firing guns or shocking our subjects.

One of my undergraduate students, Nicholas Brow, conducted an honor's thesis study similar to Travis's (1925) in which Nic evaluated stress by examining pitch increases in subjects who stuttered and those who didn't in two conditions, a stressful condition after being asked to give a speech that would be evaluated by several judges and the other in a neutral condition. The State Trait Anxiety Inventory (Iverach et al., 2009) was used to assess temperamental reactivity. The results showed that although a control group showed no more pitch increases than a group of stuttering individuals, in the stress situation, the stuttering group did show a significant positive relationship between degree of reactive temperament and pitch increase during stress, whereas the control group did not. This suggests that those in the stuttering group who did have higher temperamental reactivity were more stress-reactive in terms of laryngeal tension.

Laryngeal tension as a result of threat has been indirectly suggested by a researcher interested in species-specific defense reactions. Fanselow (1994) indicates that in animals experiencing threat, the amygdala sends a signal to the periaqueductal area of the brain that triggers physically tense immobility (freezing). The periaqueductal area is known to be richly connected to laryngeal muscles (Jurgens, 1994) and is active for expression of emotion in animals (Jurgens, 1979). Turk et al. (2021) discussed the role of dopamine in laryngeal behavior and it seems possible that excess dopamine production in basal ganglia may cause disruption in the smooth co-contractions of laryngeal muscles in stuttering. In my discussion of the types of core behaviors that characterize stuttering, in Chapter 1, I mentioned that many researchers believed that excess laryngeal tension occurs once stuttering blocks appear. I think increased laryngeal tension may occur to some extent in repetitions and prolongations as well.

The just-mentioned increases in physical tension may be part of a larger defensive response that is triggered more easily in individuals with reactive temperaments. In describing his **behavioral inhibition system**, Gray (1987) proposes that when individuals experience fear (threat), their innate response is freezing (ie, widespread muscular contractions that produce tense and silent immobility), flight (ie, speeded up activity to escape), or avoidance. Gray indicates that these unconditioned responses may occur rapidly without intervening autonomic arousal, arising from the central nervous system substrate underlying the increased muscle tension, increased tempo, and escape behaviors and avoidance behaviors (these behaviors seem to me to capture exactly what characterizes secondary stuttering). It is notable also that Gray suggests that the way an individual's behavioral inhibition system affects behavior is influenced by temperament. The more reactive individuals are, the more they will engage in freezing, flight, or avoidance responses when experiencing fear. LeDoux (2015), commenting on Gray's behavior inhibition system, suggests that, in his view, rapid defensive responses are made to nonconscious threat rather than conscious fear. LeDoux makes this distinction because he believes that the response is nonconscious, whereas responses to fear are conscious. Nonconscious responses are part of the individual's innate repertoire to enable survival and are thus very rapid. Conscious fear responses, which take longer because they require conscious processing, can create anxiety when there is uncertainty about a threat.

Further evidence of a neurological substrate underlying the characteristics of secondary behavior is provided by the research of Davidson (1984), Kinsbourne (1989), and Kinsbourne and Bemporad (1984), which was described in Chapter 3. They propose that the right hemisphere is specialized for emotions that accompany avoidance, withdrawal, and arrest of ongoing behavior, whereas the left hemisphere is specialized for emotions that are associated with approach, exploration, and release of ongoing behavior. Thus, it can be argued that individuals who stutter and are more reactive are more prone to behaviors regulated by right-hemisphere emotions. This argument is supported by the findings of Calkins and Fox (1994) and Davidson (1995) who reported that sensitive children (nonstutterers) are right hemisphere dominant for emotion. Their research may also explain why secondary behaviors develop in the forms they do in many stutterers. Those beginning stutterers who develop tension responses may be more sensitive individuals whose innate defensive mechanisms are triggered more easily because of their right-hemisphere dominance for emotions. It is possible that some of the excess activity seen in the right hemisphere of those who stutter, described in Chapter 2, may be related to activation of behavioral inhibition. Some support for this idea comes from brain imaging research by Neef et al. (2017). These researchers demonstrated that the nucleus accumbens in the right hemisphere is larger in individuals who stutter than in matched controls. Because the nucleus accumbens is considered a bridge between limbic and motor systems (Mogenson et al., 1980), the larger nucleus accumbens in those who stutter could be a link between reactive temperament and motor dysfunction in stuttering—as either a precipitator or consequence of experiences of stuttering.

The notion of greater emotional reactivity in children who stutter is supported by a study of 65 children who stuttered and 56 children who did not by Karrass et al. (2006). Those researchers found that compared to nonstuttering children, children who stutter have greater emotional reactivity, less emotional regulation, and poorer attention regulation. These authors suggest that this combination of traits contributes to the development of stuttering in a "reverberant" fashion. Reacting to their primary stuttering, these children have a strong emotional response to their primary stutters and they are unable to regulate this emotion. This in turn makes them stutter more (and more severely), and they have even stronger emotional responses to the more severe stutters and on and on.

A study related to emotional reactivity in children was conducted by Ntourou et al. (2020), reporting on a new measure of behavior inhibition in children, the Short Behavioral Inhibition Scale (SBIS). The scale was found to be valid and reliable and is reprinted in the chapter on diagnosis and assessment. In a sample of 179 children who stuttered and 198 children who did not, between ages 3;0 and 6;3, the children who stuttered were found to score as significantly ($p = .002$) more behaviorally inhibited than the children who did not. Moreover, scores on the SBIS were significantly predictive of stuttering frequency ($p = .049$) and stuttering severity ($p = .003$). These findings are supported for the hypothesis that emotional reactivity contributes to more frequent and more severe stuttering.

The importance of emotion in secondary (persistent) childhood stuttering is also supported by genetic evidence. As I indicated in Chapter 2, mutations in several genes, including GNPTG, have been linked to persistent stuttering, and it is also known that this same gene influences the development of the cerebellum and the hippocampus (Kang et al., 2010). The cerebellum is known for its role in motor control and in emotional regulation (eg, Schmahmann & Caplan, 2006). The hippocampus is also a structure that influences emotion and is a key component of Gray's behavioral inhibition system, described previously. Thus, many lines of evidence converge on the link between secondary stuttering and emotion.

I've described many of the temperamental and emotional factors related to secondary stuttering as though they were completely within the child. But of course, the child interacts with a complex environment, and this influences temperament and emotion, which in turn influence stuttering. An example that comes to mind is a girl and her mother in a study of parent-child interaction that we published many years ago (Guitar et al., 1992). We computed correlations between several variables in the mother's talking and the girl's primary stuttering and secondary stuttering. What we found led us to recognize that different aspects of the mother's conversation affected the two types of stutters differentially. The mother's speech rate was highly correlated with the girl's primary stutters but not with her secondary stutters. On the other hand, the mother's nonaccepting comments were highly correlated with the girl's secondary stuttering but not her primary stuttering. We speculated that when her mother made nonaccepting comments to her, the girl reacted with negative emotion (nonconscious response to threat), triggering secondary stuttering. We also speculated that when the mother talked fast, the girl tried to keep up, but because of an inefficient speech processing system, she stuttered with the easy repetitions of primary stuttering.

Learning

Even though I described learning factors in stuttering in Chapter 5, here I will recap the role of learning to include it in this theoretical perspective on stuttering.

The preceding information on temperament suggested that some children who begin to stutter are more reactive or sensitive than others. This reactivity may contribute to why learning affects some individuals more than others. For all of us, emotional arousal enhances learning. Emotional events are etched into the brain more strongly than neutral ones. Think about how well you can remember what you were doing when you found out about a very exciting or upsetting event. For example, many people in their 20s and 30s and older can remember vividly what they were doing when they heard about the planes crashing into the twin towers of the World Trade Center in New York City on September 11, 2001. The strength of emotional memories is enhanced even further in people with more reactive limbic systems, which may account for why some people suffer posttraumatic stress syndrome and others do not (eg, LeDoux, 2002, 2015).

This link between reactivity and learning has been shown in adults who stutter. A small but important study by Arenas and Zebrowski (2013) demonstrated the link between emotional reactivity, classical conditioning, and effects on speech production. Three individuals who stuttered were compared with three who were typical speakers in a paradigm that assessed the **autonomic reactivity** of subjects (skin conductance response) and their susceptibility to classical conditioning (reaction to stimuli linked to a loud noise). The individuals who stuttered had a significantly greater autonomic response to the aversive stimulus and they showed significantly greater susceptibility to classical conditioning. Moreover, the subjects who stuttered (but not the typical speakers) demonstrated speech production anomalies in acoustic measures taken in speech probes during the conditioning. These findings suggest that individuals who stutter may be emotionally reactive, highly conditionable, and likely to show disturbances in their vulnerable speech production systems.

Returning to children just beginning to stutter, it seems to me that children with reactive temperaments are more likely to respond to the multiple repetitions of primary stuttering with tension, escape, and avoidance and are also much more likely to store their stuttering memories indelibly. Such reactions and memories can snowball. Children's natural defensive response to a repetition that feels out of control (or to parent reactions that are perceived as negative) is to tense their muscles. This increased tension soon makes the stutter last longer, which increases their feeling that they are helpless, and then that triggers a bigger threat response that includes more tension. Children's reactive amygdala mediates the storage of unpleasant memories of stuttering, largely on a nonconscious level. At the same time, another part of the limbic system, the hippocampus, stores information about the situations in which stuttering occurs (eg, to whom the child was talking, what word was being said, where it happened). These contextual cues cause stuttering to spread rapidly from isolated experiences to more and more repeated experiences in similar contexts and eventually to many other situations.

I suggest that children with reactive temperaments are not only more likely to learn to increase tension when they anticipate or experience stuttering but are also more likely to engage in other components of the behavioral inhibition system. These include increases in tempo, other aspects of escape behaviors, and a wide array of avoidances. Thus, these children quickly develop secondary symptoms, such as eye blinks and changing words, to escape from the moment of stuttering or to avoid anticipated stuttering.

Classical conditioning occurs rapidly in these children, but unlearning is a much slower and more difficult process. There is evidence that emotional memories are stored permanently, and even when new behaviors replace them, the original emotions and learned behaviors may reappear under stress (Ayres, 1998). When clinicians work with individuals who have secondary stuttering, they need to keep in mind the strength and persistence of behaviors learned through classical conditioning. They should also keep in mind that learning is highly contextual (eg, Bouton, 2016). New behaviors will have to be learned as new responses to the stimuli that elicited the old responses. And new behaviors will have to be carefully generalized to many different contexts.

Two Predispositions for Stuttering

This is a recap to remind you that primary and secondary stuttering may have two constitutional predispositions: one for primary stuttering and one for secondary stuttering. Figure 6.9 depicts the major components of this perspective. As may be evident, the most common occurrence is for a child to have a predisposition for primary stuttering that is resolved through neural maturation or reorganization—this accounts for the 70% or so of children who recover naturally. It is also possible for a child's primary stuttering to continue into adulthood and for secondary behaviors never to emerge. Think about the evidence that some individuals have great delays in myelination of white matter tracts in speech production areas of the brain. But some of them may have very nonreactive temperaments. These adults may simply be considered highly disfluent, rather than people who stutter. But other individuals who develop stuttering instead of high levels of typical disfluency may have been born with more reactive temperaments and thus may respond strongly to primary stuttering are at the mercy of classical conditioning, increased tension in their stutters, and the vagaries of the environment. The increased stuttering leads to the operant and avoidance conditioning underlying escape and avoidance behaviors that characterize secondary stuttering. I believe that neither of these predispositions is "all or nothing." For instance, an adolescent may have a substantial number of repetitions in his speech but only occasionally show tension, escape, or avoidance behaviors. Or a child may start stuttering suddenly at age 3, with severe repetitive stutters that quickly result in struggle, tension, escape, and avoidance. Perhaps that child has only a little predisposition for primary stuttering but a substantial predisposition for secondary stuttering. This continuum for stuttering agrees with most clinicians' observations that we see a wide range of severity, from mild to very severe, with some who stutter having little avoidance and others having a great deal. I also notice that outside the clinic, there are many individuals whose "stuttering" is so mild that they don't recognize it in themselves and other lay persons don't notice it either.

The possibility of two predispositions for stuttering may also shed light on such phenomena as neurogenic stuttering, which are the disfluencies that sometimes appear in persons with neurological diseases or injuries. The changes in the brain that may occur as part of neurological lesion(s) may give rise to a dyssynchrony in speech and language production processing that is similar to that of primary stuttering. On the other hand, the changes in temperament that sometimes occur with brain injury (eg, Kinsbourne, 1989) may, in a few cases, give rise to disfluencies that are more characteristic of secondary stuttering.

There is support in genetic research for two (or more) predispositions in individuals who do not naturally recover from stuttering. After an analysis of many children who stutter for some period of time in their lives, Ambrose et al. (1997) concluded that persistent and recovered stuttering are not two different forms of the disorder. Both persistent and recovered stutterers appear to have genetic factors related to the onset of stuttering. Those children who persisted in stuttering (ie, continued to stutter for more than three years), however, have additional genetic factors, related to the persistency of the disorder. The additional genetic contributions may be related to the delayed rate of maturation in the white matter tracts interconnecting speech motor areas. But also, the additional genetic factors may result in a reactive temperament, making it more likely that these children will become frustrated, have other emotional reactions to their stuttering, and thus develop secondary/persistent stuttering. This connection between a child reacting to his stuttering and the persistence of the stuttering is reflected in Van Riper's beliefs that "...most children who begin to stutter become fluent perhaps because of maturation or because they do not react to their... repetitions, or prolongations by struggle and avoidance... [while] those who struggle or avoid because of frustration or penalties will probably continue to stutter all the rest of their lives no matter what kind of therapy they receive" (Van Riper, 1990, p. 317).

Indeed, as Ambrose et al. (1997) suggested, there may be more than two predispositions in stuttering. The factors that cause a child to have a threat-based defensive reaction (tension response) to primary stuttering may also cause another child to react the same way to lack of intelligibility or difficulties in word finding, for example. Communicative failures may lead to anticipatory struggle (Bloodstein et al., 2021), as described earlier in this chapter. However, no matter how many predispositions a child may have, the chance of his actually developing primary or secondary stuttering may be enhanced or diminished by both developmental and environmental factors.

Interactions With Developmental Factors

In this section, I describe three ways in which aspects of children's development may interact with the two predispositions to trigger or exacerbate stuttering. You will see elements of the capacities and demands theory of stuttering in this section.

The first interaction is with the demands of language development and a predisposition for primary stuttering. Consider children who begin to acquire speech with dysfunctional or inefficient speech and language networks. The functional plasticity of the children's brains may allow these pathways to reorganize or repair themselves so that the children process spoken language more efficiently as they strive to communicate. However, the exponential growth of the children's speech and language at this very time may compete for cerebral and other brain resources, straining or exceeding the children's capacity to handle the demands of both reorganization and advancing language, at the same time. To see what this may be like, imagine yourself as a student who has let part of the semester slip by without studying. After messing up the first two exams, you resolve to reorganize your study habits and catch up, but just then, your professors decide to pile on even more work than before. Like the children, you may or may not be able to accommodate the professor's increasing demands at the same time you are spending energy to reorganize.

A second interaction will be the maturation of the brain with a predisposition for primary stuttering. Some individuals will have an earlier maturation of the brain or a natural flexibility to respond to anomalies in the wiring for spoken language. Girls, for example, are more likely to recover from early stuttering—either naturally or with treatment—probably because of their inherently greater organizational plasticity and their more widely distributed language centers (Guitar et al., 2015; Shaywitz et al., 1995). Some males may also be genetically endowed with more flexibility than average for reorganizing their cerebral circuitry and thus may recover more readily than others.

The third type of interaction will occur when children have normal neural circuitry for spoken language but a constitutionally inhibited temperament. Typical developmental challenges for most children include some frustration at not being able to speak as fast or with the same complexity as adults and older children in the family. The children may not only be frustrated but embarrassed at their inability to produce more advanced speech and language. Social-emotional development takes the children through some stressful times. All of these typical experiences may produce increased tension, speeding up, escape, and avoidance behaviors associated with speech. Based on my clinical experience, I suspect that some children fitting this description might be hesitant to speak and may be referred for a stuttering evaluation but would not manifest the typical signs of stuttering. Their hesitancies may consist of long pauses, phrase repetitions, or both when their right-hemisphere proclivity toward avoidance, withdrawal, and arrest of ongoing behavior manifests itself while they are speaking. Such hesitancies may diminish in time as myelination of neural circuits and systems serving speech production continues.

Interactions With Environmental Factors

Here I consider the influence of the environment on anomalous speech and language neural networks (predisposition for primary stuttering) and on constitutional predispositions for inhibited temperaments and their effect on learning (predisposition for secondary stuttering).

Interactions of Anomalous Neural Networks With Environmental Factors

As children's developing central nervous systems adapt to the inherited or acquired differences in their neural substrates for speech and language, the environment plays a role through various listeners' responses to children's emerging speech and language skills. Obviously, their family will have the most opportunities to provide acceptance and support. The accommodations they can provide, such as accepting reactions toward the child's stuttering, using slower speech rates, fewer interruptions, and dedicated one-on-one listening time, may foster adaptations of children's inefficient, dyssynchronous neural networks. At least this environment will not stress children's speech and language production system and will probably enable children to develop their own adapted rate of speech and language output. In contrast, an environment with evident disapproval of children's stuttering, many interruptions, rapid conversational give and take, demands for recitations, and little time for children to talk may "overdrive" the children's immature speech and language production system, produce an excess of disfluencies, and inhibit the successful adaptation of the children's system to its original anomalous wiring.

Interactions of Temperament With Environmental Factors

The work of Calkins (1994), Kagan and Snidman (1991), and others (eg, Norona-Zhou & Tung, 2021; Zhang et al., 2021) suggested that families can have a strong influence on temperament. As Calkins and Fox (1994) expressed it, "the child's interactions with a parent provide the context for learning skills and strategies for managing emotional reactivity." In addition, the environmental factors that I have called "life events" can also influence the development of temperament. As noted earlier, Kagan (1994b) suggested that certain life events could cause a child who is not particularly reactive to become more reactive and inhibited.

Individual Differences

Before I discuss the treatment implications for this integrated perspective, I would like to emphasize that each child, adolescent, or adult you work with is unique. As Van Riper (1982a), Alm (2004), Smith (1999), and many others have said, each person who stutters is doing so because of a multitude of interacting factors, some of which had their effect in the past, others of which are operating today. Your job is to figure out which factors you can help to change. Getting to know and understand the individual is vital, especially if you work on this through a supportive, insightful relationship with them. Try to relinquish your preconceptions about what approach must be used, and remember to keep asking yourself, "What does this client need and how can I arrange it?"

Implications for Treatment

In some ways, this section will mirror the implications for treatment described in Chapter 5 where I discussed the unlearning that must take place for treatment to be effective. However, here we also consider treatment of primary stuttering that is not so much unlearning as it is prevention of the learning that creates secondary stuttering.

Preschool Children

Preschool children often have a milder form of stuttering—or at least stuttering that has not been subjected to years of learning. Much of stuttering at this age is primary stuttering that results from the dyssynchronies in brain development described earlier.

The first aim of treatment for this age should be to maximize these children's fluent speech, by creating an environment filled with models of slower speaking rate, including appropriate pauses. Additionally, the environment should reduce pressure on children's speech by asking fewer questions, not interrupting, and giving children adequate attention when they are speaking. These strategies can help children take the time needed to coordinate the elements of speech with the components of language to produce a fluent utterance.

The second aim in treating preschoolers is to prevent children from having a defensive reaction to their disfluencies. Such a reaction would trigger the tension response. Preventing this should be done by helping both the parents or caregivers and the child to be comfortable with and accepting of the repetitive stuttering. The parents can be guided to understand that most children recover from their stuttering and that even those children who don't recover completely can be given treatment that will minimize its effect. Parents, in turn, can reassure children if they seem frustrated or upset by their stuttering. Just a casual comment like "It's ok. Lots of kids get stuck sometimes on words" may be enough. Parents' demeanor at this moment can be relaxed and convey, "It's no big deal."

School-Age Children

Treatment for a school-age children should begin with an assessment of how much tension the children have added to their stuttering. Are their moments of stuttering often characterized by tense postures and physical struggle that are the result of them reacting to the threat of runaway repetitions by fear of being "trapped" in a stutter? Do they use extra movements or sounds to break free of their stutters? Do you hear and see "starters" or other behaviors before stutters or do they talk "all around Robin Hood's barn" to dodge possible stutters? Excess physical tension, as well as escape and avoidance behaviors, suggest that they are reacting to their stuttering, probably with both nonconscious defensive reactions and conscious fear of stuttering. If this is the case, treatment should focus on reducing the fear of stuttering to reduce reactions to it. On the other hand, if their stuttering is mostly tension free and there are few, if any, escape or avoidance behaviors, treatment can focus on helping children practice fluent speech and develop confidence in themselves as communicators. Even with children who are reacting to their stuttering, creating fluency facilitating conditions and experiencing successful communication is vital also. In both cases, generalization of new responses must be assiduously pursued to ensure that increased fluency and confidence are maintained.

Adolescents and Adults

Adolescents or adults who need treatment will probably stutter with excess physical tension, accompanied by escape and avoidance behaviors. At some point, some of these individuals benefit from training in being aware of and increasing their fluent speech. But perhaps one of the most important things is for them to be in an accepting and supportive clinical relationship with a clinician who truly understands stuttering. In that relationship, the first goal (and a continuing goal) would be to help clients develop more positive views of their ability to communicate effectively. As that is going on, they can be helped to diminish their defensive reactions and fear that trigger the excess tension and the escape and avoidance behaviors. This will take time and the clinician must be both firm and accepting as well as being able to demonstrate for the client, with voluntary stuttering, how to connect with listeners and remain calm despite stuttering. The clinician must help clients understand that what they do, think, and feel about stuttering is essentially learned behavior and can be unlearned. The clinician guides the adolescents or adults to stutter easily, without avoidances prior to the speech attempt, without the excess physical tension, and without trying to "blast out" of the moment of stuttering but instead remain relaxed as they ease the word out. The clinician also helps clients learn that most listeners are patient rather than rejecting. Some of this learning occurs when the clinician accepts whatever stuttering happens as they are working on it together. Some occurs because the clinician accepts the client as they are. And some occurs when the clinician pseudo-stutters in public and client can see for themselves that listeners are able to accept stuttering and that the person stuttering can be calm as they stutter. Much more detail is given in Sections II and III of this textbook on treatment.

Accounting for the Evidence

Let us now turn to the research findings and clinical observations for which these views of stuttering must account.

Stuttering Occurs in All Cultures

The fact that stuttering is universal should not be unexpected because it depends largely on basic biological variations of the human brain. Many other disorders, such as dyslexia and specific language impairment, as well as such personality differences as sensitive temperament, are associated with atypical activity of the central nervous system and are also universal (eg, Ziegler et al., 2003). Children's responses to their primary stuttering may be slightly different in cultures that are more or less accepting of differences, especially. But in general, children in most cultures would show reactions when their articulators suddenly go out of control.

Stuttering Is a Low-Incidence Disorder

The prevalence of stuttering may be relatively low if indeed chronic stuttering results from a combination of at least two biological predispositions (**anomalous neural organization** for speech and sensitive temperament). In addition, evidence suggests that the predisposition related to the development of neural circuitry for speech often resolves because of neural growth.

Stuttering Does Not Begin With the Onset of Speech

Why does stuttering usually begin only after fluency at the one- and two-word stage has been achieved? Most researchers agree that stuttering emerges first from disruptions caused by a child's inefficient neural networks for speech and language processing. Perhaps these networks can handle the relatively simple processing required for simple words and phrases. But once children begin to reorganize their language functions from a lexical to a grammatical focus as they try out more complicated syntax, their inefficient neural organization breaks down. An added demand on their planning system is that the shift from one- to two-word utterances requires the use of a more complex prosody that is a bigger challenge to those inefficient networks (Kent, 1984; Packman & Attanasio, 2010; Perkins et al., 1991; Wingate, 1988).

Stuttering Sometimes Begins With Tense Blocks, but More Often With Repetitions

There are children who begin to stutter with tense blocks that did not follow a period of repetitions and occasional prolongations. With a few children, the act of speech becomes so threatening that a dramatic tension response (a block) is the first sign of stuttering. In other cases, repetitions change so quickly to tense blocks that listeners don't remember that the repetitions occurred first. A few years ago, I worked with a 2-year-old girl who showed excessive squeezing and tension in her stutters after only a few hours of stuttering in a repetitive pattern. Still, in general, the first sign of stuttering is repetition of sounds, syllables, or single-syllable words. As we have said earlier, these repetitions appear to be the result of anomalies in the neural networks for speech production that are not able to have the next syllable or word ready "to go out the door." Thus, the preceding unit is repeated until the system is ready to produce the following one.

Stuttering Severity Changes Over Time

The course of development of stuttering seems to be determined in part by the biological responses of the child to uncontrollable repetitions and the classical and operant learning that follow. In more severe children, there may be a neuroanatomical basis for more frequent and persistent disfluencies (Chow & Chang, 2017) to which these responses are made. Details on the development of stuttering will be discussed in Chapter 7.

Stuttering Appears as Repetitions, Prolongations, and Blocks

Very often, the earliest signs of childhood stuttering are relatively loose repetitions of syllables. These may arise from a breakdown in the function of neural circuits for sensorimotor control of speech output. Repetitions may occur simply because there is a lag in the readiness of the next part of a word or sentence, although the impulse or pressure to continue speaking is strong. The repetitions sometimes become more rapid and end in prolongations, as the child responds—with increases in speed and tension—to the threat of being unable to speak. As the child tries to cope—consciously and nonconsciously—with being unable to continue speaking, tension increases and prolongations begin to show increases in pitch. Not long after, the tension results in momentary blockages of speech altogether.

When the earliest signs of stuttering are characterized by tension and blocking (Van Riper, 1982a), an emotional response may be primary. As Van Riper suggested, these may be children whose onset is very sudden, resulting usually after an emotionally difficult period or traumatic emotional stress.

Not All Stutterers Have Relatives Who Stuttered

How do we account for both the genetic transmission of stuttering and that evidence of genetic transmission is lacking in some cases? Genetic transmission of stuttering in many cases may be through the two factors I just described: anomalous neural organization for speech and sensitive temperament. In some cases of childhood stuttering, genetic transmission may seem unlikely because no other family members seem to be affected. However, it may occur because persistent stuttering appears to require both predisposing factors. Some family members may inherit one factor and some the other, but unless both factors are inherited by the same individual, persistent stuttering may not develop. Another reason for the absence of stuttering in other family members may be that the predisposing factors were the result not of genetic inheritance but of environmental factors affecting fetal or early childhood development that created the neural substrate for stuttering. Moreover, such anomalous speech and language circuitry may create language, learning, or phonological problems in other family members. Remember that the unfolding of the genetic blueprint is extensively influenced by environmental factors and by chance. Thus, the anomalous circuitry in one child may result in stuttering, but in an uncle or grandmother, it may have resulted in an articulation disorder or learning problem.

Stuttering Is More Common in Boys Than in Girls

I suspect that the reason more boys stutter than girls is that the genetic blueprints for neural organization of speech and language differ between boys and girls and may be more flexible in females (Burman et al., 2008; Shaywitz et al., 1995). Neuroplasticity of the human brain is greatest in the first few years of life, and this neuroplasticity probably diminishes after puberty. Neuroplasticity permits reorganization of neural pathways and, in many cases, recovery. Karlin (1947) advanced another explanation of why more girls recover early from stuttering. He postulated that delayed myelinization of nerve fibers in speech processing areas was a possible explanation of stuttering and cited research that myelinization of nerve fibers is more advanced in girls than in boys of the same age. The research by Choo et al. (2016) confirms Karlin's hypothesis, demonstrating a relationship between deficiencies in language performance and less dense white matter tracts in the left hemisphere (less myelination) in boys who stutter but not girls.

Many Conditions Reduce or Eliminate Stuttering

Conditions that temporarily ameliorate stuttering, such as singing or speaking rhythmically, probably improve fluency by giving speech and language processes more time or a supplemental organizing stimulus to aid speech production. These conditions may also involve other parts of the brain rather than those anomalous networks used inefficiently for typically spoken language. Research using neuroimaging has shown that speech-language areas of the brain that are typically dysfunctional during stuttering actually function normally during conditions that ameliorate fluency (eg, Chang et al., 2009; Toyomura et al., 2011).

Individuals Who Stutter Often Have Poorer Performance on Sensory and Motor Tasks

How about differences in performance between groups of stutterers and nonstutterers? As suggested earlier in this chapter, the wide range of performance on language tests, school achievement tests, and tests of sensorimotor ability by groups of stutterers may reflect the generally lower, but wide range of delays and deviations in the neural substrates for these abilities that led to their inefficient processing of speech and language. In fact, the neural substrates of these performance differences were demonstrated to be associated with poorer white matter integrity (less myelination) in left hemisphere auditory-motor areas (Choo et al., 2016).

Other Research Findings and Clinical Observations That Should Be Accounted for

Other characteristics of stuttering that I have said should be explained by any view of stuttering, such as the influence of developmental and environmental factors, are explicitly addressed in earlier parts of this chapter. Some characteristics, findings, and observations are explained more easily than others. Those that are not accounted for in detail (such as the strong effect of rhythmic stimuli on stuttering) should not be ignored. They are a reality and are hard-edged facts that should reshape any theoretical view until it is more fully explanatory. Can you think of any more?

SUMMARY

- Several theoretical perspectives have been proposed to account for constitutional factors in stuttering. They include views of stuttering: (1) as an **anomaly** of how the brain is organized for speech and language; (2) as a disorder of timing of the sequential movements for speech; (3) as a dysfunction of the **corticobasal ganglia thalamocortical loop**; (4) as a result of deficits in the internal modeling process used to control speech production; (5) as a disorder of spoken language production; and (6) as a multifactorial dynamic disorder.
- Current theoretical perspectives concerning developmental and environmental factors include (1) the anticipatory struggle theory, which suggests that children may develop stuttering as a result of negative anticipation of speaking after they have had frustrating or embarrassing experiences in communicating, and (2) the capacities and demands theory, which postulates that stuttering arises when children's capacities for rapid, fluent utterances are unequal to the demands within the children themselves or within the environment.
- In this chapter, I elaborated a two-stage etiological model of stuttering that I first proposed in a chapter on children's stuttering and emotions (Guitar, 1997) and that owes much to Bluemel (1957), Brutten and Shoemaker (1967), and Van Riper (1982a, 1990). The first stage is primary stuttering, which involves repetitions that are frequently the first signs of stuttering. These signs are thought to be the result of a constitutional factor: a dyssynchrony at some level of the speech and language production process. The second stage is secondary stuttering, which involves the tension, struggle, escape, and avoidance behaviors that are often present in persistent stuttering. These behaviors are proposed to be the result of a separate constitutional factor—a reactive temperament that triggers a defense response from the behavioral inhibition system and that makes the individual more emotionally conditionable than the average speaker.

STUDY QUESTIONS

1. What are the differences between the Geschwind and Galaburda (1985) theory of stuttering and the Webster (1993a) view?
2. Compare Kent's (1984) view of stuttering as a disorder of timing with the Geschwind and Galaburda (1985) theory.
3. In Chang and Guenther's (2020) view, where in the BG loop do dysfunctions occur?
4. Both Neilson and Neilson's (1987) view of stuttering and one of Max et al.'s (2004) hypotheses about stuttering suggest that repetitions occur because of a problem with the internal models used for speech production. What is the difference between the cause of repetitions in each view?
5. The study by Kelly et al. (1995) reviewed in this chapter suggested that tremors don't appear in younger children who stutter but do appear in older children. Why would this be?

6. Table 6.1 lists experiences that may generate stuttering in some children because the experiences have led children to believe speaking is difficult. Add as many other hypothetical experiences as you can to this list.
7. A capacities and demands view of stuttering in children would lead to a therapy strategy of enhancing a child's capacities (in addition to reducing demands). What are some examples of capacities in a child that you could strengthen to reduce stuttering? Describe how you would do this.
8. What is the relationship between a sensitive temperament and a notable ability to be conditioned?
9. I have suggested there may be two predispositions for persistent stuttering—one for primary stuttering and one for secondary stuttering. How, according to this view, would primary stuttering lead to secondary stuttering?
10. There is strong evidence that girls are more likely than boys to recover from stuttering and are, therefore, less likely to become persistent stutterers. Is this because girls are more likely to recover quickly from primary stuttering or because their primary stuttering is less likely to trigger secondary stuttering?

SUGGESTED PROJECTS

1. The view of stuttering as a problem of the "internal modeling" process in speech production is a complex idea. Read the article by Max et al. (2004) and make a class presentation about their full theoretical model, explaining it in as clear and simple a way as possible.
2. Read the article entitled "Resources—A Theoretical Stone Soup" (Navon, 1984) and use the arguments in it to evaluate the capacities and demands theory in this chapter.
3. Wendell Johnson's "diagnosogenic" view of stuttering led to a master's thesis that tried to create stuttering in orphans in 1939. In 2003, this thesis was the topic of a controversy that centered on the ethics of trying to induce stuttering in children. Using the internet, research this controversy, using "Monster Study" as a keyword. Make a presentation or write a paper on the ethics of this research, given the fact that it was conducted more than 80 years ago when the ethical climate was markedly different than it is now.
4. Pick a theory of stuttering—either one described in the first two sections of this chapter or one you have found elsewhere—and evaluate how it can account for the basic facts about stuttering enumerated in Chapter 1.
5. Go to Guitar and McCauley (2010b) and read two chapters concerning specific interventions related to a specific age group of people who stutter. Identify which theories addressed here are cited and how they appear to impact the developers of each intervention approach.

SUGGESTED READINGS

Alm, P. (2004). Stuttering and the basal ganglia circuits: A critical review of possible relations. *Journal of Communication Disorders, 37*, 325–396.

This journal article presents the first thorough argument that the BG loop—the circuitry that is responsible for the sequencing of planning and execution of spoken syllables—may be a critical piece of the stuttering puzzle.

Chang, S. E. and Guenther, F. H. (2020). Involvement of the cortico-basal ganglia-thalamocortical loop in developmental stuttering. *Frontiers in Psychology, 10*, 1–15.

This article builds on Alm's (2004) publication about the BG loop and cites a huge array of studies that support this hypothesis. The authors delineate three possible hypotheses about where in the BG loop dysfunctions may occur and acknowledge that different individuals who stutter may have problems in different areas of the BG loop.

Denworth, L. (2021, August 1). The stuttering mind. *Scientific American*.

This is a lay person's interesting update on stuttering, with some personal touches.

Gray, J. A. (1987). *The psychology of fear and stress* (2nd ed.). Cambridge University Press.

Gray's experimental work and his theoretical model of a behavioral inhibition system are clearly described here. Some of the book (those parts dealing with the effects of pharmacological agents on the brain) is for specialized readers. Much of it, however, is a readable exposition on the biological basis of learning, stress, and fear.

Guitar, B., & McCauley, R. (2010). How to use this book. In B. Guitar, & R. McCauley (Eds.), *Treatment of stuttering*. Lippincott Williams & Wilkins.

This chapter describes in user-friendly language what a theory is and how it can help researchers and clinicians.

Kagan, J., Reznick, J. S., & Snidman, N. (1987). The physiology and psychology of behavioral inhibition in children. *Child Development, 58*, 1459–1473.

This article discusses the findings of Kagan and his colleagues that behaviorally inhibited children show high levels of laryngeal tension. Neurophysiological mechanisms are also discussed, as well as possible genetic and environmental contributions. This article is recommended for those interested in the hypothesis that behavioral inhibition may be a component in some stuttering.

LeDoux, J. (1996). *The emotional brain: The mysterious underpinnings of emotional life*. Simon & Schuster.

LeDoux, a highly respected brain researcher, brings together a great deal of evidence about how the brain processes experiences that we consider emotional. His explanations of emotional learning are very clear and relevant to stuttering.

LeDoux, J. (2015). *Anxious: Using the brain to understand and treat fear and anxiety*. Viking.

Although I listed this book in Suggested Readings for the previous chapter on learning, I think it is important enough to suggest it again here for this chapter on theories. This book advances his views on fear and anxiety and their treatment. From his perspective, fear is not a basic response to threat, but a cognitively synthesized emotion. Fear and anxiety derive from nonconscious responses to threat. These low-level defensive automatic responses include hypertonic behaviors such as freezing. I think our understanding of stuttering may be improved if we take these into consideration.

Packman, A., & Attanasio, J. (2017). *Theoretical issues in stuttering* (2nd ed.). Routledge Press.

The authors review current and past theories of stuttering and evaluate them in terms of testability, explanatory power, parsimony, and heuristic power. This book effectively teaches the reader what a theory should be expected to do.

7

Typical Disfluency and the Development of Stuttering

Chapter Outline

Chapter Objectives

After studying this chapter, readers should be able to:

- Describe and explain the typical (1) core behaviors, (2) secondary behaviors, (3) feelings and attitudes, and (4) underlying processes for the following age and developmental levels, as well as exceptions and variations:
  - Typical disfluency
  - Stuttering in younger preschool children: borderline stuttering
  - Stuttering in older preschool children: beginning stuttering
  - Stuttering in school-age children: intermediate stuttering
  - Stuttering in older teens and adults: advanced stuttering

Key Terms

Age/developmental levels: These levels reflect both the age of the individual (eg, younger preschooler, older preschooler, etc.) and the severity of the stuttering (eg, borderline, beginning, etc.)

Antiexpectancy devices: An unusual way of speaking or acting that seems to reduce stuttering, like laughing and pretending that most things said were a joke. Another example is speaking with an accent that the speaker pretends to have. An avoidance

Avoidance conditioning: A type of learning that occurs when a person avoids something they think will be unpleasant. The avoidance is rewarded by the fact that the unpleasantness doesn't happen. Avoidance conditioning is important in thinking about stuttering development and interventions because it can be difficult to combat. See Chapter 5, on learning, to read more about avoidance conditioning

Circumlocutions: Rather than stutter on a word, a person who stutters might use a different way of saying something, such as "My father was in the N...n...he served aboard ships in the armed forces." Again, another avoidance

Covert Stuttering: Stuttering that the individual hides from listeners, usually by avoiding sounds, words, and situations that might precipitate stuttering. It is typically associated with deep shame about stuttering

Dysrhythmic phonation: A sound prolongation, broken word, or other instance of ongoing phonation being stopped, extended, or distorted

Levels of Stuttering: *Borderline stuttering*: This is the earliest or lowest level of stuttering, usually seen in children ages 2 to 3.5. This type of stuttering is characterized by more frequent part-word and single-syllable whole-word repetitions than children who are developing typically have, but without awareness or concern on the part of the child. *Beginning stuttering*: This level of stuttering is usually seen in children between ages 3.5 and 6, although it may occur before and after those ages. It is characterized by more tension and hurry in disfluencies than that seen in borderline stuttering. Stuttering at this level usually consists of repetitions and prolongations, but some children will also exhibit blocks. Escape and even some avoidance behaviors appear in this level of stuttering. *Intermediate stuttering*: Typical of children in their school-age years, this level of stuttering will abound in repetitions and prolongations, but blocks will also be frequent. In addition to escape behaviors, avoidances will be frequent at this level because there is fear of being "stuck" in a stutter and fear of listener reactions. *Advanced stuttering*: This level is characteristic of older teens and adults who have been stuttering since childhood. Their stuttering pattern, especially behaviors associated with avoidance and ways of coping with blocks, is quite ingrained

Postponements: This is like a starter, but usually it just involves waiting a few beats before saying a feared word as in "Back then I use to drink a lot of......soda." An avoidance

Starters: Words or sounds used by someone who stutters to get started speaking when blocked or when anticipating a block. For example, a person who stutters might say "My name is, uh, Barry." Starters are a type of avoidance behavior because they are used before the individual is in a moment of stuttering

"Stuttering-like" disfluencies: Short segment repetitions (ie, part-word and monosyllabic whole-word repetitions), as well as sound prolongations and blocks. These are disfluencies that are typically judged by listeners as stuttering.

Substitutions: The substitution of an "easier" word for a "harder" word on which a stutterer expects to stutter. For example, a stutterer who often stuttered on words beginning with "p" and who had a dog named "Pluto" might generally substitute "my dog" for the dog's name when talking about him. These are a type of avoidance

Typical disfluency: These are the disfluencies in the speech of individuals who do not stutter. They are more prevalent in younger children (eg, ages 2 to 4), but appear in the speech of all talkers. Some examples are (1) multisyllable word repetitions, (2) revisions, (3) incomplete phrases, and (4) interjections

Underlying processes: These are speculations about the process that may cause disfluencies or stuttering at each developmental level. These processes help us understand why stuttering often changes from borderline to beginning to intermediate to advanced levels

"Within-word" disfluencies: Disfluencies that occur within a word boundary such as repetitions of parts of words, prolongations, or blocks. Stuttered speech is said to contain a higher proportion of within-word disfluencies (as opposed to disfluencies that happen between words and across words, such as hesitations, fillers, and repetitions of whole words) compared to typical disfluency. Note that some disfluencies of children who are developing typically may also include within-word disfluencies, li-like this

OVERVIEW

This chapter describes the development of stuttering and what it is like at various ages. It is designed to help you understand why, once stuttering has emerged, it often (but not always) progresses from a few relaxed repetitions in preschool children to frequent stuttering accompanied by tension, avoidance, and many negative feelings and beliefs in older children or adults. This chapter will also help you understand how to match treatment procedures to the underlying dynamics of stuttering, as well as to the age of the client. To accomplish these goals, I have organized the content into five levels that reflect not only age groupings but also stages of development of stuttering and important characteristics of each stage of stuttering to guide your selection of a therapy approach (Fig. 7.1).

The five age groupings/developmental levels are given in Table 7.1. In subsequent sections of this chapter, I will describe each level in detail and then discuss key attributes of each level in terms of core behaviors, secondary behaviors, and feelings and attitudes, as well as underlying processes. This last attribute of each level—**underlying processes**—explains why symptoms change from level to level. My explanations are hypotheses based on evidence from studies of animal and human behavior that may help us understand how stuttering behaviors become more severe and complex. The material in the "underlying processes" subcategory should help you understand the nature of the symptoms as well as the rationales for the treatments presented in the second section of this book.

The **levels of stuttering** are based primarily on age and the degree to which the stuttering has advanced, developmentally. Developmental advancement captures not only severity of stuttering but also the accompanying behaviors that reflect cognitive and emotional responses to stuttering. Specifically, as individuals' stuttering progresses and becomes more of a burden to them, they increase tension and struggle, escape maneuvers to terminate the moments of stuttering, and avoidance behaviors to try not to stutter.

Specific age groupings (younger preschool, older preschool, school age, and teens and adults) are used for different levels because age is often critical in selecting the appropriate treatment. Let me give two examples. No matter how severely a preschool child stutters, treatment should always involve their parents and family. Conversely, a school-age child—whether stuttering is mild or severe—needs an approach that involves teachers and classmates as well as parents and family. Also, treatment helps children of this age to discuss their stuttering and their feelings about it. In general, the cognitive-emotional level of clients at different ages should be considered when choosing a therapy strategy. In other words, younger preschool children don't need extensive work on their feelings about stuttering; their parents or caregivers can reassure them when needed. School-age children, adolescents, and adults, however, may need some treatment focus on what they think and feel about their stuttering.

Exceptions and Variations

The **age/developmental levels** presented in this chapter do not characterize absolutely everyone who stutters. For example, some older preschool children may be stuttering so mildly and be so relatively unaware of it that they might best be treated by an approach described for younger preschool children. Clinicians should feel free to borrow or combine treatment strategies if an individual's stuttering does not fit the pattern described for their age. Apart from a few exceptions, however, clinicians should stay with a specific approach if it appears to be working. In my experience, it is rarely beneficial to haphazardly take procedures from several different approaches.

Another qualification of the hierarchy presented here concerns the implication that all individuals who stutter pass through each stage in sequence. This is generally true, but there are exceptions. Children may show only typical disfluencies one day and beginning or intermediate stuttering on another day. They may stop stuttering without apparent reason a week later, or they may continue stuttering unless treated. One 3-year-old boy I knew changed overnight from borderline to severe beginning stuttering after a change in his allergy medication. As soon as he resumed taking his original

Age Groupings/Developmental Levels
Typical Disfluency
Da - Da - Dad
Younger Preschool Child:
Borderline Stuttering
Wa - Wa -
Wa - Wa - Watch
my car go
Older Preschool Child:
Beginning Stuttering
C-C-C... Can I
go out to
p-p-p... play?
School-age Child:
Intermediate Stuttering
I-I-I, uh, uh,
don't, uh,
know.
Adult and Adolescent:
Advanced Stuttering
C... C... Could
y... you make
a ph... ph... phone
call for me?

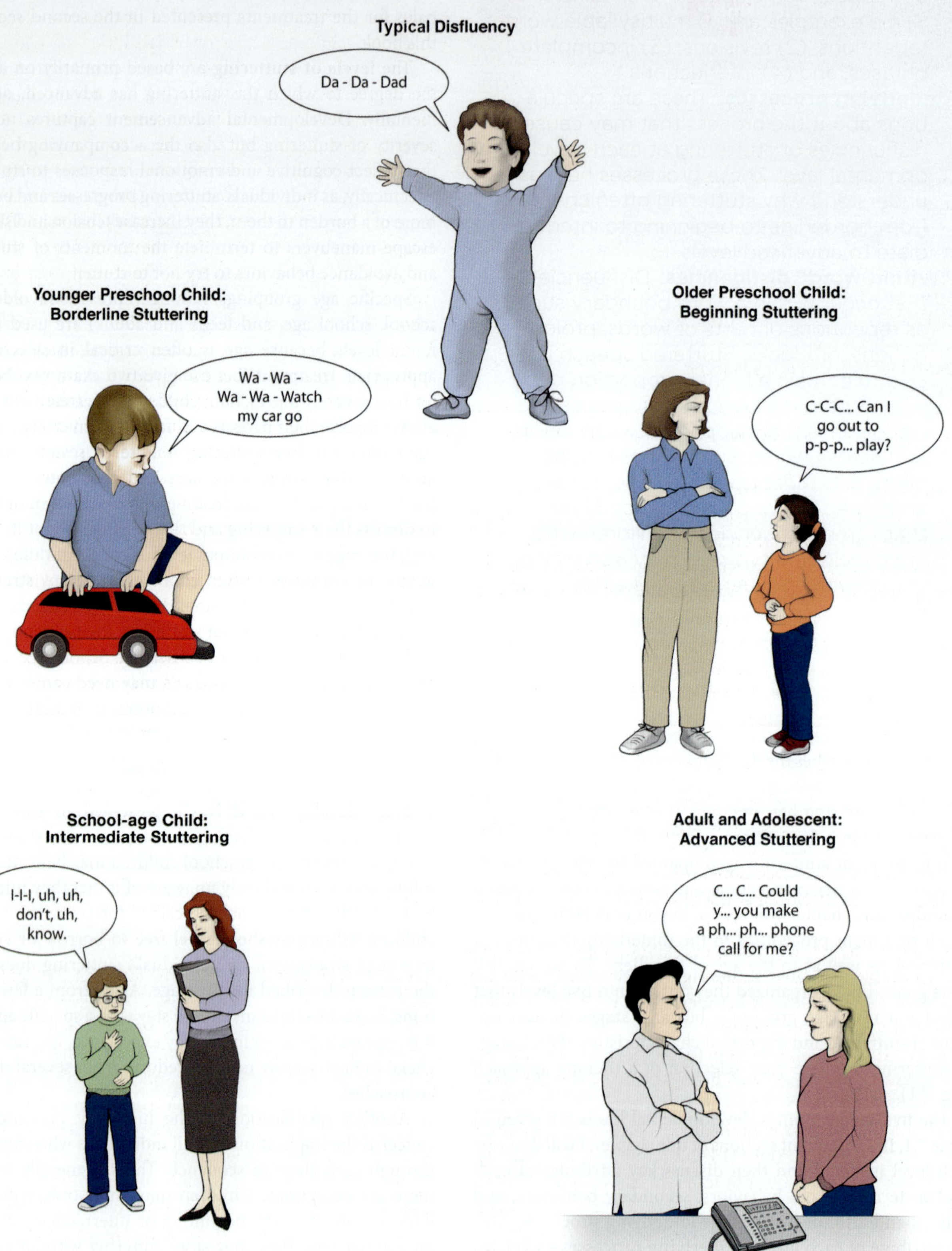

Figure 7.1 Overview of Chapter 7.

TABLE 7.1 Developmental/Treatment Levels of Stuttering

Developmental/Treatment Level	Typical Age Range (Years)
Typical disfluency	1.5–6[a]
Younger preschoolers: borderline stuttering	1.5–3.5
Older preschoolers: beginning stuttering	3.5–6
School age: intermediate stuttering	6–13
Older teens and adults: advanced stuttering	≥14

[a]A small amount of typical disfluency continues in mature speech.

prescription, he became a borderline stutterer again and then recovered completely without treatment. There are many unsolved mysteries in stuttering.

Two clinical researchers who wrote extensively about the development of stuttering, Van Riper (1982a) and Bloodstein (1960a, 1960b, 1961b), agreed that a simple sequence of stages could never capture every individual's pattern. Bloodstein (1960b) proposed a series of four stages of stuttering development, which he described as "typical, not universal" (Bloodstein et al., 2021, p. 31). He also cautioned that although stuttering near onset is often characterized by repetitions without awareness or by a lack of concern, some children at this stage show considerable effort and strain in their stuttering as well as crying from frustration at their inability to produce speech easily (Bloodstein, 1960a).

Van Riper (1982a) also noted the presence of forcing and struggle in some children at the onset of stuttering, and like Bloodstein, he was struck by the fact that most children, especially in their early years, oscillate between remissions and recurrences of their stuttering, between mild stuttering and **typical disfluency**, or between more advanced and less advanced stages of development.

In addition to such swings in the progression of stuttering development, there may also be different paths of development, which different individuals may follow. After searching his clinical files on many individuals whom he had followed for several years, Van Riper (1982a) found that his data suggested there are subgroups of individuals who stutter. These subgroups are characterized by different onsets and different trajectories of development. He proposed that there are four distinctive "tracks" that an individual may follow. The most common track consists of children with stuttering onset between 2 and 4 years of age, whose stuttering begins as repetitions, progresses to include prolongations, and then gradually develops into blocks with more and more tension as well as fears and avoidances. The next most common track comprises children whose onset is a little later and is sometimes accompanied by delayed speech development, articulation problems, or very rapid speech. An interesting aspect of this track is that these children seem to have had difficulty hearing their own speech, perhaps as a result of auditory processing problems. This is particularly interesting in light of findings from brain imaging studies of adults who stutter (eg, Foundas et al., 2001), indicating that some have anatomical anomalies that might produce difficulty with more complex auditory processing. A third track—far less common that the first two—includes children who have a sudden onset of stuttering with a great deal of tension that results in tight, laryngeal blocks. Finally, a fourth track consists of individuals whose disfluency appears to have psychological components at onset. This type of stuttering used to be called "psychogenic" stuttering but is now frequently referred to as "functional" stuttering because that term is more acceptable to clients. This track is characterized by late onset and by a stereotyped pattern of stuttering that is accompanied by few avoidances and changes very little with age.

Van Riper's four tracks serve as a warning to us that there is much diversity in the evolution of stuttering. Another clinical researcher, Yairi (2007), reviewed past attempts to subtype individuals who stutter. Yairi discussed Van Riper's tracks of stuttering development as well as other authors' attempts to identify subgroups of individuals who stutter, including variations in the progression of symptoms.

Keeping these variations, exceptions, and limitations in mind, I will now begin a detailed description of the levels of stuttering development and treatment, starting with a group of behaviors that is really not stuttering at all but appears in typical speech.

TYPICAL DISFLUENCY

Children vary a great deal in how disfluent they are as they learn to communicate. Some pass their milestones of speech and language development with relatively few disfluencies. Others stumble along, repeating, interjecting, and revising as they try to master new forms of speech and language on their way to adult competence. Most are somewhere between the extremes of exceptional fluency and excessive disfluency, such as the 2-year-old shown in Figure 7.2.

A video clip with an example of a child with typical disfluency is available on Lippincott Connect ("Normal Disfluency and the Development of Stuttering." She is the first child on this video, Annie). Notice the many different types of disfluencies in her speech, as well as her lack of concern and her happy demeanor even during her disfluencies. I have

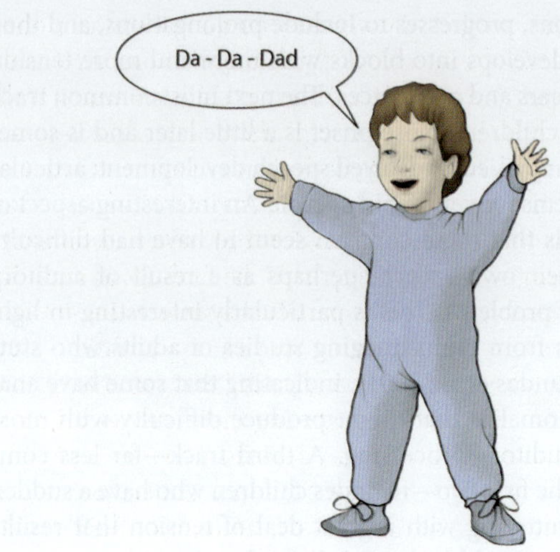

Figure 7.2 Child who may be typically disfluent.

selected a portion of her conversation that has an unusually large amount of disfluency to show that some moments of a typically disfluent child's speech can seem a lot like stuttering.

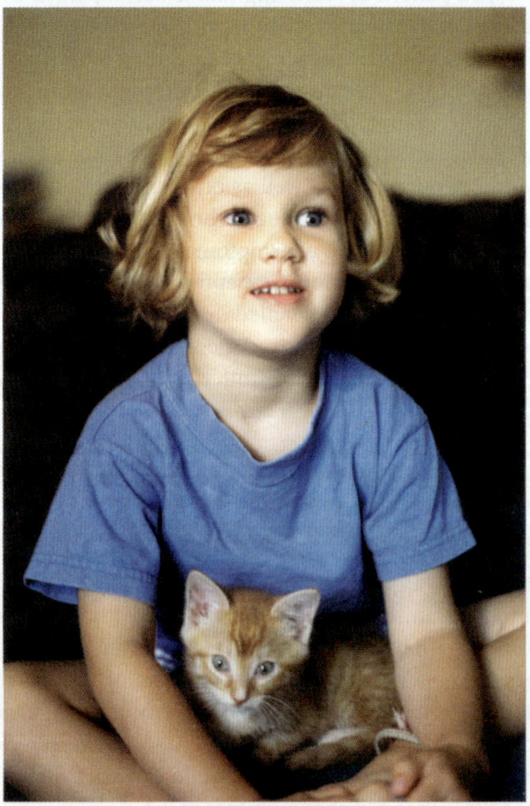

Often, disfluent children swing back and forth in the degree of their disfluency. Some days they are more fluent and other days less fluent. Such swings in disfluency may be associated with language development, motor learning, or other developmental or environmental influences mentioned in the preceding chapters. In the following sections, I discuss factors that may influence disfluency, specific behaviors that I categorize as typical disfluency, and the reactions that some children may have to their disfluency. I also highlight aspects of typical disfluency that distinguish it from early stuttering, because one of my aims in this chapter is to prepare you to make this distinction.

Core Behaviors

Typical disfluencies have been cataloged by several authors who generally agree about what constitutes disfluency (Bloodstein, 1987; Colburn & Mysak, 1982a, 1982b; Juste & Furquim de Andrade, 2011; Williams et al., 1968; Yairi, 1982, 1983, 1997a; Yairi & Ambrose, 2005). Table 7.2 lists eight commonly used categories of disfluency. The first two (part-word repetitions and single-syllable whole-word repetitions) and the last two (prolongations and tense pauses) have been labeled "stuttering-like disfluencies" (Yairi & Ambrose, 2005). "Tense pauses" are moments when the child is not producing speech but shows muscle tension in those parts of the speech mechanism that can be observed, such as the lips or jaw. However, in some cases, tension is confined to the laryngeal structures and may not be clearly visible to the observer. The other categories (multisyllable word repetitions, phrase repetitions, interjections, and revision-incomplete phrase) are believed, by most experts, to be not stuttering disfluencies but, instead, typical disfluencies. Note that some typically developing children will have a few stuttering-like disfluencies mixed in with their greater number of nonstuttering-like disfluencies.

TABLE 7.2 Categories of Disfluencies

Type of Disfluency	Example
Part-word repetition[a]	"mi-milk"
Single-syllable word repetition[a]	"I...I want that"
Multisyllable word repetition	"Lassie...Lassie is a good dog"
Phrase repetition	"I want a...I want a ice-ceem comb"
Interjection	"He went to the...uh...circus"
Revision-incomplete phrase	"I lost my...Where's Mommy going?"
Prolongation[a]	"I'm Tiiiiiiimmy Thompson"
Tense pause[a]	"Can I have some more (lips together, no sound) milk?"

[a]Stutterlike disfluencies.

The speech of typically developing children has other characteristics (besides these categories). These include the amount of disfluency and the number of units of repetitions and interjections, especially in relation to the age of the child.

Let's begin with the amount of disfluency. This is often measured as the number of disfluencies per 100 words or syllables, rather than "percentage disfluencies." "Percentage disfluencies" implies that the disfluencies are associated with the production of particular words. For example, if you said that a child had 10% disfluent words, it would be assumed that 10% of the words spoken were spoken disfluently. However, many disfluencies, such as revisions, interjections, or phrase repetitions, are composed of several words or occur between words. For example, a child may say "Mommy, can you…can you…um…can you buy me that?" It's inaccurate to say that some of these words were spoken disfluently, because the disfluencies were the repetition of the phrase "can you" and the interjection of "um." Were the disfluencies on the words actually spoken, or did they (eg, a phrase repetition) occur because the child was having trouble formulating the remainder of the sentence? In this case, we say that the child spoke six words ("Mommy can you buy me that?") and had two disfluencies (a phrase repetition and an interjection). Hence, we calculate the number of disfluencies that occur when the child speaks 100 words. More details on counting disfluencies are given in chapters on assessment.

Although many researchers have measured disfluencies per number of words spoken, a good argument can be made for measuring disfluencies per number of syllables spoken. Andrews and Ingham (1971) first recommended the practice of assessing frequency of stuttering in relation to syllables spoken because some multisyllabic words may have more than one disfluency, like "S-S-S-Sept-te-te-tember" or "di-dinosa-sa-saur." These examples would be one disfluency each if disfluent words were counted, but two if disfluent syllables were counted. In line with this, Yairi (1997a) noted that as children get older, they are more likely to use multisyllable words. To keep the count equitable between younger and older children, Yairi has assessed disfluencies in children as the number per 100 syllables attempted (Hubbard & Yairi, 1988; Yairi & Ambrose, 1996; Yairi & Lewis, 1984).

When the frequency of all of a child's disfluencies is measured, we need to know how many disfluencies are typical disfluencies. Some of the earliest research on disfluency was conducted by Wendell Johnson at the University of Iowa. He assembled a team of researchers in the 1950s to examine the evidence for his "diagnosogenic" theory of stuttering. As indicated in Chapter 6 about theories, Johnson hypothesized that at the time a child is first "diagnosed" as stuttering by his or her parents, the child's disfluencies do not differ from those of children who do not stutter. One of the research team's projects was to record children identified by their parents as children who stutter and compare the disfluency in their speech with that of children who do not stutter (Johnson et al., 1959). One part of this study compared 68 male children who stuttered with 68 male children who didn't. The results showed that although there was some overlap, the stuttering children had more than twice the amount of disfluency (on average, 18 disfluencies per 100 words) than did the children who did not stutter (only seven disfluencies per 100 words). Johnson interpreted the findings as showing that the two groups were essentially the same because there was so much overlap in both amount and type of disfluency. Researchers following Johnson (eg, McDearmon, 1968) have reinterpreted these data as indicating there are two different groups, as I discussed in the last chapter.

Other researchers who have examined the disfluencies in children who do not stutter put the amount of their disfluencies at about the same level as Johnson and his colleagues reported (DeJoy & Gregory, 1985; Hubbard & Yairi, 1988; Wexler & Mysack, 1982; Yairi, 1981; Yairi & Ambrose, 1996; Yairi & Lewis, 1984; Zebrowski, 1991). A study by Tumanova et al. (2014) examined the conversational speech of 244 children who did not stutter (ages 36 to 71 months) and found that the mean number of total disfluencies (both nonstuttered and stuttered disfluencies) was 4.28 (SD = 2.3) per 100 words. This figure may be lower than those in other studies because these researchers did not include children younger than 36 months (eg, between 24 and 36 months) when disfluencies could be quite high.

Bringing all these studies together, we can estimate that normally speaking preschool children, if you include ages 2 to 3, have on average about 6 to 10 disfluencies for every 100 words spoken. If measured in terms of syllables, it would be closer to five disfluencies per 100 syllables.

The range in frequency of typical disfluency is important to note also, especially if the frequency of disfluency is used to make clinical decisions. Johnson et al. (1959) and Yairi (1981) found that, although many children who do not stutter have only one or two disfluencies per 100 words, at least one child in their samples had slightly more than 25 disfluencies per 100 words. All of these nonstuttering children were categorized as typically speaking children by their parents and by an experienced speech-language pathologist. Thus, the frequency of disfluencies is not a definitive clinical measure by itself.

Another distinguishing characteristic of typical disfluency is the number of units that occur in each repetition or interjection. Yairi's (1981) data suggest that typical repetitions usually consist of only one extra unit. For example, a child might say "That my-my ball." Interjections are likely to be just a single unit, such as "I want some…uh…juice." Instances of multiple repetitions were occasionally observed in these children, but they were the exception. The rule of thumb is that in typical disfluencies, there is one and sometimes two units per repetition or interjection. This agrees with the findings of Johnson et al. (1959) that children who do not stutter have one- or two-unit repetitions.

Another major characteristic of typical disfluency is the type of disfluency that is most common. Johnson et al. (1959) found that interjections, revisions, and whole-word repetitions were the most common disfluency types among the 68 nonstuttering males, who ranged in age from 2.5 to 8 years of age. Yairi's (1981) study of 33 typically developing 2-year-old children found that there were two clusters of common disfluency types. One cluster involved repetitions of speech segments of one syllable or less (one-syllable words or parts of words were repeated). The second cluster consisted of interjections and revisions.

The most common disfluency type seems to change as a child grows older. In a follow-up to his earlier study, Yairi (1982) found that as typically disfluent children matured between 2 and 3.5 years, they gradually increased their frequency of revisions and phrase repetitions but decreased their frequency of part-word repetitions and interjections. He suggested that these data indicate that as typical children mature, part-word repetitions decline, even if other disfluency types increase. Thus, an increase in part-word repetitions as a child is observed longitudinally may be a sign that this child's speech warrants concern.

Although the research is far from complete, we can characterize typical disfluency types as follows:

- Revisions are common in typical development and may continue to account for a major portion of their disfluencies as children grow older.
- Interjections are also common but usually decline after 3 years of age.
- Repetitions may also be a frequent type of disfluency around 2 to 3 years of age, especially single-syllable word repetitions having fewer than two extra units. Repetitions are also more likely to involve longer segments (eg, phrases) as a child grows older.

Table 7.3 summarizes the major characteristics of typical disfluency.

Secondary Behaviors

Children who are typically disfluent generally have no secondary behaviors. They have not developed any reactions to their disfluencies, such as escape or avoidance behaviors. Although research suggests that some typical children occasionally display "tense pauses" (some muscle tension evident during the pause), such tension does not appear to be a reaction to their disfluencies. If children have what appear to be typical disfluencies, such as single-word repetitions, but consistently display pauses or interjections of "uh" immediately before or during disfluencies, they should be carefully evaluated for possible stuttering.

TABLE 7.3 Characteristics of Typical Disfluency in the Average Nonstuttering Child

1. No more than 10 disfluencies per 100 words
2. Typically, one-unit repetitions; occasionally two
3. Most common disfluency types are interjections, revisions, and whole word repetitions. As children mature past age 3, use of part-word repetitions will decline

Feelings and Attitudes

Typically disfluent children rarely notice their disfluencies, even though they may be apparent to others. Just as all children may stumble when walking but regain their balance and continue walking without complaint, children with typical development who repeat, interject, or revise usually continue talking after a disfluency without evidence of frustration or embarrassment.

Underlying Processes

First, let's review the behaviors for which we are trying to account. Typical disfluency occurs throughout childhood and adulthood. It may begin earlier than 18 months of age and peak between ages 2 and 3.5 years. It slowly diminishes, thereafter, but also changes in form. Most adults have some disfluencies, but there is a real range of fluency. The most fluent speaker I've ever heard in person is the linguist Noam Chomsky. You can find some of his talks on Google. When you listen to him, notice that where you think there should be an "um," he just keeps talking.

Some types of disfluency, such as repetitions, decrease after 3.5 years, but other types, such as revisions, may increase. Episodic increases and decreases in disfluency are also common throughout childhood (and probably adulthood, depending on stress). What causes these changes? Why are there ups and downs and changes in form? The answer, I suggest, is that like most natural phenomena, multiple forces probably have an impact at any given moment, but specific forces may predominate at certain times. In Chapter 4, I talked about developmental and environmental influences on stuttering and typical disfluency, and I will review these influences as I discuss studies of children with typical disfluencies.

The integrated perspective on stuttering described in Chapter 6 has implications for typical disfluency as well. This view suggests that breakdowns in speech fluency may occur when some of the neural pathways critical for sensorimotor control of speech production are immature or inefficient, perhaps because of delayed myelination. In fact, overall connectivity in speech production networks may be impaired, resulting in many impairments in fluency. Serious delays may result in stuttering, but minor delays and slow to develop neural networks may result in typical disfluencies, especially when children are learning to integrate all the subcomponents of spoken language at increasingly faster rates with increasingly greater options for vocabulary, syntax, and prosody.

These rapid developments in language are—as you know—the context in which disfluencies often first appear. As you have learned, children tend to be most disfluent at the beginning of syntactic units (Bernstein Ratner, 1981; Bloodstein, 1974, 1995; Silverman, 1974) and when the length or complexity of their utterances increases (DeJoy & Gregory, 1973; Gordon et al., 1986; Hall et al., 2007; Pearl & Bernthal, 1980; Zackheim & Conture, 2003). Bloodstein et al. (2021) have an excellent summary and discussion of the loci of disfluencies in typically disfluent children. Taken together, these findings suggest that disfluency is greatest when a child is busy planning long or complex language structures. Typically, children will begin speaking even before all the planning for the phrase is finished. This puts a heavy load on cerebral resources. It seems likely that producing newly learned language structures would be hardest of all because more attention must be devoted to them. It would follow, then, that disfluencies occur more frequently on children's most recently acquired forms. However, evidence gathered in a study of four children between 2 and 4 years of age suggests that typical disfluency may be greatest on structures that have been learned but perhaps not fully automated, thereby requiring more cerebral resources for their production. These extra resources may not be readily available—hence disfluencies occur (Colburn & Mysak, 1982a, 1982b).

Pragmatics may influence disfluency, too. Studies by Davis (1940), Meyers and Freeman (1985a, 1985b), and Newman and Smit (1989) indicate that children's disfluency increases under certain pragmatic conditions, such as when interrupting, when directing another's activity, or when responding to requests/demands to change their own activity, and when the listener's response time is very fast. Mastering such pragmatic skills, especially those involving more complex social interactions, creates yet another challenge for typically developing children. The pressures of language acquisition, interacting with other factors, can be seen as competing for cerebral resources, which leaves fewer remaining resources available for fluent speech production.

In addition to language acquisition, another likely influence on disfluency is speech-motor control. Most children—as they mature between ages 2 and 5—learn to produce almost all the segmental and suprasegmental targets of their native language, as well as learn to increase their speech rates as they produce longer and longer utterances. These maturational changes must keep average children fairly busy, although the demanding nature of these changes may not be obvious. Children are automatically scanning their parents' and older siblings' speech, acquiring information about talking. They are also continuously modifying their own productions to make them more and more like the speech they hear. This period—from 2 to 5 years—also encompasses an intensive refinement of nonspeech-motor skills. It is at this age that children are learning to skip, run, jump, and take part in numerous games requiring skill and speed (Gabbard, 2016). Thus, children are mastering a myriad of other motor tasks at the same time they are acquiring the ability to speak in rapid, complex, fluent sequences. With all these competing demands, no wonder that almost all children have disfluencies.

Besides the continuing demands of typical development, there are also episodic stresses in children's environments that may temporarily increase typical disfluency. An experiment by Hill (1954) demonstrated that conditioned fear could elicit disfluency in typical adults' speech. It is easy to imagine, therefore, that there are many psychological stresses in typical children's lives that would also increase disfluency. Clinically, I have observed many situations that seem to increase typical disfluency. Among them are the stress of a move from one home to another, parents' separation or divorce, the birth of a sibling, and other events that may decrease a child's sense of security.

We have also seen increases in typical disfluency during periods of excitement, such as holidays, vacations, and visits by relatives. Disfluency increases especially when excitement combines with competition to be heard, such as during dinner table conversations when everyone is talking at once or after school when several children are competing to tell Mom what happened during the day. As I speculated in Chapter 6, emotions may have an especially strong influence on fluency in young children. This happens after interactions between right and left hemispheres develop during children's first 2 years (Fox & Davidson, 1984), and overflow activity from emotional arousal in the right hemisphere may disrupt vulnerable, immature language production networks in the left.

Summary of Typical Disfluency

Between ages 2 and 5, most children pass through periods of increased disfluency. Repetitions, interjections, revisions, prolongations, and pauses are commonly heard. When typically developing children are between 2 and 3.5 years old, disfluencies reach six per 100 words spoken and may occur even more frequently in some typically disfluent children.

Repetitions are probably the most common type of typical disfluency in younger children, whereas revisions are a more common type of typical disfluency in older children.

Despite the fact that children's disfluencies may occasionally attract some adult attention, typically disfluent children seem generally unaware of the disfluencies in their own speech and don't react to them or engage in secondary behaviors to escape or avoid them as a consequence.

Some factors thought to contribute to increases in typical disfluencies include the demands of language acquisition, inefficient speech-motor control skills, interpersonal stress associated with growing up in a typical family, and threats to security from such events as relocation, family breakup, or hospitalization. Disfluencies may also increase under the ordinary daily pressures of competition and excitement while speaking. A small amount of disfluency can be seen in most typically developing older children and in adults.

YOUNGER PRESCHOOL CHILDREN: BORDERLINE STUTTERING

Stuttering in preschool children between the ages of 2 and 3.5 resembles typical disfluency but differs in several important ways. The most obvious—the thing that gets parents' attention—is that these children have more disfluencies than typically developing children (eg, Tumanova et al., 2014). We will discuss other key differences in the following sections. Sometimes diagnosis is difficult, because a child may drift back and forth between typical disfluency and borderline stuttering over a period of weeks or months. Most children with borderline stuttering gradually lose their stuttering and grow up without a trace of it. A small number develop more stuttering symptoms and progress through levels of beginning, intermediate, and advanced stuttering. Still others may continue to show borderline stuttering throughout their lives but may never seek treatment because their disfluency is so mild. They may not have as serious brain dysfunctions as those who are more severe and/or they may have particularly resilient temperaments and be unbothered by their disfluencies. A speech sample of a younger preschool child with borderline stuttering is depicted in Figure 7.3.

A video clip of a child with borderline stuttering is available on *Lippincott Connect*. ("Normal Disfluency and the Development of Stuttering." Watch the clip of the second child on the video, Ashley.) Note that although Ashley has fairly relaxed repetitions and seems relatively unaffected by them, she does stop in the midst of saying "coo-coo-coo-coo-coo-cookie" and just continues on with the rest of her utterance without finishing the word. Specifically, she says, "coo-coo-coo-coo-coo....she knocked the plant down." This is a mild escape behavior. Ashley received indirect therapy soon after this clip was filmed and has made a full recovery.

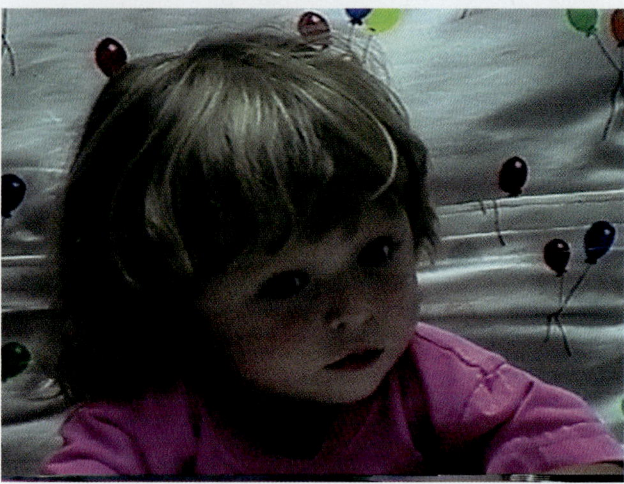

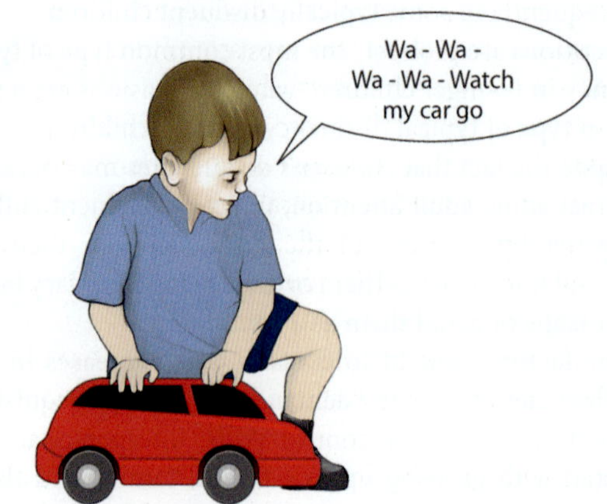

Figure 7.3 Child who may be a borderline stutterer.

In describing the behaviors of borderline stuttering, I will begin to define my view of how stuttering differs from typical disfluency. The distinction has been of great interest to theorists for many years. Some theorists (eg, Johnson, 1955; Johnson et al., 1942) suggested, as was noted previously, that a stuttering child developed symptoms only after his parents mislabeled his typical disfluencies as stuttering. That is, a child's first "stuttering" symptoms were actually just typical speech disfluencies.

An opposing view maintains that there are objective differences between the speech of a typically disfluent child and the speech of a child who is stuttering, even before a parent or someone else labels behaviors as stuttering. Although I hold this latter view, I also agree that there is much overlap between the disfluencies of stuttering children and the disfluencies of typically disfluent children. Moreover, as previously stated, children with borderline stuttering often go back and forth between stuttering and typical disfluency over a period of months. For this reason, we use the term "borderline" to indicate that these children are neither entirely normally disfluent nor undeniably stuttering.

Core Behaviors

No single core behavior distinguishes borderline stuttering from typical disfluency. However, many researchers and clinicians have suggested three elements that are useful for making this distinction. The *frequency of disfluencies* is one important aspect to consider. As we indicated in our description of typical disfluencies, children who do not stutter between 2 and 5 years may go through periods of increased disfluency. Even so, their level of disfluency averages about six per 100 words. Typically, if children have many more disfluencies per 100 words (eg, 10 or more), we consider them borderline.

Another feature that can help identify borderline stuttering rather than typical disfluency is the *proportion of certain types of disfluencies*. The study we cited earlier by Johnson et al. (1959) suggested that, compared to children who don't stutter, those who stutter had significantly more sound and syllable repetitions, single-syllable word repetitions, broken words (ie, phonation or airflow is abnormally stopped within a word), and prolonged sounds. There were no significant differences between the groups in their number of interjections, revisions, or incomplete phrases.

More information on types of disfluencies was provided by Young (1984), who reviewed a large number of studies that had assessed which types of disfluencies were identified as stuttering and which were not by the researchers who published the studies. His summary impression was that repetitions of parts of words, and, to a lesser extent, prolongations, are the disfluency types that are most likely to be classified as stuttering. Bloodstein et al. (2021) and Conture (1982, 1990, 2001a) generally concurred with other writers, suggesting that **"within-word" disfluencies** (ie, part-word repetitions and audible as well as inaudible prolongations including blocks) are the types of disfluencies most frequently heard in children who stutter.

Yairi and colleagues (eg, Yairi, 1997a, 1997b; Yairi & Ambrose, 1996) proposed that children who stutter can be distinguished from children with typical disfluencies using a grouping of **"*stuttering-like*" disfluencies**. Included in this grouping were short-segment repetitions (part-word and monosyllabic word repetitions); tense pauses (stoppage of speech with muscular tightening both within and between words); and a category introduced by Williams et al. (1968) called "**dysrhythmic phonation**" (any distortion, prolongation, or break in phonation within a word). Yairi (1997a, 1997b) notes that when many previous studies of children who stutter and children who do not stutter are reanalyzed using this grouping, the proportion of stuttering-like disfluencies in children who do not stutter is always less than 50% of the total number of disfluencies. Thus, if children's total disfluency amount is more than 50% stuttering-like disfluencies, they can be considered to be stuttering.

In summary, we can say that one measure that will help us distinguish a child with borderline stuttering from a normally disfluent child is a higher proportion of part-word and monosyllabic whole-word repetitions and prolongations compared with multisyllabic word and phrase repetitions. In the next section, we will see that children who show regular tension in their disfluencies that leads to abrupt repetitions, pitch rise, blocks, broken words, and dysrhythmic phonations are beginning rather than borderline stutterers.

Another sign that distinguishes children who stutter from their normally disfluent peers is the number of times a word or sound is repeated in a part-word or monosyllable word repetitive disfluency. In Yairi's (1981) sample of 33 children who did not stutter, repetitions typically involved only one or two extra units of repetition (eg, one extra unit would be li-like this). Other studies comparing children who stutter and children who do not stutter (Ambrose & Yairi, 1995; Johnson et al., 1959; Yairi & Lewis, 1984; Zebrowski, 1991) have found that the repetitive disfluencies of nonstuttering children average 1.13 extra units and that of stuttering children 1.51. Thus, the frequent occurrence of repetitions having more than one extra unit is a warning sign of borderline stuttering. Of course, when there are many repetition units, li-li-li-li-li-li-li-like this, it is much more likely children are demonstrating stuttering rather than typical disfluency.

We have said that borderline stuttering consists primarily of effortless repetitions and occasional prolongations. However, as Van Riper (1971, 1982a) and Bloodstein (1995) note, these young children are often highly variable in their stuttering. Although they show the core behaviors of borderline stuttering, they may have brief periods of fluency as well as days when they show signs of slightly more advanced stuttering.

Secondary Behaviors

A younger preschool child with borderline stuttering has few, if any, secondary behaviors. The degree of tension may sometimes seem to be slightly greater than normal, but these children generally don't increase tension and struggle like older preschool children do when they stutter. Children with borderline stuttering also do not exhibit accessory movements before, during, or after stutters. In fact, there is often nothing in their behavior to indicate that they are aware of their stutters. Some children with predominantly borderline stuttering may go through periods in which their stuttering suddenly escalates to the level of beginning stuttering, with tension and some other secondary behaviors, but then it falls back again to the borderline level.

Feelings and Attitudes

Because children with borderline stuttering seem to have little awareness of their stutters, they do not show concern or embarrassment. When they repeat a sound or a syllable, even five or six or more times, they usually go on talking as though nothing has happened. One exception, however, is that once in a while, children with borderline stuttering might appear surprised or frustrated when they are repeating a syllable several times and are unable to finish a word. Then, they may stop and cry out, "Mommy, I can't say that word," or otherwise demonstrate brief alarm or surprise. But in general, these younger preschool children show little or no evidence of awareness that they have disfluencies that are different from those of their peers. Moreover, at this age (2 to 3.5 years), peers usually don't react to the child's stuttering. Table 7.4 summarizes the major characteristics of younger preschool children's borderline stuttering.

TABLE 7.4 Characteristics of Borderline Stuttering in a Younger Preschool Child

1. More than 6-10 disfluencies per 100 words
2. Often more than two units in repetition
3. More repetitions and prolongations than revisions or incomplete phrases
4. Disfluencies loose and relaxed
5. Rare for child to react to their disfluencies

Underlying Processes

I hypothesize that the symptoms of borderline stuttering result from the constitutional, developmental, and environmental factors described in Chapters 2, 3, and 4. The constitutional factors associated with borderline stuttering (anomalies in the development of neural pathways for speech) often first show their effects as an excess of typical disfluencies. As I mentioned earlier, environmental and developmental pressures may be great between 2 and 3.5 years, and it is during this period that borderline stuttering typically emerges. The converging demands of expressive language and motor speech development ordinarily peak about this time "when an explosive growth in language ability outstrips a still-immature speech motor apparatus" (Andrews et al., 1983, p. 239). This age is also filled with psychosocial conflicts as a child copes with security needs as an infant while striving to become more independent as a toddler. The child may be ready to explore but is also fearful. The birth of a new brother or sister may trigger the child's insecurity with the threat of being overlooked. A still older sibling (eg, a preteen) may turn belligerent toward the child because of the older child's own need to express aggression as a prelude to puberty. Just as these stresses wax and wane in strength during preschool years, so does the child's stuttering.

As children mature, certain developmental stresses may taper off. After age 5, children may feel more integrated within themselves and within their families. Articulation and language skills, although still not at adult levels, have been mastered sufficiently for most children to say what's on their mind and to be understood. They have also mastered other motor skills, such as walking and running, as well as riding a tricycle or a bike with training wheels. They may have adjusted to a new, younger sibling as well and made at least temporary peace with an older one.

By now, the capacities of many of the children who had modest predispositions to stutter can easily meet most environmental demands. Therefore, many of those who were borderline stutterers will have acquired typical fluency skills by the time they are 4 or 5 years old. Others may still have many disfluencies at this age but will eventually outgrow them. This may happen because neural pathways will have matured enough to allow the child to speak fluently. These children may also have relatively robust (rather than reactive) temperaments and do not respond to disfluencies by increasing physical tension or speaking rate. In general, they are functioning well, feel accepted, and can use their resources to compensate for whatever difficulties in speaking remain.

Some children, of course, do not outgrow borderline stuttering. They may continue to stutter, and their symptoms may worsen. They may be children who have substantial predispositions to stutter, which cannot be offset by a "good enough" environment (Winnicott, 1971). Their ability to produce speech and language at the rate and level of complexity used by parents and peers may be insufficient. And their continuing efforts to meet advanced speech and language targets may result in excess disfluency that does not diminish as they pass their third and fourth birthdays. Their frustration tolerance for the repetitions that 2- and 3-year-olds have may be low, as a result of a reactive temperament. Rather than shrugging off their disfluencies, they may begin struggling to produce flawless speech, thereby placing greater demands on their speech production and emotional resources. Still other children may continue to stutter because environmental and developmental stresses do not diminish. Their insecurity may continue from sibling rivalry, breakup of the family, or a parent's death. They may have language or articulation problems, as well as stuttering, which limit their communication abilities throughout their preschool years.

Deficits in the processes underlying speech and language development, plus the frustration of being unable to communicate easily, may be devastating to fluency. This may result in the increased tension we see in older preschool children with beginning stuttering. A child in this situation is unlikely to outgrow stuttering unless parents and professionals provide extensive support.

Summary of Borderline Stuttering

Younger preschool children with borderline stuttering usually exhibit a greater amount of disfluency than do typical children—more than six disfluencies per 100 words. Using another measure of frequency, the proportion of stuttering-like disfluencies relative to all disfluencies may be greater than half. Children with borderline stuttering, in contrast to typically developing children, are also likely to repeat units more than once in many of their part-word and monosyllabic word repetitions and to have many more part-word and monosyllabic word repetitions and prolongations than multisyllabic word and phrase repetitions, revisions, and interjections.

At the same time, their disfluencies, like those of children who do not stutter, are usually loose and relaxed appearing. Also, like children who do not stutter, children with borderline stuttering show little or no awareness of their speaking difficulty. Only rarely do they express frustration about it. Among the underlying processes behind borderline stuttering are probably some of the neural speech and language-processing anomalies described in the earlier chapter on constitutional origins of stuttering. Such deficits in resources may interact with the demands of speech and language development, the pressure from higher rates of speech, more complex language, competitive speaking situations, and other attributes of a typical home. In addition, some of the psychosocial conflicts described earlier that increase typical disfluency are likely to be active in creating borderline stuttering.

OLDER PRESCHOOL CHILDREN: BEGINNING STUTTERING

In older preschool children (Fig. 7.4), stuttering usually has more tension and hurry than stuttering in younger children. It may have evolved over a period of months or a year or two from the borderline stuttering that these children manifested earlier. Or it may appear suddenly in older preschool children during a time of stress or excitement. The tense and hurried stuttering may alternate with looser, easier disfluencies. Gradually, this more advanced type of stuttering will become commonplace. I described this change as the appearance of "secondary stuttering" in Chapter 6. Both learning and temperament play a major role as children respond defensively to their multiple repetitions, increasing tension and hurry. Soon, these children become impatient with their stuttering as it is happening—perhaps even embarrassed—and they may begin to use a variety of escape behaviors or even avoidances as a consequence. For example, they may try to end long repetitions by using an eye blink or head nod. Or these children may respond to being stuck in a block by going back to an earlier word in the sentence and starting the phrase over. Periods of increased stuttering may last for several months, but periods of fluency may last only a few days. As these signs occur more consistently, tension increases and struggle is more evident. Classical and operant conditioning processes increase the frequency of struggle behaviors, complicate these children's pattern of stuttering, and spread the symptoms to many more situations.

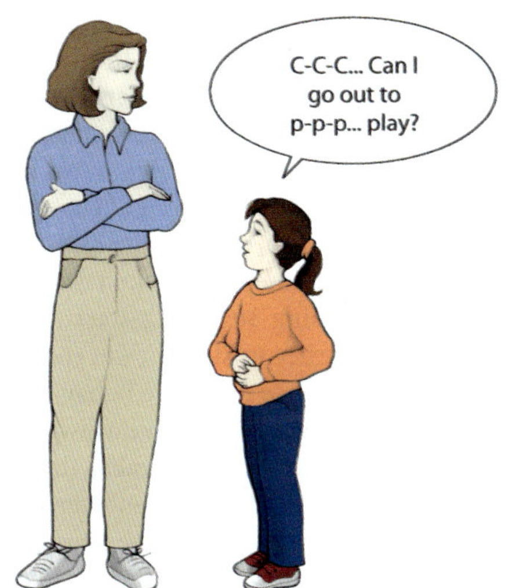

Figure 7.4 Child who may be a beginning stutterer.

As mentioned, some children exhibit beginning stuttering at onset, without passing through a stage of borderline stuttering. Van Riper (1971, 1982a) described several different profiles of stuttering with tense blockages at onset. Many of the children he depicted as more severe at onset were relatively older (eg, 4, 5, or 6 years old) when their stuttering first appeared. Onset in these children seemed to be related to one of two factors: delayed language development or emotional events. In a study of the onset of stuttering, Yairi and Ambrose (1992b) described onsets of stuttering that were characterized by the signs I described for beginning stuttering in 28% of their sample of 87 children. Many of these children had relatively sudden onsets, with typical disfluency changing to beginning stuttering within 1 day or at most 1 week.

A video sample of a child with beginning stuttering is available on *Lippincott Connect* ("Normal Disfluency and the Development of Stuttering"). The third child on this video, Katherine, has severe beginning stuttering. She shows tense blocks as well as escape behaviors. One escape maneuver that she uses is stopping in the middle of a block and restarting with the word preceding the stuttered word ("...yes, yes, I want to put it back in [block on "here"]...i-i-iiin here"). Another escape behavior that Katherine uses is to hit her mother several times to try to release the block. This sample is limited to her more severe stutters and is not entirely representative of her overall speech at this time. She received treatment beginning shortly after the video was made. Because her stuttering was severe, treatment took longer than usual—almost a year. She recovered completely and showed no sign of stuttering in her 5-year follow-up.

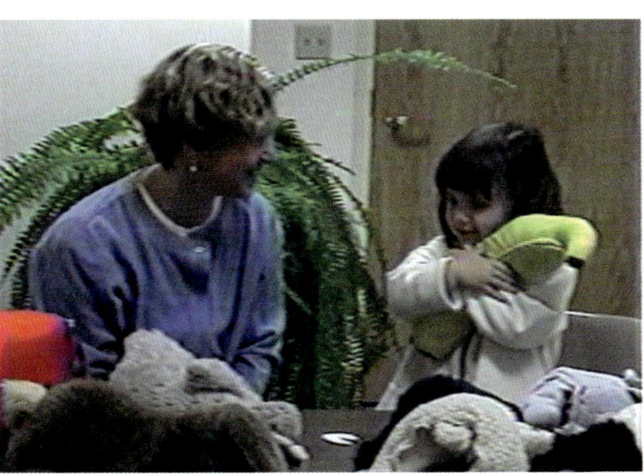

Core Behaviors

The core behaviors of beginning stuttering differ from those of borderline stuttering in several ways. Repetitions are tense, rapid, and irregular. The final segment of a repeated syllable often sounds abrupt. If it is a vowel, it will sound as if it were suddenly cut off or were a neutral or schwa vowel ("uh") that had been substituted for the appropriate one, as in "luh-luh-luh-like" instead of "li-li-li-like." Repetitions are also produced more rapidly, sometimes with an irregular rhythm. Rather than patiently repeating a syllable as a borderline stutterer does, a child with beginning stuttering hurries through repetitive stutters, as though juggling a hot potato.

As symptoms progress, children with beginning stuttering increase tension throughout their speech mechanism. Stuttering is sometimes accompanied by a rise in vocal pitch, resulting from increased tension in the vocal folds. Rising pitch may first appear toward the end of a string of repeated syllables, but over time will appear earlier in the repetitions. Rising pitch both within the stuttered iterations (liii-li-like this) and between them (li-li-li-like this) seems to be a more definitive sign of beginning stuttering. One of my students, Naomi Hertsberg Rodgers, wrote her honors thesis on a study of children between ages 2;9 and 5;4 (years;months), examining the repetitions of four typically developing children and four children diagnosed with beginning stuttering. She found that the children with beginning stuttering displayed more instances of pitch rise in their disfluencies than the typical children, that there was a moderate positive correlation between percent syllables stuttered and proportion of disfluencies with pitch rise, and that the children with beginning stuttering had greater differences between their average pitch during fluency and their pitch during disfluency, compared to the typical children. Follow-up research is needed to determine whether pitch rise during disfluencies is predictive of persistent stuttering.

Prolongations of sounds is also a hallmark for children with beginning stuttering. These children sometimes prolong sounds that they might have previously repeated. Initially, they may prolong the first sounds of syllables, but as stuttering grows more severe, they may also prolong middle sounds, and these sounds too may be accompanied by an increase in pitch.

As beginning stuttering progresses, blocks begin to replace repetitions and prolongations. These are significant landmarks, which indicate that children are stopping the flow of air or voice at one or more places (Van Riper, 1982a). They may inappropriately jam their vocal folds closed or wide open, interrupting or possibly delaying the onset of phonation (Conture, 1990). Shutting off the airway is usually heard as a momentary stoppage of sound in children's speech and is sometimes accompanied by visual cues; children may seem momentarily unable to move their mouth or may make groping movements with their mouth as they try to get air flow or voice going again. When the stoppage of movement, voice, or airflow first begins, it may be so fleeting that we don't notice it unless we are listening and watching carefully. As these blocks worsen, they become so obvious that they may overshadow the repetitions and prolongations that may remain.

The age at which most beginning stuttering occurs (3.5 to 6 years) is also when children may be showing behaviors that predict persistent stuttering. High frequency of core behaviors of stutterlike disfluencies (part-word repetitions, single-syllable word repetitions, prolongations, broken words, or hard attacks) has been shown to be predictive of persistence (Singer et al., 2020; Walsh et al., 2020, 2021). More details of this measurement and extensive discussion of other predictors of persistence/recovery will be given in the chapter on assessment.

Secondary Behaviors

As these older preschool children's symptoms progress, secondary behaviors are added. They are called secondary because they appear to be responses to the runaway repetitions and increased muscle tension that have emerged. It is not clear how voluntary they are. Many begin as almost reflexive responses, like the common eye blinks or eye squeezing that occur when a child is stuck in a stutter. They may disappear when treatment helps the individuals reduce their fear of stuttering. If these behaviors don't disappear, the individuals may reduce or eliminate them as they become more and more conscious of them as a result of treatment. A client in one of Van Riper's therapy groups told me that he had a habit of pursing his lips when he thought he would stutter. It somehow gave him a start on getting the word out. Van Riper made him go to a pet store and stand in front of the goldfish tank and purse his lips while watching the goldfish do the same as they breathed. That experience made his lip-pursing "starter" so notable to him that he soon got rid of it.

Among the earliest of the secondary symptoms are "escape" behaviors, which are maneuvers used to end a stutter and finish a word. Children with beginning stuttering often show escape behaviors after several repetitions of a syllable. They may nod their heads, squint their eyes, or blink just as they try to push a word out. This extra effort often seems to help—in the short run. For the moment, they escape from the punishing repetition, prolongation, or block. Alternatively, they may insert a filler, such as "uh" or "um," after a string of fruitless repetitions. The "um" seems to release the word, perhaps by relaxing the tightly squeezed larynx or by unlocking the lips. The "um" can usually be said fluently, and once uttered, phonation and movement for the word often begin. The fillers work like a little push you might give your sled if it were stuck in the snow as you start down a hill; the "um" gets children going again when they are stuck in a stutter.

Children with beginning stuttering start to use escape behaviors earlier and earlier in stutters. Let me give you an example: the first appearance of escape behaviors is usually after children have repeated a sound quite a few times and are thoroughly frustrated about it. It may sound this way: "Luh-Luh-Luh-Luh-Luh-umLet's go!" Soon, however, children will not wait until they have tried to say the sound five times. They find themselves about to say a word, feel convinced it won't come out, and then perhaps instinctively use escape behaviors when they are first starting to stutter: "L-umLet's go!" Such "starters" may even appear before the first sound of the word, in this fashion: "umLet's go!" This is really an avoidance behavior (because it is deployed to avoid a stutter before being stuck in one). These escape-avoidance behaviors are more common among children with intermediate stuttering, even though these behaviors occasionally appear in the speech of a child with beginning stuttering.

Feelings and Attitudes

Older preschool children with beginning stuttering have stuttered many times. They are aware of stuttering when it happens. The feelings beginning stutterers have just before, during, and after stutters are often strong. Frequently, frustration is a major feeling. Children may stop in the middle of a stutter and say, "Mommy, why can't I talk?" However, such momentary frustration grows into fear when a word or sound is stuck for several seconds, and the child feels helpless and out of control.

Although children with beginning stuttering are conscious that they have some "trouble" when they talk, they have not yet developed a belief that they are defective speakers. This lack of a negative self-image may be attributed, as Bloodstein (1987), Zebrowski (2003), and Van Riper (1982a) have suggested, to the "episodic" nature of beginning stuttering. Sometimes it's there; sometimes it's not. Sometimes children feel that they have problems when they talk; other times they forget about it. The essential characteristics of beginning stutterers are presented in Table 7.5.

Underlying Processes

The signs and symptoms of beginning stuttering in older preschool children can be recognized by any experienced clinician. But the processes underlying these behaviors are not so easy to see. In Chapters 5 and 6, I suggested that beginning stuttering may result from the interplay between constitutional and environmental factors, especially in children with a reactive temperament. In the next sections, I review my speculations about the core behaviors of beginning stuttering as well as the learning processes that are likely to perpetuate the core behaviors and children's secondary reactions.

TABLE 7.5 Characteristics of Beginning Stuttering in an Older Preschool Child

1. Signs of muscle tension and hurry appear in stuttering. Repetitions are rapid and irregular with abrupt terminations of each element.
2. Pitch rise may be present toward the end of a repetition or prolongation.
3. Fixed articulatory postures are sometimes evident when the child is momentarily unable to begin a word, apparently as a result of tension in speech musculature.
4. Escape behaviors are sometimes present in beginning stuttering. These include, among other things, eye blinks, head nods, and "ums."
5. Awareness of difficulty and feelings of frustration are present, but there are no strong negative feelings about self as speaker.

Increases in Muscle Tension and Tempo

One of the first signs of beginning stuttering in older preschool children is the appearance of excess muscular tension in repetitions and prolongations and increased tempo or rate in repetitive stutters (Boey et al., 2007; Van Riper, 1982a). Why do these changes occur? Oliver Bloodstein (Bloodstein, 1987; Bloodstein et al., 2021) suggested that facial tension and strained glottal attacks in the speech of young children who stutter may reflect the extra muscular effort that emerges when they anticipate difficulty. Conture (1990) offered a related view. He sees the increased articulatory and laryngeal muscle tension as children's attempts to control sound-syllable repetitions, which are so distressing to them and to some listeners. We have described such tension as children's efforts to control a frustrating and scary behavior of their own body, an attempt to stiffen the speech muscles and brace themselves against the perturbations of seemingly involuntary, runaway repetitions (Guitar et al., 1988). One can imagine this taking place in the same way that children who are learning to skate may respond to the threat of falling by stiffening and assuming a less than ideal stance for continued forward movement. I've speculated in Chapters 5 and 6 that the initial increases in tension are nonconscious.

The other early sign of beginning stuttering— increases in the rate of repetitive stutters—is cited by a number of authors as an indication that stuttering is worsening. Van Riper (1982a), in describing the developmental course of the majority of children whose stuttering persists, stated "the tempo changes as the disorder develops. The repetitive syllables become irregular and are often spoken more rapidly than other fluent syllables." Starkweather (1987) explained this increase in the speed of repetitions as a product of the pressure that children feel as they become more aware of the extra time it takes them to produce an utterance.

But why are these increases in tension and tempo so common in the development of stuttering, and why are they so difficult to change in therapy? In Chapter 6, I described my view that children in whom stuttering persists may be especially sensitive to certain kinds of experiences. Faced with frustration or fear, they react to this threat with a type of freezing or flight response, increasing muscle tension and hurry, turning their frustrating or frightening repetitive disfluencies into abrupt, tense repetitions, blocks, or prolongations. As I have mentioned, some children appear to show tense blocks at the onset of their stuttering. These may be children who have high degrees of emotional sensitivity and whose very first manifestation of stuttering (tense blocks) may result from defensive responses mediated by the amygdala.

Research bears out the speculation that at least some adults who stutter contract their muscles in such a way that movement and phonation are immobilized. Freeman and Ushijima's (1978) and Shapiro and DeCicco's (1982) studies indicate that stuttering is associated with abnormal muscle co-contraction of adductor and abductor muscles in the larynx. Such co-contraction could produce stiffening of the phonatory structures and silencing of vocal output. Other studies of stuttering have confirmed this co-contraction in articulatory structures (Fibiger, 1971; Guitar et al., 1988; Platt & Basili, 1973), which could also produce immobility and silence.

Unfortunately, little research directly supports the notion that the increased rate of repetitions reflects the flight response. We have some preliminary evidence that stutterers have more rapid productions during repetitions than do children who do not stutter. An unpublished study (Allen, 1988) carried out in our clinical laboratory and described in an earlier edition of this textbook indicated that the durations of beginning stutterers' repeated segments and the silences between them were shorter than the durations in similar disfluencies of children matched for age who did not stutter. This finding has been confirmed in the work of Throneberg and Yairi (1994), who replicated our work and also found that the silent intervals and the total durations of repetition disfluencies were significantly shorter in stuttering children compared with those of children who did not stutter. Such shortening of segments results in a faster speech rate, at least for the stuttered elements and may reflect the "great increase in activity" seen in the flight response (Gray, 1987), although these particular data do not exclude the possibility that stuttering children were more rapid speakers to begin with. It may be relevant at this point to note that Kloth et al. (1995) found that rapid speaking rate was a predictor of which young children who were fluent at the time of testing but had family histories of stuttering would eventually stutter. The rapid rate in these children might be related to a reactive limbic system, although no evidence indicates that speech rate is related to such reactivity.

The possibility that increased muscle tension and rapid repetitions are a result of biologically based freezing and flight responses is highly speculative at this time. If these responses are part of humans' neural wiring designed for survival, this may be a potential explanation of why some children develop stuttering so rapidly and why tension responses are so difficult to change. The work of Bolles (1970) and LeDoux (2015) has influenced my thinking on this.

Effects of Learning on Stuttering

I presented a detailed account of the effect of learning on the development of stuttering in Chapter 5. Here is a quick overview: Once children with beginning stuttering react to their "runaway" repetitions with increased tension because they are threatening (they feel out of control), the repetitions themselves elicit the tension response. Through classical conditioning, the repetitions themselves become a conditioned stimulus that elicits the conditioned response of tension. The repetitions then become more abrupt and more rapid and gradually turn into prolongations and blocks, as tension increases. Classical conditioning also generalizes the tense stuttering to any stimuli that are paired with the children's stuttering. People, places, words, sounds, and the pragmatics of speaking situations become conditioned stimuli that elicit the tense stuttering.

As classical conditioning continues its work, operant conditioning becomes important as well. When children are frustrated or embarrassed by a moment of stuttering, they will often employ an escape behavior (such as facial squeezing or eye blinking) to get out of the stutter and finish the word. Because escaping the stutter and finishing the word reward the behavior, it is likely to increase in frequency. Soon, children with beginning stuttering are using a variety of "moves" to get out of the stutter. These should be enumerated during a diagnostic evaluation. They don't necessarily need to be addressed directly in treatment, however. If all goes well, they will disappear as children replace their stuttering with fluency.

Avoidance conditioning may occur to some extent in beginning stuttering but will be more evident in intermediate and advanced stuttering (school age, adolescent, and adults). This learning process also combines classical and operant conditioning. Classical conditioning turns cues—both nonconscious and conscious—into conditioned stimuli. These cues may be proprioceptive information from muscles that are beginning to tighten as a stutter looms ahead. Or they may be conscious knowledge that "words beginning with/b/ are hard to say." Because these cues have been followed repeatedly by the experience of stuttering with all its attendant threat and fear, they induce threat and fear. When children sense these cues, they experience threat and fear. But if they substitute another word for the feared word or refuse to talk, the threat and fear are reduced and they are rewarded. Several years ago, I saw avoidance conditioning in a 2-and-a-half-year-old. For a week after the onset of her repetitions, she kept trying to talk despite a high frequency of stuttering. But, in the second week, she'd had enough. She then refused to talk and only pointed to what she wanted. In very young children like this, avoidances will usually disappear after a few months of treatment. Hers did.

Summary of Beginning Stuttering

Borderline stuttering seen in younger preschool children compared with beginning stuttering that is common in older preschool children shows five principal differences:

1. First, older children with beginning stuttering show more tension and hurry in their repetitions. This is often manifested in abruptly ended syllable repetitions, irregular

rhythms of repetitions, evident stoppages of phonation, and momentarily fixated articulatory postures. Older preschool children also show such secondary behaviors as escape devices (eye blinks, head nods) and starters such as "uh" (a type of avoidance). In addition, children with beginning stuttering sometimes see themselves as persons who have trouble talking. This comes and goes, but as their stuttering is more frequently present and they use escape and avoidance behaviors, the more their self-image is that of someone who can't talk right.

2. Second, a major factor underlying beginning stuttering appears to be a child's having a reactive or sensitive temperament, which may result in the experience of threat, triggering tension responses.
3. Third, classical conditioning then links such unconditioned response sensitivity (the feeling of being threatened) to disfluency. When children are disfluent, they experience threat because the disfluencies feel out of control. This experience of threat, in turn, leads to the rapid, tense disfluencies that appear in beginning stuttering. These may be freezing or flight responses to threat. After repeated pairings of the disfluency and threat, classical conditioning results in the disfluency itself, rather than the emotion related to threat. Classical conditioning elicits increased tension and increased rate. Classical conditioning also links children's disfluency to more and more people and places.
4. A fourth factor in beginning stuttering in older preschool children is operant conditioning. This results in the increased frequency and maintenance of escape devices. These escape behaviors are negatively reinforced by reduction in frustration and positively reinforced when children are then able to finish the stuck word and to complete their communication.
5. Avoidance conditioning can also appear in beginning stuttering. Using "um" or a similar extra sound as a "starter" is one example. Avoidances are rewarded by the relief felt when children are able to get the word out and avoidances are triggered by the association made to a word or sound that has been stuttered in the past.

SCHOOL-AGE CHILDREN: INTERMEDIATE STUTTERING

School-age children with intermediate stuttering (Fig. 7.5), who are typically between ages 6 and 13 years, are consciously aware of their stuttering and may have strong feelings about it. Frustration, embarrassment, and fear during the moment of stuttering become stronger as stuttering develops and persists. These feelings motivate escape and avoidance behaviors. Both behaviors can be seen in the video clip of "David" on *Lippincott Connect* (he is the fourth individual in "Normal Disfluency and the Development of Stuttering"). In this clip, David is explaining a board game to his clinician. It starts with him just ending a sentence, saying, "...land here. He-he-he goes home auto..." (voicing cuts out, perhaps as the larynx abducts or adducts, then a silent block occurs on /m/ and David rocks back in his chair and comes forward in an escape behavior to help him finish the word "automatically." He continues, "...matically because...um...("tsk" sound made with tongue)...because he he i...is on the shortcut." Note that the "um" and perhaps the "tsk" sound are starters (avoidances). His repetition of "he" is also a starter. All these starters are probably motivated by his fear of stuttering on "is."

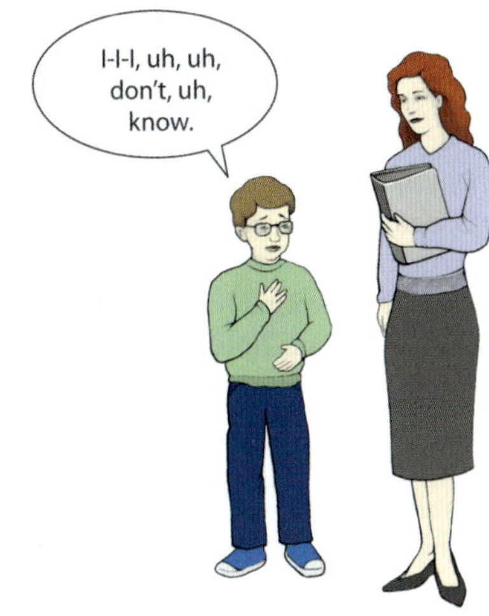

Figure 7.5 Child who may be an intermediate stutterer.

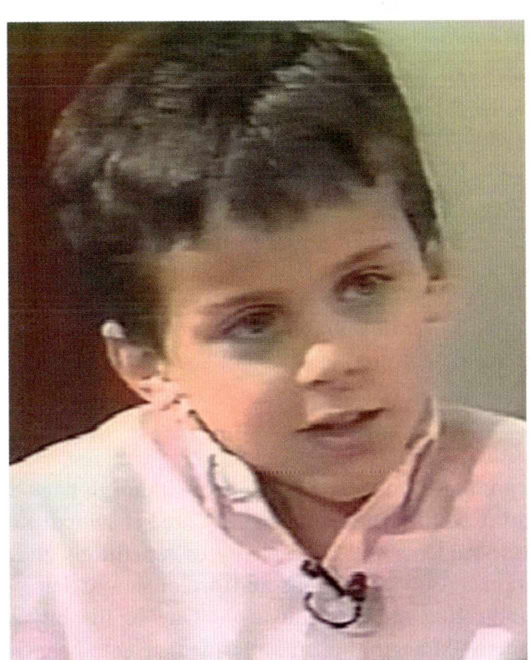

The fear felt by students with intermediate stuttering may be attached at first to the sounds and words on which they stutter most. They become convinced that these sounds are harder to say. Then they begin to scan ahead to see whether they might have to say them. When they anticipate the sounds they may stutter on, they try to avoid them. For example, children may say, "I don't know" to questions that a teacher asks them in class, or they may substitute "my sister" for their sister's name when talking about her. Sometimes, they may start a sentence, realize a feared word is coming up, then switch the sentence around to avoid stuttering, and end up producing a maze of half-finished sentences. With tactful questioning, radiating an accepting attitude, the clinician can verify these avoidances. They can also explore the escape behaviors—those things a child does to finish a word they are stuttering on. It is essential that as the clinician talks to students about their pattern of core behaviors, escapes and avoidances, they adopt an approach that helps the students feel accepted, "warts and all." Much will be conveyed by a warm tone of voice. It's as if they say, "Yes you do have some things you've learned to do to try to deal with your stuttering. It's ok. But we'll work together to try to make talking easier so you don't have to use all these extra things to talk."

The fear of stuttering felt by most students with intermediate stuttering may be associated not only with sounds and words they often stutter on but with situations as well. The youngsters may find that they stutter more in some situations than in others. At first, they approach these situations with dread, but later, they may go to great lengths to avoid them. Van Riper (1982a) suggested that the development of such situational fears and avoidances depends on listener reactions. I think peer reactions may be particularly important. Unfortunately, being bullied is not uncommon for students who stutter, but a number of clinician-authors have described helpful approaches to deal with bullying (eg, Hughes, 2014; Murphy et al., 2007). As these publications describe, students can be helped to deal with negative peer reactions, by learning to be open about their stuttering with their class, their peers, and by talking with the clinician about some people's reactions. Sometimes a small group of students who stutter can join together and can share their wounds inflicted by unhelpful or even belligerent peers and gain strength and stuttering pride through these discussions.

With this overview in mind, we'll now get into the details of intermediate stuttering in school-age children.

Core Behaviors

What are these students' moments of stuttering like—when they don't avoid them? What are the core behaviors?

These students still have plenty of repetitions and prolongations. Many repetitions and prolongations have pitch rise, indicating increasing tension. One of the big differences between beginning and intermediate core behaviors is the frequency of blocks. The blocks of students with intermediate stuttering seem to result from the cycle of threat/fear → tension → longer, more struggled blocks → more threat/fear → more tension. Individuals at the intermediate level often stutter by stopping airflow, voicing, movement of articulators, or all three, and then struggling to get their speech going again. Their stutters seem to surprise them less than when they were beginning stutterers. Instead, as evidenced by their voice and manner in certain situations, they anticipate stutters.

I have the impression that the blocks in intermediate stuttering are frequently characterized by excessive laryngeal tension (Van Riper, 1974). Of course, tension is often seen elsewhere as well. Students may squeeze their lips together, jam their tongues against the roof of their mouth, or hold their breath. Even though they are not highly conscious of just what they're doing during a block, they have a vivid awareness that they are stuck, that they feel helpless, and that the words they want to say just won't seem to come out. Because this happens when they are talking to someone, the connection to that person seems to be fractured when they get stuck. As a result, students often project their own worst thoughts on the listener and imagine rejection.

David (the school age child you may have just seen on *Lippincott Connect*) described his feeling of being blocked as like "a rock stuck in my throat." When he was lucky, he said, a little army of men would come into his throat and break the rock into little pieces, breaking the block so that sounds would come out. In that description, he was recounting the experience he felt of first being totally stuck and then rapidly repeating the first segment of the sound as he fought his way out of the block. A common example is the "…uh-uh-uh-I" that you will hear when someone is blocked on "I" and tries to push through it. At first, there is a moment of silence and then the rapid, staccato first segment of the sound as children who stutter get their larynx vibrating while maintaining a static articulatory posture. The larynx is still very tense; vibration stops and starts again and again. The vowel—either at the beginning or end of the syllable—is often the "schwa" or neutral vowel. In fact, it is only the first, brief segment of the intended vowel, which is cut off too abruptly to be perceived as the sound normally used in the word. Inexperienced clinicians sometimes mistakenly categorize these repeated parts of blocks as repetitions, not realizing the stuttering has advanced from repetitions to blocks.

In addition to repetitions of parts of sounds, blocks can have prolongations in them. Sometimes, as they are pushing through a block, students will momentarily prolong a continuant sound as in "[m]…mmm…mmmm…my." Again, this probably results from an individual's larynx vibrating momentarily, then seizing up again, and then vibrating again. I categorize these events as blocks rather than prolongations, because I think the core behavior is a complete stoppage of speech, even though it is mixed with momentary releases of laryngeal vibration. This confusing situation probably results from the fact that the sequence of repetitions, prolongations, and blocks reflects basically similar behaviors along a continuum of increasing tension, particularly in the larynx, as stuttering progresses. When you analyze the speech of school-age children with intermediate stuttering, try to discriminate which stutters are really repetitions and prolongations on their own, versus parts of the struggle behavior in blocks. The presence of blocks may mean that the young people's stuttering behaviors are affected by threat and fear, and this must be dealt with in treatment.

Secondary Behaviors

The blocks just described can be devastating to students who stutter. They are frustrated not only with their inability to make a sound but they are often faced with surprised and uncomfortable listeners as well. Even patient listeners may not know what to do. They may interrupt, look away, or fidget, leaving the children to conclude that they are doing something very wrong and should try to escape or avoid these painful moments.

The escape behaviors that speakers use to free themselves from stutters are present in preschool children with beginning stuttering, but they occur far more frequently in school-age children with intermediate stuttering. They are often more complex, too. Children with intermediate stuttering may blink their eyes and nod their head in an effort to escape a block. Sometimes, they may do both, and if they are still unable to say the word, they may resort to yet another device, such as slapping their legs. As these patterns grow more complex, they may also become disguised to look like natural movements and are performed more rapidly.

A video clip of Richard, showing an escape behavior, is available on Lippincott Connect. The clip is in the Chapter 7 videos and is titled "Rich—Intermediate with Escape and Avoidance Behaviors."

Notice that when Richard is first talking with the clinician, you can see movement of his right arm as he speaks. Later, when he answers the clinician's question "Where do you usually fish?" Richard brings his arm up near his mouth. What is he doing to escape from his moments of stuttering? Do you think his gesture becomes an avoidance behavior when he seems to bring his arm up before beginning the first word in his reply? Richard is now in his 30s and is Operations Manager for one of the largest automobile auction companies in the country. He uses his speech extensively to work with the 30 employees who work for him, and he is constantly on the phone with dealers despite a little residual stuttering.

In addition to escape behaviors, students at the intermediate level develop both word and situation avoidances, as previously mentioned. Word avoidances appear after students have repeated difficulty with a particular word or sound and have discovered how to take evasive action before they have to say it. For example, a young client in our clinic had been asked his name by a particularly stern teacher. He blocked severely on it and subsequently became fearful of saying his name, as well as other words starting with the same sound. He could usually think up synonyms for other words but what could he substitute for his name? So, he learned to get a running start in saying his name by beginning with "My name is..." whenever he was asked his name. This permitted him to avoid stuttering about half of the time. It is a subtle form of avoidance that many clinicians call "starters." More obvious examples of avoidances are given in the following paragraph.

Van Riper's (1982a) catalog of word avoidance techniques included **starters** (beginning a word by saying another word or sound, such as "well" or "uh" just before saying it); **substitutions** (substituting a word or phrase for another when stuttering is expected, as in "he's my unc-unc-unc...my father's brother"); **circumlocutions** (talking all around a word or phrase when anticipating stuttering, as in "well, I went to... yes, I really had a good time there, I saw the Empire State Building"); **postponements** (waiting a few beats or putting in filler words before starting a word on which stuttering is expected, as in "My name is.........Bill"); and **antiexpectancy devices** (using an odd manner or funny voice to avoid stuttering when it's anticipated). I had a client when I worked in Australia who could only tell jokes fluently if he put on an accent that sounded like he came from Alabama.

Like escape behaviors, word avoidance techniques often become more rapid and more subtle with time. Indeed, some individuals can disguise word avoidances to look like typical behavior. For example, they may put on pensive facial expressions and appear to search for a word while postponing their attempt to say a feared sound. Experienced clinicians learn to pick up subtle cues in the rate and manner of speaking that tip them off to the use of such avoidances. These avoidances can be explored, in an accepting way, by the clinician and client at the appropriate moment in treatment.

Situational fears and avoidances are also common in the school-age child with intermediate stuttering. Past stuttering in specific places or with specific people are the seeds from which situational fears grow. In school, students who stutter usually have trouble reading aloud or giving oral reports. Most people who stutter, and even many who don't, dread those classes in which teachers call on students by going up and down the rows. As in an earlier example, students' fears steadily mount as a teacher goes down the row, getting closer and closer to calling on them. Then, if called on, they may say "I don't know" even when they do. Or they may take a failing grade rather than give the oral report. In contrast, other school situations, especially casual ones like gym class or lunch period, are likely to hold less fear or expectation of stuttering for them.

Situational fears quickly generate situation avoidances. Students who fear talking aloud in class may try to slouch low in their seat in hopes of being overlooked. A person who stutters who is afraid of making introductions will contrive ways of having other people make them. In junior high school, I coped with my fear of ordering in restaurants by ducking into the bathroom when the waitress approached our table, asking my friends to order a cheeseburger for me. Every person who stutters has his or her own pattern of situation avoidances, which may provide an important focus for therapy.

Feelings and Attitudes

Students with intermediate stuttering have gone well beyond the momentary frustration and embarrassment experienced by those with beginning stuttering. They have felt the helplessness of being caught in many blocks and runaway repetitions. The anticipation of stuttering and subsequent listener penalties has been fulfilled many times. These experiences pile up like cars in a demolition derby to create an entanglement of fear, embarrassment, and shame that accompanies stuttering. These feelings may not be pervasive or dog a stutterer all the time. However, stuttering has now changed from an annoyance to a serious problem.

A major influence on such students' feelings is increased cognitive maturity, starting at age 3 or 4, that enables them to compare themselves with their peers. Once these students begin school, peers have a greater and greater influence on them. They may stutter more as they encounter new people and new situations, and, as they do stutter more, peers may begin to ask them why they talk the way they do and to make comments about their stuttering or tease them about it. As a result, increasingly negative self-awareness about their speech leads to feelings of embarrassment, shame, and guilt.

The Stuttering Foundation pages "Kids' Letters and Drawings" (www.stutteringhelp.org/kids) have had several comments by school-age children that vividly depict their feelings about stuttering: "When I stutter, I feel like I am an idiot and dumb." "I stutter a lot and when I stutter, I feel like I am trapped in a box with no door. I am trying to break down the walls with an axe." "My stuttering feels like a volcano." On the bright side, many of the students who made these comments also expressed very positive feelings about their progress in treatment. They also expressed their own growing confidence as they work on their speech: "I am a stuttering hero!" "Stuttering has never stopped me from being who I am." And they appreciate the help they get: "I love my speech teacher!"

Many intermediate stutterers express their feelings in the documentary film, "My Beautiful Stutter." You can get a sense of how powerful this film is by watching the trailer for it, available on Google. The film takes place at camp for children and teens who stutter between ages 8 and 18, Camp Say, that is run every summer. Information is available at campsay.org.

For those who aren't able to get therapy, negative feelings may grow and soon affect behavior. Students may look away from listeners when they are stuttering and flush with embarrassment immediately afterward. They may become stiff and uneasy at the prospect of speaking. Their stuttering patterns include an increasing number of avoidance devices, and they are beginning to evade situations in which they anticipate that they may stutter. These are all signs that their feelings and attitudes are becoming suffused with fear. Table 7.6 gives the characteristics of intermediate stutterers.

The emotions I have described, especially embarrassment and shame, may be mixed with hope as treatment begins. Figure 7.6 was drawn by a young man in his first few weeks of therapy. It reflects his extensive negative feelings on the left side—he has drawn himself in a jail cell with tears/rain falling around him and the key just out of reach. On the right side of the drawing, he shows himself as he hopes he will be after therapy, escaping from jail, running in the sunshine with grass underfoot and a flower in the background.

TABLE 7.6 Characteristics of Intermediate Stuttering in a School-Age Child

1. Frequent core behaviors are blocks in which the child shuts off sound or voice. They will also probably have many repetitions and prolongations.
2. Child uses escape behaviors to terminate blocks.
3. Child appears to anticipate blocks, often using avoidance behaviors prior to feared words. They also anticipate difficult situations and sometimes avoids them.
4. Fear before stuttering, embarrassment during stuttering, and shame after stuttering characterize this level, especially fear.

Underlying Processes

Many of the symptoms of intermediate stuttering result from the same processes that underlie those of beginning stuttering. There are important differences, however. In intermediate stuttering, classically conditioned tension responses are more evident, conditioned emotion is now turning into a more intense conscious threat/fear reaction, and avoidance conditioning has become a big factor in shaping stuttering behaviors.

Avoidance conditioning transforms escape behaviors, such as the use of "um" to escape from a stuttering block, into avoidances, such as saying "um" before saying a word on which stuttering is expected. This learning process (classical conditioning plus operant conditioning) also teaches students with intermediate stuttering to avoid words, to change sentences around, and to avoid speaking situations entirely. Avoidance learning also generalizes from one word to another and from one situation to another.

Avoidance conditioning may proceed very quickly in people with persistent stuttering because they may have a genetic or congenital bias toward right hemisphere, emotionally based behaviors, as we described in Chapters 2, 3, 5, and 6. The threat of stuttering may elicit "prepared" defensive reactions, such as avoidances of words or situations. Such avoidances are strongly maintained because individuals who have developed them use them when they anticipate stuttering, which decreases or eliminates the threat/fear. Thus, avoidances are maintained by negative reinforcement. By avoiding the stuttering, individuals who stutter never have the opportunity to discover that stuttering is not so painful after all.

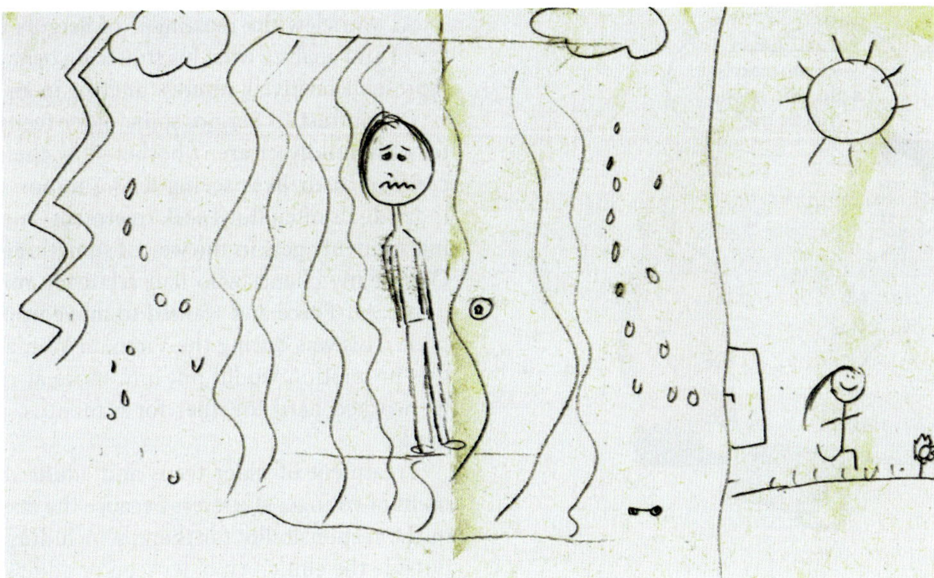

Figure 7.6 A young man's drawing of himself as he begins therapy **(left side)** and his hopes for a happy outcome **(right side)**. (Drawn by Marcel Etienne.)

Some intermediate level stutterers develop avoidances that are almost masterpieces of listener- and self-deception. This may lead them develop covert stuttering—to be discussed more fully in the section on core behaviors in advanced stuttering.

For more typical intermediate stutterers who do show some stuttering but also have many avoidances, therapy can help to reduce avoidances. To begin, the clinician must build a trusting relationship with these children, so they feel accepted as they are—stutters, avoidances, and everything else. Parents should be invited to observe and participate *only* with the children's permission. Gradually, the clinician can structure situations to help the students learn that the moment of stuttering can be tolerated and threat/fear can be reduced by resisting the impulse to push through the stuttering—a behavior that rewards tension and struggle. As you will see in the chapter on treatment of intermediate stuttering, the clinician—again, with the children's permission—can pretend to stutter and show that they are comfortable with it and gradually have the children join in. As that has started and continues, the clinician should help the children learn new behaviors to substitute for the old avoidances. Specific strategies such as having children share with their class that they stutter and even offer to show volunteers how to stutter in various ways that actually associate stuttering with fun. Then easier ways of stuttering, such as using easy onsets and slow pullouts, combined with reduction of fear and tension in the moment of stuttering, can provide students who stutter with new tools that will increase their confidence and have them actually look forward to stuttering so they can modify it. What better feeling for the students to have about their stuttering than "Bring it on!"

Summary of Intermediate Stuttering

Three characteristics differentiate intermediate stuttering in school-age children from beginning stuttering in preschool children:

1. There are increasingly tense blocks, repetitions, and prolongations. The increased tension results from feelings of frustration, threat/fear, and helplessness. These feelings trigger further tension responses, which interfere with fluency and in turn produce more frustration, threat/fear, and feelings of helplessness. As tension mounts, this vicious cycle continues. Blocks are longer and more noticeable, more listeners react with surprise and impatience, and students' feelings of threat and fear increases in response to these reactions from listeners.
2. The increasing presence of fear and anticipation of bad experiences spurs students to develop avoidance behaviors in addition to the escape behaviors they may be already using. Avoidance conditioning is difficult to undo. Unless the threat and fear that underlies avoidance is markedly reduced, relapse lurks close by.
3. The child with intermediate stuttering increasingly feels embarrassment, shame, and guilt as they realize that their speech is markedly different from that of their peers.

OLDER TEENS AND ADULTS: ADVANCED STUTTERING

Individuals whose stuttering has persisted into older adolescence and adulthood (Fig. 7.7) typically have a deeply ingrained pattern of core and secondary behaviors. Often,

C... C... Could
y... you make
a ph... ph... phone
call for me?

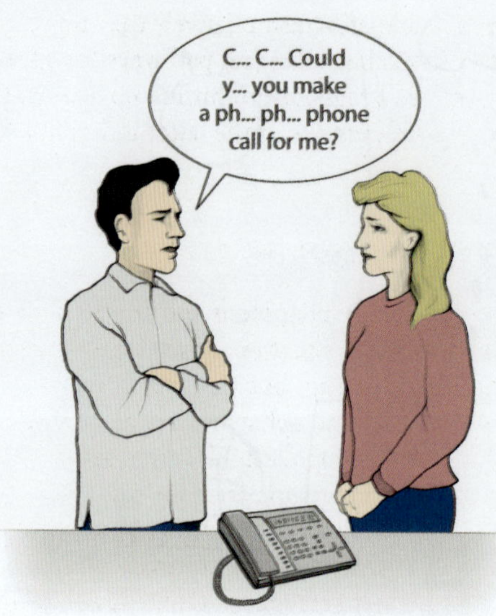

Figure 7.7 Individual who may be an advanced stutterer.

stuttering is a major player in their school, work, and social lives. They may avoid talking in class, decline job opportunities, and limit their social activities from fear of stuttering. This describes me at age 20.

A clip of "Sergio"—an adult who stutters—is the fifth and last sample on *Lippincott Connect* video section titled "Normal Disfluency and the Development of Stuttering." This video clip starts with Sergio answering my question, "How has your speech been lately?" Sergio begins with a silent block accompanied by jaw tremor and then says, "A lot of my bad habits are back." He is fairly fluent on this sentence, but we see some eye closures associated with his Tourette syndrome, which he has had, along with stuttering, since childhood. I then suggest, "Why don't you talk a little about what those bad habits are." Sergio responds with "uuuuuh," accompanied by a facial grimace used probably to release a laryngeal block. He then says, "I'm-I'm-I'm using mu- (note schwa or truncated vowel)-my (here Sergio makes a facial grimace to escape from the block) eyes to uh to get the words out."

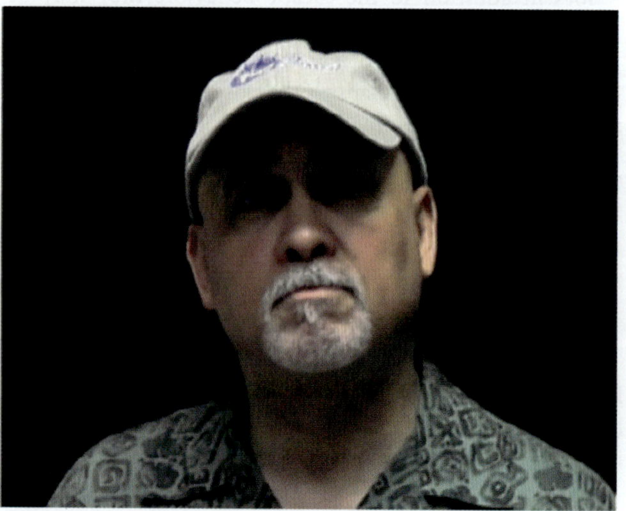

As you view the remainder of Sergio's clip, make a transcript and analyze what his stuttering behaviors are. This clip represents relatively severe stuttering in an adult.

In contrast to Sergio, some older teens and adults stutter only mildly or aren't bothered by their stuttering. They carry on their lives seeing it as a minor annoyance. These individuals often don't seek treatment—unless their stuttering suddenly gets in the way of something they want to do. One of my clients who had relatively mild stuttering was in the Air Force and wanted to move up from navigator to pilot. This was during the Vietnam War, and I worried that this promotion would put him more at risk. Nevertheless, we worked hard together for 6 months, and he made the grade.

Treatment of older teens and adults differs from treatment of younger stutterers because the client can take much of the responsibility for therapy including substantial work outside the clinic. An older teen or adult's increased capacity for independent work may compensate for another characteristic of this level—a long history of stuttering. Patterns of stuttering with tension, escape, and avoidance behaviors are now firmly established. Emotions such as frustration, fear, guilt, and hostility have built up over many years of being unable to speak like other people and many bad experiences with thoughtless, uninformed, or momentarily startled listeners. Beliefs are usually distorted by the conviction that other people are impatient or disgusted by the speaker's stuttering.

After many years of stuttering, adults and adolescents who stutter increasingly think of themselves primarily as "stutterers" rather than as people who have occasional difficulty speaking. Except for a few safe situations in which they may be relatively fluent, they have some fear of most speaking situations, and they shape their lives accordingly. They may believe that their stuttering is as noticeable to others as though they had two heads—and nearly as unacceptable.

Core Behaviors

Core behaviors in advanced stuttering include repetitions and prolongations, but the most notable are struggled and tension-filled blocks—the stoppages of sound and movement that are most confusing and surprising to listeners. Advanced stutterers may block and then release a little sound only to fall back into the block again. It might sound like this: "[silence]...m-m-m...[silence]...m-m-muh...[silence]... my [said with a sudden effort]...name is Barry." Such behaviors may be longer and display more struggle in clients with advanced stuttering than in school-age youngsters who have intermediate stuttering, but they are essentially similar. However, blocks now may be associated with tremors. During blocks, tremors of the lips, jaw, or tongue may be apparent. Tremors appear in those individuals who have been stuttering for several years and may occur when stuttering is accompanied by strong emotion.

Van Riper (1982a) described the effects of tremors on the person who stutters:

> *Tremors affect the stutterer strongly. They make him feel helpless. He cannot understand why they persist or how they begin or are maintained. They violate the integrity of the self for they are sensed as being involuntary. The stutterer feels that he has lost control (p. 126).*

The video clip of "Sergio" referred to earlier has examples of tremors, such as when he makes his first attempt to say "patience."

In a small number of advanced stutterers, blocks are hardly evident. These individuals may have honed their avoidances to such a fine edge that their stutters are scarcely noticeable. If stuttering does occur, it usually feels devastating to them. Consequently, much of their energy is spent anticipating blocks that never happen and mustering avoidances to keep anxiety at bay. These individuals are usually referred to as "covert" stutterers. Their motivation to hide their stuttering often comes from particularly devastating listener reactions, such as being rejected by an acquaintance or being fired from a job. They often use extensive avoidance behaviors, such as changing words or refusing to participate in certain speaking situations that may expose their stuttering. Some of these individuals avoid stuttering by successfully using techniques sometimes taught in therapy, such as slowing their speech or relaxing muscles before saying a feared word. Sometimes the burden of hiding their stuttering becomes great enough that they will seek treatment. A very knowledgeable and accepting therapist can help them become more open about their stuttering and guide them to learn ways to stutter more easily and openly. Meeting others who stutter, especially in a self-help or support group, can provide a pathway to change. There are some excellent publications describing **covert stuttering**, including Constantino et al. (2017), Douglas and Quarrington (1952), and Douglass et al. (2018).

One individual with covert stuttering was a delightful woman I knew and whom I'll call "Lenore," who said she had stuttered since childhood. Yet, she almost never had a repetition, prolongation, or block that I witnessed. Lenore was highly competent at everything she did, but she severely limited her life because of her fear that she would stutter. In particular, she often felt she came across as far less articulate than she might have because of the frequency with which she substituted words to avoid stuttering.

Returning to the typical stuttering behaviors of older teens and adults with advanced stuttering, these individuals will have repetitions as well as blocks. These are usually not the easy, regular repetitions of borderline stuttering but are more like those of beginning stuttering—tense, with a rapid, irregular tempo. They may be repetitions of syllables, luh-luh-luh-like this, or words, like I-I-I-I. As I've indicated earlier, some apparent repetitions are actually components of blocks. The latter look as if the speaker recoils from a momentary fixation and then gets stuck again. In an evaluation, and throughout therapy, be sure to distinguish relatively easy repetitions that emerge from anomalies in neural pathways for speech from those that are recoil reactions to hitting up against the hard wall of a block. An example of the latter is Sergio's "mu-mu-my eyes."

Secondary Behaviors

Advanced stuttering in older teens and adults involves many of the same word and situational avoidances that are seen in intermediate stuttering, but the avoidances are likely to be more extensive. Some behaviors are more obvious than others. When I was in high school, I used several avoidance devices that often didn't work, such as "uh...well...you see" and a gasp of air, followed by a block of long duration filled with unsuccessful escape attempts before I finally released the blocked word with great effort. Other advanced stutterers may approach feared words cautiously and use subtle mannerisms, such as appearing to think just before saying the feared word, so that most listeners don't realize they are stuttering. These stutterers are usually on guard much of the time, scanning ahead with their verbal early-warning systems.

Many individuals with advanced stuttering also control their environments carefully so that they can avoid situations in which they are likely to stutter. They may feign sickness when they have to give a speech, use answering machines rather than answering the telephone, or arrange to have their spouses or children deal with store clerks. Often, with careful questioning of individuals with advanced stuttering who use avoidances a great deal, you can learn what occurs when avoidances don't work. Even the most skillful avoiders are sometimes caught with their defenses down and become stuck in a block. Core behaviors may also be elicited by asking some stutterers to stutter openly without using secondary behaviors. Individuals who can do this, especially those who can do it without excessive discomfort, are more amenable to change.

Feelings and Attitudes

The feelings and attitudes of older teens and adults, like their stuttering behaviors, have been shaped by years of conditioning. Over and over, they have learned that much of their stuttering is unpredictable. When it is predictable, it comes when they want it least—when they want more than anything to be fluent. As a result, they often feel out of control. Figure 7.8 reflects one individual's depictions of his own feelings of being "locked up" and out of control when stuttering. Note the iron band clamping his head, his jammed-up teeth, and clenching of his abdomen.

These uncomfortable feelings are often buttressed by individuals' perceptions of how others see them. Listeners' reactions look overwhelmingly negative to them. Even when listeners say nothing, their faces appear, to the stutterer, to say everything. It is as though stuttering is a rattletrap car

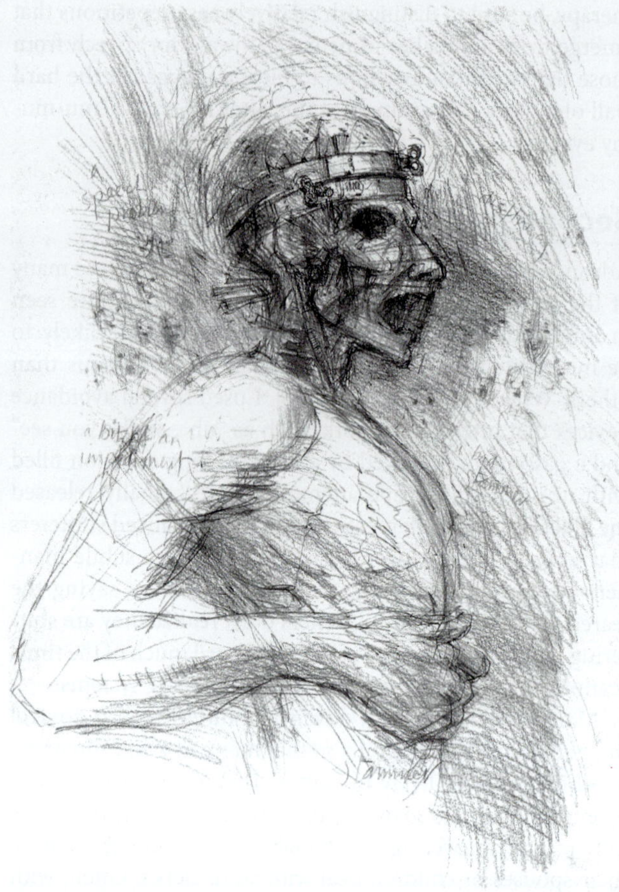

Figure 7.8 "How I feel when I stutter" by Mike Peace. (Courtesy of Dr. Trudy Stewart.)

that always stalls in heavy traffic amid honking drivers. Such experiences gradually shape the attitudes of those with advanced stuttering toward feelings of helplessness, frustration, anger, and hopelessness.

Of course, individuals' responses to stuttering vary greatly. If a person who stutters has many talents and abilities for which they are recognized and if they have an assertive personality, they may be less devastated by stuttering. The former CEO of General Electric, Jack Welch, is a good example. In talking about his stuttering, he said that his mother taught him that if it bothers anyone, that's their problem. Welch was an aggressive manager and became known for his strong and successful leadership style. Might that aggression may have been a defense for an underlying more sensitive temperament? If an individual who stutters has a sensitive nature that is not deeply defended, their feelings and attitudes about stuttering may be an important component of their problem. The movie "The King's Speech" suggested that Bertie, who was to become the King of England, George VI, was a sensitive soul who was debilitated by his stuttering until he received some very confidence-building treatment from Lionel Logue, his unorthodox Australian clinician.

The point is that by the time a person who stutters is an adult, they have had years of experiencing stuttering, feeling frustrated and helpless, and have developed techniques to minimize pain. Unless they have a strong personality to compensate, they are likely to feel that stuttering is a big part of who they are to other people. It is a part that they hate, a part on which they blame many other troubles, and a part they want desperately to eliminate.

Some people who stutter, however, who reach the advanced level have become reconciled to their stuttering. If they are in their 20s, 30s, or beyond, there may be some natural resistance to treatment, because stuttering has become part of their identities. After years of doubt and turmoil, they've grown accustomed to themselves as someone who stutters. To consider treatment is to reject a part of themselves, to open old wounds. Those who risk change, enter treatment, and succeed will find the risk to have been worthwhile. But those who enter treatment and do not succeed may suffer twice from the pain of failure as well as the loss of the denial or reluctant acceptance of stuttering that had been in place before the attempt at treatment but was given up. I saw this happen with many of the clients we treated in a behavioral therapy program focused on slow speech. When I followed them for several years after their therapy, many were doing fine, but many were not. They had become quite fluent while they were in treatment, but relapsed precipitously in the months and years afterward, and blamed themselves for the loss of their fluency.

Table 7.7 lists the major characteristics of advanced stutterers.

Underlying Processes

Advanced stuttering, unlike milder levels of stuttering, is influenced less by its original constitutional, developmental, and environmental factors than by early classical

TABLE 7.7 Characteristics of Advanced Stuttering in Older Teens and Adults

1. Most frequent core behaviors are longer, tense blocks, often with tremors of the lips, tongue, or jaw. Individual will also probably have repetitions and prolongations.
2. Stuttering may be suppressed in some individuals through extensive avoidance behaviors.
3. Complex patterns of avoidance and escape behaviors characterize the stutterer. These may be very rapid and so well habituated that the stutterer may not be aware of what they do.
4. Emotions of fear, embarrassment, and shame are very strong. The individual has negative feelings about themselves as a person who is helpless and inept when they stutter. This self-concept may be pervasive.

conditioning of the tension response, as well as by these individuals' emotional reactions to their stuttering. That is not to say that anomalies in neural pathways are having no effect. It is likely that individuals with more inefficient neural pathways will still experience the effect on their fluency. However, it seems likely that the influences of home environments and developmental pressures of speech and language have been somewhat diminished by maturation and learning. But conditioned responses that were learned in reaction to disfluencies caused by constitutional factors are stronger than ever. Their effects have been magnified by years of experience, and the way the brain operates in speech has probably been modified as a consequence. Moreover, an individual's characteristic patterns of tension, escape, and avoidance have become almost automatic through years of practice. For example, the individual with advanced stuttering may exhibit a string of avoidance and escape behaviors but only remember that "the word got stuck."

As I described in Chapter 5 on Learning, classically conditioned responses—such as the tension response to threat and fear in stuttering—stay in memory essentially forever. This is an important underlying process to help us understand why, even when stuttering has become milder for a while, it may come back with severe symptoms. When, for example, the individual has received stuttering therapy and the stuttering is "under control," the passage of time after the classically conditioned response is extinguished and the change in context (the clinic and the clinician are no longer present) will often cause the tension response to reappear.

Older teen and adults' stuttering is affected by higher-level explicit learning, as well. They have developed a self-concept as an impaired speaker, which carries highly negative connotations for most. Self-concepts begin to be formed during preschool years and are based initially on what one can do, rather than what one is (Clarke-Stewart & Friedman, 1987). More enduring traits are added as a result of social interactions in later childhood, adolescence, and beyond (Roessler & Bolton, 1978). Thus, the self-concept of individuals who stutter is determined, in part, by their perception of how they talk. In children's early years, their impression of stuttering may be a fleeting awareness that they sometimes have difficulty talking. In later levels of development, the reactions of significant listeners—parents, peer group, other adults—have a major impact. By the time individuals who stutter are teens or adults, their self-concepts may become filled with relatively enduring negative perceptions as a result of listeners' impatience and rejection. A negative self-concept is formed not only by perceptions of listeners' reactions but, in a continuing spiral, the negative self-concept also affects those perceptions.

To return to research, studies of the psychology of disability suggested that "one's perception of self influences one's perception of others' views of oneself, rendering social interaction more difficult" (Roessler & Bolton, 1978). Applied to clients with advanced stuttering, this suggests that they are likely to project their own rejections of stuttering onto listeners, thereby affecting their interactions with them. This cycle may be stopped when an outsider helps a person who stutters test the reality of his perceptions. As the clinician and client work together to explore the client's stuttering, they can reexamine the client's assumptions about whether stuttering is actually bad and whether people actually respond to it negatively. The clinician can, with the client's ok, pseudo-stutter to strangers and have the client observe the listener's reaction. When the client is ready, they can switch roles and let the client discover whether listeners are really responding badly to their stutters.

As suggested earlier, there is a growing awareness that people who stutter—in fact all people with any kind of difference—can experience a blossoming of their resilience and celebrate their differences (eg, Runswick-Cole and Goodley, 2013). We see this vividly in these films: "For Kids, By Kids," "For Kids, By Kids: All Grown Up," and "My Beautiful Stutter." Another documentary, "When I Stutter," is more focused on advanced stuttering and captures the miserable experiences that many stutterers suffered as they grew up. However, the film also portrays the joy that accompanies gains made with successful therapy. More information on these films is given at the end of the chapter.

In addition to working on cognitive aspects of the problem, therapy for advanced stuttering also must deal directly with the avoidances that such clients have learned so well. As mentioned in the discussion of intermediate stuttering, as avoidance conditioning progresses, individuals fear not only words and situations but also stuttering itself. By reducing this fear—helping the client feel that stuttering is ok—and changing avoidances into approaches, treatment enables individuals who stutter to stutter with less fear by associating the clinician's approval and their own successes with a calmer, more relaxed way of stuttering. Gradually, tension and hurry fade from disfluencies, they feel more in control, and their fears diminish even further as a result.

Summary of Advanced Stuttering

The category of advanced stuttering in older teens and adults describes a developmental level and implies a particular treatment orientation as characterized by the following:

1. Treatment may be easier because the client can assume much of the responsibility for generalization beyond the clinic.
2. On the other hand, treatment is more challenging because the client with advanced stuttering has more deeply habituated patterns of behavior than at earlier levels. The individual's core behaviors often consist of long blocks with considerable tension and at times visible tremors. Secondary behaviors may consist of long chains of word avoidance and escape behaviors. Situational avoidance is common.

TABLE 7.8 Characteristics of Five Developmental/Treatment Levels

Developmental/ Treatment Level	Core Behaviors	Secondary Behaviors	Feelings and Attitudes	Underlying Processes
Typical disfluency	10 or fewer disfluencies per 100 words; one-unit repetitions; mostly repetitions, interjections, and revisions	None	Not aware; no concern	Typical stresses of speech/language and psychosocial development
Borderline stuttering	≥11 disfluencies per 100 words; more than two units in repetitions; more repetitions and prolongations than revisions or interjections	None	Generally not aware; may occasionally show momentary surprise or mild frustration	Stresses of speech/ language and psychosocial development interacting with constitutional predisposition
Beginning stuttering	Rapid, irregular, and tense repetitions may have fixed articulatory posture in blocks	Escape behaviors such as eye blinks, increases in pitch or loudness as disfluency progresses	Aware of disfluency, may express frustration	Conditioned emotional reactions causing excess tension; instrumental/ operant conditioning resulting in escape behaviors
Intermediate stuttering	Blocks in which sound and airflow are shut off	Escape and avoidance behaviors	Fear, frustration, embarrassment, and shame	Above processes, plus avoidance conditioning
Advanced stuttering	Long, tense blocks; some with tremor	Escape and avoidance behaviors	Fear, frustration, embarrassment, and shame; negative self-concept	Above processes, plus cognitive learning

3. Some older teens and adult stutterers may hide and disguise their stuttering well enough to avoid detection by many listeners, but this is at the cost of constant vigilance. If this behavior is pervasive, it can become covert stuttering. This can be difficult to treat because the individual may strongly resist bringing the stuttering out into the open so that they may modify it.
4. Feelings of frustration and helplessness usually accumulate over the years, leading to coping behaviors and a lifestyle that may be highly constrained. Such responses create a self-concept of an inept speaker whose stuttering is unacceptable to listeners. This in turn affects the stutterer's perceptions of the listener's reactions.

SUMMARY

- Table 7.8 summarizes the characteristics of the five developmental/treatment levels described in this chapter.
- Individuals who stutter will each have their own course of development, influenced by the interaction of constitutional (including temperamental), environmental, and learning factors.
- Clinicians need to use their understanding of the underlying processes to design procedures to treat each individual's core behaviors, secondary behaviors, and feelings and attitudes.
- Because much of stuttering is influenced by learning, treatment may appear to extinguish many stuttering behaviors, but the passage of time and the change of context after treatment ends will cause many behaviors to reappear. Treatment must prepare the client to deal with this relapse.

STUDY QUESTIONS

1. In the "Exceptions and Variations" section of this chapter's Overview, different types of stuttering onset and development are described. What factors might cause these differences?

2. In discussing typical disfluency, it is suggested that "if a child shows what appears to be typical disfluencies, such as single-word repetitions, but consistently displays pauses or interjections of 'uh' immediately before or during disfluencies, they should be carefully evaluated as possibly stuttering." What might be going on? What might these pauses or interjections signify?
3. The idea of a dyssynchrony in the timing of the elements of spoken language production is suggested as an underlying process of typical disfluency. It is also used to account for primary stuttering. How can both types of disfluency be accounted for by the same process?
4. What is the difference between core behaviors and secondary behaviors?
5. At what ages is typical disfluency likely to be most frequent?
6. Name three influences that may cause typical disfluency to increase.
7. What are three ways in which core behaviors of typical disfluency differ from those of borderline stuttering?
8. Describe the core behaviors of the beginning stutterer.
9. What causes greater muscle tension in beginning stuttering compared to borderline stuttering?
10. Describe why escape behaviors are used by stutterers. Give examples.
11. What is a major secondary behavior that differentiates the intermediate from the beginning stutterer?
12. Compare the feelings and attitudes of the borderline, beginning, and intermediate levels of stuttering.
13. Describe the role of the listener in the development of the advanced stutterer's self-concept.

SUGGESTED PROJECTS

1. Visit *Lippincott Connect* and watch the video clips of speakers who are representative of each level of stuttering (typical disfluency, borderline, beginning, intermediate, and advanced), and play them in random order for your class. See how many of your fellow students can correctly identify each level.
2. Make audio or video recordings of a number of nonstuttering students in a class, and determine which of them are more disfluent and which are less disfluent. Is there a gradual continuum between more disfluent and less disfluent, or are there two distinct groups? Are any of the "typically disfluent" students who show a high frequency of disfluencies actually showing borderline stuttering? Should the term "borderline stutterer" be used only for preschoolers?
3. See pages 31–34 of Bloodstein et al. (2021) (see Suggested Readings). Under the title "Guitar's Classification Schema," the authors discussed the stuttering levels described in this chapter. Compare this classification system with those of Bloodstein and Van Riper, both of which are described in these pages of Bloodstein et al. What are the advantages and disadvantages of Guitar's Classification Schema, compared to the other two classification systems.

SUGGESTED VIEWING

"When I Stutter." *This is a powerful documentary featuring many advanced stutterers who recount their life experiences with severe stuttering. Throughout much of the film we observe treatment for an adult stutterer who makes great improvement over the course of several months. In addition to sharing many stuttering stories, the documentary provides a large number of samples of stuttering that can be analyzed by students to hone their skills at identifying core and secondary behaviors.*

"My Beautiful Stutter." *The trailer is available by Googling this title, and other opportunities for viewing the entire movie are described. This is an emotionally joyful documentary capturing the experiences of several children between 9 and 18 years old who, after years of being dissed and bullied for their stuttering, get to meet other kids who stutter at a summer camp and learn to feel "stuttering pride" about their speech.*

"For Kids, By Kids." A Stuttering Foundation video available on YouTube by searching for "Stuttering Kids." A follow-up video was made of four of the youngsters, 11 years later, showing their success: "For Kids, By Kids: All Grown Up."

The original 12-minute video is full of excellent cameos of kids who stutter and what it's like for them. It is an excellent resource for understanding children who stutter and for viewing many different types of stuttering to hone your skills in analyzing stuttering.

SUGGESTED READINGS

Bloodstein, O., Ratner, N., & Brundage, S. (2021). *A handbook on stuttering* (7th ed.). Plural Publishing, Inc.

In this book, the section of Chapter 1 titled "Stuttering Over the Lifespan: Phases, Stages, 'Tracks,' and the Possibility of Subtypes" covers some of the material in the current chapter. As indicated in "Suggested Projects," the classification system used in the book you are reading is compared with other classification systems.

Gray, J. A. (1987). *The psychology of fear and stress*. Cambridge University Press.

This is a very readable exposition of findings about innate fears, conditioning, and brain processes involved with escape and avoidance learning. Gray also describes his concept of the "behavioral inhibition system," a model of the effect that conditioning, language, the limbic system, and anxiety have on behavior.

Luper, H. L., & Mulder, R. L. (1964). *Stuttering: Therapy for children.* Prentice-Hall.

An excellent treatment text that describes four developmental levels of stuttering similar to the levels described here. Although out of print, this book is available for as little as $3 at http://www.AbeBooks.com.

Stuttering Foundation. www.stutteringhelp.org

Much information is available here for kids, teens, Speech-Language Pathologists (SLPs) parents, teachers, and pediatricians. The Kids' Letters and Drawings pages are constantly updated and a good place for your young clients to have their comments and their illustrations "published."

Van Riper, C. (1982b). The development of stuttering. In: *The nature of stuttering* (pp. 88–110). Prentice-Hall.

In this chapter, Van Riper describes four developmental tracks of stuttering, three of which depart substantially from our stages of stuttering development. This chapter gives the reader a good sense of individual variability in stuttering.

8

Atypical Disfluency

Chapter Outline

Chapter Objectives

After studying this chapter, readers should be able to:

- Describe the multiple possible etiologies and speech characteristics associated with acquired neurogenic stuttering
- Describe the nature of stuttering associated with stress and injuries while in the military
- Describe the conditions that may give rise to functional stuttering
- Describe the speech characteristics of functional stuttering
- Describe the nature of stuttering seen in instances of malingering
- Describe the nature of cluttering

Key Terms

Adaptation: The phenomenon of repeated reading of a passage resulting in stuttering becoming less and less frequent with each reading

Delayed auditory feedback (DAF): Hearing one's own voice, via a microphone and headphones, a half-second or so after speaking. This was once done via an electromechanical device but is now usually done via a computer program. It typically forces a client to speak more slowly and reduces stuttering dramatically. It can cause a normal speaker to have repetitions of words and syllables

Fluency-inducing or fluency-enhancing conditions: Stimuli that usually cause a person who stutters to speak much more fluently. Examples are speaking in a rhythmic or staccato manner, speaking under loud masking noise so the client can't hear his own voice, and speaking while very relaxed

Mazing: A disorder of spoken language characterized by false starts, hesitations, and revisions that make the speaker's message difficult to understand

Pacing: A treatment technique in which each individual syllable is spoken separately, sometimes accompanied by physical movement such as tapping a finger as each syllable is spoken

Posttraumatic stress disorder (PTSD): An anxiety disorder that occurs after a person has experienced or witnessed a terrifying event. Reminders of the event can bring back traumatic memories that trigger emotional and physical responses

Prolonged speech: A treatment for stuttering that induces the client to stretch out sounds, start words with a gentle onset of phonation, and touch the articulators lightly when producing consonants

Traumatic brain injury (TBI): An injury to the brain from an external force. This may be either an injury that penetrates the skull (such as a bullet shot into the head) or a closed-head injury (such as a bomb concussion close to a person) where penetration does not occur

Trial therapy: A brief treatment of stuttering carried out during the evaluation to determine which treatment techniques are most effective

OVERVIEW

This chapter discusses three fluency disorders that are different from "developmental" stuttering. These disorders—neurogenic stuttering, functional (previously "psychogenic" stuttering), and cluttering—are similar to developmental stuttering in some ways but are generally distinctly different in etiology, symptoms, and treatment. Figure 8.1 gives an overview of the chapter.

ACQUIRED NEUROGENIC STUTTERING

Nature

The term "acquired neurogenic stuttering" (ANS) denotes stuttering that appears to be caused or exacerbated by neurological disease or damage. It is typically acquired after childhood, and its etiology may be stroke, head trauma, tumor, disease processes such as Parkinson's, or drug toxicity. Additional, though rare, causes are dialysis dementia, seizure disorders, bilateral thalamotomy, or thalamic stimulation (Duffy, 2019). Demyelination of the corpus callosum has also been identified as a cause of stuttering (Decker et al., 2018). ANS has also been seen in active-duty service members and veterans with combat-related brain injury (traumatic brain injury, TBI) and co-occurring **posttraumatic stress disorder (PTSD)**.

For more than a hundred years, clinicians have described cases of ANS and some have suggested that understanding neurogenic stuttering may help us understand some aspects of typical or "developmental" stuttering (Pick, 1899). Another important reason for learning about ANS is that it may be an early diagnostic sign of a neurological problem in some patients. Helm-Estabrooks (1999) described this eloquently: "Fluent speaking is, perhaps, the most refined motor act performed by humans, requiring complex coordination of many different muscle groups. It can be sensitive, therefore, to even small changes in neurological status, which may be why stuttering occurs in a wide range of neurological disorders, from Parkinson disease to closed head injury. If this fact is ignored, clinicians may be overlooking an important early indicator of neurological disease" (p. 265).

Some writers prefer to use the term "neurogenic disfluency," because they don't consider neurogenic stuttering to be true stuttering. Such usage may, however, blur the distinction between two different phenomena that may occur with neurological insults. One is an increase in typical types of disfluencies (eg, whole-word and phrase repetitions, revisions, interjections, and pauses); the other is a speech disorder presenting stutterlike disfluencies (ie, part-word repetitions, prolongations, and blocks), that are, sometimes, but not very often, accompanied by tension, struggle, escape, and avoidance behaviors. In this chapter, I will be focused primarily on the second type, the disorder with stutterlike disfluencies.

Although much of the literature on ANS consists of single-case studies (eg, Bijleveld et al., 1994; Decker et al., 2018; Dinoto et al., 2018; Sudo et al., 2018; Tani & Wada, 2018), there have been several attempts by clinician-researchers to summarize their findings on multiple cases and thereby develop a clearer picture of the disorder. Canter (1971) wrote a seminal article that went beyond case studies to suggest a possible way of categorizing types of ANS. He proposed three subgroups. One is dysarthric stuttering—seen, for example, in individuals who have Parkinson disease or have a cerebellar lesion—in which stuttering appears to emerge from the same lack of neuromotor control as the primary dysarthric disorder. The second is apraxic stuttering, in which stuttering may arise from a basic problem in motor planning. Both silent blocks and repetitions occur as the speaker struggles to sequence the appropriate speech movements. The third subgroup is dysnomic stuttering, which sometimes accompanies aphasia. Stuttering symptoms occur as an individual

I-I recently-ly had a st-st-stroke
Neurogenic Stuttering

I've j....(silent block)...j ust ex-ex-ex-experienced an e....(silent block) ..... e motionally upsetting event
Psychogenic Stuttering

Why-why uh does everyone...you know..uh...tell me ... ask me ..uh...to...uh...to repeat....well.... to repeat what I've....what I've....uh....just said?
Cluttering

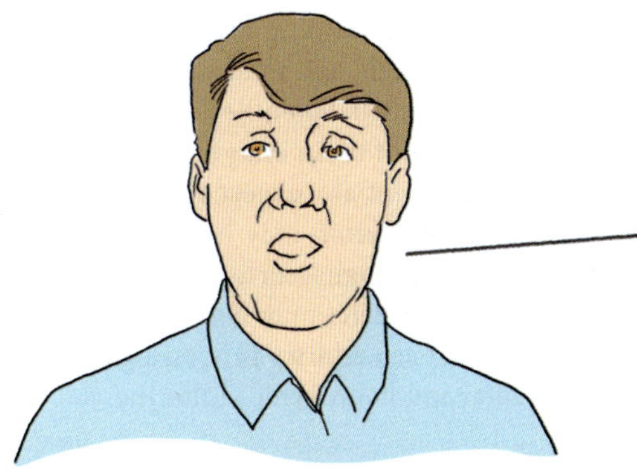

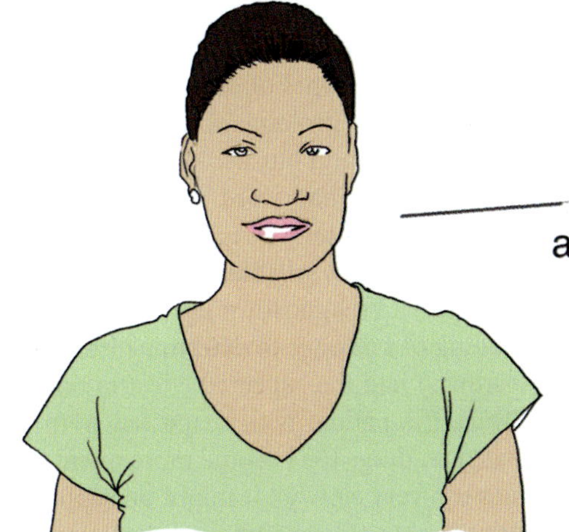

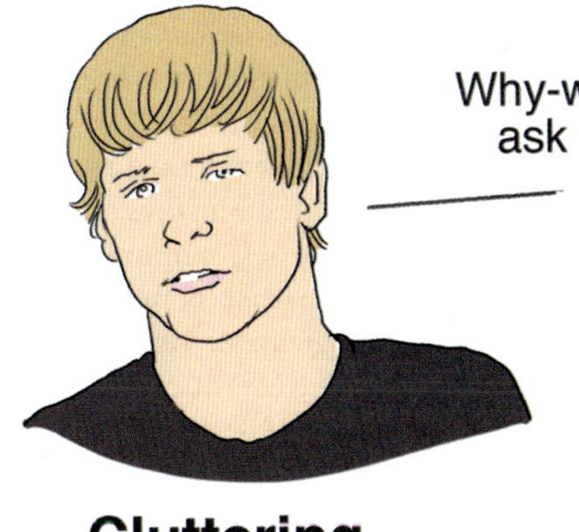

Figure 8.1 Overview of the chapter.

searches for the word they are having trouble retrieving. Canter speculated that there may be a parallel to this type of stuttering in children who have word-retrieval problems and who develop stuttering as a result of their emotional reactions to the word-retrieval difficulty. Canter seemed to believe that acquired stuttering (AS) following neurological disease or insult is closely related to, or is caused by, the neuropathologies underlying dysarthria, apraxia of speech, or difficulty remembering words (dysnomia). Later studies take a different view—that ANS may often be a separate disorder, related to deficits in the neural circuitry underlying developmental stuttering.

Rosenbek (1984) also summarized findings from multiple cases. He made the point that ANS should be distinguished from other disfluent behaviors that are associated with neurological problems, such as palilalia (word and phrase repetitions produced with increasing rate and decreasing loudness). It should also be distinguished from repetitions that some patients make as they try to correct their motor speech or linguistic errors. Observations of his own patients led Rosenbek to suggest that stuttering following nervous system damage is characterized primarily by involuntary repetitions of correct sounds and syllables, not those produced in error that occur at any place in a word (initial, medial, final). Clearly, his view differed from that of Canter (1971). But Rosenbek was distressed by the lack of detail in clinicians' descriptions of patients with this disorder and called for a moratorium on the use of the term "neurogenic stuttering" until more is known about it. Despite his call for a moratorium, case studies of "neurogenic stuttering" have continued to flow forth in the literature.

Several studies of ANS, long after Rosenbek's (1984) critical publication, have questioned the long-accepted hypothesized differences between persistent developmental stuttering (PDS) and ANS. Krishnan and Tiwari (2013) reviewed the literature on the effects of fluency-enhancing conditions (such as choral reading and singing) on ANS versus PDS and concluded that there is not a clear distinction between their responses. This casts doubt on the use of fluency-enhancing stimuli to definitively distinguish ANS from PDS. Another supposed difference between ANS and PDS is the loci within an utterance where stuttering was likely to occur, including such variables as word length and word class. Max et al. (2019) compared a group of ANS individuals with a group of PDS individuals and found few differences between the groups. This suggests the possibility that ANS may be very similar to PDS in many ways, perhaps even anatomically, as intimated below.

Sites of Anatomical Lesion in ANS-Stroke

Theys et al. (2013) studied a relatively large group of stroke patients with neurogenic stuttering, distinguishing between those with a substantial number of stutterlike disfluencies ($n = 20$) and those with more typical disfluencies ($n = 17$). Using statistical analysis of brain scans made soon after the strokes, they found differences between the two groups in both gray and white matter areas. Specifically, they identified nine affected areas of the left hemisphere corticobasal ganglia-cortex neural network that distinguished patients who had numerous stutterlike disfluencies from the control group. Affected areas included inferior frontal cortex, superior temporal cortex, intraparietal cortex, basal ganglia, superior longitudinal fasciculus, and internal capsule. This circuitry is thought to have important sensory and motor functions in typical speech production, including articulatory planning, auditory monitoring of speech, and internal timing (eg, Alm, 2004; Chang & Guenther, 2020; Guenther, 2007; Guenther et al., 2006). Citing a number of brain imaging studies of developmental stuttering, Theys et al. suggest that both developmental and neurogenic stuttering may have their origins in deficits in the corticobasal ganglia-cortical circuitry. They go on to suggest that these deficits may also give rise to concomitant problems (such as auditory processing difficulties) in both developmental and neurogenic stuttering.

Disfluency Characteristics of ANS-Stroke

In one of the most detailed studies of ANS-stroke, De Nil et al. (2017) reviewed 53 studies published between 1996 and 2013, which included 127 patients with ANS-stroke. They found that the most common types of disfluencies were repetitions. Many had repetitions, prolongations, and blocks, but none had *only* prolongations and blocks. Most of the repetitions were word-initial; some had word-medial repetitions, but few had word-final repetitions. Frequency of stuttering was highly variable: 0.5% to 20% syllables stuttered in conversation. Of special interest for diagnostic purposes, **adaptation** tasks (repeated reading of a passage to determine if stuttering decreases over readings) had the expected effect in only half of the patients. Thus, if a patient with suspected ANS does *not* adapt to repeated readings (or become more fluent when singing or talking very, very slowly), it might be support for an ANS diagnosis rather than developmental stuttering.

DeNil et al. (2017) also reported that 50% of their ANS-stroke patients showed some sort of secondary stuttering behaviors such as eye blinks, facial grimaces, and other signs of struggle. The same proportion of patients studied in Theys et al. (2008) showed secondary stuttering behaviors. This suggests to me that patients with secondary behaviors were experiencing frustration or even more serious emotional reactions to their speech difficulty. This possibility is borne out by findings both in the DeNil et al. and the Theys et al. studies that many patients did have negative emotional reactions to their stuttering, as indicated in questionnaires they completed, such as the Erickson S-24 Scale of Communication Attitudes.

The information on ANS-stroke is probably relevant to other types of ANS, although more studies are needed to detail the speech behaviors of ANS with etiologies other than stroke. The next section, on ANS resulting from military stress and injury, provides at least initial descriptions of this stuttering etiology.

STUTTERING AS A RESULT OF STRESS AND INJURIES WHILE IN THE MILITARY

This is a special section for those readers who are or will be working with active-duty military service members or veterans whose stuttering appeared as the result of stress or injuries while in combat. It combines information relevant to the preceding material on ANS and foreshadows the upcoming section on functional (formerly "psychogenic") stuttering.

Roth et al. (2011) summarized the behaviors and symptoms of sudden-onset stuttering appearing in military personnel who have been in combat and who have sustained **traumatic brain injury (TBI)** and/or PTSD. They found that these individuals' stuttering behaviors can include initial syllable or whole-word repetitions, prolongations, tension with facial grimaces, posturing of articulators or whispering before starting speech, hesitations, and/or blocking before initial sounds. These speech behaviors may be accompanied (and exacerbated) by attention problems, slow speed of processing, and word-retrieval problems. Other signs of TBI/PTSD may be present such as problems sleeping, nightmares, or difficulty concentrating.

In a publication going beyond TBI and PTSD as etiologies of stuttering, Norman et al. (2018) studied 235 veterans of the wars in Iraq and Afghanistan who had been diagnosed with sudden-onset stuttering following combat. These individuals were more likely to show AS if they also had been diagnosed with TBI *and* posttraumatic stress disorder (PTSD) (43.4%). However, some had AS with TBI only (5.6%), a sizeable number had AS with PTSD only (30.6%), and some had AS with neither TBI nor PTSD (20.4%). The authors were particularly interested in the sizeable proportion of those with AS who had been given medications that were known to affect fluency (66%) in contrast to the proportion given medications who were without AS (35%). The medications given to the veterans included those that may (1) increase dopamine levels (this may cause stuttering—see Chapter 2), (2) reduce Gamma-aminobutyric acid, a primary inhibitory neurotransmitter in the brain (this blocks neurotransmitters), and (3) those with anticholinergic properties (this blocks the important neurotransmitter acetylcholine). All of these effects have the potential to result in stuttering. Most of the drugs given were to reduce anxiety. This may be the only study that provides evidence—although circumstantial—that medications given to reduce the effects of TBI and PTSD may themselves contribute to AS. Their recommendations for evaluation and treatment are included in Chapter 16.

A comparison of the characteristics of ANS with the characteristics of developmental stuttering is given in Table 8.1.

FUNCTIONAL (PREVIOUSLY TERMED "PSYCHOGENIC") STUTTERING

It has been suggested that the formerly common label psychogenic stuttering be renamed as functional stuttering (FS) and considered to be part of a group of other functional speech disorders, such as dysphonia and prosodic disorders, that appear to be caused by psychological factors, including stress and emotional trauma (eg, Duffy, 2015; Duffy, 2019; Edwards et al., 2014). Clinicians who see patients with what have been called psychogenic disorders are now convinced that this term is demeaning to these patients and makes them feel as though they are in effect, being called "crazy" (Peacock, 2020) or told that it is "all in their heads." The result of this is that the very real suffering they experience may seem to be minimized or even ignored by the clinicians who work with them.

Nature

Functional stuttering, like neurogenic stuttering, is often, but not always, a late-onset disorder. Van Riper (1982a) describes FS (he does not use this new terminology) as it sometimes occurs in children, categorizing it as Track IV, in his chapter on the development of stuttering. In his view, there are four different developmental trajectories in children who stutter and this track is the rarest, actually seen more often in adult-onset stuttering. Some of its characteristics are a very consistent, stereotyped behavior that seems to be done almost on purpose, to manipulate parents or others. These stuttering behaviors are exaggerated and are more often blocks than repetitions. Van Riper says that he has seen children manifest this pattern and continue it into adulthood without change. A number of other authors have described its features when it is seen in adults, particularly after a prolonged period of stress or after a traumatic event (Baumgartner, 1999; Duffy, 2013, 2016; Mahr & Leith, 1992; Roth et al., 1989). It has sometimes been characterized as a conversion symptom (ie, a physical or behavioral expression of a psychological conflict) (Lazare, 1981).

When it occurs in adults, FS often resembles developmental stuttering in terms of core behaviors (ie, repetitions, prolongations, and blocks), but in some cases, secondary behaviors may be unusual and occur independently of attempts to produce words (Baumgartner, 1999). FS may occur alone or together with signs of neurological involvement. The latter phenomenon sometimes makes it difficult to be certain that psychological factors alone were responsible for the stuttering. Strict definitions of FS exclude cases in which childhood stuttering had been initially resolved but then reappeared under prolonged or sudden stress.

Duffy (2019) noted several aspects of FS that help to differentiate it from neurogenic AS. FS can be highly variable, with extended periods of fluency alternating with periods of severe stuttering. However, when FS is manifest, stuttering may occur on almost every word, rather than intermittently. Struggle behavior can be obvious, including facial grimacing and twisting of the head and neck. Duffy suggested that with FS, the client usually does not also have aphasia, dysarthria, or apraxia of speech. Another phenomenon that may characterize FS and distinguish it from neurogenic or developmental stuttering is the potential for rapid response to treatment. I will give more extensive details in Chapter 16 about management, but **trial therapy** should be attempted in the evaluation. The clinician should explain to the client

TABLE 8.1 Characteristics of Acquired Neurogenic Stuttering Compared With Characteristics of Developmental Stuttering

Characteristic	Neurogenic Stuttering	Developmental Stuttering
Etiology	Specific injuries or disease processes in neural pathways for speech	Deficits in the speech production areas of the brain
Onset	Often in adulthood, after brain injury or disease process	Usually in early childhood between ages 2 and 5 years
Development or change over time	Stuttering symptoms are quite stable following diagnosis	If it does not disappear in early childhood, stuttering usually gets gradually more severe during childhood and adolescence
Types of stuttering behavior	Most often repetitions, but sometimes also prolongations or blocks	Repetitions, prolongations, and blocks
Frequency of stuttering	Similar to frequency of developmental stuttering	From mild to severe. Almost always below 45% syllables stuttered
Secondary behaviors	Typically, very few secondary behaviors but, in some cases, stuttering is accompanied by tension, struggle, escape, and avoidance behaviors	Beyond early childhood, tension and struggle often observed, along with escape and avoidance behaviors
Emotional response to stuttering	Usually little emotional response to stuttering, except occasional frustration	Beyond early childhood, frequently notable emotional reactions such as struggle, embarrassment, and shame
Locus of stutters	Stutters occur at many locations in words and phrases Stutters may occur just as often on function as on content words	Stutters tend to occur on syllables at beginnings of words and at beginnings of phrases More stuttering on content words than function words
Response to fluency-inducing conditions such as swinging arm or choral reading	Sometimes no improvement with fluency-inducing conditions	Stuttering markedly reduced in fluency-inducing conditions
Adaptation effect: repeated reading of a passage	Adaptation often does not change the frequency or severity of stuttering	Adaptation frequently seen—stuttering frequency and severity decrease with repeated reading of passage

with confidence that the following steps will provide fluent speech:

1. Have the client say single words with a pattern expected to eliminate stuttering, such as speaking in a slow, prolonged fashion, using the clinician's model to guide the client.
2. Gradually expand the length of slow, prolonged utterances, providing enthusiastic approval for changes.
3. If needed and with their permission, touch the client's face (or put your hand near their face), as you guide them to try slow, **prolonged speech**.

As Duffy (2019) has described, this approach very often works with FS during the evaluation and can be built on in subsequent sessions. Sometimes, just the trial therapy during the evaluation is enough, but one or two follow-up treatment sessions are advised.

In light of some work on AS, the possibility of individuals with prolonged stress or sudden trauma being given medications known to affect fluency should be investigated in cases of FS. The study of veterans of the wars in Iran and Afghanistan who developed stuttering presented strong evidence that many were given anxiolytic drugs that had been known to bring on stuttering (Norman et al., 2018). Evaluations of patients with FS should include examination of the medications they were given to reduce stress or the effects of trauma. When FS patients are found to be on medications known to be associated with stuttering, perhaps other appropriate medications can be substituted for them and the results observed.

TABLE 8.2 Characteristics of Functional Stuttering Compared With Those of Developmental Stuttering

Characteristic	Functional Stuttering	Developmental Stuttering
Etiology	Response to emotional stress	Deficits in the speech production areas of the brain
Onset	Late childhood or adulthood, soon after emotional stress	Usually in early childhood between ages 2 and 5 years
Development or change over time	Stuttering symptoms are quite stable following diagnosis	If it does not disappear in early childhood, stuttering usually gets gradually more severe during childhood and adolescence
Types of stuttering behavior	May be similar to developmental stuttering. Alternatively, may consist of very rapid repetitions. Unusually steady eye contact is sometimes evident	Repetitions, prolongations, and blocks
Frequency of stuttering	Varies a lot. When it occurs, stuttering may be on every word, but long periods of fluency may alternate with stuttering	From mild to severe. Almost always below 45% syllables stuttered
Secondary behaviors	May consist of unusual or severe blocks	Beyond early childhood, tension and struggle often observed, along with escape and avoidance behaviors
Emotional response to stuttering	Usually, little emotional response to stuttering. In some cases, client may smile during stuttering	Beyond early childhood, frequently notable emotional reactions such as struggle, embarrassment, and shame
Locus of stutters	Stutters occur at many locations in words and phrases Stutters may occur just as often on function as on content words	Stutters tend to occur on syllables at beginnings of words and at beginnings of phrasesMore stuttering on content words than function words
Response to fluency-inducing conditions such as swinging arm or choral reading	Sometimes, no improvement with fluency-inducing conditions. In some cases, stuttering becomes more severe	Stuttering markedly reduced in fluency-inducing conditions
Adaptation effect: repeated reading of a passage	Adaptation often does not change the frequency or severity of stuttering	Adaptation frequently seen—stuttering frequency and severity decrease with repeated reading of passage

Table 8.2 lists the characteristics of FS compared with the characteristics of developmental stuttering.

MALINGERING

Although malingering (pretending to have a disorder to receive some benefit) is not technically psychogenic, I think it would be helpful for me to describe this manifestation of stuttering in close proximity to my discussion of neurogenic and psychogenic stuttering because all three of these will usually occur with adult onset, which makes it important to differentially diagnose them. Also, who knows? You may someday be asked to testify in court if malingered stuttering is suspected.

Case reports by Shirkey (1987) and Seery (2005) describe protocols that they used to attempt to distinguish between developmental, neurogenic, and psychogenic stuttering, versus malingering. In each case, the person in question had been accused of a crime during which they spoke fluently but claimed they were innocent because they stuttered so severely that they could not have been that individual. Their approaches to evaluation were similar and the suggestions given in Chapter 16 on evaluation and treatment combine their reports. An additional report by the neuropsychologists Binder et al. (2012) detailed three cases of possible

TABLE 8.3 Comparative Characteristics of Malingering Compared With Developmental Stuttering

Characteristic	Malingering	Developmental Stuttering
Etiology	Attempt to gain benefit by appearing to stutter. May fake more severe stuttering than is actually the case	Deficits in the speech production areas of the brain
Onset	Adulthood, sometimes after an accident to claim compensation or after a crime to claim innocence	Usually in early childhood between ages 2 and 5 years
Development or change over time	Stuttering usually remains similar to what it was like when diagnosis was made	If it does not disappear in early childhood, stuttering usually gets gradually more severe during childhood and adolescence
Types of stuttering behavior	May be similar to developmental stuttering, but also may have unusual symptoms	Repetitions, prolongations, and blocks
Frequency of stuttering	Sometimes, high frequency of stuttering	From mild to severe. Almost always below 45% syllables stuttered
Secondary behaviors	May appear like developmental, but also may be very rote, with the same type of stutter in each instance	Beyond early childhood, tension and struggle often observed, along with escape and avoidance behaviors
Emotional response to stuttering	Typically, little emotional response to stuttering. No shame or embarrassment	Beyond early childhood, frequently notable emotional reactions such as struggle, embarrassment, and shame
Locus of stutters	Stutters occur at many locations in words and phrases Stutters may occur just as often on function as on content words	Stutters tend to occur on syllables at beginnings of words and at beginnings of phrases More stuttering on content words than function words
Response to fluency-inducing conditions such as swinging arm or choral reading	Usually, no improvement with fluency-inducing conditions	Stuttering markedly reduced in fluency-inducing conditions
Adaptation effect: repeated reading of a passage	Adaptation often does not change the frequency or severity of stuttering	Adaptation frequently seen—stuttering frequency and severity decrease with repeated reading of passage

malingered, neurogenic, or psychogenic stuttering that were evaluated after mild brain injury resulted in lawsuits or workers' compensation claims. Seery's protocol was used, along with other neuropsychological assessment procedures, to evaluate the claims of these clients.

Characteristics of malingered stuttering—compared with developmental stuttering—are given in Table 8.3.

Not all cases of individuals deliberately stuttering are true malingering if malingering is strictly defined as knowingly pretending to have a disorder to receive a benefit. A report by Bolat and Yalcin (2017) described two adolescents evaluated separately in a Turkish psychiatric clinic who were found to be pretending to stutter, and each had comorbid depression. These individuals had begun to stutter not long before the referral, with prolongations and repetitions of the first syllable of words. They were suspected of manifesting "factitious disorder," defined as pretending to have a disorder, sometimes *without benefit or reward*. Each adolescent in this report was confronted empathetically when the clinicians felt they were ready to admit to deliberately stuttering and each admitted they were only pretending to stutter. Both adolescents gradually became fluent after several sessions of treatment for depression. Follow-ups indicated that neither individual relapsed when examined months after treatment. To declare that they pretended to stutter without anticipated benefit may miss the fact that their pretended stuttering could have been a cry for help, which, in both cases, was answered.

CLUTTERING

Nature

Many years ago, cluttering was described as "...a torrent of half-articulated words, following each other like peas running out of a spout" (Van Riper, 1954, p. 25). The essence of cluttering, as this quote suggests, is rapid speaking that is difficult to understand. Words may be collapsed, syllables may be omitted, or sounds may be slurred. Cluttering is often accompanied by disfluencies that differ from those typically heard in stuttering; instead of blocks, prolongations, and repetitions, individuals who clutter may produce fillers, incomplete phrases, word and phrase repetitions, revisions, and hesitations—all usually without tension. The speaking rate of a person who clutters is not continuously rapid, however, but gives the impression of coming in sudden impulsive bursts that are filled with misarticulations and disfluencies. In contrast to people who stutter, individuals who clutter become more fluent—as well as slower and more intelligible—when they make an effort to control their disorder. This rarely happens, unfortunately, because most people who clutter are often not aware they are "cluttering" unless someone brings it to their attention.

A widely accepted description of cluttering was termed "Lowest Common Denominator" definition of the disorder in that it reflected common symptoms agreed upon by experts and minimizes other variables sometimes seen in individuals who clutter (Scaler Scott, 2020; St. Louis & Schulte, 2011).

> *According to Scaler Scott, this definition primarily includes "perceived rapid and/or irregular speech rate and one or more of the following symptoms: 1. excessive 'normal' disfluencies; 2. excessive overcoarticulation (i.e., collapsing word syllables such as 'tephone' for 'telephone') or deletion of syllables; 3. abnormal speech rhythm, pausing or syllable stress."*

Using the above description of cluttering, Scaler Scott (2020) compared eight school-aged boys diagnosed with cluttering with matched controls speaking in three contexts: conversation, monologue, and expository discourse. The author found that only overcoarticulated words were seen in the boys with cluttering in *all* contexts, but more normal disfluencies were seen only in the monologue by the cluttering boys. Follow-up studies involving girls who clutter are obviously needed.

Several excellent publications on cluttering have described the disorder as manifesting the above speech characteristics but also as being characterized by, in many cases, language and learning problems (St. Louis, 1996; St. Louis et al., 2003, 2007; Ward & Scott, 2011). The language problems were first recognized by Weiss (1964), who described cluttering as a problem of "central language imbalance" that may reflect a disorganized formulation process. If he used the current parlance, Weiss would say it's a language disorder. The person who clutters seems to be unable to put his thoughts into coherent sentences and link them together in a logical way. Such language behavior is sometimes termed "**mazing**," a metaphor for repeated false starts, hesitations, and revisions that leave listeners puzzled about a speaker's verbal destination. The concomitant problems of people with cluttering may include distractibility, hyperactivity, learning difficulties, articulation problems, and auditory processing problems. Cluttering is sometimes accompanied by stuttering.

Cluttering, then, seems to be a disorder whose core signs or symptoms are rapid and irregular speech rate that is often unintelligible and replete with typical nonstuttering-like disfluencies. Language is often disorganized and the individual often lacks awareness of his difficulty and of listener cues signaling lack of understanding. Neuropsychological problems may or may not be present.

There is not a lot of information about the prevalence of cluttering. However, a report by Van Zaalen and Reichel (2017) suggested among 219 adolescents in Netherlands, 1.1% cluttered and among 85 adolescents in Germany 1.2% cluttered. A more extensive study by Sommer et al. (2021) examined a German health insurance company's sample of 585,551 patients of all ages who had speech or language disorders and found that cluttering had been diagnosed in 1,800 patients (3%). Of these, 71.5% were male and 28.5% female, giving a 2.5:1 ratio for males to females. This ratio is slightly smaller (less difference between the sexes) than the sex ratio for stuttering, which is 3:1 (younger children) to 5:1 (older children). The peak ages for diagnosing cluttering in the Sommer et al. sample was 4 to 6 years, but note that their overall sample comprised all ages. In an aside, the authors indicate that in the population of *stutterers* that were identified, 1.2% also cluttered.

Speculation about the neurophysiological basis of the disorder suggests abnormalities in the basal ganglia (Alm, 2004; Kent, 2000). More precise information was reported by Ward et al. (2015), who conducted a functional MRI study of 17 individuals with cluttering and 17 typically speaking individuals matched for age and sex. They found that the group with cluttering had the following characteristics compared with controls: greater activity in premotor cortex bilaterally and pre-supplementary motor area (SMA), greater activity in caudate nucleus and putamen of the basal ganglia, and reduced activity in lateral anterior cerebellum. No abnormal activity was seen

TABLE 8.4 Comparison of Cluttering With Developmental Stuttering

Characteristic	Cluttering	Developmental Stuttering
Etiology	Neurological anomalies appear to consist of overactivity in premotor cortex pre-SMA and basal ganglia. These suggest a problem in planning and execution of speech-motor control	Probably neurophysiological (anomalies in left hemisphere) exacerbated by temperament and environment
Typical onset	May be present in preschool years, but often not diagnosed until problem interferes with school performance	Usually ages 2-5, with some onsets in school years
Speech characteristics	Excess of normal disfluencies, lack of intelligibility, especially during rapid bursts of speech. May slur syllables and leave out others entirely	Single-syllable whole-word repetitions, part-word repetitions, prolongations, and blocks. Frequency is usually more than 3% syllables stuttered. Secondary behaviors (escape and avoidance) common. Pattern varies somewhat
Client's level of concern	Frequently unaware of problem, except when listeners tell them they can't understand what they said	Client typically shows frustration and embarrassment about stuttering, as well as fear of speaking
Other diagnostic information	Often accompanied by stuttering, as well as language, attention, auditory processing, writing, and reading problems, and other learning disabilities	Frequency and severity are often variable from day to day and situation to situation

SMA, supplementary motor area.

in higher language areas. They surmised that these findings suggest that the major problem in cluttering is difficulty with both planning and execution in speech-motor control.

Summary of Cluttering

Cluttering is a speech disorder characterized by the appearance of rapid speech rate that results from the speaker collapsing syllables and making them briefer and less intelligible. Cluttered speech often occurs in bursts with numerous nonstuttered disfluencies. Individuals who clutter are often unaware of their difficulty and are referred for therapy by family members or friends. The speaking style of cluttering sometimes gives the impression of accompanying language difficulty, but brain imaging suggests no abnormalities in higher language areas. However, there appear to be abnormalities in the corticobasal ganglia-cortex loops, including premotor planning of speech.

Table 8.4 provides a comparison of the characteristics of cluttering with the characteristics of stuttering.

SUMMARY

This chapter focuses on fluency disorders apart from developmental stuttering. ANS, FS, and malingering usually don't occur until adulthood or late teens. Cluttering may be diagnosed in older preschoolers and more mature individuals but is typically not treated until the school years when it may interfere with communication. Evaluation and treatment of these disorders is detailed in Chapter 18.

STUDY QUESTIONS

1. After reading about ANS, do you think Canter's three categories of this disorder are appropriate? Why or why not?
2. Name four characteristics of ANS that distinguish it from developmental stuttering.
3. If an adult-onset stuttering client appeared to have evidence of neurological dysfunction, would you rule out FS? Why or why not?
4. What are the two most salient problems in cluttering?
5. Why do individuals who clutter appear to have language problems?

SUGGESTED PROJECTS

1. Get together with two classmates and have one of you three practice one of these disorders: (1) ANS, (2) FS, and (3) malingered stuttering. Then make a class presentation in which you speak briefly and then have your other classmates ask questions so that they can try to identify who is (1), (2), and (3).
2. Get together with another classmate and practice imitating cluttering. Then you each work with a small group of the other students to teach them how to clutter. If the class is large, more than two students need to learn to clutter and then each teach a small group of students.

SUGGESTED READINGS

Acquired Neurogenic Stuttering

Duffy, J. (2019). *Motor speech disorders* (4th ed.). Elsevier, Mosby.

This book provides excellent coverage of the nature of neurogenic and FS as well as their management. Duffy is particularly good at describing etiologies of these disorders and the other conditions with which they may be associated. His sections on management reflect his extensive clinical experience.

Theys, C., De Nil, L. F., Thijs, V., Van Wieringen, A., & Sunaert, S. (2013). A crucial role for the cortico-striato-cortical loop in the pathogenesis of stroke-related neurogenic stuttering. *Human Brain Mapping, 34*(9), 2103-2112.

This study evaluated a large number of patients who had ANS after stroke. Most interesting was a comparison of those patients whose disfluencies were stutterlike and those patients whose disfluencies were similar to typical disfluencies rather than stuttering. Their anatomical findings provided evidence that the cortical-basal ganglia-cortex neural network may be an important etiological factor in both ANS and developmental stuttering.

Stuttering as a Result of Stress and Injuries While in the Military

Norman, R. S., Jaramillo, C. A., Eapen, B. C., Amuan, M. E., & Pugh, M. J. (2018). Acquired stuttering in veterans of the wars in Iraq and Afghanistan: The role of traumatic brain injury, post-traumatic stress disorder, and medications. *Military Medicine, 183*(11/12), e526.

In this publication, the authors studied veterans of the Afghanistan and Iraq wars who developed stuttering after their experiences in military combat. In their analysis, the factors of TBI, PTSD, and medications were considered. The study provides evidence for brain injury, emotional stress, and anxiolytic medications as causal factors in stuttering.

Malingering

Bolat, N., & Yalcin, O. (2017). Factitious disorder presenting with stuttering in two adolescents: The importance of psychoeducation. *Noro Psikiyatr Ars, 54*(1), 87–89.

This publication reports on two unusual cases of malingering that expand our understanding of how unconsciously motivated deliberate stuttering may be. The two adolescents in this study were suffering from depression and pretended to stutter, perhaps unwittingly, hoping to get help. They were treated in a psychiatric clinic, lessening their depression and relieving their stuttering.

Seery, C. (2005). Differential diagnosis of stuttering for forensic purposes. *American Journal of Speech-Language Pathology, 14*, 284–297.

Although this article appears to be a case study, the background and protocols for evaluation are thorough and insightful. It is a must read for anyone who will be evaluating a case of suspected malingering of stuttering.

Cluttering

Van Zaalen, Y., & Reichel, I.K. (2015). *Cluttering: Current views on its nature, diagnosis, and treatment*. iUniverse.

The authors are experienced clinicians and researchers in the area of cluttering. Although I have not read this book, the reviews suggest that it contains much detailed information about the nature of cluttering as well as its evaluation and treatment.

Ward, D. (2017). *Stuttering and cluttering: Frameworks for understanding and treatment* (2nd ed.). Taylor and Francis.

This is the second edition of a scholarly and clinical book on the nature and treatment of both cluttering and stuttering.

II

Assessment of Stuttering

9

Preliminaries to Assessment

Chapter Outline

Chapter Objectives

After studying this chapter, readers should be able to:

- Understand how to discern the client's needs and plan treatment around them
- Describe how to protect the client's right to privacy and how awareness of the client's right to privacy can facilitate trust
- Explain why multicultural awareness is important when working with clients from different cultural and linguistic backgrounds
- Describe how a clinician can demonstrate her expertise about stuttering in a way that will engender trust and motivation
- Explain why reliability in a measurement procedure is important and how reliability may be assessed
- Discuss the need for obtaining appropriate speech samples when assessing stuttering
- Explain the advantages and disadvantages of assessing frequency of stuttering and describe two different ways it can be assessed
- Explain why it can be useful to assess different types of stutters that a client may have
- Describe how duration of stutters may be important and how this can be assessed
- Discuss assessment of secondary stuttering behaviors
- Describe four tools to assess stuttering severity and explain when each might be used
- Explain why speech naturalness can be a useful measure related to fluency
- Explain why assessment of speaking rate may affect the client's communication

Key Terms

Confronting stuttering: Talking about stuttering, emulating it, and being aware of what's happening during the moment of stuttering. These activities can be engaged in by either the clinician or client, when appropriate. These activities and others are thought to reverse the tendency to run away from stuttering that may make stuttering worse

Duration: The length of time, usually in seconds, that a stutter lasts. From my perspective, the duration of a stutter includes the time when forward movement of speech is halted; therefore, the moment of the actual block, prolongation, or repetition is measured as well as the time taken by various starters, postponements, and other secondary behaviors

Empathy: The capacity to understand another's perspectives, beliefs, and emotions. Having this capacity to some degree allows the clinician to undertake appropriate treatment and to develop trust between themselves and the patient—a prerequisite for change

Evidence of reliability: Data suggesting that a procedure or measurement tool produces approximately the same result when used by different individuals or the same individual at different times

Feelings and attitudes: Feelings are the transient emotions experienced by the person who stutters, especially regarding the experience of stuttering and perceived listener responses. They can vary from one time to the next. Attitudes are more long-lasting; they reflect the stutterer's beliefs about how people perceive them and how they perceives themselves in regard to their stuttering

Health Insurance Portability and Accountability Act of 1996 (HIPAA): Legislation that created national standards to protect the privacy of patient information and still allow access to that information for the safety and proper treatment of patients

Interrater reliability: Comparison of results by different individuals using a measurement tool

Intrarater reliability: Comparison of results by an individual using a measurement tool at two or more different times

Multicultural perspective: An awareness by the clinician of differences in cultures regarding speech, language, and hearing issues as well as differences in styles of interaction between men and women, elders and younger individuals, family and strangers

Percentage of syllables stuttered: A common measure of frequency of stuttering obtained by counting the total number of syllables spoken and dividing it into the number of syllables that are stuttered

Severity: Generally, a measure of the impediment to communication caused by the stuttering. This may be an overall impression elicited from a parent or the person who stutters themselves or a compilation of stuttering frequency and duration as well as other behaviors that impede communication.

Speaking rate: How fast a person talks, usually with short pauses included. Articulation rate is with the pauses removed. Speaking rate is most often measured in syllables per minute

Speech naturalness: The extent to which speech sounds like that of a typical speaker who doesn't stutter. This measure is useful because sometimes treatment leaves the individual technically "fluent" but sounding overly slow or otherwise odd, for example, due to altered intonation patterns

Types of stutters: The different ways in which an individual may stutter. These include the categories of repetitions, prolongations, and blocks, or a combination of these

Assessment operates on many levels. On one level, there is information gathering, such as interviewing, measuring speech fluency, and administering tests and questionnaires. This requires careful planning, good observation, and thorough analysis. It begins with clients seeking help and often ends with a plan for treatment. On another level, assessment is a personal encounter. It involves getting to know another person and sometimes their family as well, trying to connect to them, and tuning your antennae to pick up the subtle signals they may be sending out about their needs and how you might help them. On this more subjective level, you are becoming aware of the entire person and family, not just the stuttering. Your clients are also getting to know you and sizing up your apparent ability to help them; thus, the first meeting may be the most critical. Although you will want to show an individual client or family that you know about stuttering and understand its treatment, you will want to spend most of your time listening to their concerns and demonstrating your desire to understand them. The two hats you will wear—that of the humanist and that of the scientist—will become a natural part of your wardrobe as you gain more experience.

THE CLIENT'S NEEDS

It is easy to say we must always consider a client's needs, but it can sometimes be difficult to put this into practice. One reason for this being a challenge is that we can develop expectations that function as blinders. Such expectations affect our perceptions of what our clients want, what caused or precipitated their stuttering, what their priorities are, and many other things. Although I know intellectually that every client is different, I have found a tendency in myself, perhaps increasing as I have become more experienced, to jump to conclusions. I sometimes think, "Ah, yes, I understand this kiddo. So much like that child I saw last month." You will find this true for yourself, too, as you work with more and more clients. We must try to listen carefully to what each client says and see each person with fresh eyes.

We must also be cautious about letting referral information, past experience, and biases cloud our ability to see all aspects of the person clearly. We must be wary of simple explanations and quick judgments about which factors are critical for a client. For instance, if parents tell us that they often ask their child to stop and start again when they stutter, that both parents work long hours outside the home, and that dinner is a noisy and confusing time, we should try not to assume that these pressures at home are a major problem for the child. They may or may not be, and other things may be more critical. We need to ask the parents more questions and explore how the child copes with their requests to stop and start over and we need to get more details about the parents' feelings and concerns, as well as how the child speaks in many different situations before we decide how to begin helping the child and their family.

Sometimes, individuals' or families' requests differ from what we think they need. An adult may say that they want "completely fluent speech," but we know this is not a likely outcome for a person who has been stuttering for 20 or 30 years. Or a family may want us to treat their 3-year-old child without their having to take part in therapy, although our preferred approach for a child this age involves parent participation. I have found it best not to feel I have to resolve such issues during a single session. I make no promises but do make a concerted effort to understand what clients and families want and why. My experience has been that after I work with a family or individual for several sessions, we build up enough trust to work together to make the changes that we mutually decide are appropriate. I vividly remember a young school-age child brought to me by his mother after years of previous therapy had failed. When we started therapy, this mom was troubled by the approach I took for therapy with her son. As I adjusted the therapy so that it was less objectionable to her but still moving in the right direction to help her son, I also spent a considerable amount of time listening to her concerns about her son's future and his difficulty in school because he was teased about his stuttering. Over the ensuing months, my graduate student and I also went to the child's classroom to help his peers understand the child's stuttering. Gradually, the mother began to trust us and became a stronger ally in the treatment of her son.

One way to begin to understand an adolescent or adult client's needs is to ask them directly about what they would like from therapy. Rebecca McCauley and I (Guitar & McCauley, 2010b) developed a questionnaire to gather this information from clients. It has been improved by Hilda Sønsterud and her colleagues at the National Support System for Special Education in Norway. The form is illustrated in Figure 9.1. It should be used as a basis for discussion of what the client's hopes and desires are in therapy, rather than for clinicians to gather the information to simply decide for themselves about what to focus on in treatment. With adolescents and adults, the course of therapy is a mutually determined process.

In this regard, I remember seeing a young man who came to our clinic from some distance away for intensive therapy. We didn't have the questionnaire for discussing aims at that time, but during the evaluation, he said he didn't want a kind of therapy he'd heard about in which the person who stutters is treated like a rat in a cage. In other words, he wanted no talk of conditioning, reinforcement, or shaping. In responding to his concerns, I talked about his stuttering with him in terms of what he felt about it, what he believed listeners thought, and why he did some of the things he did when he stuttered. Together, we designed an intensive treatment program for him that included some "fluency shaping" and "maintenance" but that made him feel respected as a human being and not treated like a laboratory animal. In the process, I also explored with him his concerns about therapy that was too "behavioral." I think that in this case, my careful and active listening to his feelings about his stuttering were key elements in his eventual success.

In trying to meet clients' needs, I consider the person as well as the problem. The clients, no matter what their age, will sense quickly whether a clinician is seeing them as individuals or only seeing their stuttering. Effective clinicians are genuinely interested and empathetic; they accept failures and reversals into older habits as well as victories and progress. The clinician's initial evaluation session with a school-age child, a teen, or an adult provides them with their first opportunity to show the client that they accept them just as they are, without rejection or fear of their stuttering. This atmosphere helps clients begin to accept themselves and their stuttering. A change takes place in the clients' feelings of frustration and fear when the clinician shows genuine curiosity and interest in what the clients do when they stutter and empathetically delve into clients' feelings about their stuttering. You can see this happening right before your eyes as you encourage your client to stutter, as you both try to collect a good sample to analyze together. As Van Riper (1982a) observes, "….in this collecting and analyzing process, [the person who stutters] soon discerns that the clinician does not reject or punish his stuttering but instead welcomes it as necessary for the analytic confrontation. Identification aids desensitization" (p. 246).

INSURANCE CONSIDERATIONS

An issue that might come up when you first talk with clients is whether their insurance will cover their stuttering evaluation and treatment sessions. You may help them get the best information about how to approach the problem by doing an internet search using the phrase "insurance coverage for

Personal aims for the stuttering treatment

I would like treatment to focus on:

[ ] the physical aspects of stuttering
[ ] the feelings associated with stuttering
[ ] both physical and emotional aspects

How important are the following goals for you?	(Rank from 1 = not important to 5 = very important)				
Very fluent speech	1	2	3	4	5
Feeling of control of stuttering	1	2	3	4	5
More positive feelings associated with stuttering	1	2	3	4	5
Ease of participation in most or all speaking situations	1	2	3	4	5
Other: ______________	1	2	3	4	5

In which situations would you particularly like to speak more easily?					
Talking on the telephone	1	2	3	4	5
Introducing myself to others	1	2	3	4	5
Conversations with family members	1	2	3	4	5
Conversations with friends	1	2	3	4	5
Conversations with strangers	1	2	3	4	5
Conversations with colleagues	1	2	3	4	5
Talking to supervisor	1	2	3	4	5
Other situations: ______________	1	2	3	4	5

Motivation and expectations	(Rank from 1 = not at all/nothing, to 5 = very much, completely)				
Answer the questions based on your personal views:					
How persistent are you at seeing tasks through, in general?	1	2	3	4	5
How motivated are you to work on your stuttering?	1	2	3	4	5
How much time can you set aside for independent training?	1	2	3	4	5
How much support or help do you expect during the treatment?	1	2	3	4	5
What is your anticipation of the success of the treatment?	1	2	3	4	5

Figure 9.1 Personal aims for stuttering treatment. This is a questionnaire filled out by a client that can provide a basis for understanding clients' hopes and desires for treatment. (Reprinted with permission from Guitar, B., & McCauley, R. J. (2010). *Treatment of stuttering: Established and emerging interventions*. Wolters Kluwer Health/Lippincott Williams & Wilkins; 2010.)

Describe, using your own words, your goals and wishes for the treatment (both short- and long-term)

____

____

____

____

What do you need in order to achieve these goals?

____

____

____

____

Other factors that are important for you in this collaboration, or that you wish to highlight:

____

____

____

____

Name of a close friend or relative who can take a role of "training partner":

____

Your name: ______________________ **E-mail:** ______________________

Phone: ______________ **Date for filling out this form:** ______________________

Figure 9.1 *(Continued)*

stuttering." Excellent advice is available online from the Stuttering Foundation (https://www.stutteringhelp.org › insurance-coverage), the American Speech-Language-Hearing Association (https://www.asha.org › private-plans › reimb_stutter_trtmnt), the National Stuttering Association (https://westutter.org/slp/insurance-advocacy-information/), and, almost certainly, other sites.

Among the tips that these sources provide are that (1) clients should read their insurance policy and talk with a representative on the phone to get details on coverage for stuttering evaluation and therapy; (2) clients should provide the insurance company with information about the neurological and genetic basis of stuttering (some websites provide examples) and that stuttering is not an educational issue or a developmental issue but a medical problem, with its onset in childhood; (3) some insurance companies require a referral from a physician for treatment; and (4) there are steps to follow to respond to a denial of coverage, via an appeal process.

CLIENTS' RIGHT TO PRIVACY

All clients should feel they can trust you to protect their privacy and confidentiality. Trust is a vital element of client-clinician relationships. It enables clients to feel that they can safely reveal personal information to you that will help you plan and carry out appropriate treatment. In many cases, the act of expressing feelings in an accepting, secure environment can be therapeutic. For example, a mother whose school-age child was not making progress told her clinician that she was feeling resentment and impatience about her child's stuttering. She talked at some length about this over several sessions, and the clinician listened empathetically. Once this mother had released these feelings, her child made remarkable progress. Although creating an accepting atmosphere for the child is the most important outcome in this scenario, this example illustrates that the parent had to trust the clinician to accept her feelings without judgment, as well as not to share this information inappropriately with other family members or the child, or, just as inappropriately, with others not involved in the child's care.

Federal and state legislation, such as the **Health Insurance Portability and Accountability Act of 1996 (HIPAA)**, helps clinicians follow best practices for protecting clients' privacy. Clinicians should familiarize themselves with these laws and guidelines and ensure that clients give their consent for video recording and observation and for sharing information about them. You can learn more from the website http://www.hhs.gov/ocr/privacy/. Here is a website that gives you resources about the client's right to privacy: https://compliancy-group.com/?s=Right+to+Privacy. When clients perceive that we are scrupulous in guarding their privacy and confidentiality, we gain a level of trust that enhances therapy. This confidentiality extends to children as well. The bond between children and clinicians will be enhanced if clinicians discuss what information children are willing to have shared with their parents and what not to share. This is especially relevant for school-age children, who should also be consulted about the extent to which they would be comfortable having their parents involved in treatment.

I should mention that there are a few rare circumstances in which confidentiality may be broken. These are the unusual situations when a client discloses plans to hurt self or others and instances of child abuse disclosed by the child.

MULTICULTURAL AND MULTILINGUAL CONSIDERATIONS

Let me begin this discussion of stuttering in other cultures and other languages by introducing you to a former client of mine, Sergio Torres. Sergio grew up in New York City in a Latino household. His parents were from Puerto Rico, and Sergio said that his father embraced an attitude of "men don't cry" and was intolerant of Sergio's stuttering. In fact, Sergio's father regularly hit him on the head with his fist when Sergio stuttered. Sergio thus learned to fear stuttering in the presence of his father, and soon his fear of stuttering generalized to most other listeners. When he came to us for treatment, we worked with him both individually and in a group. In both settings, Sergio talked at length about his father and his growing up in an environment where he was teased for his stuttering and treated badly by schoolmates. He dropped out of school at an early age and supported himself working as a musician—singing and playing a guitar. In his therapy, clinicians and group members were empathetic listeners, and, as time went by, Sergio seemed to forgive his father, explaining that his hitting him was a result of ignorance and frustration in a culture that valued manliness and regarded stuttering as weakness. Sergio gradually learned to stutter more easily and became an inspiration to students and other clients, helping out in the classroom and in our support group. Sergio is now employed as a group leader in a rehabilitation setting and also works as a musician with his own band. In a video clip, Sergio first demonstrates his old stuttering and then changes to a more fluent form of stuttering, as he talks about his recent visit with his parents and relatives. This is available on Lippincott Connect in a clip for Chapter 9 that is titled "Multicultural and Multilingual Considerations: Sergio."

When people who stutter grow up in cultures that differ from our own, our task of deeply understanding them requires an understanding of their culture as well as how that culture regards stuttering. This understanding is vital and increasingly important as the world changes. The 21st century appears to be a time of more and more migration among people from different cultures and countries. For example, my own state of Vermont has recently become home to immigrants and refugees from 23 different countries, and yet it ranks as only 48th of the 50 states in diversity. Other states like California, Texas, Hawaii, and New Jersey have much larger and more diverse populations. Many other countries besides the United States have hugely diverse populations. Some of the diversity comes from refugees who have resettled in countries other than their own. Many have experienced serious trauma that, in some cases, may have precipitated or worsened stuttering. Thus, it is vital for clinicians working with communication disorders to develop a **multicultural perspective** on assessment and therapy.

An underlying principle of this perspective is becoming sensitive to differences in communicative style in other cultures and learning how other cultures view speech and language disorders and, especially for our purpose here, stuttering. You can improve your multicultural sensitivity by reading about cultural issues related to communication disorders in general (Battle, 2012; Coleman, 2000; Taylor, 1994) and to stuttering in particular (Conrad, 1996; Cooper & Cooper, 1993; Culatta & Goldberg, 1995; Tellis & Tellis, 2003; Watson & Kayser, 1994). Insights into cultural differences can change the way treatment is organized. For example, Tellis and Tellis (2003) reported that families from India often feel that stuttering is a reflection on the entire family. This perception may strongly influence family members' responses to a child's stuttering. It would be important to listen to family members' perspectives on stuttering and, in the process, gently let them know about the latest scientific findings about stuttering, about high-achieving individuals who stutter, and about remediation for stuttering. This may lead to the family being more accepting of a family member's stuttering. Tellis and Tellis suggested that the clinician ask "open-ended culturally specific questions that address the beliefs, attitudes, and values of the client" (p. 23), in ascertaining how best to work with the client or family.

The University of Minnesota at Mankato has long supported The Stuttering Home Page—an information source about fluency disorders for the public and professionals. However, since 2022, what used to be the Stuttering Home Page is now called "Information about Stuttering" and is available at Mankato's Department of Communication Sciences and Disorders. On this department's website are a wide variety of interesting papers that are accessible from a web page titled "Stuttering in Other Countries/Cultures." It also contains resources in many other languages. In addition, on a different website from the University of Buffalo, there are a series of monographs about working with people with disabilities from other cultures, available from http://cirrie-sphhp.webapps.buffalo.edu/culture/monographs/.

In addition to these readings, a special issue of *Perspectives on Fluency and Fluency Disorders*[1] contains several articles on multicultural issues in stuttering. In that issue, Daniels (2008) and Ramos-Heinrichs (2008) suggested that, as we have said before, finding out about the client's and/or family's attitudes about stuttering is crucial. Many of the questionnaires to assess attitudes and feelings that will be presented later in this chapter can tap into perceptions of stuttering behaviors and how much stuttering impedes an individual's communication, but these questionnaires don't plumb the client's culture's views of stuttering. To help clinicians learn about Hispanic American clients' beliefs about stuttering, Tellis (2008) created a questionnaire that taps into many cultural values that may be different from those in the dominant culture. The Stuttering Inventory for Hispanic Americans may be adaptable for cultures other than Hispanic, with minor changes. Culturally sensitive questionnaires should be administered in a way that makes the client feel safe in responding honestly and fully. Right from the beginning, the clinician should begin to establish a relationship in which the client feels accepted for who they are and trusts that the clinician is open-minded and genuinely curious about the client's culture.

As you work with clients from other cultures, here are a few issues that may be important as you explore the client's stuttering and help them become more fluent:

1. *Eye contact.* Most treatments for stuttering encourage clients to improve their eye contact when speaking. A major reason for this is that many people who stutter look away from the listener when they stutter, increasing the perceived abnormality of the symptom and further disrupting communication, in cultures that value eye contact between speaker and listener. However, in some cultures, eye contact with a listener may be inappropriate, depending on the status of the listener and the context. Among some Native Americans, for example, not looking at the listener is a sign of respect. Thus, a person from such a culture who stutters may look away from listeners but not necessarily because of shame or embarrassment. The clinician should become aware of situations in which eye contact while speaking is appropriate and when it is not.
2. *Physical contact.* During an evaluation or in treatment, many clinicians may touch clients to help them identify points of tension or to signal them to make a change in their stuttering as it is happening. However, many individuals may regard being touched during an evaluation as an invasion of their personal space. It is important to ask permission before touching someone. You might say, for example, "I'd like you to try to catch a stutter and keep it going without finishing the word. Is it OK if I touch your arm to signal you to stay in the stutter?" In cultures where touching is considered especially intimate, you may want to refrain from touching the client at all.

   This cultural difference became clear to me when I gave a stuttering treatment workshop in Saudi Arabia. Typically, in the United States, I have a volunteer come to the front of the room where I would have them pretend to stutter with tightly pursed lips. Using my hand, I would coach them to loosen their lips and slowly finish the stuttered word. In Saudi Arabia, where it was customary for women to wear a *naqib* to cover their faces in the presence of a man, I volunteered my own face to demonstrate this slow loosening of a stutter.
3. *Nature of reinforcers.* Some approaches to treatment use praise as a reinforcer that is given immediately after a child has spoken fluently. Cultures differ in the amount and type of praise they give children. A clinician I know working in a suburb of Sydney, Australia, a city rich in new immigrants, adapts her treatment contingencies to fit many different cultures. One family from the Middle East was adamantly against giving verbal praise to their child. Instead, they developed a special signal that the father gave to his son to reinforce fluent speech.
4. *Family interactions.* Children with borderline stuttering are often helped when families change their interaction patterns. One such change that families can make is to speak more slowly and pause between conversational

[1]This is a publication by the Fluency and Fluency Disorders Special Interest Group 4 of the American Speech-Language-Hearing Association.

turns when speaking with the child (eg, Stephanson-Opsal & Bernstein Ratner, 1988, and our own treatment of borderline stuttering described in Chapter 11). However, in some cultures, particularly in urban areas of the eastern United States, families speak quickly and often overlap each other while talking. For these families, slowing speaking rate and not interrupting each other may seem so unnatural that they are unable to sustain this new interaction pattern. For their children, an operant conditioning approach in daily one-on-one conversations with a parent may be more appropriate.

5. *Intentional stuttering.* Sometimes I ask the person I am working with in therapy to stutter on purpose, thereby decreasing their tendency to avoid and be afraid of stuttering. But in some cultures, stuttering is regarded so negatively that stuttering on purpose would be unthinkable, at least in the early stages of treatment. It is important for you to become aware of how stuttering is viewed in different cultures and to understand when and where voluntary stuttering might be helpful and acceptable to your clients. Sometimes, the cultural stigma of stuttering makes it difficult for individuals and families to even discuss it.
6. *Conversational style.* Sensitive evaluations and treatment take into consideration not only the culture's view of stuttering but also the culture's style of verbal and nonverbal interaction. Taylor (1986) described a number of cultural differences in communication style that are relevant to evaluations of stuttering. For example, interruptions of one speaker by another may be expected among African Americans, so trying to change that style of interaction in a family may meet with resistance. In addition, people from African American and Native American cultures may feel uncomfortable responding to the personal questions often asked in an initial interview, and people from a Hispanic culture may feel it is rude to get down to business before greetings and pleasantries are exchanged.
7. *Modes of address.* The clinician should find out how to address individuals involved in the assessment and treatment, including proper pronunciation. Also, discuss how they'd like to address you. A family from India that I worked with preferred to address me as "Dr. Barry," rather than simply calling me by my first name, which I invite all of my clients to do, even children.

These cultural considerations are summarized in Table 9.1. It may not be possible for a clinician to know all relevant aspects of each new client's culture. But clinicians can be aware of the importance of culture in a person's response to stuttering, as well as the differences in communication styles between their own cultures and those of their clients. Such awareness can come from reading about a client's culture and discussing it with the client, if appropriate.

Similar sensitivity should be extended to different social groups within the clinician's own larger culture. Understanding and respecting class differences in such areas as vocabulary and values are crucial. Sometimes, working with people from other cultures increases our respect for group or class differences within our own culture. When I worked in Australia, I often attended grand rounds in a Sydney hospital. One particular case presentation involved a working-class Australian woman who had been mutilating herself with needles. Some of the staff and medical residents were highly unsympathetic to her condition, but a psychiatrist, renowned for his work in other cultures, shifted their attitudes. He spoke passionately about how we fail to understand people when we are blinded by our own values and beliefs and that trying to learn about this woman's circumstances would go a lot further in helping her than our simple condemnations of her self-mutilating behavior.

Some clients will not only be from a different culture or different social class but they will also speak a different language, one that the clinician neither speaks nor understands. In this case, an interpreter is necessary, if a referral to a clinician who speaks the client's language is not available. Because interpreters are often from the same culture as that of the client, they may help not only in translating but also in providing information about important aspects of the culture to aid the clinician's understanding. In the process of translating sensitive or complex messages, interpreters sometimes need to change the clinician's message to the client. When a message is rephrased by an interpreter to a more culturally appropriate style, therapeutic interaction will be facilitated. However, if an interpreter doesn't understand the intent of a question or statement, they may inadvertently convey wrong information. A friend of mine who was working with non-English–speaking Haitian immigrants in Boston understood just enough French to realize that the interpreter was providing wrong information to a client. She rectified the situation by giving the interpreter a brief overview of what she wanted to discuss with the Haitian family and why certain elements were vital, which immediately improved communication.

Special considerations apply when clients are both bicultural and bilingual. Bilingual clients, in fact, are not uncommon; there is evidence of an increased risk for stuttering in bilingual individuals (Howell & Van Borsel, 2011; Karniol, 1992; Mattes & Omark, 1991; Roberts & Shenker, 2007; Van Borsel et al., 2001). In these cases, one challenge for clinicians is to determine if the "stuttering" is really stuttering or is simply an increase in disfluency as a result of limited proficiency in a second language. Making this determination may be aided by careful observation of whether there are secondary symptoms (such as eye blinks or signs of increased tension) and cognitive or emotional responses to the suspected stuttering. For example, does the client feel ashamed of their disfluencies? Do they anticipate them? Are they consistently on the same words or same sounds? Another clue is that the

TABLE 9.1 Cultural and Interpersonal Considerations in Assessment and Treatment

Issue	Cultural or Interpersonal Concern	Possible Solution
Eye contact is sometimes a target of treatment.	In some cultures, direct eye contact may be disrespectful.	Discuss the role of eye contact in the client's culture and whether there are contexts in which a lack of eye contact may pose a problem.
Clinician may touch a client to make a point, such as helping client tune into excess tension.	For some individuals, physical contact is unwelcome.	Ask permission before touching a client.
Clinician may use or advocate reinforcers such as candy or praise.	Some families do not choose to use these reinforcers.	Explore with the family what would be acceptable reward for the child.
Clinician may try to change family interaction style.	Family may value their interaction style and not welcome changing it.	Clinician should talk with family about rationale for suggesting a particular change but should accept that family may prefer not to change interaction style.
Clinician may try to teach client to use voluntary stuttering.	Some clients or their families may find stuttering so unacceptable that they will terminate treatment rather than use voluntary stuttering.	Clinician should proceed slowly and tactfully in helping client learn and adopt voluntary stuttering. Some clients will never use it, which is reasonable but may require a work-around such as coaching the client in varying or playing with their stuttering.
Clinician may not use appropriate conversational style with client.	Some modes of conversational style (such as asking personal questions) may offend some clients.	Clinician should become aware of conversational style preferences when client is from a different culture than her own.
Clinician may not use appropriate mode of address.	Clients may be offended by insensitive mode of address (eg, use of first name) or mispronunciation of name.	Clinician should become sensitive to client's preferred way of being addressed and proper pronunciation of client and family names.

disfluencies may be stuttering if there is a history of stuttering in the client's family.

There is some debate in the literature about the extent to which stuttering occurs in one or more languages of a bilingual speaker. The excellent review of stuttering and bilingualism by Van Borsel et al. (2001) discusses the evidence on this issue, concluding that although stuttering may occur in one or both languages, it is more likely to occur in both. In some speakers, stuttering may be more severe in one language than the other, so that careful analysis of stuttering in both languages will enable clinicians to decide whether to apply treatment to both, if stuttering remains in the other language after the clinician treats stuttering in the language the client uses. Analysis of stuttering in a language not spoken by the clinician is likely to be more accurate if a native speaker of that language, such as a family member or friend of the client, can work with the clinician to identify stutters. In adults, the client themself will be able to help identify stuttering in the language unfamiliar to the clinician. This topic is more thoroughly discussed in the many good chapters on multilingual aspects of stuttering in Howell and Van Borsel (2011).

Even the evaluation of stuttering in bi- or multilingual speakers can be a problem. Bilingual speakers evaluated by SLPs—even those who speak the languages of the client—may be mistakenly identified as stuttering because of the criteria used to quantify stuttering. Measures that count sound, syllable, and word *repetitions* as stutters, such as Ambrose and Yairi's (1999) refined analysis of stuttering-like disfluencies (SLD) that included part-word repetitions single-syllable word repetitions as well as the Stuttering Severity Instrument (SSI) (Riley, 2009), may create false positives (identifying repetitions in a fluent speaker as stuttering) in bilingual or multilingual speakers because these speakers may produce more repetitive disfluencies as they try to choose the correct word or phrase in the language they are trying to use (Byrd et al., 2015; Byrd et al., 2020; Eggers et al., 2020).

In terms of treatment of bilingual speakers, Findlay and Shenker (2014) demonstrated that bilingual/bicultural children take essentially the same amount of time to achieve fluency as monolingual children. It should be kept in mind, however, that there are probably widely different bilingual/bicultural groups of individuals. Some have grown up in an environment where their dual language and culture are the norm and the individuals feel accepted. The children in the study by Findlay and Shenker may be an example of that—the children in this study were from Montreal where many grow up in bilingual homes. In other cases, children may be refugees who are learning a new language outside of their home and may not feel part of the new environment, thus being perhaps more anxious and insecure and more at risk for stuttering, and may take longer in treatment.

THE CLINICIAN'S EXPERTISE

During an assessment, clinicians have a chance to demonstrate not only their **empathy** with clients' feelings but also their mastery of evaluating and treating stuttering. Adolescents and adults who stutter and their family members often come into treatment with feelings of frustration, fear, and helplessness. They are looking for someone they can trust and someone who can successfully guide them through the often-difficult process of change. One of the first things that clinicians can do to establish trust and credibility is to show that they not only know about stuttering but are comfortable asking questions about it, duplicating it in their own speech and exploring it empathetically. This provides both clients and family members with an ally, someone who is unafraid of the problem that is so troubling to them.

This process can begin with clinicians asking older school-age children, adolescents, or adult clients how they feel about their stuttering and appropriately indicating that those feelings are very typical and acceptable for people who stutter at the beginning of treatment. Clinicians may also speak about other clients they have seen who have similar feelings, and describe those feelings. In some cases, clinicians may ask clients specific questions about avoidance behaviors and explain to clients why they use them and why they may be only temporarily helpful. This same credibility can be achieved in the evaluation of preschool children if clinicians ask these children's families about the **types of stutters** that the children have and demonstrate various possible types such as repetitions, prolongations, and blocks. With younger school-age children, once clinicians have gotten to know the children a little—this may take a few sessions of working together—clinicians can tell children they have worked with other kids who stutter but they need to learn about the client's particular ways of stuttering. Then clinicians can ask them if it's OK if they interrupt them when they stutter to have the client show them how they stutter. This requires tact, a sense of timing, and even humor to be sure children feel comfortable **confronting stuttering**, but it can convey the clinicians' expertise and thus engender trust.

The clinician's statements and questions also convey her expertise. For example, as they interview older children, the clinician can show that they know about stuttering by making empathetic comments, such as "Giving reports in front of class can sometimes be really hard." This allows children to respond without the pressure of a direct question but also lets children appreciate that their clinician is someone who has experience with stuttering. When talking with families, clinicians can intersperse questions with such statements as "When children keep repeating a sound that won't come out, their voices sometimes rise in pitch as the repetition continues." The family can then confirm whether or not they have noticed this in their child's speech and at the same time recognize that the clinician is knowledgeable about children's stuttering. Obviously, these kinds of comments and questions are easier for experienced clinicians, but even beginning clinicians can rely on their reading, their all-too-brief practicum experiences, and their intuition to convey their interest and understanding.

Because it has risks as well as rewards, the approach to interviewing clients and families that was just described should be used carefully. By making comments based on past experience, we may inhibit some individuals and families from telling us about experiences that differ from those offered by the clinician. It is an art to find the balance between showing understanding and leading the witness. As your clinical judgment develops, you will learn which clients will be helped by this approach and when.

I also caution that demonstrating your expertise should be secondary to acquiring an understanding of clients' needs. A clinician's first task is to discern what an individual or family would like from her. The second task is to understand the stuttering problem. In the normal course of accomplishing these two tasks—with attentive listening, empathetic comments, and perceptive questions—clinicians' expertise will emerge naturally.

ASSESSING STUTTERING BEHAVIOR

Assessment of stuttering behaviors is a broad topic that can be divided into several different areas for evaluation, such as frequency, type, **duration**, and **severity**. In some situations, it may also be important to assess **speech naturalness**, speech rate, and concomitant or associated behaviors. The importance of each of these is slightly different, depending on the age of the client and the type of treatment you expect to use. Before describing how to assess stuttering, I will clarify what behaviors are considered stuttering. As I mentioned in Chapter 7, a number of authors (eg, Brundage et al., 2021; Conture, 2001; Yairi & Ambrose, 1992a) have discussed which types of disfluencies distinguish stuttering from nonstuttering children. Borrowing from their discussions, the consensus appears to be that the following behaviors should be counted as stutters: part-word repetitions, monosyllabic whole-word repetitions, sound prolongations, and blockages of sound or airflow. The latter category (blockages of sound or airflow) can sometimes be quite subtle, occurring in the middle of a word (as in "cooo-kie" in which a glottal stop appears to break the word in half) or just before a word is produced. I also count successful avoidance behaviors as stutters if they are unequivocally an avoidance. Pay special attention to the section on assessing frequency for a further description of deciding on unequivocal avoidances because such avoidances can be a little tricky, particularly for beginning clinicians.

Reliability

Whenever a procedure is used to assess a behavior or a trait, it is important to know how reliable the procedure is. For example, if a police officer pulls you over for speeding because the radar gun has clocked you going 40 mph in a 25-mph zone, you might want to know how reliable the radar gun was. When this happened to me several years ago, I went to court to contest the ticket. Many factors, I figured, could affect the accuracy of the radar gun's measurement of my speed: the weather, the age of the gun, and whether it was adjusted properly. Fortunately, the judge asked the officer for **evidence of reliability** of the radar gun to prove that it could repeatedly, dependably, and consistently measure the speed of a car. Unfortunately for me, the officer was able to provide the judge with evidence of the radar gun's recent reliability check, and I shelled out $85 for the fine.

Reliability is an important characteristic of both formal and informal measures related to stuttering. In the case of formal measures—the most formal of which are usually referred to as tests or scales, the measure's developers have an ethical obligation to examine and report on the reliability and validity of the measure, where reliability refers to the ability of the measure to return consistent findings regardless of factors such as who is giving the test, the characteristics of the person (eg, age, gender, and other demographic characteristics). Validity refers to the extent to which the measure is actually measuring what it claims to measure. For the purposes of this book, we will trust that readers have had some training in evaluating the evidence presented for such measures of both reliability and validity (eg, interrater reliability; construct validity). Here, we will discuss only the concept of reliability as it relates to direct clinician-made measurements, usually from conversational, reading, or other samples of the client's speech. This phenomenon and its consequences are described by Cordes (1994) in her seminal article about reliability:

> *Perceptions, judgments, and observations are affected by variables attributed to the observers, to the instrumentation or coding procedures, to the situation or conditions of observation, to the subjects being observed, and to interactions among all of these. Consequently, researchers using direct observation methods are currently expected to provide evidence that their findings are not simply the results of situational influences or observer idiosyncrasies. They are expected, in other words, to provide evidence that their data are reliable (p. 264).*

The same caveat is true for clinical work. Despite our good intentions, observations of clients' stuttering before and after treatment may be influenced by our desires to see them improve. Measurements may also be affected by random fluctuations in stuttering apart from treatment effects—by the setting in which the client is assessed, by length and type of sample taken, and by the particular dimension of stuttering, such as frequency, severity, duration, or type that is chosen for assessment. It is important for clinicians to learn to assess stuttering reliably and to provide evidence that they have done so.

When human judgment is involved, as it usually is with measures of stuttering made from a speech sample, reliability is checked first by demonstrating that the observer makes the same judgment when observing the same behavior a second time from a video recording, usually several weeks later so that the second observation is fresh and not affected by memories of the earlier judgment. This is called ***intrarater reliability***. Reliability is also checked by comparing the original judgment with the judgment of a second observer who rates the sample independently of the first observer. This is called ***interrater reliability***.

Remeasurement of the data does not have to include the entire sample, although doing so would certainly be the most rigorous approach (eg, O'Brian et al., 2004). It is common for clinical researchers in stuttering to remeasure a randomly selected portion (10% to 25%) of samples taken (eg, Hakim & Bernstein Ratner, 2004; O'Brian et al., 2004). When reliability of judgments is to be established for measurements made on clients who increase their fluency over the course of a treatment regimen, samples should be randomly selected from various points in therapy, which will likely include both less fluent and more fluent samples. Cordes (1994) notes that 80% agreement is commonly thought of as the lower limit for the measurement of a sample to be considered sufficiently reliable.

Measures of reliability are usually selected according to what behavior is being measured. In situations where evaluation and treatment depend on accurate identification of stuttering moments (such as whether a word or syllable is stuttered or not), reliability can be measured using what is commonly called "point-by-point agreement." A videotaped sample (eg, 400 syllables of conversational speech) can be transcribed, and each stutter can be identified and marked on the transcript by an original judge or rater. Sometime later, the rater can return to the sample and again identify stutters by marking a fresh copy of the transcript. The two transcripts are then compared syllable by syllable, and the rater determines how many syllables are agreed upon as stuttered and how many are agreed upon as fluent. This total is termed "number of agreements." The number of disagreements (syllables that were determined to be stuttered in the first rating but not stuttered in the second rating or vice versa) is totaled and termed "number of disagreements." The reliability measure is then the number of agreements divided by the total number of agreements plus disagreements multiplied by 100. Figure 9.2 gives an example of a point-by-point assessment of reliability.

Point-by-point agreement is appropriate when it is important to judge whether stuttering is present or absent on each syllable. It is also a good tool for new clinicians to use to assess their ability to accurately judge stuttering. However, other procedures are called for when assessment requires quantification rather than presence or absence. An example would be measurement of the duration of stutters. An appropriate measure of reliability would be percent error, obtained by remeasuring at least 10% of the data. In this case, it is appropriate to begin by (1) obtaining the absolute differences between each first judgment and each second judgment (change all negative numbers to positive so they become absolute differences), (2) summing the absolute differences together, (3) dividing by the total number of comparisons to get the average, and finally (4) dividing the average absolute difference by the average of the first judgments. Table 9.2 gives an example.

A third method of assessing intra- and interrater reliability can be used when measuring the amount of stuttering in cases when point-by-point agreement is not critical. One example would be when you are assessing frequency of stuttering to use as a measure of week-by-week progress. This procedure involves calculating both the correlation between the first rating and a second rating (either the individual rater's first and second ratings or the rating of the first rater and the second rater) for multiple samples, as well as a test of significant differences between the means of the ratings, such as a paired sample *t* test. Correlations and *t* tests should be done for both intrarater and interrater reliability. Correlations should be above 80%. Also, *t* tests should show no significant difference between the samples to confirm the similarity of the two raters

Observer 1:

You wish to know all about my grandfather. Well, he is nearly ninety-three years old; yet he still thinks as swiftly as ever. He dresses himself in an old black frock coat, usually several buttons missing. A long beard clings to his chin, giving those who observe him a pronounced feeling of the utmost respect. When he speaks his voice is just a bit cracked and quivers a trifle. Twice each day he plays skillfully and with zest upon our small organ. Except in the winter when the snow or ice prevents, he slowly takes a short walk in the open air each day. We have often urged him to walk more and smoke less, but he always answers, "Banana oil!" Grandfather likes to be modern in his language.

Observer 2:

You wish to know all about my grandfather. Well, he is nearly ninety-three years old; yet he still thinks as swiftly as ever. He dresses himself in an old black frock coat, usually several buttons missing. A long beard clings to his chin, giving those who observe him a pronounced feeling of the utmost respect. When he speaks his voice is just a bit cracked and quivers a trifle. Twice each day he plays skillfully and with zest upon our small organ. Except in the winter when the snow or ice prevents, he slowly takes a short walk in the open air each day. We have often urged him to walk more and smoke less, but he always answers, "Banana oil!" Grandfather likes to be modern in his language.

There are approximately 14 syllables upon which the observers did not agree. There are approximately 156 syllables upon which they agreed were either stuttered or were fluent. The simple point-by-point agreement (rather than the kappa statistic) would be calculated as agreements (156) divided by agreements plus disagreements (170), or 92 percent.

Figure 9.2 An example showing how to calculate point-by-point agreement. An initial observer has marked the reading passage by underlining syllables on which stuttering was judged to occur. A second observer has marked the second passage. Point-by-point agreement can be calculated by comparing the total number of agreements with the agreements plus disagreements.

TABLE 9.2 An Example of Assessment of Reliability by Calculating Percent Error of Duration Measurements

	Time 1	Time 2	Absolute Difference
	3.5	3.0	0.5
	4.0	4.0	0.0
	0.5	0.7	0.2
	0.4	0.3	0.1
Mean	2.1		0.2

NOTE: Duration of stuttering (in seconds) measured by an observer at time 1 and remeasured at time 2. Percent error = 0.2/2.1 = 9.5%.

or the single rater's two sets of measures. Table 9.3 depicts correlations and *t* tests for 12 pairs of measurements by two observers. A similar table could depict correlations for 12 pairs of measurements made two times by a single observer.

As a final comment about reliability, I would suggest that although different measures of reliability can be used for different purposes, beginning clinicians should establish their reliability using a point-by-point agreement procedure, both during their initial training and to recheck their reliability periodically as they gain more experience. This may help them develop relatively consistent and agreed-upon definitions of what a stutter is and is not.

A summary of reliability measures is given in Table 9.4. Although I believe that examining stuttering with methods described are important, there has historically been dissatisfaction that levels of agreement are not as high as they should be. This has contributed to recent arguments that such external definitions of stuttering should be supplanted by those that capture the experiences of those who stutter or parents of children who stutter instead (O'Brian et al., 2020; Onslow et al., 2018).

Speech Sample

Because of the variability of stuttering, a single speech sample will often not be sufficient to provide a clear understanding of the phenomenon. The size and number of samples depend on the purpose of the assessment. In a first assessment, it would be wise to have at least two samples: one recorded in the clinic and one recorded in the client's typical environment. Before I see a preschool child for an evaluation, I ask the parents to send in a video of the child in conversation at home. It may be convenient for one family member to engage the child in conversation while another records the child's speech via cell phone video. When video recording is not possible, audiotaping is still useful. With a school-age child, a sample collected in the school would be important. Practically speaking, of course, a sample could be most easily recorded in the therapy room at school. A second sample from home would also be very helpful, but it is not always obtainable. When evaluating an adolescent or adult, I recommend that a sample be taken in the treatment room and a sample be taken from work or home. It is often convenient for adolescents or adults to audio record telephone conversations on their cell phones. I ensure that the client knows how to record only their own voice and not that of the listener, unless they have gotten permission, which is usually easy to do.

An important consideration in obtaining samples is that, as we have said before, stuttering varies. It differs in frequency and severity from month to month, week to week, day to day, and situation to situation within the same day. Such variability affects both children and adults but is most apparent with young children who stutter. Sometimes, a preschool child is stuttering severely, and then 3 weeks later

TABLE 9.3 Assessing Interrater Reliability by Calculating Correlations and *t* Tests

Observer 1	Observer 2
12	11
10	9
15	10
4	6
8	5
2	2
14	12
7	9
3	4
6	6
5	3
1	3

NOTE: (Online help for making these calculations can be found at https://www.meta-calculator.com/statistics-calculator.php.) Measures are percentages of syllables stuttered measured by observer 1 and observer 2. Pearson $r = 0.90$; paired $t = 0.92$; df = 11; $P = .38$. These calculations suggest that substantial interrater reliability exists because the ratings are highly correlated, and no significant difference is observed between the means.

TABLE 9.4 Measures of Reliability

Type of Reliability	Brief Description	When to Use
Point by point	Transcript of speech sample made; original judge and another observer mark whether a syllable is stuttered. Reliability is assessed by counting the number of syllables that were agreed upon by both observers as stuttered and dividing that number by the total number of syllables in the sample (agreements plus disagreements).	Use when it is important to ascertain whether stuttering has occurred on each individual syllable, as in an experiment that consequates individual stutters. Also useful for new clinicians or clinicians who feel they might have gotten rusty to assess their accuracy at judging stuttering.
Percentage error	Experimenter assesses the difference between the first observer's judgment and the second observation on at least 10% of the sample. Expressed as absolute difference (all numbers made positive). Then these differences are averaged (average absolute difference), and this figure is divided by the average of the first observer's measures.	Use when assessing reliability of a continuous variable like duration of stutters.
Correlation and *t* test	Pearson product-moment correlation used to see the extent to which initial observations of behavior are related to second observations. In addition, the *t* test is used to assess whether the mean of the second observations is significantly different from the mean of the initial observations.	Use when an overall measure of variable (eg, percent syllables stuttered) is used and when it is not important to show agreement on individual syllables.

during the evaluation, the child is entirely fluent. Therefore, it is important to discuss with the client or family whether the sample you have obtained is representative of the stuttering and if not, whether more samples should be taken, maybe in other situations and at other times.

After the initial sample, when further assessment is done to measure progress in therapy, it is crucial to ensure that any reduction in stuttering is not confined to the therapy room. Thus, ongoing assessments should include measures taken in the client's real world, outside the treatment situation.

For any sample in which severity of stuttering is to be rated, or any sample for research purposes, video recording is essential. Many subtleties of stuttering would be missed if only an audiotape were used; thus, video recording allows better assessment of observer reliability than audio recording. Sometimes online (while the client is talking) scoring can be done without either video or audio recording. For example, online scoring is appropriate when the clinician samples severity of stuttering at the beginning of every session for clinical rather than research purposes.

The length of the sample must be long enough for it to be representative of the speaker's typical stuttering. A sample that's too short won't include enough stuttering to see the range of severity and types of stuttering, and a sample that's too long would take time away from other assessment activities and would be tedious to score. For a client who reads, I usually like to take a sample of 300 to 400 syllables of conversational speech (where there is likely to be more variability) and 200 syllables of a reading passage (where there is likely to be less variability). Using a typical figure of 1.5 syllables per word (Williams et al., 1978), these samples would be equivalent to approximately 200 to 265 words and 130 words, respectively.

When obtaining a reading sample, it is important to ensure that the reading passage is at or below the client's reading level. A client's stuttering is likely to worsen when reading a passage that is difficult, giving a false impression of typical stuttering during reading. Reading passages in the Stuttering Severity Instrument-4 (SSI-4) (Riley, 2009) are designed for third, fifth, and seventh grade levels, as well as for an adult reading level. If you want to write your own passage and check what grade level it works for, use Google to search for tools that assess the grade level of a reading passage. When obtaining a speaking sample, it would be wise to select topics that are not emotional unless it is desirable to elicit a maximal amount of stuttering, as you might do with clients who say they stutter but are not demonstrating any during the evaluation. I usually ask children and adolescents to talk about their favorite weekend or after-school activities, sports, hobbies, or pets. With adults, I ask them to talk about their favorite activities, sports, hobbies, work, or school.

When making a formal assessment or when first learning to assess stuttering, it is very useful to make a written transcript of the spoken material, including all words and even those nonmeaningful utterances, such as "uh." However, you should not indicate on the original transcript which syllables are stuttered, so that you, at a later date, or another rater, on a separate occasion, can re-score a copy of the transcript to check for reliability without being influenced by the notations indicating which syllables were stuttered. Using your recording of the spoken material and an unmarked transcript, you can note where the stutters are, with details of how the individual stuttered. Write out each element of a repeated sound or syllable, the sounds that were prolonged, and the sounds on which blocks occurred. Describe escape and avoidance behaviors accompanying each moment of stuttering. Mark those moments of stuttering that seem longer than most. For a complete assessment, you will want to return to the longer stutters and time how long each one was to determine the average length of the three longest stutters. You will also want to count the words or syllables spoken, although it is often most accurate to count syllables from recordings because some speakers omit syllables in longer words. This can be done with software, such as the Computerized Scoring of Stuttering Severity (CSSS) software that accompanies the SSI-4 (Riley & Bakker, 2009).

Assessing Frequency

As I'll mention again, the next four attributes of stuttering—frequency, types of stuttering, duration of stutters, and secondary behaviors—all contribute to the overall severity of stuttering. The first of these attributes, frequency of stuttering, is a simple, acceptably reliable measure (Andrews & Ingham, 1971) that can be used for a variety of purposes. It is important in an initial assessment to help distinguish a normally disfluent child from a child with borderline stuttering. It is a vital part of composite ratings, such as the SSI-4 (Riley & Bakker, 2009), that provide a multidimensional view of stuttering. Frequency of stuttering is also useful as a "snapshot" measure of progress during treatment. In the first place, it is highly correlated with severity (Young, 1961). If used alone, however, frequency has the limitation that it doesn't reflect the duration of stutters or physical tension associated with stuttering. Decreases in these variables are often signs of improvement.

Frequency of stuttering is most commonly reported as **percentage of syllables stuttered**, although some use percentage of words stuttered or number of stutters per 100 words. I prefer to use percentage of syllables stuttered, following the logic of Minifie and Cooker (1964), because it can capture instances when a speaker stutters on more than one syllable of a multisyllable word. Moreover, when counting syllables and stutters online, syllables can be counted more easily than words by counting the syllable beats as the client talks.

Here are some guidelines for counting stutters:

- Each syllable can be counted only once. Thus, multiple repetitions, like "Where is my ba-ba-ba-basketball?" are counted as only one stutter.
- The total number of syllables are only those that would have been produced if the speaker had been fluent. Thus, "Where is my ba-ba-ba-basketball?" is totaled as six syllables. Each syllable that would have been produced if the speaker had been fluent is counted as either stuttered or fluent.
- Don't count interjections that you judge to be part of the stutter as syllables or as separate stutters. In the sentence "Where is my...my...uh...well ba-ba-ba-ba-basketball?" there would be a total of six syllables and one stutter.
- If a speaker seems to be using a particular word or sound as an avoidance behavior, I will count the next syllable as stuttered even if no overt stuttering occurred. For example, a speaker may say "Where is my...uh...uh...uh basketball?" In this case, the speaker seems to be using "uh" to postpone starting the word "basketball" on which they anticipate stuttering. And they keeps saying "uh" until they feel they can say "basketball" fluently and then rushes to say "basketball" after saying the last "uh." When I am fairly certain that a speaker has used a sound or word as a (successful) avoidance behavior like this, I count the next syllable as stuttered. Note that I do not count each utterance of the sound or word that is used as an avoidance; instead, I count the next syllable in the utterance as stuttered. When I am in doubt about whether an avoidance has occurred in anticipation of a stutter, I count it as fluent.
- When assessing the speech of someone who can read, I find it helpful to compare the frequency of stuttering in reading to that in speaking. If stuttering is markedly greater in the reading task, this may be because the speaker is avoiding words that they expect to stutter on in the speaking task, but they can't do this when reading. In most cases, I talk about my hypothesis with the client to see if they agree.

A variety of instruments designed for counting stutters are available. A free online counter that you can use by pressing keyboard keys to count stuttered syllables and fluent syllables and calculates percent syllables stuttered and speech rate is available at http://www.natke-verlag.de/silbenzaehler/index_en.html/.[2]

Assessing Types of Stutters

When assessing the speech of preschool children, it is often useful to count the total number of disfluencies, both those that are considered types of stutters and those considered typical disfluencies. As you will remember from Chapter 7, disfluencies that are not considered stutter-like include multisyllable word repetitions, phrase repetitions, interjections, and revisions in which a phrase is incomplete. Stutter-like disfluencies are part-word repetitions, single-syllable word repetitions, prolongations, broken words, or hard attacks. Remember that stutters can sometimes be complex and include multisyllable word repetitions that turn into blocks. When both stutter-like and not SLDs are counted, you can use the proportion of total disfluencies that are stutter-like to help you decide whether a child is stuttering or normally disfluent. If a child's speech has more than 3% SLDs, this can be considered stuttering (Bloodstein et al., 2021).

[2]I thank Julie Pera for recommending this online tool.

Caution must be used with any single measure used alone. Conture (2001) noted that a child he had recently evaluated was, in his opinion, stuttering severely even though the child's proportion of SLDs was only 34% of the total disfluencies. Clearly, Conture had relied on several other measures of stuttering in concluding that the child was a severe stutterer.

Another measure involving the type of disfluencies that a child produces is the number of SLDs per 100 words. In summarizing his findings on disfluencies in stuttering and nonstuttering children, Yairi (1997b) noted that children who stutter have more than three SLDs per 100 words, whereas normally disfluent children have fewer. In this same chapter, Yairi reviewed research about the gradual decline in some types of disfluencies as children grow older. Perhaps the most important finding is that part-word repetitions show a steady decline in normally disfluent children by age 4 and thereafter. Thus, if a child shows a plateau or increase in part-word repetitions in later preschool years, the child may be showing stuttering rather than normal disfluency.

Assessing Duration

In a thorough assessment, measures of the duration of a clients' longest stutters can give us important information about how much their stuttering may be interfering with their communication. Van Riper (1982a, p. 208) noted in his inimitable prose that "The duration of the individual moments of stuttering is one of the basic components of any adequate index of severity. Like tapeworms, longer stutterings are worse than shorter ones."

A common practice is to average the duration of the three longest stutters in a speech sample (Myers, 1978; Preus, 1981; Riley, 2009; Van Riper, 1982a). One way to do it is to use a digital stopwatch while watching a video recording of the client speaking. With a little practice, you can turn the stopwatch on at the moment the stutter begins and turn it off when it ends and measure the moment of stuttering to the nearest half-second. Any delays in starting the stopwatch at the beginning of stutters are compensated for by similar delays when you stop it at the end. I recommend using duration as part of a more complete assessment of severity, such as the SSI-4 (Riley, 2009), when making an initial assessment of a client's progress and when you want to give a detailed description of a client's stuttering in a report. The software accompanying the SSI-4 provides a means to automatically calculate the mean of the three longest stutters by holding down the mouse key for the duration of each stutter as it is being counted.

Many applications are available on the internet to assess stuttering using your cell phone or other connected devices. But buyers beware: read the reviews of various apps using a search engine, as well as Google Scholar before purchasing. In a later section of this chapter, I'll discuss a free website for assessing stuttering that is part of FluencyBank (http://fluency.talkbank.org).

Assessing Secondary Behaviors

To the person who stutters, stuttering feels like being in the grip of an unseen hand damming up the flow of your speech. Or as one of my young clients said, it is like having "a rock jammed in your throat." You struggle to keep going, squeezing your lips, blinking your eyes, and twisting your shoulders in the process. Such behaviors add to the abnormality of stuttering and reflect an important aspect of its development. Reducing or eliminating these behaviors may be a vital goal for therapy.

Secondary behaviors are also referred to as "concomitant," "associated," or "accessory" behaviors. They are most often escape behaviors that are used to break out of a stutter once it has started, but secondary behaviors may also be avoidance behaviors that are used in an attempt to keep from stuttering (see Chapters 1, 5, and 7 for further discussion of these terms). These behaviors may be physical movements (eg, eye blink), extra sounds (eg, "uh," tongue clicks or other sounds not typically part of the speaker's language), or changes in the way speech is produced (eg, pitch rise). They are often signs that stuttering has progressed to a more advanced stage (eg, escape behaviors distinguish beginning from borderline stuttering), but they may in a few cases appear very close to the onset of stuttering.

Conture (2001) briefly reviewed the limited research on secondary behaviors and noted that most are just more frequent and more exaggerated versions of behaviors seen in normal speakers. Zebrowski and Kelly (2002) suggested that the most common behaviors involve the eyes, particularly blinking, squeezing, lateral and vertical eye movements, and loss of eye contact. These authors and Shapiro (2011) also pointed out that the presence of secondary behaviors can be an important diagnostic sign that may distinguish normally disfluent children from those who are beginning to stutter. A perceptive and detailed description of secondary behaviors is given in the 7th edition of *A Handbook on Stuttering* (Bloodstein et al., 2021). The authors noted that secondary behaviors may begin as conscious actions to limit the frustrating and embarrassing experiences of stuttering (such as a head nod to end a stutter and finish a word). Soon, however, secondary behaviors may become automatic and are incorporated into the individual's byzantine stuttering pattern. The description in Bloodstein et al. (2021) includes the following suggestion for seeing examples of secondary behaviors:

> *It is challenging to illustrate the varied nature of secondary behaviors using the written word. Readers can explore some of these features by watching John Gomez's 2017 award-winning film, When I Stutter, or by viewing interviews with adults and children who stutter at the Voices Project at FluencyBank (https://fluency.talkbank.org/teaching/)—often used in teaching future clinicians about the ABCs of stuttering. (p. 11).*

Some clinicians enumerate these secondary behaviors as part of their assessment, particularly when they will use a treatment approach that helps clients gradually modify their stuttering behaviors. Standardized measures, such as the SSI-4 (Riley, 2009), include ratings of these behaviors as part of an overall severity assessment. We will consider this assessment next.

Assessing Severity

Measures of severity may be the most clinically relevant assessment of overt stuttering behaviors. Severity reflects an overall impression that listeners may have when they listen to an individual who stutters. Thus, it is an important measure for assessing the outcome of treatment. It is also an important yardstick of progress during therapy because many treatments gradually reduce the severity of stuttering rather than eliminate it.

The most commonly used measure of severity is the SSI, which was first published in the Journal of Speech and Hearing Disorders (Riley, 1972). A recent version, the SSI-4, is illustrated in Figure 9.3. It is available with forms and a manual from ProEd (to find it on the internet, Google "SSI-4"). In my mind, it is the best measure of severity available, but like its predecessors, the SSI-4 has some drawbacks. The sample of children and adults on which it was normed is not well described, its reliability evidence is not particularly strong, and its validity has not been convincingly demonstrated (McCauley, 1996). Despite these limitations, the SSI is easy to use and captures the severity of overt stuttering behaviors as a composite of three important dimensions: frequency, duration, and physical concomitants. In addition, because there are no perfect measures, the goal in choosing a measure is to choose the one that seems to have the best evidence of those available. The SSI-4 is one of the few measures of stuttering for a broad age range that has standardized procedures for gathering and scoring speech samples and is the only measure that includes the three dimensions just cited.

The total overall score for the SSI is the sum of the three subcomponents measured.

1. *Frequency* is assessed as the percentages of syllables stuttered on a speaking task and a reading task. For nonreaders, the speaking task is given twice the weight in the scoring procedures. Riley originally used percentage of words stuttered but currently uses the percentage of syllables stuttered, which is converted to a "task score" on the form for the Frequency Score.
2. *Duration* is assessed by measuring the length of the three longest stutters, calculating their mean duration, and finding the appropriate "scale score" on the form for the Duration Score.
3. *Physical concomitants* are assessed by adding the scale values of each subcomponent (ie, distracting sounds, facial grimaces, head movements, and movements of the extremities) and deriving a Physical Concomitants Score.

The values for frequency, duration, and physical concomitants are then added together to provide a total overall score. Percentiles and severity ratings (eg, mild, moderate, and severe) based on total overall scores are given on the form. Clinicians should carefully read Riley's directions in the manual of the SSI-4 before administering this measure.

Clients should be video recorded, and the SSI-4 should be calculated from the recording because duration measures and assessment of physical concomitants cannot be done easily online and the frequency count will be more accurate if equivocal stutters are replayed repeatedly until a decision can be reached. The CSSS software accompanying the SSI-4 allows computer-aided calculation of stuttering frequency and duration for the overall severity score.

Another measure of severity, the Test of Childhood Stuttering (TOCS) (Gillam et al., 2009), can be used with children ages 4 to 12. It can be obtained from PRO-ED (http://www.proedinc.com). The TOCS consists of several subparts:

1. A Speech Fluency Measure, which is based on scores obtained during four tasks: (1) rapid picture naming, (2) modeled sentences, (3) structured conversation, and (4) narration.
2. An Observational Rating Scale to be used by the clinician, teacher, or caregiver. This component provides information from the observer about (1) how often the child has various stuttering behaviors and (2) how often the child has negative responses to his own stuttering, such as showing such secondary reactions as concomitant physical behaviors and avoidance of speaking.
3. A Supplemental Clinical Assessment, which allows a more detailed analysis of the stuttering frequency, duration, types, and associated behaviors, as well as speech naturalness. This measure can help to decide if the child stutters and how severe the child is. It can also be used for assessment before and after treatment.

In a review of TOCS in *Mental Measurements Yearbook*, Shapely and Guyette (2010) commented favorably on the instrument's validity and reliability but suggested caution in interpreting the test's index scores and percentile ranks because of limited sample sizes used in standardization and in validity and reliability assessment. Tumanova et al. (2018) used the TOCS observational rating scales from this measure to compare ratings of parents who showed concern about their child's stuttering (n = 91) with parents who showed little or no concern (n = 92). Results indicated that the more concerned parents had higher rating scores than the less concerned parents, suggesting their concerns were justified. The higher scores of the concerned parents were validated by assessments of stuttering during clinician-child conversational interactions. Interestingly, the children with more stuttering showed shorter mean lengths of utterance in the interaction, independent of their language ability, suggesting they may have been limiting their conversation to avoid stuttering. Thus, for children with concerned parents and with higher parent rating scores, assessment of stuttering should take place in several different settings, especially those in which the child feels more comfortable talking.

A fourth measure of severity in children is the Child Stuttering Severity Chart (also referred to as SR scale), which was developed by Onslow et al. (1990) as part of a direct treatment program for preschool children. This is simply a 0-to-10 scale that parents use to make daily ratings of their child's stuttering (0 = no stuttering, 1 = extremely mild stuttering, through 10 = extremely severe stuttering). The scale, in a format that allows for a week's ratings, is shown in Figure 9.4. At the beginning of treatment, parents are trained to accurately rate their child's severity using observations of the child's speech in the clinic. The clinician and parent compare their ratings and discuss any differences between them until the parent's ratings are within one scale value of the clinician's. Throughout treatment, a sample of the child's speech that is long enough to ensure that any stuttering is observed is taken at the beginning of each clinic meeting. Both the clinician and the parent rate this sample, ensuring continued agreement.

This SR scale has also been used with school-age children who stutter. These older children often rate themselves in a

Stuttering Severity Instrument–4

SSI–4

Examiner Record Form

Glyndon D. Riley

Identifying Information

Name ______ Female ☐ Male ☐
Grade ______ Date of Birth ______
Date of testing ______ Age ______
School ______ Examiner ______
Preschool ☐ School Age ☐ Adult ☐ Reader ☐ Nonreader ☐

Frequency (Use Readers Table or Nonreaders Table, not both)

Readers Table				Nonreaders Table	
1. Reading Task		2. Speaking Task		3. Speaking Task	
%SS	Task Score	%SS	Task Score	%SS	Task Score
1	2	1	2	1	4
2	4	2	3	2	6
3–4	5	3	4	3	8
5–7	6	4–5	5	4–5	10
8–12	7	6–7	6	6–7	12
13–20	8	8–11	7	8–11	14
21 & up	9	12–21	8	12–21	16
		22 & up	9	22 & up	18

Frequency Score (use 1 + 2 or 3) ☐

Duration

Average length of three longest stuttering events timed to the nearest 1/10th second		Scale Score
Fleeting	(.5 sec or less)	2
Half-second	(.5–.9 sec)	4
1 full second	(1.0–1.9 sec)	6
2 seconds	(2.0–2.9 sec)	8
3 seconds	(3.0–4.9 sec)	10
5 seconds	(5.0–9.9 sec)	12
10 seconds	(10.0–29.9 sec)	14
30 seconds	(30.0–59.9 sec)	16
1 minute	(60 sec or more)	18

Duration Score ☐

Physical Concomitants

Evaluating Scale
0 = none
1 = not noticeable unless looking for it
2 = barely noticeable to casual observer
3 = distracting
4 = very distracting
5 = severe and painful looking

Distracting Sounds:	Noisy breathing, whistling, sniffing, blowing, clicking sounds	0 1 2 3 4 5 ___
Facial Grimaces:	Jaw jerking, tongue protruding, lip pressing, jaw muscles tense	0 1 2 3 4 5 ___
Head Movements:	Back, forward, turning away, poor eye contact, constant looking around	0 1 2 3 4 5 ___
Movements of the Extremities.	Arm and hand movement, hands about face, torso movement, leg movements, foot-tapping, or swinging	0 1 2 3 4 5 ___

Physical Concomitants Score ☐

Total Score

Frequency ______ + Duration ______ + Physical Concomitants ______ = ☐ Percentile ______ Severity ______

2 3 4 5 6 7 8 9 10 17 16 15 14 13 12 11 10 09 08

Additional copies of this form (#13027) may be purchased from PRO-ED, 8700 Shoal Creek Blvd., Austin, TX 78757-6897 800/897-3202, Fax 800/397-7633, www.proedinc.com

Figure 9.3 The Stuttering Severity Instrument-4. (From SSI-4 Stuttering Severity Instrument-4: Examiner Record Form (pp. 1-2), by Riley, G. D. (2009), Austin, TX: PRO-ED. Copyright © 2009 by PRO-ED, Inc. Used with permission. No further duplication may be made without written permission from PRO-ED, Inc.)

Table 2.2

Percentile Ranks and Severity Equivalents of SSI–4 Total Scores for Preschool-Age Children (*N* = 72)

Total score	Percentile rank	Severity equivalent
0–8	1–4	Very mild
9–10	5–11	
11–12	12–23	Mild
13–16	24–40	
17–23	41–60	Moderate
24–26	61–77	
27–28	78–88	Severe
29–31	89–95	
32 and up	96–99	Very severe

Table 2.3

Percentile Ranks and Severity Equivalents of SSI–4 Total Scores for School-Age Children (*N* = 139)

Total score	Percentile rank	Severity equivalent
6–8	1–4	Very mild
9–10	5–11	
11–15	12–23	Mild
16–20	24–40	
21–23	41–60	Moderate
24–27	61–77	
28–31	78–88	Severe
32–35	89–95	
36 and up	96–99	Very severe

Table 2.4

Percentile Ranks and Severity Equivalents of SSI–4 Total Scores for Adults (*N* = 60)

Total score	Percentile rank	Severity equivalent
10–12	1–4	Very mild
13–17	5–11	
18–20	12–23	Mild
21–24	24–40	
25–27	41–60	Moderate
28–31	61– 77	
32–34	78– 88	Severe
35–36	89– 95	
37–46	96– 99	Very severe

Figure 9.3 *(Continued)*

version of the Lidcombe Program developed for older children. Research on this SR scale has shown it to be a valid and reliable tool for conveniently obtaining information on a child's stuttering outside of the treatment environment (Onslow et al., 1990; Onslow et al., 2002). In a recent article, a cohort of clinical researchers has published a strong argument espousing use of the SR scale for clinical research (Onslow et al., 2018). They suggested that the SR scale is easier to use than measuring frequency of stuttering using percent syllables stuttered. In my own mind, both measures are useful, but the SR scale is far easier to use for constant assessment (ie, daily ratings) of a child's progress or problems in treatment. Assessing stuttering severity with detailed measures, such as the SSI-4 or the nine-point stuttering severity scale used by the Lidcombe Program, can be important for assessing progress, comparing scores at the beginning and end of treatment.

ASSESSING SPEECH NATURALNESS

Many years ago, clinical scientists became concerned that treatments that produce fluency may not always result in natural-sounding speech. As Schiavetti and Metz (1997) warned, "Some stutterers may reduce their number of stutters at the expense of a speech pattern that is stutter-free but not really fluent." Thus, some stuttering treatments may get rid of stuttering but leave an individual with speech that sounds odd, unusual, or unnatural. This concern about natural-sounding speech was more important in the 1970s, 80s, and 90s when operant conditioning procedures were often used for stuttering treatment (Ingham, 1999; Ryan, 1974). Most current treatments meet Bloodstein's criteria number 7 for assessing the effectiveness of treatments: "The person who stutters (PWSs) speech must sound natural and spontaneous to listeners" (Bloodstein et al., 2021, p. 418).

Historically, Martin et al. (1984) were among the first to report on concerns about speech naturalness. They found that unsophisticated listeners rated the stutter-free speech of individuals who stutter speaking under delayed auditory feedback as significantly more unnatural than the general speech of people who don't stutter. Ingham et al. (1985) used the same rating scale and found that the fluent speech of individuals treated with fluency shaping was judged to be more unnatural than that of people who don't stutter. Both investigations used a nine-point, equal-appearing interval scale to rate speakers based on judges' intuitive sense of what sounded "natural." The judges in these and most subsequent studies exhibited satisfactory levels of intrarater reliability and agreement, although between-rater reliability (interrater) was only marginally satisfactory.

A description of speech naturalness as a quality that is important in stuttering as well as other disorders can be found in a chapter by Stepp and Vojtech (2019). They discuss the use of listener perceptions of clients' speech to evaluate the extent to which the speech matches "the typical patterns in terms of intonation, voice quality, rate, rhythm, and intensity, with respect to the syntactic structure of the utterance" (p. 2). Relevant to our focus on rating clients' speech in a clinical setting, these authors imply that multiple listeners are often used for this rating. However, they also suggested that clients themselves may effectively rate the naturalness of their own speech.

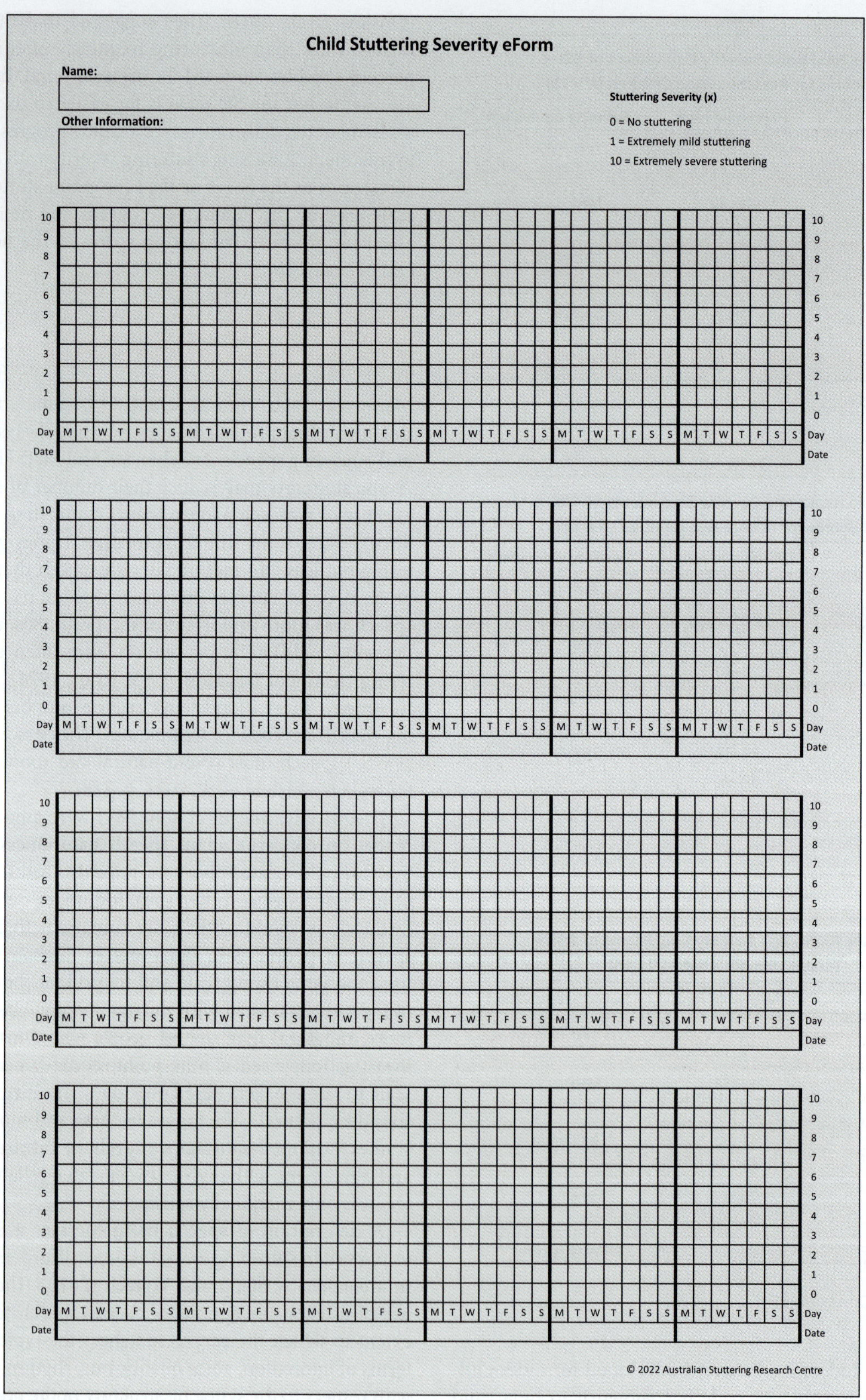
Child Stuttering Severity eForm

Name:

Other Information:

Stuttering Severity (x)

0 = No stuttering

1 = Extremely mild stuttering

10 = Extremely severe stuttering

10 9 8 7 6 5 4 3 2 1 0

Day M T W T F S S M T W T F S S M T W T F S S M T W T F S S M T W T F S S M T W T F S S Day

Date

Figure 9.4 The Child Stuttering Severity Chart (SR Scale). Rate the speaker on a ten-point scale, where 0 = no stuttering and 10 = extremely severe stuttering (the worst stuttering the speaker has produced) for the entire day. Put an X in the appropriate box at the end of each day. (Reprinted with permission from the Australian Stuttering Research Centre (2020). Child Stuttering Severity Chart, https://www.uts.edu.au/asrc/resources/lidcombe-program.)

Clinically, we need to be sure that clients sound as natural as possible after treatment. Otherwise, they are likely to abandon their fluency skills in favor of old, familiar stuttering patterns because of their own and listeners' negative reactions to their posttreatment speech. Can we rate our clients' naturalness reliably? Schiavetti and Metz (1997) indicated that clinicians who have learned to be consistent raters of speech naturalness may rely on the relative values of their ratings. Thus, they can judge when a client sounds less natural than other clients they have treated and take appropriate steps to improve that client's naturalness before releasing her from treatment. The SSI-4 incorporates a naturalness rating as part of the assessment. This rating may be all that modern clinicians need to ensure that are taking naturalness into account during their evaluation.

ASSESSING SPEAKING AND READING RATE

Many clinicians believe that speaking rate often reflects the severity of stuttering (eg, Shapiro, 1999, 2011; Starkweather, 1985, 1987). Van Riper (1982a) described studies that found correlations that ranged from 0.68 to 0.88 between reading rate and severity. In other words, stutterers who were more severe read more slowly. If a client's speaking rate is well below average for their age, communication will be affected; listeners may become impatient or lose the thread of what the speaker is saying. Speech rates that are too fast will also affect communication. A subgroup of individuals who stutter also has the disorder of cluttering, which is rapid, often unintelligible speech (as described in Chapter 8). Thus, it is useful to measure the client's rate in standard speaking and reading tasks. Table 9.5 gives average speaking rates in syllables per minute for children and adults.

TABLE 9.5 Average Speaking Rates for Children and Adults

Age (y)	Syllables per Minute (Range)	Reference
From 2-3 (girls)	169 (age 2)-205 (age 3)	Tendera et al. (2019)
From 2-3 (boys)	178 (age 2)-213 (age 3)	Tendera et al. (2019)
3	116-163	Pindzola et al. (1989)
4	117-183	Pindzola et al. (1989)
5	109-183	Pindzola et al. (1989)
6	140-175	Davis and Guitar (1976)
8	150-180	Davis and Guitar (1976)
10	165-215	Davis and Guitar (1976)
12	165-220	Davis and Guitar (1976)
Adult	162-230	Andrews and Ingham (1971)

Rate can be measured as either words or syllables per minute, depending on the clinician's preference. Some clinicians find it easier to calculate rate by using words per minute because words are easily observable units on the page. Others note that syllables per minute can be calculated more rapidly than words because clinicians can use the "beat" of syllables to count them online (ie, while a speaker is talking). The syllables-per-minute approach also accounts for the fact that some speakers use more multisyllabic words than others and might be penalized because such words take longer to produce than one-syllable words. I recommend using syllables for these reasons.

No matter which method is used, the following rules can be used for counting words or syllables for this task. Note that they are essentially the same ones described earlier for transcriptions of speech samples used for other stuttering characteristics. Count only those words or syllables that would have been said if the person had not stuttered. Thus, if a person says, "My-my-my, uh, well my name is Peter," this should be counted as four words or five syllables because it is apparent that the extra instances of "my," the "uh," and the "well" are part of the stuttering. If a person says, "When I went to Boston, I mean when I went to New York...," and it does not appear that the person was postponing or using a "trick" to avoid stuttering, this would be counted as 13 words or 14 syllables because stuttering did not interfere with the utterance. Only true words (or syllables in true words) are counted; "uh" or "um" is not counted. "Oh" or "well" are counted, unless they are used as a postponement, starter, or other component of stuttering. These distinctions may seem difficult to remember, but the main rule of thumb you should use is that you are counting syllables or words that convey information to the listener.

When syllables per minute are calculated, it is often easiest to use an inexpensive calculator to count syllables cumulatively as they are spoken, although this takes some practice. Before the speaker begins, push the "1" key and then the "+." When the speaker starts speaking, press the "=" key for each syllable spoken or read, and the cumulative total will appear in the readout window. It is easier to count syllables by reading a transcript of the conversational sample aloud slowly and pushing the "=" key for each syllable spoken; inexperienced raters should learn to count syllables first from a transcript. Experienced raters can assess conversational speech rate directly from recordings by pressing the "=" key for each syllable spoken. Some calculators will count cumulatively when the "1" is pressed, followed by repeated presses of the "+" button; I have not found an expensive calculator that will count cumulatively (a cheap one will), but the calculator that came with my PC laptop and also the one on my Mac will count cumulatively with the 1, +, = maneuver.

Some clinicians have found that they are able, with practice, to count syllables per minute as the client is speaking by using graph paper with small boxes. As the client is talking, they put a dot in each box for each syllable spoken. They also use this method to assess frequency of stuttering, by putting a check instead of a dot for each syllable stuttered.

When words per minute are calculated, a transcript is made of a client's 5-min sample of conversational speech, then the transcription is marked to indicate the 5-min endpoint. The total number of words is counted in that section of the transcript, and this figure is divided by 5 to give a per-minute conversational or reading rate. It is important to measure these samples accurately with a stopwatch or another timing device. In measuring the amount of speaking time in a conversational sample, I stop the stopwatch whenever the client is not talking but allow it to run during moments of stuttering. Short pauses of less than 2 s are incorporated into the 5 min, but formulation pauses longer than 2 s are excluded. With a little practice, starting and stopping a stopwatch during pauses and turn-switching become easy and natural.

The CSSS software that comes with the SSI-4 allows the clinician to count number of stutters and number of fluent syllables and assess total sample duration in seconds. By totaling the stuttered and fluent syllables and dividing that total by the sample duration in minutes, you can get overall speech rate in syllables per minute.

USING FLUENCYBANK TO ASSESS STUTTERING BEHAVIORS

FluencyBank is a website that hosts computational programs for analyzing samples of stuttered (and fluent) speech from your clients and research subjects, as well as a useful teaching resource. The site was developed by Nan Bernstein Ratner and Brian MacWhinney, extending the original TalkBank platform to include stuttering and cluttering (Bernstein Ratner & MacWhinney, 2018). To access the site, go to talkbank.org and, then under the "Clinical Banks" heading, choose "FluencyBank." You will see a myriad of links to help you learn to use the FluencyBank tools. FluencyBank also invites you to send audio and video samples of stuttering so that they may be used by clinicians and researchers around the world.

For our purposes, I would like to introduce you to the tools you can use to make a transcript of a speech sample from your client and then analyze it. The result of the "instant" analysis will be many bits of information that will, among other things, be helpful in deciding if a young child is normally disfluent or is stuttering. Of particular interest is the weighted SLD index. The publication by Ambrose and Yairi (1999)—particularly Figure 1—suggests why this index may be important. As I will describe in Chapter 10, I used FluencyBank to analyze a child's speech during a parent-child interaction to show how strong the quantitative evidence was that the child was stuttering rather than normally disfluent. But it should be noted that when you watch the parent-child video, your qualitative judgment should bring you to the same conclusion.

To use FluencyBank, go to www.talkbank.org and choose (under Clinical Banks) FluencyBank. On that web page, see the Speech-Language Pathologists's (SLP's) Guide to computerized language analysis (CLAN) that explains many programs but, for our purpose, tells you how to use CLAN to create a transcript and have it analyzed via FLUCALC. Also, on the FluencyBank web page, see the tutorial screencast that also describes how to use fluency calculation (FLUCALC). It takes some careful reading, viewing, and listening to digest all the steps needed to get an output, based on the transcript that you have marked with codes for various kinds of stutters. The output will be an Excel sheet that details total numbers and percentages of various stuttering behaviors and typical disfluencies. As I indicated, the weighted SLD output may be helpful indeed, despite the extra effort it may take you to master this way of detailing your client's stuttering. Obviously, it gets easier the more you do it.

ASSESSING FEELINGS AND ATTITUDES

The feelings or emotions of individuals who stutter, as well as their beliefs and attitudes about themselves, about communication, and about stuttering, are all components of stuttering, if not the central part of the experience of stuttering (eg, Tichenor & Yaruss, 2019). For most people who stutter, the experience of stuttering and the reactions of others to their stuttering have a notable effect on their behavior and on their response to therapy. Therefore, assessment of these aspects of stuttering is critical. The next two chapters focus on assessment of individuals who stutter at different age and severity levels; in these chapters, I will provide detailed information about the assessment of **feelings and attitudes**, as well as guidelines for overall assessment of these different stuttering levels.

SUMMARY

- In an assessment, the clinician has a variety of tasks. These include
- Gathering information from the client.
- Getting to know the client as an individual.
- Helping the client and/or family get to know you.
- Showing an understanding of the client's point of view and hopes for treatment.
- Demonstrating an understanding of stuttering.

- Helping the client or his family determine whether their insurance covers the assessment and treatment. If not, are there scholarships available to help them?
- Ensuring that the client/family knows about their right to privacy regarding what happens in the evaluation and treatment.
- Clinicians must develop skills and sensitivities in working with clients from cultures other than their own.
- Building a relationship with a client begins in the first meeting, which is usually the assessment. A clinician must take this opportunity to demonstrate that they know about the disorder of stuttering, is unafraid of it, and is accepting of it. At the same time, the clinician must show that they feel positively about the client's ability to change their stuttering, if this is what the client wants to do.
- Behaviors counted as stutters include part-word repetitions, single-syllable whole-word repetitions, prolongations, blocks, escape behaviors and unequivocal avoidance behaviors—or combinations of these that may occur in a single episode of stuttering.
- Samples for assessing stuttering should include a variety of situations. The initial sample and samples assessing outcome should be video recorded for more accurate scoring and measurement of reliability. These samples should include speaking and, when appropriate, reading.
- Frequency of stuttering is commonly assessed as the percentage of syllables or words stuttered.
- Different types of disfluencies can be assessed to reveal the percentage of stutter-like disfluent syllables or number of these disfluent syllables per 100 words. This information may be particularly useful in helping to decide if a preschool child needs treatment.
- Durations of moments of stuttering are useful in quantifying an aspect of the abnormality of a client's stuttering and the extent to which it may interfere with communication. Speaking and reading rates will also help to quantify this aspect of the impact of stuttering.
- Frequency and severity of secondary or concomitant behaviors associated with stuttering can be important measures of how much these behaviors call attention to themselves and distract listeners.
- Four severity scales are the SSI-4, the Scale for Rating Severity, the Lidcombe Program's SR Scale for children, and Self-Reported Stuttering Severity (O'Brian et al., 2020). The commonly used SSI-4 combines an assessment of frequency of stuttering, mean duration of the three longest stutters, and physical concomitants accompanying stuttering.
- Speech naturalness can be reliably and easily assessed. It is thought to be most important when evaluating outcomes of treatments that teach a client to use an unnatural speech pattern to initially achieve fluency.
- Various instruments have been created to assess emotions and attitudes associated with stuttering. When combined with measures of stuttering behaviors, these measures provide a multidimensional view of the disorder. These are presented in the next two chapters, with different assessments for each age and severity level.

STUDY QUESTIONS

1. What does it mean to suggest that a clinician must play two different roles during an evaluation?
2. Which types of disfluencies are counted as stutters, and which are considered typical?
3. What factors can affect the process of measuring stuttering?
4. Describe the procedures for the two measures of reliability called "point-by-point agreement" and "percent error."
5. Why is it important to obtain several samples of speech from a client when assessing stuttering, whereas a single sample might sometimes be adequate for assessing a phonological disorder?
6. Give two reasons why assessment of intra- and interrater reliability of direct measurements of stuttering is important.
7. Describe five dimensions or aspects of stuttering that may be assessed in an evaluation of a client who stutters.
8. To you, what is the most important aspect of stuttering? How a client feels about his stuttering? How much the client's speech deviates from typical fluency? How much the client avoids words and situations? Something else? Defend your choice. How do you measure it?
9. Why is it relevant to assess speech rate for a person who stutters?
10. Discuss the pros and cons of protecting the privacy of conversations between yourself and a teenage client by not sharing their contents with parents.

SUGGESTED PROJECTS

1. Research how different cultures react to stuttering and suggest how evaluation procedures in this chapter need to be changed for individuals from a culture that has very different beliefs about stuttering than those suggested in this text.
2. Make or obtain a video of a conversational and a reading sample of a person who stutters. Use two different methods of measuring the stuttering (such as percentage of syllables stuttered or duration of three longest stutters or speech rate or Scale for Rating Severity of Stuttering) and obtain intraobserver and interobserver reliability assessments for each method. Discuss why one measurement procedure is more reliable than the other.
3. Obtain a video recorded conversational sample of one or more individuals who stutter, and identify moments when you think the client has used an avoidance behavior to prevent stuttering. Discuss whether these avoidances should be counted as stutters. If need be, you can watch the videos on the Fluency Bank or the documentary *When I Stutter* to see avoidance behaviors.
4. Obtain samples of repetitive stutters from normally fluent children and from children who stutter. Compare the repetitions from both groups in terms of length of silent periods between iterations, pitch, and other acoustic variables. Videos for Chapter 1 on Lippincott Connect have both a fluent child and children who stutter.
5. Search the literature on assessment of stuttering to determine whether reliable methods have been developed for clients to assess their own stuttering during the progress of treatment.

SUGGESTED READINGS

Battle, D. (Ed.). (2012). *Communication disorders in multicultural and international populations* (4th ed.). Elsevier/Mosby.
This book provides many descriptions and insights into evaluating and treating communication disorders in many cultures not only in the United States but throughout the world.

Bloodstein, O., Ratner, N., & Brundage, S. (2021). *A handbook on stuttering* (7th ed.). Plural Publishing, Inc.
Chapter 13, on Assessment of Stuttering, provides detailed information about the evaluation of stuttering in adults, children, very early stuttering, and special populations.

Brundage, S., Ratner, N., Boyle, M., Eggers, K., Everard, R., Franken, M. C., Kefalianos, E., Marcotte, A., Millard, S., Packman, A., Vanryckeghem, M., & Yaruss, J. S. (2021). Clinical focus: Consensus guidelines for the assessments of individuals who stutter across the lifespan. *American Journal of Speech-Language Pathology, 30*, 2379–2393.
This article created a consensus of practicing speech language pathologists (the authors) specializing in clinical research on stuttering to describe and enumerate assessment procedures used in the evaluations of stutterers across the age span. The authors present procedures to use in six key areas for assessment and provide an appendix of tools and methods to use at each age level for a complete assessment.

Brutten, G., & Vanryckeghem, M. (2007). *Behavior assessment battery for school-age children who stutter*. Plural Publishing.
This set of assessment tools is designed to measure communication attitudes and reactions to specific speaking situations for school-age children who stutter.

Cordes, A. K. (1994). The reliability of observational data: I. Theories and methods for speech-language pathology. *Journal of Speech and Hearing Research, 37*, 264–278.
This article provides an excellent tutorial on the problems associated with establishing reliability of observational data in stuttering.

Guttormsen, L., Kefalianos, E., & Næss, K. (2015). Communication attitudes in children who stutter: A meta-analytic review. *Journal of Fluency Disorders, 46*, 1–14.
This is a careful review of studies assessing the communication attitudes of children (ages 3–18 years) who stutter. Some clear conclusions are drawn, and directions for future research are suggested.

Howell, P., & Van Borsel, J. (2011). *Multilingual aspects of fluency disorders*. Multilingual Matters.
An edited book that discusses stuttering in many languages and cultures as well as stuttering and bilingualism.

Rosenberry-McKibbin, C. (2018). *Multicultural students with special language needs: Practical strategies for assessment and intervention* (5th ed.). Academic Communication Associates, Inc.
This book provides many insights into evaluation of multicultural students.

Zebrowski, P., Anderson, J., & Conture. E. (Eds.). (2022). *Stuttering and related disorders of fluency* (4th ed.). Thieme.
This new edition of the classic text updates background research on the nature of stuttering and provides key information on assessment and treatment. A wide array of international experts contributed to this book.

10

Assessment of Preschool Children Who Stutter

Chapter Outline

Chapter Objectives

After studying this chapter, readers should be able to:

- Plan and carry out an evaluation of a preschool child
- Understand how to evaluate the stuttering behaviors of a preschool child
- Understand how to evaluate attitudes and feelings of a preschool child and of the client's family
- Understand how to determine appropriate follow-up to the evaluation of a preschool child

Key Terms

Accepting environment: Behavior by parents and other family members (and teachers and classmates where appropriate) that convey to the child that they accept the child and their speech

Clinician-child interaction: Play-based conversation between clinician and child in which the clinician observes the child's speech and may seek information about child's feelings about their stuttering, as well as information about child's other speech and language skills

Closing interview: A conversation at the end of an evaluation session in which the clinician informs the client or family of their findings, makes recommendations for the future, and answers any questions they have

Parent-child interaction: Play-based conversation between parent(s) and child that is often used to gather a sample of the child's speech and to assess environmental influences on a child's stuttering

Parent interview: A conversation with the parent(s) in which they are encouraged to describe their child's stuttering and express their concerns. In this interaction, the clinician elicits and gives information relevant to the child's stuttering

Preassessment: The time before the formal assessment, in which the clinician gathers key information needed for the assessment

Risk factors for persistent stuttering: Characteristics within the child or within the environment that are hypothesized to increase probability that the child will not overcome their stuttering naturally—that is, without intervention. These may also be called prognostic factors

Speech sample: A segment of speech used to assess a client's stuttering; typically, three samples are sought where a sample should be between 150 and 500 syllables (Riley, 2009). These samples—gathered from the child's home or in the clinic are meant to be representative of a client's speech in general

This chapter on preschool assessment and the preceding one on preliminaries to assessment are bridges between chapters on the nature of stuttering and chapters on treatment. My aim is to show you how to understand clients and their families and their children's stuttering problems and then to use the information you have gathered to share with the child's family to determine treatment approaches. Figure 10.1 illustrates the components of assessment and diagnosis.

STEPS IN ASSESSMENT OF PRESCHOOL CHILDREN WHO STUTTER

Preassessment

In this section, I will present a few ideas to consider before you evaluate a preschool-aged child who may be stuttering. These ideas will help you listen effectively to what the family says about the child and perhaps ask some preliminary questions before you arrange for a face-to-face meeting. For the sake of brevity, I will use the words "parents" and "family," but I also mean "other caregivers" when that is applicable.

Clinical Questions

When you assess a preschool child, you want to answer two questions: Is this child stuttering, or are they typically disfluent? And, if they are stuttering, what treatment approach will best meet their needs?

In the process of trying to answer these questions, much of the focus will be on the child. What are the amounts and types of disfluencies this child shows in various situations? Is the child reacting to their speech with frustration, fear, or other emotions? Is the child temperamentally sensitive enough that parents' alarm would influence the child to try to stop or hide their disfluencies? Or would the parent's alarm just make them more frequent and severe?

Some focus will also be on the family. With preschool children, the family's role is crucial. To respond to the family's needs and to involve them fully in planning treatment, you need to know the answers to questions like the following: How do family members feel about the child's possible stuttering? Do they feel that treatment is needed immediately? Or, do they just want to know if this is stuttering and whether it should be treated sometime? Can you tell whether family members show alarm when the child is disfluent? Do they think the child is bothered by their own disfluencies? How does the family express their concerns about the child's stuttering? What are their preferences and expectations for treatment?

Once you have gathered this information and more, you will need to form a hypothesis about the best options for the child and family: (1) no treatment, (2) watchful waiting with regular family contact, (3) clinician-guided environmental change and family counseling, and (4) direct treatment by the clinician or clinician-guided parent-delivered treatment. I say "form a hypothesis" rather than "decide" the best options for the family because you will need to involve the parents before a choice is made. In addition, you will want to determine if the child is within the normal range for language, phonology, and voice, if the parents are able to discern this.

1
Clinician reviews Case History, questionnaires, and questions to be answered. She also watches video sent by parents of the child talking at home.
2
Clinician observes parent-child interaction in clinic room with toys and records this speech sample.
3
Clinician interviews parent(s)/caregiver(s) and listens carefully to learn what their concerns are and their observations of the child's stuttering.
4
Clinician plays with child with toys and talks with child to observe child's stuttering and possibly talks about stuttering with child.
5
Clinician interprets the information gathered from parent interview and her observations of interaction with child and writes a brief summary of her impressions and recommendations.
6
Clinician offers positive comments about child and the parents' interaction with the child. Clinician gives parents her brief summary of her observations and recommendations regarding child's speech. Parents and clinician plan next steps: Treatment soon? Watchful waiting with regular communication with parents? No treatment?

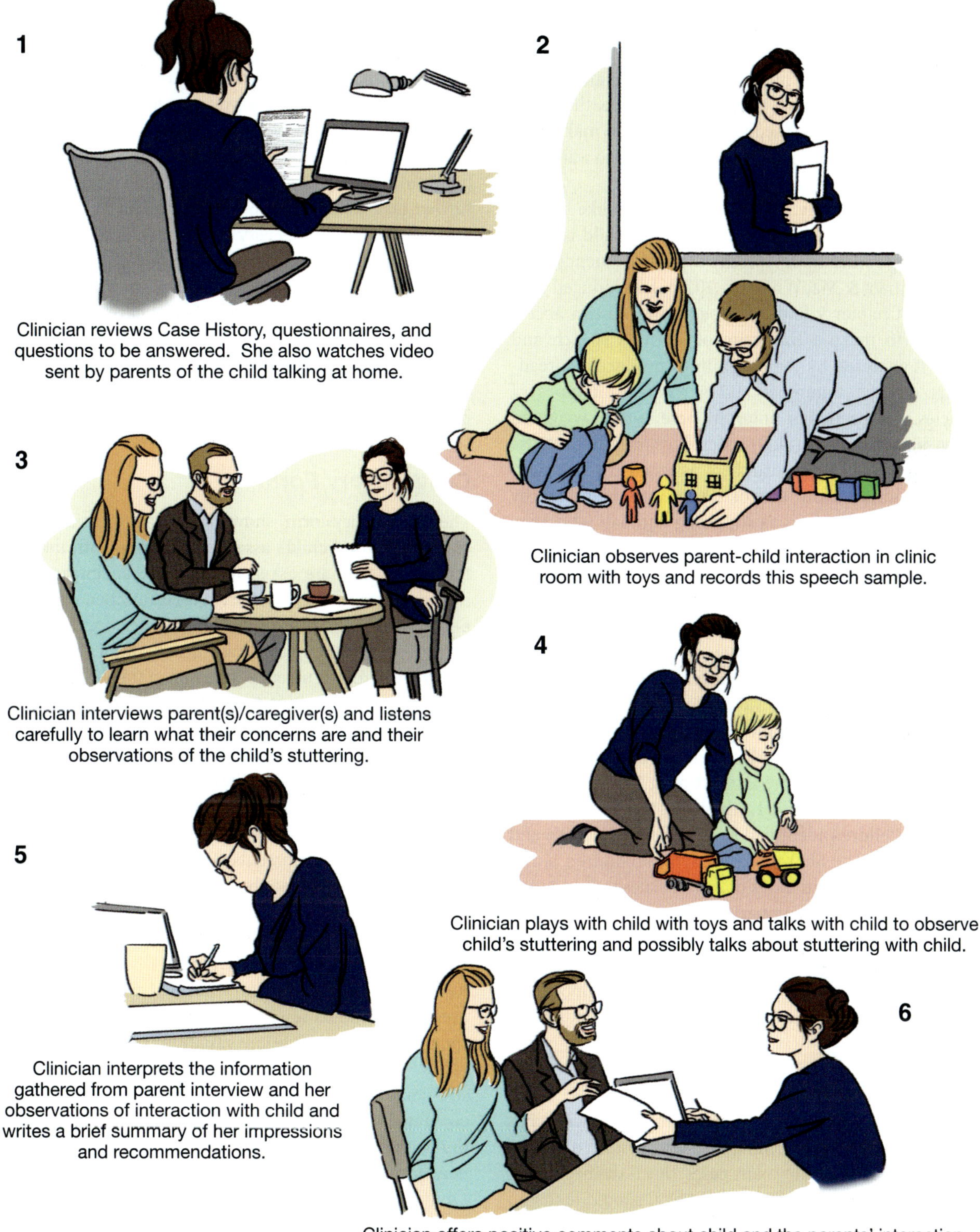

Figure 10.1 Steps in assessment of preschoolers who stutter.

In the actual evaluation, you may want to test for problems in these areas, if you suspect an issue. Finally, you will develop an initial idea of whether referral to another professional (eg, a family counselor or a learning specialist) is warranted. Like the final decision about what treatment to pursue, this decision may not be evident in the first contact(s) you make with the family, will require their input, and may need to wait until you or another clinician sees the child.

If you are statistically minded, you might like to use another tool to help you determine whether a child is likely to be stuttering rather than typically disfluent: FluencyBank (Bernstein Ratner & MacWhinney, 2018). I introduced FluencyBank in Chapter 9 and described how you can access the tutorials to make a transcript of a child's speech and then have it analyzed by the program to produce a spreadsheet that quantifies number and percentage of types of disfluencies. Of particular interest, here is the weighted stuttering-like disfluency (SLD) index developed by Amrose and Yairi (1999). Those researchers assessed the disfluencies of 90 children, about half of whom were identified by parents and the researchers as stuttering and half who were categorized as typically disfluent. The weighted SLD values for the 90 children were presented in Figure 1 of that article, in which children who were identified as stuttering were, by and large, separated statistically from the typically disfluent children. Elsewhere in this chapter, I suggest you watch a video recording of a **parent-child interaction** on Lippincott Connect called "Preschool Evaluation Identifying Stutters Part I." I used the FluencyBank transcript analysis program, FluCalc, to determine this child's weighted SLD index for her speech in the first part of the interaction. I found the value for her weighted index to be 21, which was well into the high values of the children identified as stuttering. Ambrose and Yairi suggest that the SLD index for typical children is not greater than 4 and that an index of 21 translates to "moderate stuttering." Based on this comparison, then, the child seemed appropriate for immediate treatment, which was started within a few weeks of the diagnostic evaluation. She became fluent within a year and has remained fluent through our last contact, approximately 5 years after her treatment ended.

Initial Contact

In your initial contact, the family member who has approached you will start forming a first impression of you in your early conversations. In many cases, this is the beginning of a therapeutic alliance. For your part, you should focus on understanding the family member's point of view; their concerns and hopes. Listen closely to them and let them know that you are ready to work with the family as part of a team who will, together, help the child.

Your initial contact is likely to be on the telephone. If it is, listen to the parent's voice and pay attention to the parent's level of concern. As you listen carefully, you may need to ask an occasional question to get clarification and to show your interest and expertise. When you think you have an initial understanding of the problem, set up an appointment, if appropriate. If you cannot meet with the family for several days or longer, I think it is important to give them some suggestions to get started.[1] For example, you may want a parent to rate the child's stuttering using the Lidcombe Severity Rating Scale described in Chapter 9 and shown in Figure 9.4. This will keep them from feeling as if they are in a holding pattern, awaiting further instructions. It also may be helpful to have the family set aside a few minutes every day, in which one parent can play alone with the child and give them special attention. Finally, consider letting the family know that they can contact you before the first formal meeting if they have new concerns or forgot to ask you something. Prior to an evaluation, you should let the family know what will take place in the evaluation and approximately how long it will take. A discussion of fees and payment may also be appropriate.

Case History Form

The case history form, shown in Figure 10.2, is sent to parents before their child's assessment. Along with the case history form, they are asked to complete an intake form that includes date, name, address, phone number, permission to e-mail, what the concerns are, and a note about the insurance we accept. The completed case history informs the clinician about the parents' current perception of the problem, as well as its onset and development, and the child's medical, family, and school history. Considerable detail is obtained about the child's stuttering pattern to help the clinician understand the severity and extent of core and secondary behaviors. Many families will need help understanding what the different stuttering behaviors sound and look like, so this can be part of the discussion in the meeting with the parents. This will be discussed when the actual evaluation is described, later in this chapter.

Video Recording

Along with the case history form, I ask the parents of a preschool child to send me a video recording of their child speaking in a typical home situation. I encourage parents to video 5 or 10 minutes of themselves playing with their child so I can preview the child's speech soon after the parents have contacted me. In cases in which several weeks elapse between the parents' contact and the evaluation, the child's stuttering may have diminished substantially, so during the evaluation, I may observe only a fluent cycle of the child's speech in contrast to how the child was speaking when the parents first contacted me. In addition to sampling the child's speech, the recording can help me learn a little about this family's parent-child interactions.

[1]It should be noted that some clinicians—for example, those working with direct treatment programs—prefer not to have the family make changes on their own before the evaluation meeting.

STUTTERING CASE HISTORY FORM – PRESCHOOL AND SCHOOL-AGE CHILD

Instructions: Please fill out this form in as much detail as possible. You can be assured that this information will be treated as confidential. If information is not available, please specify the reason so that we will know that the question has been considered. **Please return this form prior to your appointment.** Thank you.

Date: ______________________________

Child's Name: ______________________________

Address: ______________________________

____

Sex Assigned at Birth: __________

(This information is helpful in knowing the chances that the child will recover from stuttering naturally)

Gender: __________ Age: __________

(years: months)

Preferred Telephone: ____________________ Email Address: ____________________

Date of Birth: ____________________ Place of Birth: ____________________

Medicaid#: ____________________ Referring Physician: ____________________

Family and Others with whom Child Lives: ______________________________

____

____

____

Teacher's Name (if applicable): ______________________________

School (if applicable): ______________________________

School Placement or Grade Level (if applicable): ______________________________

Name of person completing this form: ______________________________

Relationship to child: ______________________________

FAMILY

Father:

Name: ____________________ Age: ____________________

Is he living with the family? ____________________ Occupation: ____________________

Employed by: ______________________________

Education level: ______________________________

Telephone (Home): ____________________ (Work): ____________________

Social Security#: ____________________

Mother:

Name: ____________________ Age: ____________________

Is she living with the family? ____________________ Occupation: ____________________

Employed by: ______________________________

Education level: ______________________________

Telephone (Home): ____________________ (Work): ____________________

Social Security#: ____________________

Figure 10.2 Case history form.

Brothers and Sisters:

	(Name)	(Age)		(Name)	(Age)
1.	____________	______	4.	____________	______
2.	____________	______	5.	____________	______
3.	____________	______	6.	____________	______

HISTORY OF STUTTERING

Give approximate age at which stuttering was first noticed: ____________

Who first noticed or mentioned the stuttering? ____________

In what situation was the stuttering first noticed? ____________

Describe any situations or conditions that might have been associated with the onset of stuttering:

____

____

Under what different circumstances did the stuttering continue after initial onset? ____________

____

What were the first signs of stuttering (check all that apply):

A. Repetitions of the whole word? (boy-boy-boy) ____________

B. Repetitions of the first letter? (b-b-b-boy) ____________

C. Repetitions of the first syllable? (ca-ca-cat) ____________

D. Complete blocks on the first letter? (b....oy) ____________

E. Prolongations of the vowel? (caaaaaaaat) ____________

F. Visible attempt to speak (i.e., mouth movement) but no sound forthcoming? ________

G. Other ____________

Was the stuttering always the same or did it occur in several different ways? ____________

If it occurred in different ways, how were they different from one another? Describe.

____

____

Approximately how long did each block (one word) seem to last? ____________

Was the stuttering easy or was there force at the time when the stuttering was first noticed?

____

Were stuttered words primarily at the beginning of sentences or were they scattered throughout the sentence? ____________

When stuttering first began, was there any avoidance of speaking (i.e., changing word or stopping mid-stutter, using gestures instead of speech) because of it? Give examples, if any. ____________

____

____

Figure 10.2 *(Continued)*

Assessment

I begin by greeting the family, introducing myself, and describing the activities we will be engaging in for the evaluation. In our clinic, these involve, first, our observation of the parents interacting with the child and then our interview of the parents. This is followed by my interaction with the child, then time for me to pull together the findings, and a wrap-up meeting in which I share my observations and recommendations.

Does or did the child add extra words or sounds to "get started" (i.e., hey mom, hey mom...)?
____

Does or did the child use a lot of "fillers" when they speak (i.e., uh, um)? ____________

At the time when stuttering was first noticed, what was your child's reaction?

Awareness that speech was different? ________ Surprise? ________

Indifference to it? ________ Anger or frustration? ________

Fear of stuttering again? ________ Shame? ________

Other? ________________________________

What attempts have been made to treat the stuttering problem (either at home or with a professional)? ________________________________
____

Does the child have articulation or pronunciation problems in addition to stuttering? If so, please describe. ________________________________

Does child have hand preference? Right- or left-handed or use both equally well? ________

Does child have a foot preference for kicking a ball? ________________

Does the child seem to be sensitive or have difficulty adapting to new situations? ________
____

Has the child been diagnosed with ADHD or ADD? ________________

DEVELOPMENT OF STUTTERING

Since onset, has there been any change in stuttering symptoms? Check those that are appropriate.

Increase in number of repetitions per word ________

Change in amount of force used—Increased? ________

Decreased? ________

Increase in amount of stuttering ________

Increase in length of block ________

Periods of no stuttering ________

Longer periods of stuttering ________

More precise in speech attempts ________

Lowered voice ________

Slower speech rate ________

Physical struggle (i.e., facial tension, eye blinks) ________

Looking away from the listener ________

Increase in pitch during stutters ________

Describe any of the above things the child does when he stutters (i.e., eye blinks). ________
____
____

Figure 10.2 *(Continued)*

Parent-Child Interaction

Observations of parent-child interactions are useful because they allow not only sampling of the child's speech in a natural context but also sampling of how the parent(s) interact with the child. Observations of the parent-child interaction can be done formally or informally. Some clinicians observe these interactions in the waiting room. Others

Were there any periods (weeks/months) when the stuttering disappeared? ____________________

Were there any periods (weeks/months) when stuttering increased? ____________________

Can you give any explanations for these "worse" periods? ____________________

Are there any situations that are particularly difficult? If so, describe: ____________________

____

List any situations that never cause difficulty: ____________________

____

Does the child stutter when he or she (check those that apply):

Asks questions?	______	Uses new words that are unfamiliar	______
Talks to young children?	______	Uses the telephone?	______
Says his or her name?	______	Reads out loud?	______
Answers direct questions?	______	Recites memorized material?	______
Talks to adults, teachers?	______	Talks to strangers?	______
Speaks when tired?	______	Speaks when excited?	______
Talks to family members	______	Talks to friends?	______

Do you know anyone who stutters? ____________________ Are they relatives? Friends?

Acquaintances? ____________________

Do you feel that stuttering interferes with your child's daily life? ____________________

Social relationships? ____________________

Success in school? ____________________

MEDICAL, DEVELOPMENTAL, AND FAMILY HISTORY

Describe mother's health during pregnancy and birth history (i.e., complications): ____________________

____

____

Describe any development problems during infancy or early childhood (i.e., late to walk or talk, feeding problems, food allergies): ____________________

____

Do you think the child's speech and language development was unusually rapid or delayed? If so, please describe: ____________________

____

List all significant illnesses, injuries, severe fevers, and operations:

	Date	Illness	Complications	Treatment	Physician
1.					
2.					
3					

Figure 10.2 *(Continued)*

who work in preschool or early intervention programs may visit a child's home and arrange to observe parent-child interactions while they sit quietly in the same room. Still others, myself included, video record the parents and child in a play-style interaction in a treatment room supplied with toys and games. When recording these interactions

List any medications your child is on: ____________________

List all present disabilities: ____________________

Any chronic illnesses, allergies or physical conditions?

____

Vision normal? ____________ Hearing normal? ____________

Child's eye color? ____________ Hair color? ____________

Do other members of the family have speech, language, reading problems, or learning disabilities?

If so, please describe: ____________________

____

____

____

Are any family members left-handed or use both right and left hands equally well? ____________

____

Does the child or other family members show artistic talent or interest? ____________

____

Do any family members talk very rapidly? If so, who? ____________________

____

SCHOOL AND SOCIAL HISTORY

Favorite subjects or activities in school: ____________________

Difficult subjects: ____________________

Hobbies: ____________ Sports: ____________

Leisure time activities: ____________________

Favorite toys: ____________________

What specific questions do you have about your child that you would like us to try to answer?

(Use back of sheet if necessary) ____________________

____

____

In addition, what goals would you like to see accomplished as a result of this evaluation?

____

____

____

Signature: ______________________________ Date: ____________

Please return these completed forms to us in the envelope provided. Thank you.

Figure 10.2 *(Continued)*

is possible, this sample of a child's speech can be assessed for severity and types of stuttering behavior, as described in Chapter 9.

In my practice, I like to begin with the parent-child interaction for several reasons. First, parents may be less affected by my orientation toward stuttering than if I talked with them before the observation, thereby giving me a more natural sample. Second, this interaction gives me an opportunity to see the child's stuttering firsthand (rather than via a recording). I can try to sense how much the child seems aware of their stuttering, the types of disfluencies the child has, whether or not there are escape and avoidance behaviors, and to what extent the child is reacting emotionally to their stuttering. Third, I can observe how the parents interact with their child. Do they listen to and look while the child is talking? Do they let the child do most of the talking and choose what to play with? Do they talk at a reasonably slow rate with vocabulary that is not too advanced for the child to follow? Do they interrupt? Do they correct their child? Do they talk at a fast rate or use complex vocabulary or advanced syntax? Fourth, the parent-child interaction will give me at least a larger sample of their speech so I can begin to know the child, even if they don't know me yet. Next, to help the child be more comfortable with me and gain a sample of the child's communication with unfamiliar people, I join the interaction while the parents are still playing with the child. These observations add to what I have learned from the case history and the video sample that the parents have sent before the assessment. Together, the observation of home and in-clinic samples provides a basis for the **parent interview** and for developing recommendations for treatment.

For an example of parent-child interaction with a preschool child who stutters, watch the video clip on Lippincott Connect called "Preschool Evaluation: Identifying Stutters Part I" with the Chapter 10 videos. As you watch this video clip, notice the interaction style of the mother. How does she react to her child's stutters? Does she give the child adequate time to talk? Is her speech rate slow enough for the child to process easily? Also, observe the child's stuttering. What types of stutters do they have? See if you can categorize them as repetitions, prolongations, or blocks. Are some of the "repetitions" actually responses to feeling stuck and trying to get started (ie, are they "starters")? How aware of their stutters is this child? Why do you think that?

Once you have answered these questions, watch "Preschool Evaluation: Identifying Stutters (Part II)" also with the Chapter 10 videos. Part II gives my analysis of the child's stutters and will, I hope, help you to learn to understand the different types of stutters a child may have.

Parent Interview

I usually talk with the family without the child present, giving the family an opportunity to speak about matters that they feel they would like to share in confidence. If I'm working with another clinician or a student, they play with and observe the child while I talk to the parents together. An example of this is the video on Lippincott Connect titled "Preschool Evaluation: Parent Intake Interview" with the Chapter 10 videos. If I'm working alone and both parents have come to the evaluation, I talk to each parent separately, while the other is with the child. If only one parent is present, I often arrange to have the child playing by themselves in a nearby room with the door open, if the child is comfortable with that.

I begin by asking parents to describe the problem their child is having. I ask open-ended questions, such as "Tell me about Justin's speech" or "Tell me what concerns you have about Kimberly and her speech." Open-ended questions allow parents to describe their concerns in their own words. This provides an opportunity for me to listen carefully, to be nonjudgmental, and to be comfortable with silence so that parents can express themselves fully. Listening attentively and being comfortable with silence require concentration on the clinician's part, so it is worthwhile to remind yourself of this when you are preparing for an evaluation. Often, I sit by myself for a few minutes before meeting with the family, letting my mind become quiet so that I will be open to what they have to say. In the interview, after parents have had a chance to describe the problem and appear to have no more to say at that moment, I ask about the first stages of the child's life (the child's birth and development) and then work up toward the present time. In the ensuing conversation, I try to be sure I get information indicated by the questions in the following paragraphs. This interview is not a strict question-and-answer format, but rather a discussion punctuated by both their questions and mine.

Sometimes, during an initial interview, parents ask direct questions about things they think they may be doing wrong. I let them know that, in my view, stuttering is often the result of many factors acting together and that parents do not cause it. I rarely give advice about what they should change or what they should do until after I have finished interviewing the parents and have assessed the child directly. I believe that I am more accurate, and parents are more receptive to my recommendations, if I delay a discussion of what to do until the **closing interview** when I have the most information possible. On the other hand, there may be "clinical moments" during an initial interview when parents might be most receptive to suggestions. Many times, for example, parents have asked me whether it's a good idea for them to tell their child to slow down whenever the child stutters when excited. My response is usually to ask them how the child responds to this and to build upon their answer so that we can brainstorm the best way to help the child together.

Here are some areas that I touch on during the conversation:

1. **Were there any problems with your pregnancy or the birth of this child?**
Although there is little evidence that people who stutter as a group have difficult birth histories, there is an increased incidence of stuttering among individuals who have a known history of brain injury (Boehme, 1968; Poulos & Webster, 1991). Thus, I am seeking to determine whether there is the possibility of congenital brain injury. If a difficult pregnancy or birth is reported, I might examine the child's language, motor, and cognitive development more closely. Because it is completed before the evaluation, the

case history form provides preliminary information for potential follow-up.

2. **What was your child's speech and language development like? How did it compare with siblings' development (if there are siblings) and with your expectations?** The first appearance of stuttering may be influenced by the "processing load" that language acquisition has on a child's speech production, as described in the sections on speech and language development in Chapter 4. Thus, it is important to understand the course of a child's overall speech and language development. I explore the possibility that a child's language acquisition is proceeding so rapidly that his developing motor system cannot keep up. I also examine the possibility that a child's speech and language development are delayed, making them frustrated because they find it hard to talk. As mentioned in Chapters 3 and 4, there is evidence that poorer speech and language skills may predict persistent stuttering (Singer et al., 2020; Yairi, Ambrose, Paden and Throneburg, 1996).
3. **Describe the child's motor development compared with that of their siblings or with other children you know about.** I am interested in parents' general impressions. Does their child seem to be developing motor skills like other children of their age, or do they think the child may be delayed? Some indicators of the normal range of children's gross and fine motor development, as well as their personal-social and speech-language development are shown in Figure 4.2 (child development in the first 5 years).

   In my experience, many children who stutter appear to be slightly advanced in their language and, less often, slightly delayed in their motor skills. Or, they may be well advanced in language but have completely normal motor skills. In either case, these children seem to benefit from models of speech produced at a slow rate (Guitar et al., 1992; also, see the section in Chapter 12 on indirect treatment). Other children who stutter may be delayed in several areas and may need treatment for language and phonology that is integrated with therapy for stuttering (see the section of Chapter 12, "Treatment of Concomitant Speech and Language Problems").
4. **Have any members of your family had speech or language disorders?** I ask this general question and then ask more specifically whether family members or other relatives have ever had problems related to stuttering, cluttering, speech sound development, or language disorders (see Chapter 8 for a description of cluttering). To confirm that a problem was considered significant (and was perhaps diagnosed), I ask if the person ever received treatment. I use this information when we discuss stuttering as a disorder that may have predisposing factors. Handled tactfully, a discussion of predisposing factors may help parents realize that their child's stuttering was not something they caused, which, in turn, may reduce their anxiety or guilt, making them more effective in facilitating the child's fluency.

   If a parent stutters or formerly stuttered, the parent may have strong negative feelings about the disorder, including guilt that the parent has passed it on to the child. Such feelings should be discussed in the initial interview and throughout any treatment the child receives. The way in which a parent who stutters handles their stuttering is also important, because these behaviors serve as a model for the child. It is my observation that a parent who avoids words or otherwise tries to hide stuttering is communicating an attitude that may move the child to a more advanced level faster than if the parent accepts the stuttering, comments neutrally about it in front of the child, and uses facilitating techniques to handle it.

   If any of the child's relatives stutter, it is important to find out whether they recovered. Research cited earlier found that among children who were identified within 6 months of the onset of stuttering, those with relatives who did not recover from stuttering were more likely to have persistent stuttering than those with relatives who did recover (Yairi, Ambrose, Paden and Throneburg, et al., 1996). However, see Walsh et al. (2021) for evidence that any family history of stuttering—whether the relatives recovered or not—may be predictive of persistence. I let parents know that treatment would be important whether relatives did or did not recover from stuttering. In my experience, treatment can overcome factors that suggest persistence. After obtaining this background information about family history, I turn to the onset and development of the child's stuttering.
5. **When did you first notice the child's disfluency?** I have found that if treatment begins relatively soon after a child starts to stutter (if treatment is warranted), we have a better chance of preventing negative feelings from building up for both the parents and the child. Therefore, I praise parents for bringing a child in promptly for an evaluation if they did so relatively soon after they first realized there may be a problem. Another reason I want to know how much time has passed since onset is that most of the predictive information on chronicity of stuttering is based on children identified within 6 months of onset. For example, Yairi, Ambrose, Paden and Throneburg (1996) found that children who naturally recovered began to show a steady decline in their stuttering during the first 12 months after stuttering onset, whereas children whose stuttering persisted for at least 3 years did not show such a decline. Therefore, knowing how long a child has been stuttering helps me make treatment decisions based on findings that some children are likely to recover without therapy.
6. **Was anything special going on in the child's life when the stuttering started?** This may provide some leads about the kinds of pressures to which a child may be vulnerable, which can help clinicians determine what changes parents might make to reduce stuttering. Events that may precipitate the onset of stuttering include the birth of a sibling, moving to a

new home, family travel, prolonged periods of anxiety or excitement, and growth spurts in a child's language or cognition (see Chapter 4). Often, no special circumstances have occurred at the onset of stuttering. Events surrounding the onset of stuttering should be discussed in a way that helps parents feel they are not to blame for the stuttering. For example, if parents tell me that their child first began to stutter during a busy holiday season or when they were away on a trip, I let them know that this situation at onset is not uncommon in children who stutter. I also indicate that the stuttering would probably have appeared whenever the child felt any of the kinds of stresses that are in a typical home.

7. **What was the disfluency like when it was first noticed?** Most stuttering begins with easy repetitions, although some children exhibit prolongations and blocks, as well. Some preliminary information suggests that when repetitions sound quite rapid (ie, when the pause between repetition units is brief), a child is more likely to be stuttering rather than normally disfluent (Allen, 1988; Throneberg & Yairi, 1994). In addition, rapid-sounding repetitions may be predictive of persistent stuttering (Yairi, Ambrose, Paden and Throneburg, 1996). However, the length of pauses between repetition units cannot be determined accurately without instrumentation, even though a practiced ear can help clinicians perceive the brevity of pauses between repetition units. This information should be used only to support an overall pattern of findings that will help the clinician decide whether or not to recommend treatment.

8. **What changes, if any, have been observed in the child's speech since stuttering was first noticed?** The most interesting changes include the frequency and types of disfluencies and whether and for how long the stuttering diminished greatly or disappeared altogether. As indicated in the discussion of Question 5 answered earlier, children whose frequency of core stuttering behaviors (ie, part-word and single-syllable whole-word repetitions, prolongations, and blocks) does not decrease during the 12 months after onset are at risk for becoming persistent stutterers. In my clinical experience, if a child's physical tension and struggle during stuttering are increasing, or if stuttering is becoming more consistent and less intermittent, the child is not exhibiting a borderline level of stuttering, and direct treatment should be considered.

9. **Does the child appear to be aware of their disfluency?** If a child appears to have no awareness of their disfluencies, I am more likely to categorize them as normally disfluent or as having borderline stuttering than if they notice or seem concerned about their disfluencies. If they show negative awareness, such as expressing frustration, this may be described as experiencing beginning stuttering. Note that a child may be aware of their stuttering but not particularly bothered by it; some children are even amused by it when it first occurs, though this often quickly changes to frustration. Indicators of a child's awareness include such things as their commenting about their stuttering, either when it occurs or at some other time, responding to the fact that people have brought it to their attention. Awareness is also indicated if a child stops when they are disfluent and starts again or laughs, cries, or hits themself when they stutter. Even without any of these signs, a child may still be quite aware of their stuttering. In a study of 1,096 stuttering children between the ages of 2 and 7 years, the most frequent response suggesting awareness was asking for help (Boey et al., 2009).

   In some cases, preschool children may show more than just signs of frustration. They may show negative feelings about talking and may fear using certain words. They may even comment that they wish they could speak like someone else. These signs of awareness are indications that treatment is warranted.

10. **Does the child sometimes appear to change a word because they expect to be disfluent on it?** Parents are usually able to perceive that this is happening because they can sense the child's apprehension about saying a word. I also may ask them if the child changes words in midstream; that is, do they start a word, get stuck on it, and then change it or stop talking? An example of this can be found on Lippincott Connect Chapter 1 video "A Young Preschool Child: Borderline Stuttering" when she can't finish the word "Cookie" and gives up and starts a new sentence. Such behaviors are warning signs. They suggest that the child is avoiding a possible stutter because stuttering is so distressing to them. They may be moving toward a more serious problem, indicating the importance of treatment.

11. **Does the child seem to avoid talking in some situations when she expects to be disfluent?** Again, this is something that most parents know because they sense the child's fear of talking, and like the word avoidances discussed in Question 10, this behavior may indicate a need for treatment.

12. **What do the parents believe caused the problem?** In some cases, parents may express ideas about the possible causes of their child's stuttering that I believe are appropriate and accurate. In other cases, parents' beliefs about causal factors appear to be incorrect, and I respond by providing more accurate information. I am particularly sensitive to whether or not parents blame themselves or each other for their child's stuttering. This is usually a good time to let parents know that they are not to blame. I tell them that some children may have slight differences in their neurological organization for speech, which may emerge as stuttering during the normal stresses and strains of growing up and learning to talk (see Chapters 2, 3, and 4). I may also add that sometimes differences in neurological organization may give rise to special talents, such as artistic or musical ones. In Question 6, I mentioned possible stresses related to the onset of stuttering. Sometimes, parents are deeply convinced that they caused

the child's stuttering. For example, the stress a child feels when their parents choose to divorce can sometimes trigger stuttering. I try to be honest, letting the parents know that this stress may have been related to the onset of the child's stuttering, but that the stuttering was probably dormant and would have probably appeared under other, different stresses. The parents and I then brainstorm how the child can be reassured of their love, and we discuss ways in which they can play a key role in their child's learning to deal with stuttering appropriately.

13. **How do the parents feel about the child's disfluency problem?**
The kinds of feelings and attitudes we are looking for are: Do they feel concern? Guilt? Do they assume the child will outgrow it? Parental emotions and attitudes are contagious and may influence the child to fear stuttering, particularly a sensitive child. If parents feel guilty or highly anxious, it is important to engage them in positive treatment activities as soon as possible. You will find some activities families can begin with in the section titled The Closing Interview.

14. **What, if anything, have the parents done about the child's disfluency?**
This question is aimed at finding out how the parents have responded to the child's possible stuttering. For example, have they asked the child to slow down or stop and say the word again? Knowing this will help me to decide what to do in counseling them. If parents are correcting the child, I may get them involved in therapeutic activities immediately so that they can develop more appropriate ways of responding. Either toward the end of the initial parent interview or at the end of the evaluation overall, I let parents know that direct suggestions to children about changing their speech are usually not effective in the long run. I always give them suggestions for specific things they can do instead, such as slowing their own speech without asking the child to slow their speech.

15. **Has the child been seen elsewhere for the problem? If so, what were the outcomes?**
This information can be important in planning therapy and counseling parents. For example, if their family doctor told them several years ago that the child will outgrow stuttering, this needs to be addressed because they may now be convinced that the child will not outgrow it. It is wise to comment positively or neutrally on what other professionals may have said or done. Because many children appear to overcome stuttering without treatment many doctors and nurses believe that their advice to parents to ignore the stuttering will have a good outcome. Some doctors and nurses, however, are learning to distinguish between children who are likely to recover without treatment and those who are not and will advise parents accordingly. By establishing relationships with pediatricians in the community, speech-language pathologists (SLPs) can help facilitate that process.
If the child has been in other treatment previously, knowing what advice the parents were given can be important. Sometimes, parents have been given excellent advice but were not able to follow it. If so, we need to find out why and help them overcome obstacles to helping their child. Sometimes, parents have had their child in successful therapy but have moved away and sought me out to continue the same kind of treatment. In these cases, I try to contact the previous therapist as well as explore with the parents what was done so that we can continue to work in the same direction as before. In some cases, parents come to me seeking a second opinion, and I am able to reinforce what others have said if I agree. In other cases, they may have been advised to ignore the child's stuttering, which may lead me to tactfully discuss the possibility of taking an entirely different direction now that more time has passed or indicators suggest that there may be more helpful alternatives.

16. **When and in which situations does the child exhibit the most disfluency? The least disfluency?**
This information helps to identify fluency disrupters and fluency facilitators that I will use to help parents facilitate their child's fluency. I have also found it effective to point out whenever possible all of the helpful things the parents are already doing. Just the awareness that their child's stuttering responds to environmental cues and thereby has some logic to it helps most parents feel more able to manage it.

17. **How does the child get along with their brothers and sisters and other children?**
Although I usually find that children who stutter relate fairly well to others, I want to determine whether a child's stuttering may be interfering with their relationships. Sometimes, when asking this question, I learn about pressure and competition from siblings or teasing by a sibling or by a child from outside the family who is acting as a bully in the neighborhood in preschool.

18. **What is the child's temperament like?**
Some children who stutter may be more emotionally reactive (temperamentally sensitive) than other children, and they may have less capacity for self-regulation (ie, being able to deal with that emotional reactivity). A seven-item scale, to be completed by parents or caregivers, has been shown to measure sensitive temperament in children (Ntourou et al., 2020). The scale (Short Behavioral Inhibition Scale or SBIS) has been shown to be a valid and reliable assessment of behavioral inhibition—a characteristic of children that is similar to sensitive temperament. For example, a more inhibited child might be more apt to shy away from unfamiliar people. Ntourou et al. also found that the SBIS demonstrated significantly greater behavioral inhibition in a group of children who stuttered (n = 183) compared to a group who did not (n = 201) (P = .038) (effect size $\eta^2_p = .02$).

Further analysis showed that children who stuttered who were more behaviorally inhibited showed significantly greater stuttering frequency and stuttering severity, as well as significantly more negative speech-related attitudes. This scale, which is both simple to administer to parents or caregivers and easy to interpret, can provide clinically relevant information when used in an assessment. First, it can identify children who are highly behaviorally inhibited. In my experience, these children are less likely to benefit from highly structured, direct treatments (such as the Lidcombe Program) but may do better with a less direct approach (such as parent-child interaction therapy). And the converse is true (also, in my experience but without objective data to support my impressions): less behaviorally inhibited children thrive in programs such as Lidcombe. Second, as Ntourou et al. (2020) pointed out, there is evidence that more behaviorally inhibited individuals are more susceptible to classical conditioning (cf. Arenas & Zebrowski, 2013; Holloway et al., 2014). Readers may recall that classical conditioning plays a role in the development of stuttering (see Chapters 5 and 6). In short, using the SBIS may help a clinician pinpoint those children who will be most susceptible to conditioning and then implement steps to minimize/counter the effects of negative responses by listeners or the child themselves.

19. **What is a typical day like for your child?**
It can be helpful to get an idea of how busy and rushed a family is. For one thing, it has been my experience that many children who stutter and their families benefit from having less hectic schedules, particularly if the child seems happier when the home is more tranquil. You can add this information to what the parents told you about when their child stutters most to develop a hypothesis about how much the family's schedule may be affecting the child's fluency. If the child stutters more when things are busy, frantic, and stressed, it may be appropriate to brainstorm with the parents about how everyone can have a little more "downtime." Knowledge of the family's schedule will also help you begin to consider treatment recommendations. Some treatments are demanding of parents' time and attention, and their schedule must be considered in working with them to determine the most appropriate treatment approach for their child.

20. **Is there anything else you can think of to tell me that will help me better understand your child's stuttering and your concerns?**
Sometimes, it is not possible to direct questions to all areas of concern, and this question provides parents an opportunity to provide information that I have not thought of asking about.

To see an actual parent interview, go to Lippincott Connect and watch the video titled "Preschool Evaluation: Parent Intake Interview." Observe how the clinician learns from the parents about the onset and development of the child's stuttering up to its current status.

Clinician-Child Interaction

One of the most important parts of a preschool child's evaluation is the **clinician-child interaction**. Here, the clinician can see "up close" what the child's speech is like, the extent to which the child is willing to talk about their speech, how the child responds to various cues, and how well they can modify their disfluency. I always record this interaction for later analysis because it is difficult to make notes as we interact. Video recording is preferable because visual cues are often critical in determining a child's developmental and treatment level. If audio recording alone must be used, the clinician should make notes on visual aspects of the child's disfluencies. In this section, I will also discuss the special challenges by children who may be reticent about talking about their speech.

To begin, I focus my interactions on toys or games that are suitable to the child's age. For preschoolers, the Playskool farm or airport is a good example. I play alongside the child, letting them direct the action, commenting on what they're doing or playing with. I refrain from questions as we begin and I talk in an easy, relaxed manner, much as I advise parents to do.

If a child's stuttering is like that described by the parent, I maintain the same speech style throughout the interaction. However, if a child is entirely fluent or normally disfluent and the parents have described behaviors typical of stuttering, I speak more rapidly and ask many questions. Occasionally, I interrupt the child to elicit disfluent speech, even stuttering. I do this to avoid misdiagnosing a child who is stuttering as a typically fluent speaker.

An adult client of mine described an experience that illustrates my concern. When she was 5 years old, she stuttered quite severely, and her parents were understandably concerned. Seeking the best help, her mother took her to a famous university speech clinic for an evaluation. For reasons she never understood, she was relatively fluent throughout the entire evaluation. The clinicians observed her temporary fluency and despite her mother's protestations that her daughter stuttered at home did not diagnose her stuttering and advised her mother to ignore any disfluency. Her disfluency gradually worsened, and she developed severe, chronic stuttering. Nonetheless, I realize that, even by putting pressure on the child, I may not elicit stuttering that the child displays in other settings. Thus, the parents' report and the recording they made before the evaluation are of vital importance for a full understanding of a child's speech.

Talking About Stuttering

Before interacting with a child, I try to determine from talking with a child's parents whether the child is aware of their stuttering. If I think the child isn't, I simply observe the child's speech while the child and I play. If it seems clear that the child is aware of their stuttering, I then try to determine how comfortable the child is in talking about their stuttering. Sometimes, if the child is old enough to understand, I ask the child if they know why they have come to see me. Most children answer noncommittally, but some say something like, "Because I don't talk right." This gives me an opening to discuss the stuttering. I would respond to such a comment by saying something like "It sounds like words sometimes get stuck" or another statement that acknowledges their expression of difficulty with speech. I might also say "Lots of kids that we see here have trouble getting words out. It's OK if words get stuck sometimes, but we can usually help kids and make it easier for them to talk."

Some clinicians help a child talk about their stuttering by first talking about another child who stutters (Bloodstein, personal communication, October 15, 1990). In discussing stuttering with a child, I usually try to use their vocabulary, such as "getting stuck" or "having trouble on words." If a child seems reluctant to talk about stuttering, I drop the issue for the moment and return to playing. Then, later, I will insert a few natural-sounding disfluencies in my speech and comment that I sometimes have trouble getting words out.[2] I might play some more and then insert a few more disfluencies and ask the child if they ever have trouble like this. As before, the child's response will indicate that either they remain unwilling to discuss stuttering or they will give the clinician an opening to discuss, little by little, their disfluency problem. In summary, the goals of these attempts to discuss a child's disfluency are (1) to see if they are willing to talk about their disfluencies and (2) to assure them that they are not alone with the problem and that their parents and I can help them.

A Child Who Won't Talk

At times, I encounter a preschooler who is reluctant to separate from their parents. A shy child may start to cry and cling to their parents. I don't force the child to separate, of course. It is more important to have them positively inclined toward therapy (which they will probably equate with me) than to try to elicit a few stutters. In this situation, I sit quietly while the parent and child play together. After a few minutes, I join in the play, without focusing on the child, and after a few more minutes, I'll comment on what the parent and child are doing or what I'm doing with a tractor or a farm animal or whatever I'm playing with. In most cases, the child will soon say something to me or include me in the play. This interaction, leading to at least a little speech from the child, gives me an opportunity to observe at close range any stuttering the child may have. Only after a child gets comfortable with me, do I attempt to discuss their trouble talking and only if I'm sure they are aware of their stuttering.

[2]I believe that it is appropriate for fluent clinicians to put a few disfluencies in their speech and refer to them as they talk with a child about stuttering. Everyone—even the most fluent speaker—has some disfluencies and at times they can be frustrating.

With some children, I do not attempt to discuss stuttering at all during our initial interactions, and I always take my cue from the child and go slowly in this area. A very shy child, who becomes even shyer if I produce a few easy disfluencies, may be quite turned off to therapy if I invade their space by asking about their stuttering at this point. You can infer many things about a child's feelings from observations rather than from their responses to direct questions.

A Child Who Is Entirely Fluent

Some preschool children who stutter may be entirely fluent during an evaluation. In such cases, there are several options. First, the recording I asked the parent to send me may include enough stuttering to provide a good sample for analysis. Second, if a child is in a particularly fluent period, I may reschedule their evaluation for a later time. If my recommendations to the parents enable them to change the home environment enough in the meantime so that the child remains fluent, the parents may wish to postpone the evaluation until, and if, the child's stuttering returns.

Speech Sample Analysis

With some experience, you will be able to do an accurate but quick analysis of the child's speech before the closing interview and then a more complete analysis afterward for the report that will go to the family, as well as be placed in the clinic files.

The following sections describe how to analyze samples of a preschool child's speech. You should have more than one **speech sample** to analyze from the recordings (1) that the parents sent in, (2) the parent-child interaction, and (3) the clinician-child interaction. Because you may want to use the Stuttering Severity Instrument (SSI-4) (Riley, 2009) as part of your assessment, you need to follow the procedures it recommends for this analysis. Thus, the sample obtained from the clinician-child interaction should include conversation using the pictures in the SSI-4. Riley recommended that as the child talks, the clinician should "interject questions, interruptions, and mild disagreements to simulate the pressures of normal conversation at home and elsewhere" (Riley, 2009, p. 4). The samples should be between 150 and 500 syllables long to ensure that you will have an accurate picture of the child's speech. By making transcripts of the samples, you can more easily quantify the variables described in the following section on patterns of disfluencies. I explain how below.

Patterns of Disfluencies

By analyzing the child's speech sample, I can determine whether or not the child truly stutters and, if so, their developmental/treatment level. I analyze the following six variables to begin this determination. The choice of variables owes much to six individuals who have written about the differential diagnosis of preschool stuttering (Adams, 1977; Curlee, 1984, 1993; Riley & Riley, 1979; Yairi & Ambrose, 1999). The excellent article by Brundage et al. (2021) provided further endorsement of the variables chosen.

1. *Frequency of disfluencies.* This is calculated from the entire sample and is expressed as the number of disfluencies per 100 words. Both normal disfluencies and those associated with stuttering are included in this count. Normally disfluent children have fewer than 10 disfluencies per 100 words. Frequency is also commonly assessed by calculating the percentage of stuttered syllables (rather than words) and by dividing the number of syllables stuttered by the total number of syllables spoken and multiplying by 100. Details for using both syllables and words are given in the "Assessing Frequency" section of Chapter 9.
2. *Types of disfluencies.* I described the following eight types of disfluencies in Chapter 9: part-word repetitions, single-syllable word repetitions, multisyllabic word repetitions, phrase repetitions, interjections, revisions-incomplete phrases, prolongations, and tense pauses. Children who are typically disfluent are likely to have more revisions and multisyllabic word repetitions, as well as many interjections when they are younger than 3.5 years old. Part-word repetitions, single-syllable word repetitions, prolongations, and tense pauses occur more frequently in stuttering children. Another distinguishing measure is the proportion of total disfluencies that are SLDs[3] (ie, part-word repetitions and single-syllable repetitions, prolongations, and blocks). Fewer than half of the disfluencies of normally disfluent children are SLDs, but about two-thirds of the disfluencies of children who stutter will be SLDs (Ambrose & Yairi, 1999; Yairi, 1997a).
3. *Nature of repetitions and prolongations.* This variable has several dimensions. First, normally disfluent children usually have only one extra unit in their repetitions, li-like this, but sometimes they may have two. As the number of repetition units increases, however, so does the likelihood that the child is stuttering. Second, I listen to the tempo of repetitions. If they are slow and regular, a child is more likely to be categorized appropriately as a typically disfluent speaker. If they are rapid or irregular, it is more likely that the child is stuttering. Third, I look for signs of tension in both repetitions and prolongations. Both visual and auditory cues can help here; tension can be seen in the child's facial expression and heard in their increased pitch or loudness and more staccato voice quality. Children whom I would consider typically disfluent seldom exhibit tension in their disfluencies.
4. *Starting and sustaining airflow and phonation.* The child who we usually consider as stuttering often has difficulty sustaining airflow and/or phonation when they are stuttering. You may observe abrupt onsets and offsets of words, especially repeated words, or momentary pauses with fixed articulator positions at the onset of words. Moreover, transitions between words may seem abrupt, jerky, or broken, much of the time. This may also occur during seemingly fluent speech, signaling that stuttering is just below the surface.
5. *Physical concomitants.* I look for physical gestures that accompany a child's disfluencies, such as head nods, eyeblinks, and hand or finger movements, especially gestures that coincide with the release of a disfluent sound. I also include such extra noises as a child gritting their teeth or clicking their tongue during disfluencies.
6. *Word avoidance.* Another sign I sometimes see in a disfluent preschool child, which suggests that they stutter, is word avoidance. This can be blatant, as when a child starts a word and then changes it, as in "pu-pu-pu…dog," or it may be more subtle, as when they say, "I don't know," when it's clear that they do know. I also ask about word avoidances when I interview a child's parents. When a clinician interacts with a child, they may sometimes miss avoidances in a live interaction, and it may take a viewing of the videotape to pick them out. For example, a few years ago, I noted on the videotape I watched after an evaluation a very subtle avoidance that I had completely missed during the face-to-face interaction. I had asked the child what he was going to dress as for Halloween. The child pursed their lips for a "B," but when they couldn't say the word, they used an avoidance by singing the Batman theme, "Na-na-na-na-na-na-na-nah! Batman!"

[3] SLD stands for stutter-like disfluency

In my experience, if a child shows any of the characteristics of stuttering just described, they should be considered to be at least a borderline stutterer. The presence of tension, stoppage of airflow or phonation, physical concomitants, or word avoidances would place them on a level more advanced than borderline. Further details on this placement are given in the sections on diagnosis that follow.

Patterns of Fluency

The single variable in this category is the child's speech rate. I assess preschool children's speech rate using the speech sample obtained for the SSI-4. Counting and timing procedures were described in the section on assessment of speech rate in Chapter 9. One sample of speech rates for preschool children is given in Table 9.5. If a child is stuttering and their speech rate is substantially below the range for their age, the extent to which stuttering slows their rate of speech may be a problem for both listeners and the child. Children whose rates are substantially above the norms—or who sound like they are talking too fast—may have the disorder of cluttering, which is described in more detail in Chapter 8.

Additional Tools for Analyzing Speech Characteristics

Stuttering Severity Instrument

Using the 150 to 500 syllable or longer samples gathered earlier, you should carefully follow the guidelines in the examiner's manual of the SSI-4 to determine a child's stuttering frequency, duration, and physical concomitant scores. These three scores combined result in a total score that can be used—with the "Percentile Ranks and Severity Equivalents" tables in the manual—to derive a percentile ranking for the child, which compares them to the norms for children who stutter. Severity Equivalents that range from very mild to very severe can also be derived from the total overall score. Sometimes, typically disfluent children may be rated as stuttering at the very mild level on the SSI-4. Thus, clinical judgment, informed by your analyses of the types and frequencies of disfluencies, must be used to decide which children are actually stuttering and which are not. Remember that the SSI-4 is not a tool for differentiating stuttering from normal disfluency but for assessing a child's severity.

Test of Childhood Stuttering

As described in Chapter 9, the Test of Childhood Stuttering (Gillam, Logan, and Pearson, 2009) can be used for children ages 4 to 12 years and is thus appropriate for older preschool children. This instrument evaluates the child's stuttering in a variety of speaking situations and provides a more in-depth analysis of the child's stuttering but takes more time to administer than the SSI-4. Although I have not used it often, I am aware that it provides additional information about stuttering types, speech rate and naturalness, and the effect of time stress on picture naming.

Feelings and Attitudes

In addition to obtaining information about the child's feelings and attitudes from the case history, parent interview, and my own interactions with the child, I might use the Impact of Stuttering on Preschoolers and Parents questionnaire (Langevin et al., 2010; see Chapter 9) to gather initial information about the child's (and parents') feelings and attitudes about stuttering. However, if the child shows signs of struggle and tension when they stutter, or if the parents indicate that the child is aware through various examples of their frustration with their stuttering, I explore with the child their feelings about getting stuck on words.

In the previous section on "Talking About Stuttering" when I discussed the child-clinician interaction, I touched upon asking the child about why their mother or father or another caregiver has brought them to our clinic. I will revisit that topic now. Before bringing up the topic of stuttering, I get to know the child by talking with them during various play activities. Then, as we play, I insert a question about their speech, such as "Do you sometimes get stuck on words?" Both the child's verbal and nonverbal responses to a gently asked question about stuttering tell me a lot. Even beyond what I notice when we are talking, I am often able to learn a great deal by watching the video of my interaction with a child. I find that by playing a video recording of my interaction, I am able to devote my undivided attention to observing key segments of the interaction. The recording often provides a rich payload of information about a child's feelings that may not have been apparent to me in the face-to-face meeting. Some children may be quite comfortable answering my question about getting stuck on words, while others are embarrassed, look away, or don't make clear responses. Still others emphatically deny they have any problem talking. If the stuttering is very mild and the child matter-of-factly says they don't get stuck, I may tentatively conclude that they really aren't aware.

Assessment of the feelings and attitudes of a preschooler leads me to conclude tentatively whether a child (1) is unaware of their disfluencies; (2) is occasionally aware of them and, even then, is seldom and only transiently bothered by them; (3) is aware and frustrated by them; or (4) is highly aware, frustrated, and afraid of them. The levels of awareness and emotion that a child has about their stuttering are an important consideration in planning treatment, as we shall see.

In addition, the questionnaire for parents described earlier in this chapter and shown in Figure 10.3—SBIS (Ntourou et al., 2020)—can be used to learn about how sensitive the child is. Children who are very sensitive will often be reluctant to talk about stuttering, and the approach to this topic should be gradual.

Other Speech and Language Behaviors

When I evaluate a preschool child's speech for stuttering, I also screen for possible speech sound, language, and voice problems. In addition, I make sure that the child's hearing has been checked recently and if not, arrange to have a hearing screening. Note that some aspects of the child's speech—including severity of stuttering and speech sound production—may be variables that suggest future recovery or persistence of stuttering. These are discussed in the upcoming section on **Risk Factors for Persistent Stuttering**.

A child's expressive language and articulation problems can usually be detected in the recorded parent-child or clinician-child interactions, although receptive language problems sometimes may be less obvious but might be revealed through the case history or parent interview. When I suspect problems in these areas, I administer formal tests. You may wish to consult Bernthal et al. (2022) and Velleman (2015) for testing articulatory and phonological disorders and Paul et al. (2018) for assessing language disorders. I will discuss the management of concomitant articulation and language disorders in Chapter 14 that deals with beginning stuttering.

My view of the relationship between language and stuttering, which I described in Chapters 3 and 4, is that one of the pressures on a child who stutters may result from language development that is much more advanced than motor development. Thus, in evaluating a child's language and articulation, I explore the possibility that their language exceeds age expectations. In addition, I observe their language usage and motor abilities and question parents about the child's general motor development and the intelligibility of their speech.

When language development outstrips motor development, there may be a risk that a child will try to produce long sentences at a relatively fast pace with a speech system that, at this age, is better suited to a slower rate. A child's motivation to speak quickly may come from their own eagerness to express complex thoughts, from their parents' pleasure at their adultlike speech, or just from the fact that adult speech rate models affect the child. We have demonstrated this with typically developing children—typical in both language and fluency (Guitar & Marchinkowski, 2001). We found that if a mother talks at her typical rate, then slows down her rate, and then repeats that sequence, the child will change their speech to match their mother's.

For a child who stutters and who also has advanced expressive language abilities for their age, rate of speech production may be an important factor to target in treatment. How rate is targeted in intervention depends on the child's level of stuttering. If the child is relatively unaware of their stuttering and does not seem to be reacting to it with escape or avoidance behaviors, and their frequency of stuttering is relatively low, I am likely to use an indirect treatment approach. I would train parents to use a slower, relaxed speaking style when speaking to the child as part of the treatment, with the expectation that their model of a slower speaking rate will influence the child to speak more slowly, thereby putting fluency within their reach. In such cases, I also explore ways in which the family may be putting pressure inadvertently on the child's language skills by expecting a higher level of language development than the child can achieve.

Verbal activities that some parents may particularly enjoy with their children, such as puns, wordplay, and teaching the child multisyllabic words, may convey to a child that the parents place high value on verbal ability. For most children, this would be an incentive to develop their verbal skills. But, for children vulnerable to fluency breakdowns, their parents' pride in their verbal proficiency may stress their ability to perform, resulting in increased disfluency. For those children who are really struggling with stuttering, parents' focus on verbal performance may create in the children's feelings of shame at their verbal ineptitude.

It is useful to compare a child's language (syntax) scores with their vocabulary scores. Researchers (eg, Anderson & Conture, 2000; Choo et al., 2016; Conture, 2001) have shown that many children who stutter have a disparity between syntax and vocabulary scores that is greater than that for peers who are typically developing. Interestingly, it has also been shown that children who have lower language abilities, relative to peers, at the beginning of treatment show greater long-term decrease in stuttering as a result of treatment (Richels & Conture, 2010).

As I review my observations of a child's speech and language, I consider not only the possibility that a child's language is advanced relative to their speech-motor abilities but also the possibility that their motor abilities are markedly delayed. A few children have motor problems that impair their coordination of respiration, phonation, and articulation with language production. Many are aware that speech is difficult for them and have already felt frustration and shame, not just about stuttering, but about the way they speak and how they perform other fine motor tasks. Therefore, to help these children improve their feelings about themselves as talkers, the parents and I work on their speech-motor skills. These children seem to benefit especially from models of slow but normal-sounding speech as well as activities that teach them to speak more slowly.

In addition to exploring the possibility of language and articulation difficulties, I also assess a child's voice. A hoarse voice may be especially significant in a preschool child who stutters because it may be a sign that the child has increased tension in their laryngeal muscles, perhaps in an effort to cope with stuttering. I look closely at how the child is handling their blocks and listen for signs of excess laryngeal tension, such as pitch rises, increases in loudness, and hard glottal attacks. Because many of the techniques I use in treatment of stuttering result in a more relaxed style of speaking, I usually don't treat voice separately from stuttering. However, if a child has voice problems other than hoarseness, or if hoarseness does not diminish with stuttering therapy, I refer the child to an otolaryngologist for assessment and then follow treatment approaches such as those suggested by Boone et al. (2014) that are appropriate given the child's underlying pathology.

Other Factors

In Chapter 4, I described a number of possible developmental influences on stuttering. As you conduct your evaluation of a preschool child who stutters, consult Chapter 4 for descriptions of these influences so that you can consider them as you gather information. These include physical development, cognitive development, social-emotional development, and the child's speech and language environment.

Determining a Diagnosis, Prognosis, and Planning Treatment

Once I've assembled the information obtained during the evaluation process, I turn to tasks that will prepare me to communicate with the child's parents, prepare a report and begin to plan therapy, if needed. In determining an appropriate treatment for the child, I begin by trying to puzzle out if the preschool child is normally disfluent and, if not, their level of stuttering: borderline or beginning stuttering. As well, I will consider risk factors for persistence that will help me develop a reasonable hypothesis regarding prognosis in the absence of intervention. In the following paragraphs, I briefly review these levels.

Typical Disfluency

All of the following characteristics must be met for a child to be considered normally or typically disfluent. The child has fewer than 10 disfluencies per 100 words; these disfluencies

SHORT BEHAVIORAL INHIBITION SCALE

Elizabeth Oyler DeFranco, Ph.D., CCC-SLP & Katrina Ntourou, Ph.D., CCC-SLP

Name: ______________________ Date of Birth: ______________________

Date of Evaluation: ______________ Age: _______ Sex: _______ Respondent: Mother Father

Below is a list of personal traits or characteristics that describe children. Please circle the number that best describes your child compared to other children the same age. For each item, please circle one number from the 1 to 5.

1)	Retreats immediately from unfamiliar people or objects		*OR*	Approaches people and objects	
	1 usually retreats	2 retreats somewhat	3 average	4 approaches somewhat	5 easily approaches

2)	Stays close to the parent		*OR*	Easily separates from parent	
	1 difficult to separate	2 hesitant to separate	3 average	4 separates easily	5 separates very easily

3)	Takes a period of time to warm up and interact with unfamiliar people		*OR*	Quickly warms up and interacts with unfamiliar people	
	1 long time to warm up	2 somewhat hesitant to warm up	3 average	4 approaches fairly easily	5 approaches and warms up very easily

4)	Stops playing and vocalizing when unfamiliar person approaches		*OR*	Continues playing and vocalizing when unfamiliar person approaches	
	5 stops	5 quieter and hesitant	3 average	5 plays and notices	5 plays and is unaffected by one's approach

5)	Stays alone and away from other children or caregiver/teacher when in a group		*OR*	Engages and easily mixes with children or caregiver/teacher when in a group	
	1 isolates	2 quieter and hesitant	3 average	4 mixes fairly easily	5 mixes very easily

Note to User of the SBIS: The 5- item SBIS is talker- group neutral, allowing its findings to be applied to both young children who do (CWS) and do not (CWNS) stutter. Thus, determination of whether the child stutters or not should be based on standard- of- practice behavioral, diagnostic, observational, etc., testing SBIS should be used only as *augmentation* of standard- of- practice testing and neither replace no substitute for standard for standard- of- practice means for classifying children as CWS or CWNS.

Figure 10.3 Short Behavioral Inhibition Scale.

consist mostly of multisyllable word and phrase repetitions, revisions, and interjections. When disfluencies are repetitions, they will have two or fewer repeated units per repetition that are slow and regular in tempo. The ratio of SLD to total disfluencies will be less than 50%. All disfluencies will be relatively relaxed, and the child will seem to be hardly aware of them and certainly will not be upset when they are aware. If the child's speech doesn't seem to fit into the category of typical disfluency, the diagnosis of borderline or beginning stuttering is usually made, based on which category best characterizes salient features of the child's speech and their reaction to it.

Borderline Stuttering

The child I place in this category has more than 10 disfluencies per 100 words, but they are loose and relaxed. The disfluencies may be part-word repetitions and single-syllable word repetitions, as well as prolongations, and the repetitions may have more than two repeated units per instance. Stuttering-like disfluencies will be above 50% (Yairi, 1997a), and the disfluencies may cluster on adjacent sounds (LaSalle & Conture, 1995).

Beginning Stuttering

Beginning stuttering usually occurs in children between 3.5 and 6 years old. The key features at this level are the presence of tension and hurry in the child's stuttering. Disfluencies may have some of these characteristics: rapid, abrupt repetitions, pitch rises during repetitions and prolongations, difficulty starting airflow or phonation, and signs of facial tension. Just the occasional appearance of these signs would make me believe the child is a beginning stutterer. A beginning stutterer also shows that they are aware of their stuttering (in some, this may be subtle) and may be frustrated by it. They child *may* use a variety of escape behaviors, such as head nods or eyeblinks, in terminating blocks. Occasional avoidance may occur. For example, a child who has developed language to the point of using "I" instead of "me" but begins to stutter on "I" at the beginnings of sentences may begin substituting "Me" for "I" to avoid the frustration of stuttering on "I."

Some preschool children are relatively advanced in their frequency and severity for beginning stutterers. They don't qualify as intermediate stutterers because that category is for school-age children. These advanced beginning stutterers are children who avoid words and situations, and their behavior and demeanor clearly suggest some fear and shame about stuttering. For example, they may use a variety of starters to begin sentences and look away or appear embarrassed when they stutter.

Although I use information from all sources to determine a child's developmental and treatment level, I have found that my own observations of parent-child and clinician-child interactions are most useful in making this (tentative) decision about developmental and treatment level. Parents are helpful in describing long-term changes in their child's stuttering, but they frequently miss avoidance behaviors, such as starters, circumlocutions, and postponements, which are critical indicators of this more advanced level of stuttering. Parents' reports do provide, however, as much information about a child's feelings and attitudes as I usually gather in observing interactions in the clinic. Thus, parent reports plus my own observations provide valuable, complementary data. A vital adjunct to direct observations is video recordings of parent-child and clinician-child interactions. I sometimes revise my initial placement of a child in a developmental/treatment level after viewing video of the interactions I have previously directly observed.

Risk Factors for Persistent Stuttering

Risk factors may also be termed "prognostic factors"—those elements within a child or in their environment that make it more likely that they will persist in their stuttering or take longer in treatment. Table 10.1 describes several of these factors. For almost all risk factors for persistent stuttering, you'll be able to get the information you need to determine a child's risk of persistent stuttering from the case history form, questionnaires, parent interviews, observations of the child, and measures of stuttering, speech sound production accuracy, and language skills. It should be noted that all children are unique and group studies that indicate risk factors may not necessarily apply to every child. In other words, some children with multiple risk factors for persistence may eventually recover without treatment and some children with no known risk factors may persist without treatment. The findings below are only guidelines to help clinicians decide if a child should begin treatment immediately or go through a period of watchful waiting.

In a longitudinal study of 58 children 3 to 5 years old diagnosed with stuttering, Walsh et al. (2021) found several factors to be associated with persistent stuttering when they were re-evaluated approximately 3 years later. Four factors were found to be the most reliable predictors:

1. Family history of stuttering, *regardless of whether these relatives recovered or not.*
2. Reduced speech sound production accuracy on the Bankson-Bernthal Test of Phonology (Bankson & Bernthal, 1990).
3. Poorer performance on the Nonword Repetition Task (Dollaghan & Campbell, 1998).
4. More frequent and more severe stuttering as indicated by the Weighted SLD metric (Ambrose & Yairi, 1999). This measure captures the frequency, type, and extent of SLDs in one number.

Walsh et al. (2021) suggested that these factors may predict persistence; more so, if multiple factors are operating together. They also advise that in a clinical evaluation, the Nonword Repetition Task may substitute for the Bankson-Bernthal Test if time for the evaluation is limited.

Singer et al. (2021) used data from previously published longitudinal studies (Chow & Chang, 2017; Garnett et al., 2019; Singer et al., 2020; Zengin-Bolatkale et al., 2018) to study the cumulative risk for stuttering persistence in 67 children, ages 3 to 5 years. The authors found that risk of persistence increased fivefold for each additional factor listed below.

TABLE 10.1 Risk Factors for Persistent Stuttering or Extended Treatment

Possible Factors Within Child	Factors Within Environment
Family history. If child's family history indicates that one or more relatives had persistent stuttering and did not recover without treatment, the child is more likely to have persistent stuttering (Ambrose et al., 1997). A more recent study suggested children are at risk for persistent stuttering if any relatives stuttered, whether they recovered on not (Walsh et al., 2021).	**Others' reactions to stuttering.** Clinical observations suggest that if family is critical or impatient with child's stuttering, persistence is likely. More sensitive children are probably more affected by family's reactions to their stuttering.
Gender. If child is a boy, persistent stuttering is more likely (Ambrose et al., 1997).	**Family communication style.** Studies suggest that when parents' language is more complex, stuttering is more likely to persist (Kloth et al., 1998; Rommel et al, 2000).
Speech and language skills. If child's language, phonological skills, or nonverbal intelligence is below normal, they are likely to persist in stuttering (Yairi, Ambrose, Paden and Throneburg, 1996). However, some studies question whether language skills are predictive of persistence (Watkins et al., 1999). Also, if there is a disparity between child's vocabulary and syntax, child may be at risk for continued stuttering or extended treatment (Conture, 2001). Walsh et al. (2021) found that reduced speech sound production accuracy on the Bankson-Bernthal Test of Phonology (Bankson & Bernthal, 1990) and/or poorer performance on the Nonword Repetition Task (Dollaghan & Campbell, 1998) predict persistence. Singer et al. (2020) reported that lower scores on both speech sound production and expressive language measures are related to persistence of stuttering.	**Family expectations.** Clinical observations suggest that high expectations for academic, athletic, and social or verbal performance can stress children who stutter, making the stuttering more likely to be persistent.
Sensitivity/temperament. Some evidence shows that children with inhibited or sensitive temperament may take longer in treatment or not reduce stuttering as much in treatment (Richels & Conture, 2010). A good measure of sensitivity can be found in Figure 10.3, from the article by Ntourou et al. (2020).	**Life events.** Many writers (eg, Van Riper) have suggested that stressful events may, in some cases, precipitate or perpetuate stuttering. These may include birth of a sibling, death of a relative, or emotional or physical conflicts in the home or in the environment.
Reactions to stuttering. If child reacts to stuttering with emotion and secondary behaviors, treatment may take longer. It may be related to temperament because emotional reactivity may cause more learned reactions (see Chapter 6; Ntourou et al. 2020).	**Family's schedule.** Clinical observations suggest that very busy homes in which children are overscheduled can put stress on a child who stutters. However, if child is successful in hobbies, sports, and other activities, this can bolster self-confidence.
Severity of Stuttering. Both Singer et al. (2020) and Walsh et al. (2021) reported that more severe stuttering is associated with greater risk of persistence.	

The variables most powerful in predicting persistence were:

1. Time since onset of stuttering (19 months or more)
2. Speech sound production accuracy concerns (standard score of 115 or less[4])
3. Expressive language concerns (standard score of 106 or less)
4. More severe stuttering (SSI score of 17 or greater)

Combining data from the two studies cited, clinicians would be advised to assess the following variables: family history of stuttering, severity of stuttering, time since onset of stuttering, speech sound production accuracy, and expressive language ability. Earlier studies had also suggested that these additional variables might be predictive of persistence: being

[4]The term "standard score" for a speech or language test is based on a scale with a mean of 100. Typical values for average children range from about 85 to about 115. Thus, the scores predicting persistence are not far from average.

TABLE 10.2 Factors That May Be Associated With Increased Likelihood of Recovery From Stuttering Without Treatment[a]

Factor	Comment
1. Decrease in stutter-like disfluencies during the 12 months after onset	This is an important predictor of recovery. Thus, it is important to follow preschool children and continue to assess their disfluencies.
2. Female sex	Some evidence suggests that females are more likely to recover.
3. No relatives who stutter or have ever stuttered	Preliminary evidence suggests that persistent stuttering may run in families.
4. Good language and articulation skills	Both receptive and expressive language skills should be considered. Evidence of speech sound production or language problems may predict persistent stuttering.
5. Good nonverbal intelligence scores	Children with persistent stuttering had normal but slightly lower nonverbal skills.
6. Outgoing, carefree temperament	Our clinical experience suggests that these children who begin to stutter often outgrow it.

NOTE: Factors 1-5 are based on evidence cited in Andrews et al. (1983), Yairi and Ambrose (1992a, 1992b), and Yairi, Ambrose, Paden and Throneburg (1996).

[a]When a young preschool child is assessed within 1 year of stuttering onset.

a male child; family history of persistent stuttering; having a sensitive temperament; child being upset when stuttering occurs. Possible environmental factors predicting persistence are listed in Table 10.1.

In addition to risk factors for persistence of stuttering, researchers have also suggested that certain factors predict recovery without treatment in young preschool children. These factors are described in Table 10.2.

Tentative Plans for Treatment

Although final planning must involve the child's family, at least tentative plans for treatment will be suggested by the child's diagnosis, level of stuttering, and apparent risk for persistence based on the data accumulated and analyzed thus far. Three general categories for my recommendations include (1) postponing treatment as the family and I continue to observe the child's disfluencies to see if they resolve or worsen, (2) indirect therapy that involves changes in the child's environment and helping the child become comfortable with their disfluencies as we increase their fluency, and (3) direct therapy that involves working directly with the child's stuttering to decrease its frequency and severity. I will explain further what these recommendations may look like in the next section where I will focus not just on the substance of the plans, but how they may best be communicated to parents in the closing interview.

In recent years, a final part of my planning before meeting with the family to share the results of the evaluation involves preparation of a brief, one-page summary (often hand-written) of findings and recommendations. This provides a common reference as we discuss the evaluation and where to go from here. Parents can share this with other family members, and if appropriate, the family can begin to make some changes immediately, without having to wait for the formal written report, which may take several days to prepare. A sample is shown in Figure 10.4.

Closing Interview: Recommendations and Follow-up

As I begin the closing interview with the family, I remind myself to take the necessary time to listen to the family's questions that may arise at any point. When I begin, I always make some positive comments about the child and the family and then describe important characteristics of the child's stuttering that I observed in parent-child and clinician-child interactions and the **preassessment** recording, if I obtained one. I stay away from jargon and strive to be as clear and straightforward as possible. I briefly describe the child's disfluencies, such as easy, tension-free repetitions that may be typical disfluencies, or struggle behavior accompanied by avoidances that may indicate unambiguous stuttering. I refer to the important information that the parents provided in the case history and our interview, such as the child's expressions of frustration or requests for help.

Some children will not need referral for treatment, such as when the child has only a relatively few typical, tension-free repetitions (both during the evaluation and as reported at home). Other children will show these typical disfluencies

Dear Katy and Charlie,

It has been such a pleasure meeting you and Susie today. Susie is obviously very bright and talented, and her language skills are impressive. She was also a delight to play with, showing enthusiasm and creativity.

During Katy and Susie's play together, Katy's warmth and attentiveness were evident. We think it was particularly helpful that Katy kept the focus of play on what Susie was interested in and let her take the lead.

Susie has great potential for improving her speech because of your good work with her. Children her age sometimes recover without formal treatment, but we are available should formal treatment be required. We will keep in contact with you about Susie's progress toward greater fluency.

To speed her recovery, we have a few recommendations:

1) Continue your facilitating manner of interacting with Susie. This includes using a slow and relaxed speaking style when you are talking and playing with her. Also, allowing plenty of pauses in your speech will assure her that she has plenty of time to talk. If others can do this as well when talking with Susie, she will benefit.

2) When possible, reduce the number of questions you ask Susie. Instead, try to make comments such as "I wonder if this hat goes on your doll," rather than "Where does this hat go?"

3) If Susie expresses frustration with her occasional disfluencies, respond in a reassuring manner, empathizing with her and letting her know that lots of kids get hung up on words sometimes, and that talking will get easier.

Again, we want to say how much we enjoyed having you visit today. As questions and concerns arise, please contact us by phone or email.

All the best,

Alyssa Jones, Alexandra Patch, and Barry Guitar

Figure 10.4 Sample brief comments given to family at the end of meeting.

quite frequently and may have several iterations of each repeated sound or syllable, li-li-li-li-li-like this. These children may have borderline stuttering. If a preschool child has signs of tension, fixed articulatory postures (blocks), and/or clear evidence of awareness and frustration and/or escape behaviors as they try to free themselves from their stuttering, I would classify the behavior as beginning stuttering. Treatment options for these children are described in the next few paragraphs. More details about treatment approaches for preschool children are given in Chapters 13 and 14.

If stuttering is a serious concern, I say so, and if the parents have expressed feelings of guilt about their child's stuttering, I again reassure them that they are not to blame but that they will be crucial in helping to resolve it. Next, after answering questions, I describe appropriate treatment approaches, such as environmental changes, indirect treatment, and direct treatment, which will differ depending on the developmental/treatment level of the child's problem.

Recommendations for Children With Typical Disfluency

If I believe that a child's speech is typically disfluent, I deal with the family's concerns rather than the child's disfluencies. Most families benefit from knowing how I reached my tentative conclusion, so I provide them with information about typical disfluency, such as the following: "During their preschool years, many normal children pass through periods of disfluency. Interjections, revisions, pauses, repetitions, and prolongations are common during these periods, but they usually occur in fewer than 10 of every 100 words. Interjections and revisions are more common than part-word repetitions, and part-word repetitions usually have only one or two repeated units per disfluency. [Note: I explain and demonstrate all these types of disfluencies.] Children who are normally disfluent are largely unaware of their disfluencies, do not react negatively to them, and gradually outgrow them."

In most cases, I use analogies to help the family understand their child's disfluent speech. For example, I may point out that learning to speak is like learning many other skills, such as riding a tricycle or learning to skate, and that a learner falls down a lot in the early stages. I look for analogies that will fit the family's experiences and environment to help them understand why their child is disfluent and how valuable an **accepting environment** can be to help a child feel good about themself. Parents who are concerned about their child's typical disfluencies usually feel reassured when they find out that this is not uncommon. In those rare cases when parents are still not convinced that their child's speech disfluencies are not stuttering, I teach them how to slow their speaking rates and increase pausing. I sometimes use a video from YouTube of a slow and relaxed speaker (such as "Fred Rogers' 2002 Dartmouth College Commencement Address") to illustrate how it sounds. Then, I set up another appointment to discuss their progress in slowing their speech rate and explore how the child's speech is doing. If parents really are concerned and seem likely to continue worrying and perhaps correcting their child's speech, a few more sessions can be helpful if focused on the typical nature of their child's disfluencies and the changes they have made in the family's environment, with plenty of praise for their work with the child and suggestions for improvement, if needed.

Sometimes, of course, I can be wrong about my perception that the child's disfluencies are typical disfluencies and not stuttering. A colleague of mine who had a relative in a distant city referred the relative's child to a well-known stuttering expert in their city. This very knowledgeable person evaluated the child and said they thought the child was not stuttering and the parents needn't worry about it. When my colleague—who is very experienced with stuttering—saw the child on a visit to the family some weeks later, it was clear to her that the child was indeed stuttering so she found another experienced stuttering clinician in that city to help the child. The new clinician evaluated the child, found her disfluencies to be stuttering, and successfully treated her.

In case I have been mistaken in my evaluation and because the family of a typically disfluent child may remain anxious about their child's speech, I always keep the door wide open for all parents of normally disfluent children. I reassure them that I am available to talk with them if they become concerned again and will be ready to work with them if their child does begin to stutter.

Recommendations for Children With Borderline or Beginning Stuttering

My theoretical perspective on stuttering provides guidelines for the treatment of preschool children (eg, see Chapter 6). In the chapters on treatment, I have organized treatment according to age, with younger preschool children generally labelled as having borderline stuttering and older preschoolers as having beginning stuttering. For both levels, an essential aim is for the child's fluency to be enhanced. This can be done using an indirect approach in which the family uses a slower speech rate with pauses, and many positive comments, in addition to other possible changes that make it more likely the child will find it easier and more rewarding to talk.

Good examples of parent behaviors that are facilitating and those that are not can be found in videos "Preschool Evaluation: Identifying Parent Behaviors (Part I) and (Part II)" with the Chapter 10 videos. Once these behaviors have been identified, the clinician can model fluency-facilitating behaviors and then have the parent emulate them as they play with their child. These steps can be accomplished even in the evaluation. Watch the video titled "Preschool Evaluation: Fluency-Facilitating Interactions" with the Chapter 10 videos.

For older preschool children, I often (but not always) use a direct approach that is focused on rewarding fluency. Second, the child should be helped to decrease or eliminate defensive responses to their stuttering. This may be done by increasing the child's fluency and responding matter-of-factly to stuttering, as in the Lidcombe Program (see Chapter 14). For some older preschool children with beginning stuttering, however, I may use an indirect treatment approach in which both the family and the child are guided to accept the present level of stuttering as fluency is increased, as in the parent-child interaction therapy (see Chapters 12 and 13). This is particularly important for more temperamentally sensitive preschool children with beginning stuttering.

For those preschool children evaluated fewer than 12 months after the onset of stuttering, there are guidelines to help decide which children should begin treatment and which can be followed for a period of time without treatment. First, children whose SLDs (part-word and single-syllable word repetitions, prolongations, or blocks) steadily decrease during the first 12 months after onset are more likely to recover without formal treatment. Other positive prognostic factors are described in Table 10.2.

I believe that any preschool child who has borderline or beginning stuttering should be treated or followed carefully for several months because if treatment is warranted, it should begin early. I stay in contact with families of children who are close to onset whose stuttering is diminishing, who have other indicators suggesting recovery without treatment is likely, and whose families are not overly concerned. However, if families are highly concerned or the child's stuttering is not decreasing and there are only few indicators of recovery, I begin treatment as soon as possible.

When I recommend therapy, my closing interview with parents is usually the first of many sessions we will spend together. Consequently, I don't need to accomplish everything in this meeting. Because treatment of any preschool child who stutters is often focused on the home environment, we frequently begin our discussion with things the parents can do at home. The chapters on treating preschool children (Chapters 13 and 14) contain more extensive discussions and guidelines for involving the family in treatment, but I will make some initial suggestions here.

In my experience, parents who are active in the ongoing assessment process from the beginning feel more hopeful, less guilty, and more motivated to be involved in treatment (see also Zebrowski & Kelly, 2002 and Zebrowski et al., 2022). Therefore, in the closing interview, I ask parents of preschool children who will soon start treatment to begin observing and recording the day-to-day variations in their child's fluency. Having them assess fluency in the home environment also gives me a more valid indication of changes in stuttering than if assessments are done only in the clinic.

I teach parents who are beginning treatment to use the Severity Rating Scale (Fig. 9.4) (Onslow, Andrews, et al., 1990; Onslow et al., 2003, 2018)—a form they use at the end of each day to record a number from 0 (no stuttering) to 10 (extremely severe stuttering), which is their estimate of the severity of their child's stuttering condensed from observations over the course of the day. Parents begin by rating the severity of the child's stuttering during the parent-child interaction that has just taken place in this evaluation session. The clinician also rates the severity of this sample. If the parents' and clinician's ratings differ by more than one point, the parents and clinician discuss the ratings and watch the recording of the interaction to help them come to a consensus. If more than one parent or another family member will be using the Severity Rating Scale, each person should be trained until their ratings are within one point of the clinician's rating of each sample. In addition to rating the child's severity every day, parents can use this form to record comments and questions they would like to discuss when we meet at the next session.

If a child with borderline stuttering is being followed but not formally treated, severity ratings remain an important part of the monitoring process. Clinicians can obtain information about the child's stuttering via phone calls or e-mails on a regular basis, and parents can report their severity ratings as well as discuss issues of concern and ask questions. In addition to monitoring the severity of a child's stuttering, it is often helpful to brainstorm with the parents about ways in which the environment might be made as facilitating as possible for their child's speech. I will discuss this in more detail in the following paragraphs.

For the younger preschool child with borderline stuttering who is being treated (ie, a child whose parents are concerned and/or who has multiple risk factors for persistent stuttering), the closing interview is a time when further appointments may be set up and changes in the family environment can be initiated. Such changes will be determined by the clinician's observations of parent-child interactions, the parent interview, and ideas that parents may have about what they would like to change. In my experience, one of the most powerful ways that parents can facilitate fluency is to set aside 10 to 15 minutes each day, preferably in the morning, for child-directed interactions. This is a one-on-one interaction without other children interrupting. In two-parent homes, parents may need to alternate which one does the one-on-one activity so that the other parent can watch the other children. Or a parent may conduct the session when the siblings are at school or napping. During these interactions, the parent primarily listens to the child and plays whatever games the child chooses. When the parent speaks, they should use a slow rate with frequent pauses. I have found this works best if the clinician models this interaction style and then watches the parent carry it out in the clinic. More information about changing the family environment is given in the chapter on treatment of the young preschool child with borderline stuttering (Chapter 12).

I also give parents of these children reading material or a video recording to help them better understand stuttering and what they can do to help their child. The book *Stuttering and Your Child: Questions and Answers* (Guitar & Conture, 2015) gives many good suggestions and is available from the Stuttering Foundation (www.stutteringhelp.org) for very little money. The video, *Stuttering and Your Child: Help for Parents* (Guitar & Guitar, 2003, Stuttering Foundation publication No. 70), is also available from the Foundation, both inexpensively through the online store and free as a streaming video on www.stutteringhelp.org.

For older preschool children with beginning-level stuttering, I recommend starting treatment as soon as possible using either a direct or indirect approach, depending on the child's temperament. These and other options for therapy should be described to the parents, and with the clinician's guidance, they should make an informed choice about which option to choose. In some cases, the family will be able to make their decision immediately. In other cases, they may need time to consider the possibilities.

If they choose to begin treatment immediately, one or more family members should be trained in recording daily severity ratings before they leave, and the next session should be scheduled. If the session can be scheduled within a week or two, they should be asked to bring their severity ratings with them. If it has to be delayed, the clinician should be in contact with the family each week to discuss their severity ratings until formal treatment can begin. During therapy, parents will bring in their severity ratings each week to discuss them with the clinician.

If treatment cannot begin for several weeks, I ask a parent or another family member to conduct one-on-one interactions with the child like those described above for the child with borderline stuttering. If the family is able to begin treatment immediately, the clinician can start the parents on appropriate activities.

Clinicians who carry out therapy themselves with the child will probably have a parent watch the first few sessions before the parent begins direct activities at home. With children whose temperament appears robust, I use the Lidcombe Program (Harrison & Onslow, 2010), which is a parent-delivered treatment described, along with approaches, in some detail in Chapter 14. When the family and I decide to use the Lidcombe Program, I describe the first phase of this treatment program—a daily parent-child session conducted at home—to the parents. In these daily sessions at home, a parent engages the child in an activity at an appropriate linguistic level to elicit fluent speech and reinforce fluent utterances, where "appropriate" means at a level that is easy enough to almost assure fluent speech. After explaining this to the parent, I model this type of interaction and then observe the parent as they try it. The parent then begins treatment at home, with weekly meetings with the clinician.

The closing interview should end when the family seems to have a good understanding of the clinician's findings, and they and the clinician agree what the next steps should be. Because a family may come up with new questions and concerns in the days following the evaluation, it is important to conclude the interview with information about how they can contact the clinician.

SUMMARY

- In evaluating a preschool child who may be stuttering, your task is to decide:
  1. Whether their disfluencies warrant treatment.
  2. If they do, you should also find out more about the child's history, current environment, speech behaviors, and reactions.
  3. What treatment seems reasonable given these findings?
- In assessing a preschool child, the important questions to answer are as follows:
  1. Whether the child is stuttering or is typically disfluent?
  2. Whether the child seems likely to persist in stuttering based on risk and protective factors?
  3. If treatment is warranted, whether indirect or direct is best.
- It is important to obtain some information prior to the formal assessment. This includes a recording of the child's speech at home and a completed case history.

- Key elements of the assessment for a preschool child are as follows:
  1. Case History Form
  2. Observation of parent-child interaction
  3. Parent interview
  4. Clinician-child interaction
  5. Analysis of child's speech
  6. Screening of hearing. Screening of language, articulation, and voice, especially if problems are suspected
  7. Determining risk factors
  8. Deciding on the child's need for treatment
  9. Discuss findings and recommendations with family
- Whether the child is to be treated as a typically disfluent speaker or as someone who stutters depends on your observations and interpretations rather than a simple score. You must weigh what you see and hear to determine whether these findings indicate stuttering, typical disfluency, or even another disorder. From the flood of information that you have gathered, you must extract the essential characteristics that will help the family make informed decisions about the treatment recommendations you make.
- To hone your judgment, make evaluation a continuing process. The procedures I have suggested for assessment and diagnosis in this chapter will give you a good start, but stuttering is highly variable, and no individual can be completely evaluated in just an hour or two. Consequently, you will overlook an important element at times, and sometimes a vital clue will not be present in the samples of behavior you see during an initial evaluation. With good ongoing evaluation of a client, you will be able to change decisions and redirect therapy as additional information and understanding become available. You will also be able to evaluate the effectiveness of your treatment and improve it when needed and, ideally, determine when it no longer seems necessary.

STUDY QUESTIONS

1. How do you determine whether a preschool child is stuttering, typically disfluent or has another disorder?
2. Why is it useful to obtain recordings of a preschool child's stuttering before the evaluation?
3. What are some indications that parents of a preschool child who stutters feel that they are to blame? How can you help them deal with those feelings?
4. What do you tell the parent of a preschool child who asks you what causes stuttering?
5. What are the variables assessed in the speech of a preschooler to determine their developmental/treatment level?
6. What are the advantages and disadvantages of talking to a child about their stuttering?

SUGGESTED PROJECTS

1. Role-play the part of a clinician in a parent interview, having a friend or classmate play the part of a parent. Practice your listening skills by only listening and asking no questions as the "parent" describes in detail their child's stuttering problem. Switch roles and then compare your impressions of the experience both as the parent and as the clinician.
2. Find websites on the internet that contain helpful information for parents of children who stutter.
3. One of the challenges for clinicians is to get a good speech sample from a child who may be somewhat shy or reluctant to talk to someone they don't know well. If you can play with a friend's child, experiment with different ways of interacting with the child until you find a "best" method. For example, try asking lots of questions, try just playing quietly alongside the child, and try playing with the child and making comments about things you are playing with together.

SUGGESTED READINGS

Brundage, S., Ratner, N. Boyle, M., Eggers, K., Everard, R., Franken, M-C., Kefalianos, E., Marcotte, A., Millard, S., Packman, A, Van-ryckeghem, M., & Yaruss, J. S. (2021). Clinical focus: Consensus guidelines for the assessments of individuals who stutter across the lifespan. *American Journal of Speech-Language Pathology, 30*, 2379–2393.

This article created a consensus of practicing SLPs (the authors) specializing in clinical research on stuttering to describe and enumerate assessment procedures used in the evaluations of stutterers across the age span. The authors presented procedures to use in six key areas for assessment and provided an appendix of tools and methods to use at each age level for a complete assessment.

Logan, K. (2020). *Fluency disorders* (2nd ed.). Plural Publishing.

Logan, who himself is a person who stutters, provided excellent guidance in doing clinical assessments, including how to obtain valid speech samples, make detailed analyses of them, and come up with treatment recommendations.

Manning, W., & DiLillo, A. (2017). *Clinical decision making in fluency disorders* (4th ed.). Plural Publishing.

These authors have had a great deal of experience in the field of stuttering and present excellent ideas about diagnosis and evaluation.

Richels, C., & Conture, E. (2010). Indirect treatment of childhood stuttering: Diagnostic predictors of treatment outcome.

In B. Guitar, & R. McCauley (Eds.), *Treatment of stuttering: Established and emerging interventions*. Lippincott Williams & Wilkins.

This unique chapter uses the authors' Communication-Emotion Model of Childhood Stuttering as a rationale for their thorough evaluation of a child's speech and language, as well as emotional factors in the child's life. Variables measured before treatment predict short- and long-term outcomes.

Shafir, R. Z. (2000). *The Zen of listening: Mindful communication in the age of distraction*. The Theosophical Publishing House.

This is an excellent introduction to the practice of careful listening. Shafir is a Speech-Language Pathologist who has developed her ability to listen to clients and writes eloquently about the healing powers of mindful listening.

Shapiro, D. (2011). *Stuttering intervention: A collaborative journey to fluency freedom*. Pro-Ed.

This is a very fine textbook on many aspects of stuttering—its nature, assessment, and treatment, written by someone who has coped successfully with his own stuttering for many years. The chapters on (1) preschool children, (2) school-age children, and (3) adolescents, adults, and seniors who stutter have insightful sections on assessment and diagnosis, as well as treatment.

Zebrowski, P., Anderson, J., & Conture, E. (Eds.) (2022). *Stuttering and related disorders of fluency*. Thieme.

This textbook contains many chapters on the nature, assessment, and treatment of individuals who stutter. Forty-four world-class experts write clear, understandable prose to describe, among other things, diagnostic procedure to use with preschool children.

11

Assessment of School Age Children, Adolescents, and Adults Who Stutter

Chapter Outline

Chapter Objectives

After studying this chapter, readers should be able to:

- Plan and carry out an evaluation of a school-age child, adolescent, or adult

- Understand how to evaluate a client's stuttering behaviors
- Understand how to evaluate a client's attitudes and feelings (and, when appropriate, those of the client's family)
- Understand how to determine appropriate follow-up to evaluation for each age level

Key Terms

Accepting environment: Behavior by parents and other family members (and teachers and classmates where appropriate) that convey to the student that the student and the student's speech are accepted

Classroom observation: Time spent in the classroom by the clinician to assess how a student's stuttering may be affecting them in their classes

Closing interview: A conversation at the end of an evaluation session in which the clinician informs the client or family of their findings, makes recommendations for the future, and elicits questions

Fluency shaping: Ways of speaking designed to induce fluency. Examples are slowed rate as well as easy onset of voicing and light contact of the articulators

Individualized Education Program (IEP): A plan, mandated by the Individuals With Disabilities Education Act, that describes how a person with a disability will be educated to meet their individual needs

Individuals With Disabilities Education Act (IDEA 1997): A federal law that mandates the procedures for gathering information and deciding on the treatment of children with disabilities in public schools

Parent interview: A conversation with the parent(s) in which parents of a young client in which they are encouraged to describe their student's/adolescent's stuttering and express their concerns and hopes. In this interaction, the clinician elicits and gives information relevant to the young client's stuttering

Pattern of disfluencies: The types of stuttering and/or typical disfluencies shown by someone who stutters. Examples are whole-word repetitions, part-word repetitions, and prolongations, as well as escape and avoidance behaviors

Preassessment: The time before the formal assessment, in which the clinician gathers key information needed for the assessment

Speech sample: A segment of speech used to assess a client's stuttering. A sample may be limited to 300 syllables, given time constraints and the client's volubility. It may be based on spontaneous conversation or something written that is read aloud. It is meant to be representative of a client's speech in general

Stuttering modification: Ways of managing stuttering that are designed to reduce struggle and tension. Examples are cancellations, pullouts, and preparatory sets, as well as helping the client to be open and unashamed of whatever stuttering remains as treatment proceeds

Teacher interview: A conversation with a young client's classroom teacher(s) for the purpose of getting information about the client's speech and performance in the classroom. Such a conversation may also be used to enlist the teacher's help with the client's treatment

Trial therapy: A brief administration of one or more therapy strategies, used for the purpose of determining the effect on the client's speech in an evaluation

SCHOOL-AGE CHILDREN

Preassessment

Evaluation of the school-age child is different from evaluation of the preschool student because the student's stuttering will by this point probably be more severe. An individual in this age group commonly stutters with at least some tension and struggle and will be frustrated and embarrassed by it. The reactions of the student's peers—and how they affect the student—are more important as well.

Clinical Questions

As with preschool children, it is important to begin an evaluation with certain questions in mind. What is the student's stuttering like? More specifically: What is this student's frequency and severity of stuttering? What types of disfluencies do they display? Mostly repetitions? Many prolongations? A notable frequency of blocks? Escape behaviors? Avoidances? What is their speech rate (is it below average because stuttering is taking up a lot of time)? With rare exceptions, the question of whether the youngster is normally disfluent or stuttering is not an issue. By age 6, most children who stutter do so in ways that are quite different from the normal disfluencies typical for their age.

Another key question: What emotions and attitudes does the student have about stuttering and about speaking? School children with considerable fear and avoidance may need special attention to these feelings and behaviors. Information about risk factors (eg, family history, time since onset) is important but not as critical as they are for a preschool student. For example, most school children who stutter have probably been stuttering for more than 19 months since onset. By the time a student is in school, natural recovery is less likely than in the preschool years; thus, an absence of risk factors doesn't warrant withholding or delaying treatment.

Information from the student's teachers, the clinician's observations of the student's speech in class and in the treatment room, and information from their family are all required to assign the student a developmental/treatment level. Questions about treatment of children in the public schools can be answered only in the context of federal and state laws, which are considered in the next section. With any school-age child, it is important to determine the child's school performance and whether stuttering interferes with it.

Public School Considerations

The **Individuals With Disabilities Education Act (IDEA 1997**, its reauthorization in 2004 and amendment through the Every Student Succeeds Act [ESSA], Law 115-95 in 2015) and individual state laws mandate the procedures that public school clinicians must use for gathering information about a student's disability and deciding on treatment. Every state will have their own guidelines so what I write here may not be exactly what is expected in the state you practice in. Check your state's regulations, usually accessible online via the state's Office of Education. Many states use a concept called Multi-Tiered System of Supports (MTSS) to make sure that all students are getting the educational input and support they need. The tiers of support are in a hierarchy from less intense to more intense extra support.

Tier 1 is support provided by changing the educational environment for a student but remaining in the classroom. Speech-language pathologists are usually members of a team that consults with teachers and parents to determine if a student's difficulty can be resolved by making changes in the educational setting. An example of such modifications might be discussions between the student and teacher about how the teacher can facilitate the student's class participation. If stuttering continues to be a problem in the classroom after the modifications have been in place for a designated time period or if the student's stuttering is quite severe, the speech-language pathologist (SLP) can provide some therapy outside the classroom under a Tier 2 plan. If this seems to work for the student, it can be continued, but at some point, when therapy is ongoing, the student should be placed on an Education Support Team (EST) Plan. At the same time, the SLP should document changes that are occurring in response to the treatment (changes are sometimes called "response to intervention" or RTI). The support team may consist of the SLP, administrators, special educators, possibly the student's parent(s), and others. In some schools and with some children, Tier 2 therapy may be the best approach.

Tier 3 is more serious and requires—in most states—that the student's stuttering (and/or related issues) meets the state's eligibility standards and that the student's stuttering has an adverse effect on his education. The student then could be placed on an **Individualized Education Program (IEP)** and receive direct services. The step to reach Tier 3 would be a formal evaluation by the multidisciplinary team to determine if the student meets all the requirements. As part of this evaluation, the clinician discreetly observes the student in the classroom and confirms (or disconfirms) that the student is stuttering. The clinician then discusses the student's problem with the teacher and the school's special education administrator. Next, the clinician, teacher, or administrator contacts the student's parents to ask permission to do a formal evaluation of the student. If permission is given, the clinician gathers information on as many dimensions of the student's stuttering as possible. Typically, this will include the frequency, severity, and types of stuttering observed in two or more situations, the student's feelings and attitudes about stuttering and speaking, concomitant speech or language problems, and overall communicative performance. The clinician uses standardized measures such as the SSI-4, observations, and interviews with the student and his family as well as with his teachers and others at school who know the student. After this information is gathered, a team composed of the clinician, teacher, special education administrator, and the parents meets to decide two issues. The first is whether the student's stuttering problems meet the state's criteria for eligibility, and the second is whether the student's stuttering adversely affects his educational performance. These two issues are discussed in detail later in this chapter, under the heading "Public School Setting," after the sections on the parent, teacher, and student interview.

Initial Contact With Parents

Whether contact is made because the student has been referred to the school clinician or because the parents have made an appointment at a private or university clinic, the clinician's most important task is to listen and try to understand the parents' point of view. If the school clinician is telephoning the parents for permission to evaluate their student, the clinician should describe the process by which the student was identified and convey the clinician's and the school's desire to help the student achieve their potential as an effective communicator. It will be helpful to briefly describe the disfluencies that identified the student as stuttering and to find out if the parents have also noticed them. The clinician should calmly convey their interest in the student and their stuttering in an accepting tone of voice, particularly because parents may fear that they are being blamed for the student's stuttering. It may help also to comment that current views suggest that stuttering may be the result of how the student's brain is organized, although its exact cause is unknown. The evaluation process should be described and permission sought. If the parents agree to an evaluation, this is a good time to ask them to fill out a case history form and, if possible, send a video recording of the student's speech, ideally with some stuttering, if the student stutters at home. It may be beneficial for the clinician to talk to the student as well and ask their permission to have their parents video record their speech at home. In some cases, the home video is easier to obtain once the clinician has gotten to know the student and has conveyed their acceptance and interest in the student and their stuttering.

When the evaluation will take place in a clinic rather than school, the clinician should call the parents and let them know what will take place in the evaluation, get some preliminary information about the student and their stuttering, let the parents know they will receive a case history form to complete and return, and request a video from home prior to the evaluation. As with the school clinician's telephone call, the parents' point of view about stuttering must be understood. Even though they will have a chance to talk over their concerns in person, they may also want to talk and ask questions in this preliminary telephone call.

Case History Form

The form used for this age group is the same one used for preschool children (Fig. 10.2). Some of the questions about speech and language development may be difficult for parents to recall. This is not critical for evaluating a school-age child, but it is important to probe for other speech and language problems that may be contributing factors in the school-age child's stuttering. An important section on this form deals with how the problem has changed since it was first noticed, what has been done about it, and how others have reacted to it. In addition, the section on educational history may let us know if the student is having problems in school.

Video Recording

Obtaining a video recording of the student speaking at home or elsewhere will help clinicians prepare for the evaluation because they can get a preview of the student's pattern of stuttering, analyze the sample ahead of time, and plan the assessment more carefully. For example, if a sample from home has little or no stuttering, the clinician may want to obtain another sample in a more difficult speaking situation. Up to a point, more varied samples of a student's speech lead to a more valid assessment. If a pre-evaluation sample has lots of avoidance behaviors in it, clinicians can prepare questions to ask the student about what they do when they expect to stutter, and explore in other ways the student's worry about and avoidance of stuttering. For example, the clinician can suggest that stuttering can be scary and many kids have figured out how to get around stuttering. At this point, the student may volunteer their ways of avoiding stuttering. If not, the clinician can ask the student how they handle stutters.

Assessment

Parent-Child Interaction

When I conduct an evaluation in a clinic, I usually first observe the student's speech with his parents while they are involved in an activity that promotes speech, such as how their favorite sports team is doing or describing a book or movie that they liked. I video record this with the participants' permission for later analyses and then pay close attention to both the student's stuttering behaviors and the parents' responses and interaction style.

Parent Interview

This description of the **parent interview** assumes that the parents have brought their student to a clinic for the evaluation. When the evaluation is school based, the clinician can get much of this information by telephone and follow-up with a face-to-face meeting at school.

Begin a clinic-based interview by sharing some positive observations about the student and their family and then describe the course of the evaluation. Before obtaining more background information to fill in gaps left by the case history, ask parents an open-ended question, such as requesting them to describe their concerns about their student's speech. Only after the parents or caregivers have had a chance to express their worries and observations do I ask follow-up questions. As I do with parents of preschool children, I explore the onset and development of the student's stuttering, their reactions to it, family members' reactions, and any gaps in the case history. I also ask parents of a school-age child about the child's school experiences. Does the student like school? Does their speech seem to bother them there? Do you think they participate less in school because of their stuttering? Is the student teased or bullied about their stuttering? Do you think the student stutters more at school than at home? Has the student gotten therapy at school? Has that helped? Is the student OK with the therapy?

As I ask parents questions about the student's stuttering at home and school, I listen for responses that may help me understand factors explaining why the student's stuttering has persisted into elementary school. Here are some of the questions I think about as I try to assimilate the information I am getting from the parent: is the student sensitive about their stuttering? Are the family and student comfortable talking about stuttering? Is the family supportive of the student and their ways of coping with their stuttering? Is the family motivated to participate in therapy?

Teacher Interview

The more assistance we can get from a student's teachers, the more we can help the student. We need to approach teachers respecting their heavy responsibilities and their concern for all of their students, including the one with whom we are working. But we also should anticipate that they may neither understand nor know what we do to help a student who stutters. As I conduct a **teacher interview**, I try to sense what they would like to know about stuttering and my treatment approach. The following questions serve as guidelines for the types of things I want to find out.

1. **Does the student talk in class? Does the student stutter in class? What is the student's stuttering like? How does the student seem to feel about their stuttering and about themself as a communicator?**
   Here, I am trying to determine how much the student stutters in class and whether this stuttering keeps them from talking as much as they might otherwise if they did not stutter. I may also get a flavor of how the teacher feels about the student, the student's communication abilities, and the stuttering.
2. **Does stuttering interfere with the student's performance in school?**
   This question is obviously related to the previous one about the student's stuttering in class. But it also may give us some information about how much the student may avoid speaking, especially volunteering in class. I ask about disparities between the student's oral and written performance; a large disparity may indicate that the student declines to talk or says "I don't know" even when the student knows the answers.
3. **Do other children tease them about stuttering?**
   Most school-age children who stutter are teased, at least a little, and I want to get more information about how much the student is teased (or bullied) and how it affects them. I also want to find out about any school policies that relate to bullying since teasing may be just the tip of the iceberg, and many schools are developing strategies for addressing both teasing and bullying.
4. **How do you feel about the student's stuttering, and how do you react to it?**
   I am often able to get this information indirectly, from what the teacher has already said, but if not, I ask directly. Teachers are also likely to ask how they *should* respond to a student's stuttering, which is an important issue because a teacher's response often influences how the class responds. This and other issues related to the student's speech in the classroom are discussed in the chapter on treatment of intermediate stuttering (Chapter 15).

In addition to talking with the teacher, I have used a questionnaire that they complete to report their observations on the student's communication ability in the classroom. This tool, the *Teacher Assessment of Student Communicative Competence* (TASCC; Smith et al., 2000), depicted in Figure 11.1, is designed to help determine the effect of the student's stuttering on their education. For example, one of the subscales measures approach/avoidance in the classroom based on questions about the student's class participation and volunteering to talk. Other areas that the teacher rates the student on include intelligibility, comprehension, appropriateness of communication, and pragmatic/nonverbal communication skills. I have also found the TASCC to be helpful in getting information about how a student's communication is changing over the course of treatment. The measure was tested on 69 students in grades 1 through 5 in Maine, Vermont, Texas, Virginia, and Idaho and showed high internal consistency. Cronbach's coefficient alphas (a measure of a test's reliability) for the five subscales ranged from 0.77 to 0.95, suggesting that the TASCC items were related, measuring a similar construct (Smith et al., 2000). Redundancy analysis was used to remove redundant items and combine some that were similar, leaving a 50-item scale.

Two master's theses were conducted on the TASCC to explore its use with school-age children who stutter. The first assessed 14 children who stuttered paired by gender and ethnic background with 14 who did not stutter (Sequin, 1999). Scoring of each pair of participants was obtained from teachers of children in grades 1 to 5; the participants included eight Caucasian pairs, two Hispanic pairs, and four African American pairs. Three of the pairs were females and 11 were males. The children who stuttered had significantly lower communicative competence scores ($P = .0001$) than the control children; the "approach/avoidance attitude" subscale showed the greatest difference between the groups. A second pilot study (Pierson, 2004) compared TASCC ratings of eight children who stuttered and eight children who did not (grades 1-5) matched for age, gender, grade, cultural background, and academic performance. Again, the children who stuttered had significantly

TEACHER ASSESSMENT OF STUDENT COMMUNICATIVE COMPETENCE (TASCC)

Student's Name ________________ **Age** ____ **Gender** _____ **Ethnicity** ________

Below are a series of items that describe a student's communicative competency. Use the following scale to rate a student in your grade whom you consider to have communication competency issues. For each item, circle the number that best describes the student's communication. Please answer each item as well as you can, even if the item does not seem to apply to the student.

1 = Never **2 = Seldom** **3 = Sometimes** **4 = Often** **5 = Always**

Item					
1) Student remains attentive when others communicate with him/her	1	2	3	4	5
2) Student verbally relates thoughts in an age-appropriate meaningful manner to adults	1	2	3	4	5
3) Student adjusts style and content of speech according to communication partner and situation	1	2	3	4	5
4) Student appears to nonverbally relate feelings in an age-appropriate meaningful manner (e.g., facial glare, smile)	1	2	3	4	5
5) Student demonstrates age-appropriate nonverbal requests for message repetition (e.g., makes a "puzzled" face)	1	2	3	4	5
6) Student participates in age-appropriate turn-taking in conversations and class discussions	1	2	3	4	5
7) Student demonstrates age-appropriate verbal requests for message repetition (e.g., "Could you say that again?" or "What?")	1	2	3	4	5
8) Student uses appropriate voice inflection when speaking (e.g., intonation with questions)	1	2	3	4	5
9) Student uses appropriate eye contact when speaking to adults	1	2	3	4	5
10) Student gets the listener's attention before the student introduces a topic	1	2	3	4	5
11) Student uses age-appropriate opening and closing communication comments in conversations with peers (e.g., "Hello, see you later.")	1	2	3	4	5
12) Student's speech is understandable even when the topic is unknown	1	2	3	4	5
13) Student participates in story-description/retell interactions	1	2	3	4	5
14) Student verbally relates thoughts in an age-appropriate meaningful manner to peers	1	2	3	4	5
15) Student sticks up for his/her own views when confronted by group pressure	1	2	3	4	5
16) Student's overall speech is understandable (e.g., clear voice, clear articulation)	1	2	3	4	5

Figure 11.1 Teacher assessment of student's communicative competence.

17) Student nonverbally expresses frustration toward peers when appropriate	1	2	3	4	5
18) Student responds within an appropriate time frame to remarks, questions, requests	1	2	3	4	5
19) Student joins into conversations with peers easily	1	2	3	4	5
20) Student uses vocabulary that is relevant to the conversation	1	2	3	4	5
21) Student appropriately engages in group discussions	1	2	3	4	5
22) Student uses appropriate rate of speech for situation	1	2	3	4	5
23) Student initiates topics of conversation in one-to-one situations with adults	1	2	3	4	5
24) Student initiates topics of conversation in one-to-one situations with peers	1	2	3	4	5
25) Student adjusts vocal intensity to account for distance and noise variables	1	2	3	4	5
26) Student freely volunteers answers to questions in class	1	2	3	4	5
27) Student uses speech effectively in directing peer's actions when intended	1	2	3	4	5
28) Student's speech is understood by unfamiliar listeners	1	2	3	4	5
29) Student uses appropriate eye contact when speaking to peers	1	2	3	4	5
30) Student uses age-appropriate humor within peer conversations	1	2	3	4	5
31) Student uses age-appropriate verbal communication to gain attention	1	2	3	4	5
32) Student nonverbally expresses frustration toward adults when appropriate	1	2	3	4	5
33) Student uses a variety of age-appropriate (or better) vocabulary	1	2	3	4	5
34) Student seems to understand age-appropriate humor within peer conversations	1	2	3	4	5
35) Student clarifies and/or rephrases when verbal communication is not understood by the listener	1	2	3	4	5
36) Student uses age-appropriate (or better) sentence length when answering questions in class	1	2	3	4	5
37) Student is able to shift to different topics within conversations	1	2	3	4	5
38) Student links his/her words together with age-appropriate (or better) grammatical structures	1	2	3	4	5
39) Student follows three-step instructions with minimal need for repetitions or visual cues	1	2	3	4	5
40) Student's speech is understood even when the speech becomes more complex (e.g., longer sentences, change in topic)	1	2	3	4	5

Figure 11.1 *(Continued)*

41) Student verbally or nonverbally indicates that he/she understands the speaker's message	1	2	3	4	5
42) Student is able to integrate information presented auditorily (e.g., lessons, stories, a sequence of directions) and comprehend the meaning	1	2	3	4	5
43) Student identifies characters/people in conversations	1	2	3	4	5
44) Student uses age-appropriate (or better) sentence length when having a conversation	1	2	3	4	5
45) Student uses the environment to get a message across when the student's verbal communication is not understood (e.g., points to relevant objects or people)	1	2	3	4	5
46) Student seems to understand nonverbal communication (e.g., gestures)	1	2	3	4	5
47) Student uses age-appropriate nonverbal communication to gain the attention of adults	1	2	3	4	5
48) Peers and adults seem to understand what the student says to them	1	2	3	4	5
49) Student interacts with a variety of peers and adults	1	2	3	4	5
50) Student uses age-appropriate nonverbal communication to gain the attention of peers (e.g., wave, gentle tap)	1	2	3	4	5

TASCC SUBSCALES

The TASCC is divided into five subscales. The following information indicates which items, distributed randomly, belong to which subscales.

Subscale	Item #s
I. Intelligibility	8, 12, 16, 22, 25, 40, 48
II. Appropriateness of Communication	2, 3, 6, 10, 11, 13, 14, 18, 20, 27, 30, 31, 33, 36, 37, 38, 44
III. Comprehension (of input) and Clarification or Repair (of output)	7, 34, 35, 39, 41, 42, 43, 46
IV. Pragmatic/Nonverbal	1, 4, 5, 9, 17, 29, 32, 45, 47, 50
V. Approach/Avoidance Attitude	15, 19, 21, 23, 24, 26, 49

Figure 11.1 *(Continued)*

lower communicative competence scores (P = .002). The approach/avoidance attitude subscale was not found to be significantly different between the groups, but the following three scales were, with the differences between the groups in this rank order: (1) intelligibility > (2) appropriateness of communication > (3) clarification/repair (of output)/comprehension (of input) > (4) pragmatic/nonverbal communication. Clinically, I have found it useful to know what subscales are most deviant for a student in a classroom. In one instance, a student who was rated deviant on the intelligibility subscale benefited from learning to speak more slowly and loudly, even when he stuttered.

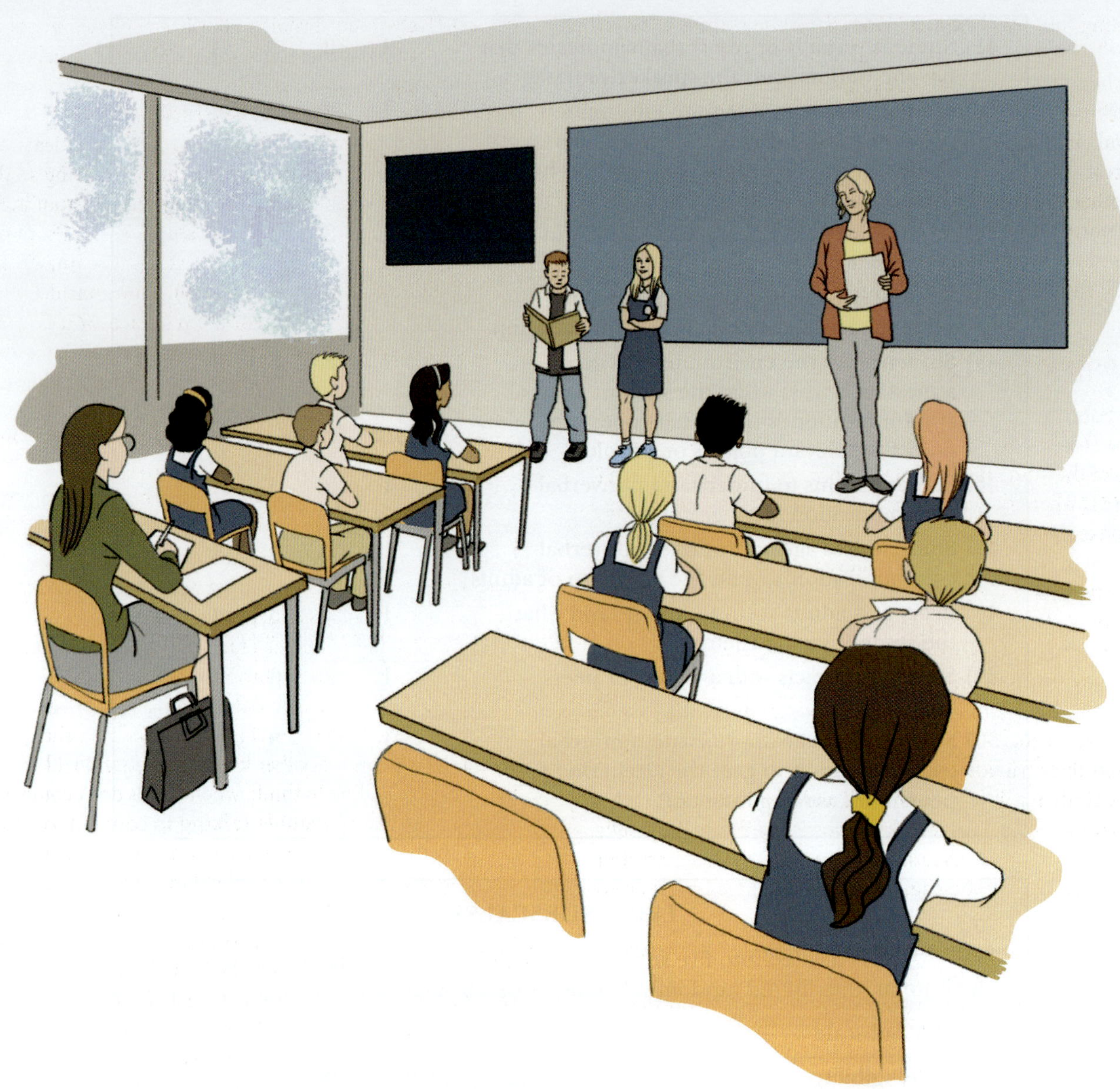

Figure 11.2 Classroom observation by SLP.

Classroom Observation

In addition to the information obtained from teacher and parent interviews and the TASCC, direct **classroom observation** can help clinicians understand the severity of a student's stuttering and the degree to which it interferes with their academic adjustment. If a student is to receive services in the school, the clinician must establish that the student's stuttering is interfering with their education. One way to verify this is by firsthand observation of a student in the classroom.

You should arrange with the teacher to come to the classroom at a time when the student will have opportunities to participate in class and observe the class as unobtrusively as you can. By observing the class when many students are participating, not just when the student you are evaluating is talking, you will not call as much attention to them. Figure 11.2 depicts how this observation may take place. Most school-age children want to be like their peers and dread being singled out. For more on this, read the very funny essay by David Sedaris about being pulled out of class to work on his lisp. This essay can be found by Googling "Go Carolina pdf."[1] When I observe a student in a class, I let the student know beforehand that I will not be interacting with them when I come to class, so no one will know I am there to observe them. I let the student know that I only want to hear their speech in class. Notice whether the student participates in class discussion. If called on, does the student speak in a straightforward manner or does the student hesitate or deploy any postponement devices, such as

[1]David Sedaris exaggerates his descriptions of some of his characters, so don't take his depiction of the speech-language pathologist in this essay too seriously.

repeating "uh" several times? Does the student answer "I don't know?" This is a reply many children who stutter (including me, when I was in school) use to avoid speaking and thus risk stuttering—even when they know the answer. If the student does talk in class and happens to stutter, notice how other children react to the student's stuttering. Do they giggle and look at each other and make comments under their breaths, or do they seem normally attentive? Because the classroom is the arena where children learn, socialize, and develop communication skills, it should be a target of assessment and treatment.

Student Interview

After I obtain parents' consent to evaluate a student, I arrange for the student to come to the treatment room. Here, I work to make the student feel that my room is an **accepting environment** where they can have fun and also discover how they can make their speech much easier. School-age clients sometimes tell me that it helps just to have someone to talk to about stuttering and other things that are bothering them. This can occur only after a trusting relationship is established, and the initial interview is the beginning of building that relationship.

During our first encounter, it is important for a student to feel that I am genuinely interested in them as well as their stuttering. I usually begin by asking what the student likes to do, who their friends are, and who is in their family. Then, I tell the student a little about myself and how I work with other kids who sometimes get stuck on words. As the student talks, I note whether or not they stutter or not and how they stutter. When a student's body language and behavior tell me they are comfortable in the session, I talk to them about their speech. The following questions are not asked one right after another but over a session or two. Often, it is more effective to make the question a comment, such as phrasing the first question below as "Sometimes kids have trouble getting words out. Their words just seem to stick a little bit." Then, leave some silence to see if the youngster will talk about his own speech. Whatever you do, don't ask the questions "bang-bang-bang," one right after the other. The questions I list below are just to give you ideas for talking to the student about their experiences and feelings. For most children, talking about their stuttering will make them anxious so you need to do things that relieve their feelings as they talk. Playing a game while you talk is helpful as long as it isn't so engrossing that talking about their speech annoys them because it distracts them from the game.

1. **Do you ever think that you have any trouble talking?**
I rarely see school children who stutter who are unaware of their difficulty. However, if a student regards their problem as minor or seems genuinely unaware of the problem, I avoid giving it undue emphasis or creating an unfavorable attitude about it. Thus, my first talk with a student is usually low-key, and if they truly don't seem to be bothered by their stuttering, although their parents and teachers are, I respect the student's perception and try to treat it as a relatively minor problem, but I remain aware that the student may be bothered by their stuttering much more than they wish to let on at first.
2. **What happens when words get stuck for you?**
I am looking for several things here. One is to learn the words the student uses to describe their stuttering so that I can use them when talking with the student about it. For example, they may say they "get stuck" or are "jammed up." I also want to find out if the student is unaware of some of their stuttering behaviors, if they consider these behaviors to be too painful for them to face, or if they just don't like talking about them. Even more important, these questions let a student know that the clinician really wants to understand their problem.
3. **Have you learned to use any helpers to get words out? Do you sometimes avoid certain words?**
With this question, I can convey that I understand what some kids do when they stutter. I can also let a student know that I am nonjudgmental about the dodges they use to avoid stuttering by conveying my acceptance and interest in their descriptions. Occasionally I might comment that the student is clever to think of that way of avoiding stutters. In addition, I am also exploring which level the student's stuttering has reached by determining if they are using escape and avoidance behaviors. It may help to share with the student things that other kids who stutter do, like looking away, pretending to think, when words don't come out.
4. **Do you have more trouble talking in some places than in others? Or with some people compared to others?**
These questions help me understand what a student is experiencing while conveying my understanding.
5. **Most kids who stutter get teased or picked on about their speech. Do you ever get teased about your stuttering? (*Follow-up questions if needed:* What do you do when that happens? How does it make you feel?)**
Many children who stutter are teased about their speech but are not willing to talk about it straightaway with someone they don't know well. So, this question is a "feeler," and if the student denies being teased, I won't dwell on it now.
6. **How do you feel about your speech?**
To help a student express their feelings about stuttering, I can suggest some possibilities by asking, "Does it make you mad sometimes?" or "Do you wish you didn't get stuck?" Don't be surprised, however, if a student says it doesn't bother them because their feelings may have been rejected, perhaps unintentionally, by adults. Adults may say, for instance, "You shouldn't feel that way," or "Why do you let it bother you?" An effective clinician will show the student that whatever feelings they have are OK and that the clinician is really trying to understand. More in-depth discussions of feelings probably won't begin until a student has learned to trust the clinician deeply. However, in this first interview, I may be able to infer what some of the student's feelings are and, from that, understand how far their stuttering has advanced.

Another avenue for eliciting feelings is through drawing pictures. For some children, drawing makes it easier to talk about feelings. The student doesn't have to look directly at the clinician, and their self-consciousness may be decreased by their focus on drawing. I usually suggest to a student that both of us draw whatever we would like, and as we are drawing, I talk about feelings. If this goes well, I bridge the gap between the drawing and talking by suggesting that the student might want to draw a picture of what stuttering is like or what they feel like when they stutter. I have found that this technique can make extensive discussion of feelings much easier for some children. In some cases, children have used their drawings when they talked about stuttering with their class once therapy has helped them feel more comfortable with themselves and their speech.

Some of the activities in the workbook titled *The School-Age Child Who Stutters: Working Effectively With Attitudes and Emotions* (Chmela & Reardon, 2001) are helpful in exploring a student's emotions in both evaluation and treatment. I will discuss some of these a little later.

7. **How do your mom and dad (or other caregivers) feel about your speech? Do they ever say anything or give you advice?**
   This helps me determine what sorts of experiences the student may have been going through at home. One parent may be much less accepting of a student's stuttering than the other. Whatever I find out may help me enlist the parents' participation in treatment.
8. **Can you think of anything else important for me to know about you or about the trouble you sometimes have when you talk?**

This lets the student know that I am interested in them and that their ideas are important to me.

Speech Samples

Preliminaries

With a school-age child, I video record them talking for 10 minutes about school and other activities in the therapy room. I prefer not to turn on the recorder the moment the student walks into the room. Instead, after talking for a few minutes, I ask the student if they would mind my recording our conversation as we talk. If it's OK with the student, I record a sample that optimally includes 300 to 400 syllables of his speech. For those few children who are reluctant at first, I explain that I need a recording of their speech to understand their stuttering better. In rare cases, I might need to postpone recording until the student is more comfortable with me. After recording the **speech sample**, I ask the student to read approximately 200 syllables of age-appropriate material. I often use the SSI-4 examiner's manual that has 200-syllable reading passages at the third, fifth, and seventh grade levels.

If possible, I also obtain a video recording from home for a second sample. In some instances, you may not be able to get a second recorded sample from home or elsewhere. Even if you are not able to record a second sample, write down your impressions of the student's stuttering, including the amount of stuttering and the core and secondary behaviors you observed.

Pattern of Disfluencies

A school-age student is likely to show beginning or intermediate stuttering, so you want to know as much as possible about the amount of tension in the student's stuttering, the escape behaviors they use, and the extent to which they avoid words and situations. You can obtain this information directly by observation or indirectly through parent and teacher interviews. As with adults or adolescents who stutter, I use this information not only to decide at which developmental/treatment level to place the student but also, when appropriate, to plan the process of unlearning conditioned responses, which, once having been brought into play, now maintain the student's pattern of stuttering.

Stuttering Severity Instrument (SSI-4)

Samples of conversational speech and reading are needed to calculate scores on the SSI-4. Administration and scoring of the SSI-4 were described in Chapter 9 (see Fig. 9.3).

Speech Rate

The samples you collect for rating severity with the SSI-4 can also be used to assess the student's speaking rate. The purpose of assessing speech rate is to get some idea of how much the student's stuttering interferes with the rate of speech they normally use. Most (but not all) children who stutter have a slightly reduced speech rate. As I help the student manage their stuttering, I expect a steady increase in his speech rate toward typical levels.

Typical speech rates for schoolchildren measured in syllables per minute were given in Table 9.5. The rates for school children, listed as Davis and Guitar (1976), were obtained from children's conversations with a clinician (in Vermont) about holidays, hobbies, school, and home activities. They were calculated by including typical pauses in their conversation but excluding pauses longer than 2 seconds. It is reasonable to expect that children's speech rates in other states will be similar.

Trial Therapy

Trial therapy with a school-age child will help me understand how easily a student can talk about his stuttering, including about his feelings. If the student is able to make even small changes in his stuttering, though they will be only temporary in this trial therapy, they will gain hope and motivation for the fluency work we embark on as part of the student's treatment.

I usually begin by asking the student to identify moments of voluntary stuttering in my own speech. I explain that I will be putting stutters in my speech and want to see if they can catch me. It's more fun if I can use a small reward for their successes. For example, I might give them tokens to be cashed in later for an activity that they would find really cool, like throwing a ball to knock down a pyramid of cans. I then tell them about my favorite recent movie or television show (something they can later also talk about themselves) and put in a variety of stutters in my speech. As I talk and encourage them to catch my stutters, I let them know how good they are when they catch one of my stutters without my help and hand them a token, a piece of candy or a sip of soda. After a few successful catches, we switch roles and I ask them to put in some stutters—pretend or real—as they talk about a movie, TV show, or any other handy topic, and I try to "catch them." Each time I catch a stutter of theirs (with their permission), I make a positive comment about their stutter and give them a reward. Rewarding stutters of school-age children causes no harm; in fact, it reduces negative emotion, which is a very positive step in treatment.

As the student becomes tuned in to their stutters by my catching them and commenting interestedly on them, I begin to explore with them both what they do when they stutter and how they feel. For example, after I have commented on a stutter, I might say, "OK, let's see what was going on there. Seems like you were squeezing pretty hard with your lips," if that was what they seemed to be doing. "Did you feel that? Let me try it." Then, I would try to emulate what they had done on the sound they had stuttered on. "Did I have that right? Can you make it happen again? Can you stutter on the same word?" I encourage them to pretend to stutter if they don't have a real one when they try again. If they do stutter on it again or pretend to, I say, "Wow. That was great. You really did that stutter well!" If they don't want to stutter again, I let it go and try again later, after we do something more fun for the student.

Take a look at the video clip of me working with a student when we both practice stuttering on the word "apple." It's in the Trial Therapy segment of the series of video clips ("CM Trial Therapy") on *Lippincott Connect* on evaluation of school-age children. Note how I coach the student to try to stay in the moment of stuttering and finish the stutter with less tension. After a few tries, this student does a pretty good job of staying in the beginning sound and easing off on his tension before finishing the words. Throughout, I praise his stuttering, letting counterconditioning (associating something positive—my praise—with something that has been frustrating and even fearful for years) reduce his negative emotions.

Because emotions are such a large part of stuttering, it is important to explore how the student feels about their stuttering as well as what they do. The student and I have been talking about the student's moments of stuttering and so I begin to ask them about how one of those stutters feels. After the student has stuttered, I show my interest and curiosity and then ask them, "How did it feel when you stuttered that time? I mean, how did it feel inside of you?" If the student seems not to quite understand, I might suggest, "Lots of kids tell me that stutters feel bad, like they wish they didn't stutter. Is that about how it feels to you?" After a little bit of talking about how the student's stutter feels to them, I might ask them to draw their stutter. With some encouragement, and with me offering to draw something of mine I don't like, a student will usually draw a picture that we can then discuss.

For some children, you can sense when they've done enough. That's a time to stop and do something different. If the student seems like they can deal with a little more, I might see if they can make a little change in their stuttering by not just blasting through it but instead staying in the stutter and letting some of the tension go. As always, I first demonstrate what I'm asking the student to do. I have the student signal me by pointing to me when they want me to stutter and make me hold on to the stutter for several seconds by continuing to keep their finger pointing at me. Then, we reverse roles and I coach them to hold onto either voluntary or real stutters. Coaching is essential because it will be unnatural for them to hold onto a stutter and they may need some practice until they can do it. I also coach them, while they're holding on to the stutter, to let it go slowly and loosely when their ready to move on. Typically, my models of holding onto a stutter, my enthusiasm, and the reinforcements I use enable most children to be able to carry out these activities. Note that if the student cannot do these activities, it suggests a higher level of fear or an inability to focus on the task. These possibilities usually mean that a student needs a slower approach, and I will consider helping them reduce fear of stuttering before attempting to hold onto stutters.

In the rare case that the student doesn't seem to have much or any negative emotion associated with his stuttering, I might try teaching the student a few fluency skills such as those described in Chapter 14 on treatment of stuttering in school-age children. This approach doesn't deal directly with any tension or fear about stuttering. It simply teaches the student to talk in a way that is likely to engender fluency. I use a word list and give the student an example by producing each word myself before they try it, using a slow rate and gentle onset of voicing. The severity of the student's stuttering will determine how slowly I begin the word; my aim is to use modeling of slow rate and easy onset to produce fluency in the student. Once they can say words after me in that slow fashion, I then ask them to say each of several words again, but without my model. If they can do this, I create sentences beginning with those words said slowly and with an easy onset (but with the remainder of the sentence produced at a near-normal rate) and again assess whether they can repeat them fluently with my model and then without.

These exercises help me determine how well the student can make changes in their speech and their stutters. By using a large amount of modeling and appropriate reinforcement, I can often take the student quite far along in the time I have.

Feelings and Attitudes

One of the best assessments of a student's feelings and attitudes about their stuttering is the clinician's judgment. In the trial therapy and just by observing the student's stuttering, the astute clinician can usually tell if the student has mild, moderate, or severe negative feelings and attitudes about their stuttering. Watch how the student responds when asked about their stuttering, and note how much they avoid stuttering. When the student does stutter, observe if they are calm and how consistent their eye contact is.

After the clinician has gotten to know the student a bit, they may want to administer a paper-and-pencil assessment of attitude. Figure 11.3 depicts the A-19 scale (Guitar & Grims, 1977), a measure developed to assess children's communication attitudes. This scale consists of questions that were found to distinguish children who stutter from those who do not, but the differences were not great. Hence, if treatment is effective, a student's attitude about communication may change, although this has not been established by research. One of the best uses of such measures is as a starting place for discussions about how a student's stuttering is affecting them.

In addition to the A-19, the Communication Attitude Test (CAT), which was developed by Brutten and his colleagues,

Establish rapport with the student, and make sure that he or she is physically comfortable before beginning administration. Explain the task to the student, and make sure he or she understands what is required. Some simple directions might be used:

"I am going to ask you some questions. Listen carefully, and then tell me what you think: true or false. There is no right or wrong answer. I just want to know what you think." To begin the scale, ask the questions in a natural manner. Do not urge the student to respond before he or she is ready, and repeat the question if the student did not hear it or you feel that he or she did not understand it.

Do not reword the question unless you feel it is absolutely necessary, and then write the question you asked under that item.

Circle the answer that corresponds to the student's response. Be accepting of the student's response because there is no right or wrong answer. If all the student will say is "I don't know," even after prompting, record that response next to the question. For the younger children (kindergarten and first grade), it might be necessary to give a few simple examples to ensure comprehension of the requited task:

a. Are you a boy?	Yes	No
b. Do you have black hair?	Yes	No

Similar, obvious questions may be inserted, if necessary, to reassure the examiner that the student is actively cooperating at all times. Adequately praise the student for listening, and assure him or her that a good job is being done.

It is important to be familiar with the questions so that they can be read in a natural manner.

The student is given 1 point for each answer that matches those given below. The higher a student's score, the more probable it is that he or she has developed negative attitudes toward communication. In our study, the mean score of the K through fourth grade stutterers (N = 28) was 9.07 (S.D. = 2.44), and for the 28 matched controls, it was 8.17 (S.D. = 1.80).

Score 1 point for each answer that matches these:

1. Yes	11. No
2. Yes	12. No
3. No	13. Yes
4. No	14. Yes
5. No	15. Yes
6. Yes	16. No
7. No	17. No
8. Yes	18. Yes
9. Yes	19. Yes
10. No	

Figure 11.3 A-19 scale of children's attitudes by Susan Andre and Barry Guitar (University of Vermont). (Reprinted from Susan Andre, with permission.)

A-19 SCALE

Name____________________________ Date ________

1.	Is it best to keep your mouth shut when you are in trouble?	Yes	No
2.	When the teacher calls on you, do you get nervous?	Yes	No
3.	Do you ask a lot of questions in class?	Yes	No
4.	Do you like to talk on the phone?	Yes	No
5.	If you did not know a person, would you tell your name?	Yes	No
6.	Is it hard to talk to your teacher?	Yes	No
7.	Would you go up to a new boy or girl in your class?	Yes	No
8.	Is it hard to keep control of your voice when talking?	Yes	No
9.	Even when you know the right answer, are you afraid to say it?	Yes	No
10.	Do you like to tell other children what to do?	Yes	No
11.	Is it fun to talk to your dad?	Yes	No
12.	Do you like to tell stories to your classmates?	Yes	No
13.	Do you wish you could say things as clearly as the other kids do?	Yes	No
14.	Would you rather look at a comic book than talk to a friend?	Yes	No
15.	Are you upset when someone interrupts you?	Yes	No
16.	When you want to say something, do you just say it?	Yes	No
17.	Is talking to your friends more fun than playing by yourself?	Yes	No
18.	Are you sometimes unhappy?	Yes	No
19.	Are you a little afraid to talk on the phone?	Yes	No

Figure 11.3 *(Continued)*

has been shown to be a reliable and appropriate tool to measure the attitudes of children and adults who stutter. This was done in a series of studies from 1991 to 2001. Initially, in 1991, in a study of 341 children between the ages of 7 and 14 years—70 children who stuttered and 271 children who did not stutter—De Nil and Brutten (1991) found that the children who stuttered had significantly more negative communication attitudes ($P < .01$) and that this difference increased with age. Vanryckeghem and Brutten (1997) replicated this finding with children aged 6 to 13. In 1993, Vanryckeghem and Brutten affirmed the CAT's test-retest reliability using 44 school-age children; results indicated correlations of 0.86, 0.81, and 0.76 for retesting after 1, 11, and 12 weeks, respectively, indicating that it is appropriate to administer it to a student several times. In a study of 143 children who stuttered (ages 7-13), Vanryckeghem et al. (2001) examined the relationship between negative attitudes as measured by the CAT and negative emotions elicited by the questions on the CAT, as measured by a 1-to-5 scale filled out by the children. The authors found a high positive correlation ($r = 0.89$) between negative attitudes and negative emotions. Both negative attitudes and negative emotions increased with age. In summary, the CAT is a well-researched tool that can be used to determine the presence of negative attitudes in individuals ages 6 and older. It is now part of a larger assessment battery (Behavior Assessment Battery for School-Age Children Who Stutter; Brutten & Vanryckeghem, 2007), which also contains the Speech Situation Checklist that evaluates a student's reactions to a range of situations, as well as the Behavioral Checklist, which assesses a student's coping responses to his disfluency. It is important that a trusting relationship with the student has been developed before administering either the A-19 or the CAT to a school-age child.

Many informal methods of assessing feelings and attitudes are given in the workbook referred to earlier, *The School-Age Child Who Stutters: Working Effectively With Attitudes and Emotions* (Chmela & Reardon, 2001). These include such activities as a "Worry Ladder," in which a student lists their worries in a hierarchy, and "Hands Down," which elicits things the student likes and does not like about themselves. Although the reliability and validity of these tools have not been determined, they provide useful starting points for communication about feelings and attitudes.

With some children, both formal and informal methods of assessing feelings will be productive during the evaluation. But others will hold back until they have developed a trusting relationship with the clinician. Thus, clinicians should be mindful that information about a student's feelings and attitudes obtained in a first meeting may not be complete or accurate.

Other Speech and Language Disorders

In my discussion of the preschool student, I described the importance of screening speech sound production and language. The same abilities should be screened in the school-age child. You can use the Goldman-Fristoe Test of Articulation-3 (Goldman & Fristoe, 2015) and the Hodson Assessment of Phonological Patterns (HAPP-3) (3rd ed.) (Hodson, 2004) for speech sound production. For language, I would suggest the Clinical Evaluation of Language Fundamentals-5 Screening Test (Wiig et al., 2013) and the Peabody Picture Vocabulary Test 5 (Dunn, 2018) and Expressive Vocabulary Test 3 (Williams, 2019) for vocabulary. In addition to tests of oral language, for a school-age child, written language (ie, reading, writing, and spelling) may also be a concern. Reading problems will be of special interest for a student who stutters reading impairment may be wrongly diagnosed when measures of reading fluency (eg, DIBELS8, Biancarosa et al., 2020) are used as part of a reading assessment (ASHA Ad Hoc Committee on Reading Fluency for School-age Children who Stutter, 2014; Games et al., 2014). Therefore, you can play an important role in recommending appropriate accommodations if testing is done by others or avoid such measures if your practice includes the evaluation of literacy skills.

If a student has been previously diagnosed with communication disorders besides stuttering, you should seek out details of any current or previous therapy, including what therapy was conducted and what progress was made. Did his stuttering first appear or worsen during treatment? If so, the clinician should pay particular attention to indications that the student may think of themselves as a poor speaker and may believe that speaking is difficult. The interviews and questionnaires I suggested in the previous section on feelings and attitudes will help you explore this possibility, and the therapy approaches described for treatment of school-age children (Chapter 15) are designed to help a student regain confidence in his ability to speak easily and well.

Diagnosis

At this point in a clinic-based evaluation, the clinician pulls together the information collected from (1) the case history; (2) parent, teacher, and student interviews; (3) speech samples; and (4) classroom observations. This information helps the clinician determine the developmental/treatment level of the student's stuttering, which will give direction for selecting a treatment approach.

Occasionally, a school-age student is referred for stuttering, but it may not be clear whether they stutter or only have a high level of typical disfluency. You probably know some adults who are quite disfluent but don't consider themselves as stuttering and are not inhibited about talking. When a school-age child seems genuinely unbothered by their disfluency and do not avoid speaking or show excess tension or other escape behaviors, they should be given the option of therapy, but they should not be forced to accept it. I have talked with several adults who felt they were unfairly badgered about their speech and think they would have coped quite well and probably outgrown the disfluency except for the pressure on them to "do something about it." Instead, they became quite self-conscious of it and developed a serious stuttering problem. These may be real examples of the "diagnosogenic" theory of stuttering discussed in Chapter 6.

Despite the rare exceptions just described, most school-children you will see are at beginning or intermediate levels of stuttering. Beginning-level stuttering is most likely to occur in younger school-age children and is characterized by physical tension, hurry, escape behaviors, awareness of difficulty, and feelings of frustration, but lack of extensive avoidance. The intermediate level also involves tension, hurry, escape behaviors, and frustration but also includes notable avoidance behaviors as a result of fear and anticipation of stuttering. It is important that we understand whether the key stimuli for a student are only in his experience of being stuck in a stutter (escape behaviors) or are *also* in the anticipation of stuttering (avoidance behaviors). As I'll discuss in future chapters, treatment for these two levels of stuttering should be different because we need to decondition the link between anticipated stuttering and the preparatory tension that occurs when a student (or an adult) fears a stutter coming up and tries to fight it.

In addition to a student's stuttering behaviors and feelings, developmental and environmental pressures currently affecting the student must be considered in planning treatment. Such pressures can be uncovered from parent, teacher, and student interviews and the speech sample. Some pressures may result from other speech and language disorders, motor problems, or pressures in the student's home. Goals can be formulated with the parents' input for alleviating those pressures that can be changed and helping the student cope with those that can't be changed. Some pressures can be dealt with in treatment, but others may require parent counseling or referral to other professionals.

Closing Interview

When parents have been able to be involved in my evaluation of the student, the **closing interview** provides an opportunity to summarize my immediate impressions for the parents and make recommendations about treatment. It also provides an opportunity to discuss the crucial role parents can play in reducing environmental pressures. I point out the many beneficial things they have done about their student's speech and assure them that stuttering was not caused by anything they have done. Although some parents may have created conditions in which a student's predisposition to stutter has been transformed into a serious problem, it does not help to make an issue of this. Rather, we want to convince them that they are in a key position to help.

After describing clearly and simply what I observed about the student's stuttering, I summarize my thinking about appropriate treatment. I do this in only general terms because parents' main concerns at this time are not the details of treatment but the prospects for their student's future. Therefore, I rely on my experience to describe likely outcomes. For example, I might say that a combination of many factors will determine the student's outcome. These include the natural increases in fluency that occur as a student matures, feelings of self-acceptance that a student develops when they find that people accept them whether or not they have trouble with their speech, and their learning ways to speak more fluently. When I talk about the student's prognosis, I always include some aspect of the parents' role, such as their acceptance of the student's speech or their participation in treatment, as part of the formula for recovery. Sometimes, a key aspect of the parents' acceptance of stuttering is realizing they are not responsible for curing it. If I feel that there is a good chance the student will have some stuttering remaining after therapy, I talk with the parents about this possibility, indicating that many people who have some stuttering remaining lead highly successful lives. A few who come to mind are Malcolm Fraser, a very successful businessman who founded the Stuttering Foundation, Billionaire Walter Annenberg who was ambassador to Great Britain, singer Ed Sheeran, and, if they are Democrats, President Joe Biden.

After summarizing my impressions and describing some of the ingredients for recovery, I discuss some of the things the parents can do to promote recovery. Specific suggestions depend on findings from our interviews, but the sections on parent counseling in the chapter on treatment of stuttering in school-age children present general ideas for parents' involvement. Discussion of the family's involvement in therapy is the most important part of the closing interview and in fact may continue for several more meetings. If I treat the student directly and, in a clinic, rather than in a school setting, I meet with at least one parent weekly as part of treatment. In these meetings, I continue to help them explore how various changes in the home environment can facilitate their student's fluency.

The video titled "CM Wrap Up" on Lippincott Connect shows a closing interview with a school-age student and his parents that illustrates some of the points made in the preceding section.

Public School Setting

SLPs working in the public schools need to learn the regulations of the state they are in. In most cases, those regulations are online and can be accessed through the state's office of education.

The sequence indicated by MTSS (see the section on "Public School Considerations" earlier in this chapter) is that after a referral for stuttering is made, the SLP may start by informally assessing the student's speech by talking with them, visiting their classroom, and talking to their teacher. But first, before assessing the student's speech, the SLP should contact the student's family to ask permission to do so. This contact would require that the parents be told what the school's concerns are—in a general way—and it is an opportunity to find out if they have noticed the student's stuttering also and if they have their own concerns. Once permission is obtained and the student is assessed, the SLP may then start to meet the student's needs at a Tier 1 level by having the teacher try to give the student opportunities to talk in low-stress situations like in small groups. The teacher should also monitor the student's speech in class to further assess how much, if any, it interferes with their classroom participation. The teacher can also become aware of how other children are responding to the student: are other children reacting to the student's speech? Interrupting? Teasing?

It is usually important to involve the student's parents/family in treatment if possible. The SLP can meet with them and, if appropriate, include the student so that suggestions can be explored about how the family can help the student's speech. Specific ideas are given in more detail in Chapter 13, on the treatment of school-age children.

Returning to the SLP's work with the student in school, after 4 to 6 weeks of Tier 1 classroom environment modification, the student's stuttering is not improving; the SLP can move to Tier 2, which involves trial "pullout" therapy (in the SLP's room) for 4 to 6 weeks, to see if that is meeting the student's needs. If the student needs further pullout therapy, the SLP may want to involve an Education Support Team (EST) (SLP, administrator, special educator, and appropriate others). The EST can develop a plan that includes goals and objectives and could continue for some time.

If the student has other challenges, such as reading problems, or if the student's stuttering is quite severe, it may require a special education assessment and eventually an Individualized Education Program (often referred to as an IEP). If this were the case, the formal evaluation by the team would be comprised of parent input, a detailed assessment of the student's stuttering using standardized measures such as the SSI and assessment of the student's attitudes and feelings, and demonstration that the student's speech (and/or other challenges) prevents them from obtaining an adequate education. In other words, the team needs to show that the student meets eligibility standards (severe enough challenges) and that the challenges (stuttering alone or combined with other handicapping conditions) are having an adverse effect on his education.

Evidence of adverse effect can be obtained from measures of communicative functioning in school, such as the *Teacher's Assessment of Student Communication Competency* (Fig. 11.1) (Smith et al., 2000), observations of the student in the school, and interviews with teachers and parents. Lisa Scott Trautman (personal communication, July 30, 2003) noted that adverse effects can be shown by demonstrating that the student cannot meet the school district's curriculum objectives because of his stuttering. Examples of such objectives might be that students will be active in class discussions or that students must be able to speak effectively in front of a group.

If the evaluation determines that the student is eligible for services, an IEP team, often headed by the SLP, develops measurable goals and short-term objectives (also called "benchmarks") as well as services to be provided that will help the student improve his performance in all aspects of the educational setting. These goals and objectives are considered in detail in the chapters on treatment of beginning and intermediate stuttering.

I have made available a series of video clips of our evaluation of a school-age child. You can find them on *Lippincott Connect*. The evaluation of this school-age child begins with an interview of his parents. This interview is part of a video titled "CM Introduction." The student, whose name is Cameron (Cam for short), is 7 years old and, as you will see, his stuttering has been getting worse. Cam had been more fluent as the result of treatment administered by a school clinician. Recently, however, the effects of the former treatment have worn off and Cam has become increasingly upset by his stuttering. We began the interview by asking an open-ended question: "Why don't you tell me about Cam's speech?" The parents then describe Cam's stuttering and their empathetic concern about it. Interestingly, they mention that he felt better after watching the Stuttering Foundation video "For Kids by Kids." Cam refers to this video in the later clip about trial therapy. The parents also relate that Cam talked to his class about his stuttering, letting them know about it and asking them not to tease him. (Such openness about stuttering is rare in a student this age.)

In the second clip of Cam, "CM Speech Sample and Exploration," notice the things he does when he stutters. For example, when he stutters on "ink," he simply prolongs the vowel, without a great deal of struggle and no avoidance. He doesn't shut off his voicing. This suggests that for him—at this point—being stuck in a stutter is not a terrifying experience requiring a big reaction. Later in this clip, he talks openly about his accessory behaviors, such as looking up at his hair when he stutters. This openness to discuss aspects of his stuttering so matter-of-factly is a very positive prognostic sign.

In the next clip, "CM Trial Therapy," we experiment with trial therapy to see if Cam can tolerate staying in his stutter. As he talks about holding in his stutters rather than letting them out, he is unusually candid. Not many school-age children will be this open, and it usually takes some time to get them comfortable talking about their stuttering. In the trial therapy, I ask Cam to stay in the stutter and feel it loosen up. We talk about practicing in the therapy sessions and not having to do anything embarrassing with his speech in public.

The last clip is the closing interview of the evaluation, "CM Wrap-Up." This does not show everything we said and did, but you can get an idea of how we praise Cam and his family for the openness they are all showing about the stuttering. In the last few minutes, we discuss his coming to our clinic to work on his stuttering. That therapy, which Cam needed intermittently for several years, is discussed and shown in Chapter 15 on the treatment of stuttering in school-age children.

ADOLESCENT

In this assessment section, we focus on individuals between the ages of 13 and 19. As you read about assessment of adolescents, you may decide that a particular client who is slightly outside this age range is best evaluated with the procedures described here. In fact, some authors describe the age range for adolescents as from 10 to 24 years old (Sawyer et al., 2018).

Evaluation of adolescents should take into account that these young people are usually striving to become independent of their parents, that they may have had unsuccessful therapy in the past, and that they should be major players in the planning process for any therapy that the adolescent chooses to undertake (Rodgers, 2022).

Clinic Versus School Assessment

This section is written as though the evaluation is being carried out in a clinic rather than a school. When the setting is a public school, the evaluation process is determined by the Individuals with Disabilities Education Act (IDEA, 1997) and the laws of each state. Updates on the Act can be found at https://sites.ed.gov › idea.

Some guidelines for assessment were described in the previous section on evaluating a school-age child. For the adolescent, an additional consideration is his participation in the IEP process and his transition beyond high school. When a student reaches age 14, his input is sought by the IEP team, and he gradually becomes an active member of the team, not only with regard to his present situation but also in terms of his aspirations beyond secondary school. When a student reaches age 16, an individualized transition plan (ITP) is a mandated part of the IEP. At age 18, students take over responsibility from their parents for signing off on documentation.

Preassessment

Case History Form

A case history form is sent to the adolescent several weeks before their appointment. This form is shown in Figure 11.4. When possible, the adolescent should fill it out themselves to promote their independence and helps them feel

CASE HISTORY OF ADOLESCENTS AND ADULTS

Instructions: Please fill out this form in as much detail as possible. You can be assured that this information will be treated as confidential. If information is not available, please specify the reason so that we will know that the question has been considered. **Please return this form prior to your appointment.** Thank you.

Date: ______________________

Name: ______________________ Gender: ____________

Address: ______________________ Telephone: (home) ____________

______________________ (work) ____________

E-Mail Address: ______________________ Cell Phone: ____________

Date of Birth: ______________________ Place of Birth: ____________

Referring Physician: ______________________

Marital Status: ______________________

Education Level: ______________________ Occupation: ____________

Employed by: ______________________

Referred to this Center by: ______________________

Name of spouse/nearest relative: ______________________

Address: ______________________ Telephone: ____________

HISTORY OF STUTTERING

Are there other individuals in your family background or immediate family who stutter?

____

Give approximate age at which your stuttering was first noticed: ______________________

Who first noticed or mentioned the stuttering? ______________________

In what situation did this occur? ______________________

Describe any situations or conditions that you associate with the onset of stuttering:

____

____

____

What were the first signs of your stuttering? (If you don't remember, you might ask your parents or siblings.) ______________________

____

Was the stuttering always the same or did it occur in several different ways? ____________

____

If they occurred in different ways, how were they different from one another? ____________

____

Figure 11.4 Case history form for adolescents and adults.

that the clinician values what *they* want. This form allows the clinician to learn ahead of time whether the client referred for stuttering may have a different or additional disorder. The case history gives the clinician information about the extent to which stuttering affects a client's life, as well as details about onset of stuttering, and what it's like now, previous therapy and whether it has helped or not, what they do to help with their stuttering, how others react to their stuttering, and what they hope to gain from therapy.

Did the first blocks seem to be located in the tongue? lips? chest? diaphragm? or throat?

____

Approximately how long did each block (on one word) seem to last? ______________

____

Was the stuttering easy or was there force at the time when the stuttering was first noticed?

____

Were the words that were stuttered at the beginning of sentences, or were they scattered throughout the sentence being said? ______________

____

When stuttering first began, was there any avoidance of speaking because of it? Give examples, if any. ______________

____

At the time when stuttering was first noticed, what was your reaction?

Awareness that speech was different? __________ Indifference to it? __________

Surprise? __________ Anger or frustration? __________ Shame? __________

Fear of stuttering again? __________ Other? __________

What attempts have been made to treat the stuttering problem? ______________

____

DEVELOPMENT OF STUTTERING

Since the onset, have there been any changes in stuttering symptoms? Check those that are appropriate.

Increase in number of repetitions per word __________

Change in amount of force used (increased? decreased?) __________

Increase in amount of stuttering __________

Increase in length of block __________

Periods of no stuttering __________

More precise in speech attempts __________

Lowered voice loudness __________

Slower rate of speech __________

Change in location of force when stuttering, if force is present __________

Looking away from listener __________

Describe any of the above that apply ______________

____

____

Figure 11.4 *(Continued)*

Forms to Assess Attitudes and Feelings

Overall Assessment of the Speaker's Experience of Stuttering (OASES)

Another form sent to adolescents is the OASES (Fig. 11.5). If there are concerns about the adolescent's literacy, it can be done with the clinician in person. The OASES is a questionnaire designed to assess the impact of stuttering on a person's life. Based on the World Health Organization's *International Classification of Functioning, Disability, and Health* (World Health Organization, 2001), the OASES focuses on feelings about stuttering, reactions to stuttering, communication in

Were there any periods (weeks/months) when the stuttering disappeared? ______________

____

Were there any periods (weeks/months) when the stuttering increased? ______________

____

Can you give an explanation for these "worse" periods? ______________________

____

CURRENT STUTTERING

Are there any situations that are particularly difficult? If so, please describe. ____________

____

List any situations that never cause difficulty. ______________________________

____

Answer the following "yes" or "no" as they apply to your stuttering. Do you stutter when you

Talk to young children? _________ Say your name? _________

Answer direct questions? _________ Talk to adults, superiors at work, teachers? _________

Use new words that are unfamiliar? _________ Use the telephone? _________

Read aloud? _________ Recite memorized material? _________

Ask questions? _________ Talk to strangers? _________ Speak when tired? _________

Speak when excited? _________ Talk to family members? _________

Talk to friends? _________

Do you know any stutterers? _________ Describe your relationship with them. ____________

____

Do you feel that stuttering interferes with your career? _________ Social relationships? _________

Success in school? _________ Success on the job? _________ Daily life? _________

Describe what your stuttering currently looks and sounds like. ______________________

____

____

MEDICAL, DEVELOPMENTAL AND FAMILY HISTORY

If possible, describe mother's health during pregnancy and/or your birth history (i.e., complications). ____

____

____

Describe any development problems during infancy or early childhood (i.e., late to walk, feeding problems, food allergies, late to talk). ________________________________

____

Figure 11.4 *(Continued)*

daily situations, and the extent to which stuttering interferes with daily living. There are versions of the OASES for children ages 7 to 12 (OASES-S) (Yaruss et al., 2016), teens ages 13 to 17 (OASES-T) (Yaruss et al., 2016) and adults 18 and older (OASES-A) (Yaruss & Quesal, 2010, 2016). The teen form (OASES-T) is obviously the one used with adolescents.

Are you: Right-handed? __________ Left-handed? __________ Both? __________ Is there any evidence of visual, artistic abilities in your family? ______________________________

Were you sensitive as a student? ______________________________

Would you describe yourself as sensitive now? ______________________________

List your history of any significant illnesses, injuries, and/or operations:

Date	Fever	Complications	Treatment	Physician

List all present physical disabilities. ______________________________

____

Any chronic illnesses, allergies, or physical conditions? ______________________________

____

Vision normal? __________ Hearing normal? __________ List any medication you take regularly or are taking currently. ______________________________

Describe any learning or reading problems you experienced as a student or are currently experiencing. ______________________________

____

Do any members of your family have speech or language problems or learning disabilities? If so, describe.______________________________

____

SOCIAL HISTORY

Hobbies ______________________________

Leisure time activities ______________________________

Describe any previous therapy you have participated in to aid your fluency. When? Where? With whom? Length of time? The outcome? ______________________________

____

____

Add anything else you would like to include and think might be important: ______________

____

____

In addition, what goals would you like to see accomplished as a result of this evaluation? ________

____

____

Signature: ______________________________ Date: ______________

Figure 11.4 *(Continued)*

The OASES is divided into four sections: (1) General Information, (2) Reactions to Stuttering, (3) Communication in Daily Situations, and (4) Quality of Life. An "impact score" for each section as well as a "total impact score" can be calculated and then related to normative data so that a clinician can find out how severely stuttering is impacting a client's life.

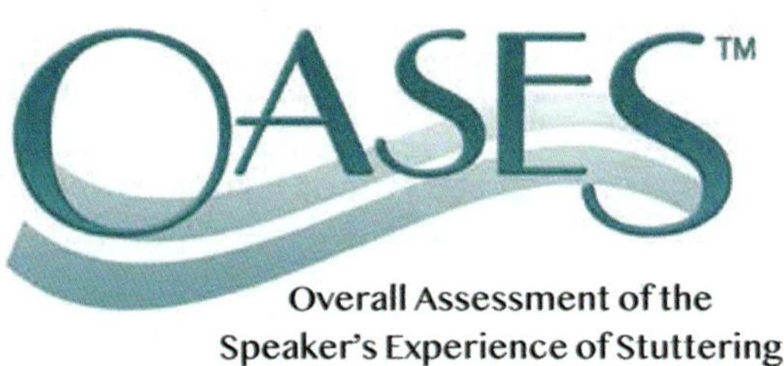

OASES-A
Response Form
Adult: Ages 18 and Above

J. Scott Yaruss, PhD, CCC-SLP, BCS-F, F-ASHA
Robert W. Quesal, PhD, CCC-SLP, BCS-F, F-ASHA

Name: ____________________

Birth Date: ____/____/____ Age: ______ Sex/Gender: ____________

Test Date: ____/____/____ ID Number: ____________

Clinician: ____________________

General Instructions:
This form includes four sections of questions that examine different aspects of your experiences with stuttering. Please complete each question in each section by circling the appropriate number. Please think about how you are *currently* feeling or speaking when answering each question. Some of the questions do not apply to everyone. If one of the questions does not apply to you, please check ❑ N/A for "Not Applicable" and go on to the next question.

Scoring: For Office Use Only

Instructions for Clinicians:

- Calculate Impact Scores for each of the four sections on the OASES-A by first summing the number of points in each section (A) and then counting the number of items completed in each section (B). Divide the total number of points (A) by the number of items completed (B) to obtain the Impact Score.
- Calculate the Overall Impact Score by summing the numbers in columns (A) and (B) at the bottom of each column. Divide the sum of (A) by the sum of (B) to obtain the Overall Impact Score.
- Impact Scores range between 1.0 and 5.0. Circle the Impact Rating that corresponds to the score for each section and for the Overall Impact.

	Impact Score			Impact Rating				
	A Points	B Items Completed	A ÷ B = Impact Score	Score 1.00–1.49	Score 1.50–2.24	Score 2.25–2.99	Score 3.00–3.74	Score 3.75–5.00
Section I: General Information	÷	=		Mild	Mild-Moderate	Moderate	Moderate-Severe	Severe
Section II: Speaker's Reactions	÷	=		Mild	Mild-Moderate	Moderate	Moderate-Severe	Severe
Section III: Daily Communication	÷	=		Mild	Mild-Moderate	Moderate	Moderate-Severe	Severe
Section IV: Quality of Life	÷	=		Mild	Mild-Moderate	Moderate	Moderate-Severe	Severe
OVERALL Impact:	÷	=		Mild	Mild-Moderate	Moderate	Moderate-Severe	Severe

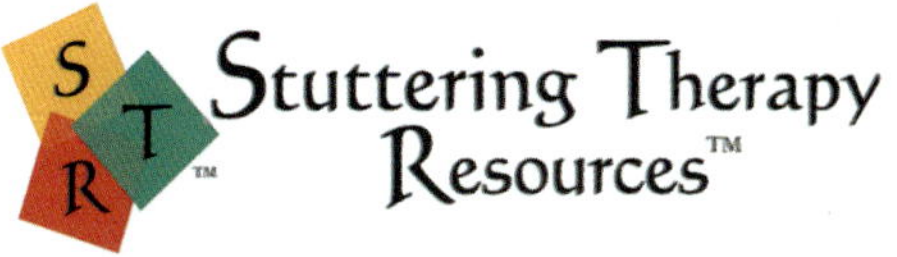

Figure 11.5 Overall assessment of the speaker's experience of stuttering. (Reprinted from OASES-A, Copyright © 2016 Stuttering Therapy Resources, Inc. All rights reserved. www.StutteringTherapyResources.com, with permission.)

The developers of the OASES published data on validity and reliability (Yaruss & Quesal, 2006) on the adult version, indicating that internal reliability within each of the four sections was high (Cronbach's alpha coefficient ranged from 0.92 to 0.97), suggesting that questions within a section were tapping into a homogenous area. In addition,

MODIFIED ERICKSON SCALE OF COMMUNICATION ATTITUDES (S-24)

Name: ____________________ Date: __________ Score: __________

Directions: Mark the "true" column with a check (✓) for each statement that is true or mostly true for you and mark the "false" column with a check (✓) for each statement which is false or not usually true for you.

	TRUE	FALSE
1. I usually feel that I am making a favorable impression when I talk.		
2. I find it easy to talk with almost anyone.		
3. I find it very easy to look at my audience while speaking to a group.		
4. A person who is my teacher or my boss is hard to talk to.		
5. Even the idea of giving a talk in public makes me afraid.		
6. Some words are harder than others for me to say.		
7. I forget all about myself shortly after I begin a speech.		
8. I am a good mixer.		
9. People sometimes seem uncomfortable when I am talking to them.		
10. I dislike introducing one person to another.		
11. I often ask questions in group discussions.		
12. I find it easy to keep control of my voice when speaking.		
13. I do not mind speaking in front of a group.		
14. I do not talk well enough to do the kind of work I'd really like to do.		
15. My speaking voice is rather pleasant and easy to listen to.		
16. I am sometimes embarrassed by the way I talk.		
17. I face most speaking situations with complete confidence.		
18. There are few people I can talk with easily.		

Figure 11.6 Erickson S-24 scale of communication attitudes. (Used with permission of American Speech-Language-Hearing Association from Andrews, G., & Cutler, J. (1974). Stuttering therapy: The relation between changes in symptom level and attitudes. *Journal of Speech and Hearing Disorders*, *39*(3), 312–319; permission conveyed through Copyright Clearance Center, Inc.)

Pearson product-moment correlations between total scores for these four sections were low enough (0.66-0.85) to indicate that the different sections were measuring different domains. Criterion-related validity was assessed by comparing an earlier version of the OASES to the Erickson S-24 Scale of Communication Attitudes (Andrews & Cutler, 1974; Erickson, 1969). Correlations suggested one section (Reactions to Stuttering) was positively and

19. I talk better than I write.
20. I often feel nervous while talking.
21. I find it hard to talk when I meet new people.
22. I feel pretty confident about my speaking ability.
23. I wish that I could say things as clearly as others do.
24. Even though I knew the right answer, I have often failed to give it because I was afraid to speak out.

Data on the "Modified Erickson Scale of Communication Attitudes"

I. Answers (Andrews & Cutler, 1974)

Score 1 point for each answer that matches this:

1. False	13. False
2. False	14. True
3. False	15. False
4. True	16. True
5. True	17. False
6. True	18. True
7. False	19. False
8. False	20. True
9. True	21. True
10. True	22. False
11. False	23. True
12. False	24. True

II. Adult Norms (Andrews & Cutler, 1974)

	Mean	Range
Stutterers	19.22	9–24
Nonstutterers	9.14	1–21

Figure 11.6 *(Continued)*

highly correlated with the S-24, whereas the other two sections (Communication in Daily Situations and Quality of Life) were moderately correlated. Test-retest reliability was assessed by giving the OASES to 14 individuals two different times, separated by 10 to 14 days without intervening treatment. Responses were identical for 77% of responses and within ±1 for 98% of responses, suggesting that it is appropriate to administer the instrument repeatedly to an individual (eg, before, during, and after treatment).

Erickson Scale of Communication Attitudes (S-24)

The Modified Erickson Scale of Communication Attitudes (S-24) (Andrews & Cutler, 1974) is a good way to obtain information about a client's communication attitudes (Fig. 11.6). This questionnaire has been normed on both individuals who stutter and individuals who don't stutter. A colleague and I (Guitar & Bass, 1978) studied a sample of 20 individuals treated by a fluency-shaping program and found that if communication attitude as measured by the S-24 does not change during treatment, the likelihood of relapse within 12 to 18 months increases. Ingham (1979) disputed this finding, but Young (1981) confirmed it using a reanalysis of the original data. Later, a study by Andrews and Craig (1988) also supported the relationship between normalizing attitudes on the S-24 and long-term treatment outcome. Thus using this measure to assess attitudes when an evaluation is done is helpful. Using it throughout treatment will show whether attitudes change, along with changes in stuttering, during and at the end of treatment. As mentioned, if attitudes don't change during treatment, relapse is more likely and treatment of attitudes should continue before the client is dismissed.

Assessment

Interview/Conversation

The initial interview with an adolescent who stutters can be a challenging but rewarding opportunity. Typically, adolescents are trying to establish themselves as individuals, independent from their parents and teachers. Therefore, if you are comfortable with this, reassure the adolescent that what you talk about with them is confidential and will not be shared with their parents or teachers.

A good way to begin is to get to know the adolescent—apart from their stuttering. Learn about their strengths and their interests. Don't be afraid to have a long conversation in which they tells you about themselves and you can show them, by your attentive listening, that you see them as much more than a walking stutter. Your knowledge of what they like and are good at will supply you with plenty of good ideas and metaphors to help them relate to ideas you may come up with if they want to stutter more easily.

Sometime during the interview, you might want to learn what the adolescent's own motivation for therapy is. You can ask, "Are you ok if we talk about your stuttering?" If the adolescent agrees, you can comment on the fact that many of the young people you see are here because their parents or a teacher wants them to get help with their stuttering, but some want help themselves. Leave some silence after saying this to see if they will respond to this implied question. During the first few minutes of the conversation, it might be good to let them know that even though they stutter—which is ok with you—they can accomplish as much as anyone. They can be whatever they want, stuttering or not. There are a lot of famous people who stutter, like the actor Bruce Willis, Elvis Presley, the singer Ed Sheeran, the man who played Darth Vader in the Star Wars movies—James Earl Jones. Just Google "List of Stutterers" and see lots of them. There is an especially long list on Wikipedia. Most of these people accomplished great things and stuttered, too.

Ensure that your adolescent client knows that stuttering is fine with you, they should be told that they can feel free to stutter as much as they want with you. Also, be sure they know that if they want you to help them, you can help them and you will work on their stuttering together.

Perhaps at this point, after you've talked a little, you could ask the young person if it's ok to video record the conversation so you can learn more about their stuttering and be able to help them more. It they give the ok, then you can begin to record them. If not, then proceed without video recording, for now.

Once the conversation is going, it will be helpful to find out if they've had help with their stuttering in the past and how that worked out for them. I might just mention to them that some kids have had help and it has been great for them, while others didn't think their therapy helped them. I can also say, "Tell me about any therapy you've already had." I might add, "Tell me some things you worked on." And "Was it helpful or not-so-helpful?" And "Are there some things you'd like to work on with me?"

In the conversation, explore with the client what effects stuttering have on their life, what are the hard parts. Is it hard to talk in school? At home? On the phone? What would they want to do differently if their stuttering wasn't a challenge anymore?

It's also important to explore what the adolescent wants to get out of therapy. To probe this, you could ask them, "What are some of your best hopes for therapy?" or "If we work together for some time and you come to think, 'wow, I'm so glad I've been working on this because I'm doing a lot better,' what would be changed?" Then to get them thinking about small steps they could start taking to get on their desired change path, you could follow up with, "How do you think you'll manage to do that?" or "What's one small thing you could start doing that would help you achieve that goal?" Getting their idea about how you—the clinician—can be helpful in their change process is also important: "How do you see me being helpful in this process? How can I best support you?"

Also, it would be useful to explore whether the client has been teased or bullied about their stuttering. You can say, "Lots of the kids I see for help with their stuttering tell me that they have been teased or bullied for their stuttering. Has this ever happened to you? You can follow this with some silence and an interested look on your face. If they are willing to talk about it, you can let them know you realize how mad that can make you. I sometimes comment about how other kids I've worked with have practiced a reply, like "Oh yeah, I bet you're not smart enough to learn to stutter like I have." This may get them thinking about responses that they can make when you talk about it again in therapy sessions.

As you wind down the conversation, be sure you ask the adolescent "Is there anything more about your stuttering and your life I should know?" At some point near the end of the interview be sure to ask, "Are there any questions about stuttering you'd like to ask me?" and "Or anything you'd like to know about me?"

Speech Sample

Collecting a sample of the client's speech will give me an opportunity—both in the moment and in my more thorough analysis later—to study and understand what the adolescent does when they stutter. It gives me insight that I can use to help them. If I haven't gotten the client's permission to video record them earlier, during our conversation, I ask again if I can record their talking so that I may learn about their stuttering and then be able to help them talk easier.

I ask the client to talk about something that is interesting to them—perhaps about their favorite sports, the best book they've ever read, the greatest movie, or the video games they play. If you ask about their favorite video games, be sure you know something about one or two, like Minecraft or Exploding Kittens. If I can get them to talk without me interrupting with questions, it's easier to analyze their stuttering. So, I give them all my attention and I am free with nods, smiles, and sounds of interest. The speaking sample you obtain should be between 150 and 500 syllables. After this sample is gathered, a reading sample is obtained. The SSI-4 has reading passages appropriate for readers up to 7th grade, then adult level passages. The SSI-4 manual gives details about scoring the frequency, duration, and physical concomitants of the stutters.

As I observe the adolescent's stuttering, I pay particular attention to the frequency and severity of core behaviors (repetitions, prolongations, and blocks) and secondary behaviors. Details are given in Chapter 7 in the sections on Intermediate and Advanced Stuttering. Secondary behaviors, as you know, include escape and avoidance behaviors. Escape behaviors (such as eye blinks or head nods to end a moment of stuttering) tend to make stuttering more obvious and are learned behaviors that often can be unlearned to reduce physical struggle. Avoidance behaviors (such as using sounds like "um" before stutters or changing words to skip over stutters) are critical. They indicate that the client's stutters are accompanied by fear that may gradually increase and make the stuttering worse and more pervasive. This fear must be addressed in treatment.

Trial Therapy

Trial therapy for adolescents can be brief if the client seems to be tired of talking about stuttering and wants to move on. However, if the client seems enthusiastic about changing his stuttering, trial therapy can be long enough so the adolescent can take away a new way of responding to their stuttering to try out. I might start out by saying to the client that I'd like to learn about their stuttering by having them teach me to stutter like they do. Curiosity is your friend here. If they are willing to do this, you should probably show them that you are not as good as they are at doing their kinds of stutters. If they have blocks, then as you are having them teach you how to block, express real interest in what they do when they block and then see if you and they can keep the block going for several seconds, beyond the time they would typically finish the stutter. If they stutter like this: M m m (silent continuing block) see if, with your model, spoken aloud as they stutter, can get them to stay in the stutter and relax until they can finish the stutter in a slow, relaxed way. A good example of this trial therapy is the video of Dean Williams working with a young adolescent, which is available on Lippincott Connect with Chapter 11 videos. Dr. Williams himself stuttered and was a renowned stuttering therapist. The brief video clip shows Williams helping a young man who stutters to be able to go into a stutter rather than avoiding it, then stay in the stutter deliberately, and finally relax so that his muscles let him finish the word.

Interview With Parents of an Adolescent

As I mentioned earlier, adolescents strive to become more and more independent of their parents, and I have found that therapy works best if an adolescent is treated as an adult. I begin fostering independence by talking first to teenage clients separately from their parents so that they can give me their own views of the situation and how they view the prospect of treatment. I ask them if they would like to be present when I talk with their parents and if there's anything the adolescent client has said to me that they would not like me to share with their parents. In the next paragraph, I'll describe an interview with the teen's parents when they have requested not to be present in the interview.

I begin the interview when the adolescent is not there by asking the parents to describe the problem as they see it and encourage them to express their fears, concerns, and frustrations, as I listen carefully. I try to get an understanding of how their student functions within the family and I usually ask such questions as "What is their stuttering like at home?" "How do they seem to feel about it—are they embarrassed or do they show fear of talking or anger about their speech?" "How do you feel about it?" "What are your and other family members' reactions to it?" "What do you do when your student stutters?" "Have they been seen anywhere else for therapy?" "If so, what were the results?" Even though I am putting some of these questions in groups, I am careful to ask one question at a time and listen carefully to the answer before I ask another question. Although parents, in an interview without the teen, may ask what can be done to help their student and what they should do, I prefer to wait until I am meeting with both the parents and the teen before answering these questions. A relatively recent orientation to help parents and adolescents work together is called Solution-Focused Brief Therapy for Stuttering (Nicholas, 2015; Rodgers et al., 2020). It helps the adolescent and parents focus on the client's strengths and hopes, rather than simply on the problem of stuttering, and is integrated into the overall therapy program. Stuttering Foundation has an excellent lecture with video examples on Solution-Focused Brief Therapy for Stuttering, entitled "What Makes You You" in their section on Virtual Learning Classes. Here is a link to help you find this class and videos: thestutteringfoundation.vhx.tv. My sense is that Solution-Focused Brief Therapy is related to modern wellness perspectives on psychotherapy and counseling that will be discussed in Chapter 12, Preliminaries to Treatment (Holland & Nelson, 2020).

Returning to my approach to working with adolescents who stutter and their parents, if I am meeting with the parents and the teen together, at some point I let the parents know that I will respect the teen's confidentiality in terms of what the teen shares with me when we are working together. In a joint meeting with parents and teen, I also try to begin with a discussion of all the good things the teen has going for them—such as his participation in sports, achievements in school, friendships, or proficiency on the internet. Remember we will be talking about the adolescent's stuttering—something the teen probably feels at least a little ashamed about. Thus, the atmosphere needs to be leavened with talk of the teen's good qualities so that both parents and adolescent feel hope about the future. Previously when I interviewed the teen, I have probably done some trial therapy, and, if the teen has given me permission, the teen and I share how well they are able to confront their stuttering (if that is the case). We might then let the parents know what sort of things the adolescent will be doing in therapy so the parents can appreciate that if stuttering spikes or becomes more evident or longer at times at home, it is all part of the plan. For example, this plan might include the teen experimenting with stutters at home, by staying in them and loosening them before finishing the word.

I meet with the parents and teenage clients together to seek mutual agreement about their respective roles in treatment. This is often an important time. It serves to let teens know that I respect their ability to work independently from the parents, and it serves to let the parents know that they can be most helpful by being supportive but not directive.

Diagnosis

After I have met with the parents and have interviewed the adolescent, I need to determine whether the client stutters and, if so, what treatment level is appropriate. At this point, I usually ask the family to wait in the clinic room while I confer with any students or colleagues involved the evaluation, in a separate room to review the gathered information: video recordings, case history, personal perspectives, and questionnaires.

I begin by considering the possibility that a teenager turns out *not* to have a problem with stuttering. In rare cases, teens who are typically but highly disfluent may be considered to be stuttering by teachers or parents. Most of these highly disfluent individuals have phrase repetitions, circumlocutions, revisions, and hesitations, which are the types of disfluencies described in Chapter 7 as typical. Sometimes, high levels of disfluencies are associated with language disorders or with attention-deficit disorders, especially during the production of longer utterances and narratives (Bangert & Finestack, 2020)—conditions that are likely to have been identified prior to a student's referral for a possible stuttering disorder.

Typical disfluencies are relatively infrequent after children's elementary school years; however, some adolescents may simply be at the disfluent end of the continuum of normal fluency.

I also keep in mind that sometimes these typical disfluencies are used intentionally to mask, or avoid, stuttering. So, if I notice a lot of these typical disfluencies in their speech, and I've established a trusting relationship with the teen, I may ask them, "I've noticed that you sometimes repeat a phrase, talk around a word, or that you sometimes hesitate before saying a word. Have you ever noticed those things? Do you have a theory about why you might do that?"

In addition to noting lots of typical disfluencies, we may not suspect stuttering if secondary behaviors and negative feelings and attitudes are absent. Our role in such cases is to explain to the individual and to the referring person (if this is a referral) that this kind of speech is not indicative of a fluency disorder. It may also be emphasized to the referring source that excessive attention to these disfluencies may be more harmful than helpful. If the client or referring person feels strongly that the disfluent speech interferes with communication, and their anxiety about speaking is low, a fluency-oriented treatment described in the chapters on treating intermediate and advanced stuttering may be offered to the client.

Another need for differential diagnosis, in addition to identifying cases of normal disfluency, is ensuring that cluttering, neurogenic disfluency, and psychogenic disfluency be identified and distinguished from "typical" or "developmental" stuttering. Moreover, it is also necessary to rule out disfluencies caused by word-finding difficulties that might be evident in a person with a learning disability.

Some of the salient features of cluttering in adolescents are rapid and sometimes unintelligible speech; frequent repetitions of syllables, words, or phrases; lack of awareness or concern about their speech; disorganized thought processes; and language problems. Cluttering often coexists with stuttering, and both disorders may respond to a highly structured, fluency-shaping approach for treatment. Evaluation and treatment procedures for cluttering are described in Chapter 18.

Neurogenic disfluency in adolescents is usually the result of stroke, head trauma, or neurological disease. Symptoms are likely to be repetitive disfluencies but may include blocks as well. Because stuttering commonly begins in childhood, if a client reports onset of stuttering after age 12, a neurogenic-based disorder is a possibility. In almost all such cases, onsets of neurogenic-based fluency problems are clearly linked to a well-defined episode of neurological damage. A section of Chapter 18 is devoted to evaluation and treatment of neurogenic stuttering.

Disfluency that begins in adolescence can also result from psychological trauma. When late-onset disfluencies are seen that are associated with psychological stress and conflict or the onset of a psychiatric condition, psychogenic disfluency should be suspected. Traditional treatments, such as those described in the chapters on treatment of intermediate and advanced stuttering, may or may not be helpful. The patient should be referred for both psychological and neurological assessments, so that treatment needed in these areas will be identified and provided. See Chapter 18 for more information.

When a clinician determines that stuttering treatment would be appropriate for a client, whether the stuttering had a typical onset during early childhood or has another etiology, the focus turns to a consideration of what level of treatment to select for the client. As I indicated earlier, adolescents are most likely to be at advanced developmental and treatment levels. Signs of this level include the core behaviors of repetitions, prolongations, and blocks, all with tension; the secondary behaviors of escape and especially *avoidance*; and strong negative feelings and attitudes about communication in general and stuttering in particular.

Determining Developmental and Treatment Level

The determination of a developmental/treatment level for an adolescent is based largely on the client's age. Intermediate and advanced treatment approaches are well suited for clients whose core behaviors are blocks, who have escape and avoidance behaviors as secondary symptoms, and whose attitudes about speech are relatively negative. Clients suited to the advanced-level treatment will usually have more entrenched negative attitudes about speech and themselves as a speaker simply because they have been stuttering longer. It's possible that someone who is at the advanced level will have developed an extensive repertoire of avoidance behaviors so that actual stuttering behaviors are rare, but the individual's life is highly constrained by their efforts to avoid and hide his stuttering. The major difference between intermediate and advanced treatment levels is that more independence and responsibility are required of clients for treatment at the advanced level. Consequently, before deciding on a treatment approach for an adolescent, the clinician must consider how much responsibility they can take for self-therapy.

Intermediate Stuttering

A client whose stuttering is at the intermediate level will probably be younger than midteens, perhaps 13 or 14. Their stuttering pattern will be characterized by escape and avoidance behaviors and considerable tension on blocks, prolongations, and repetitions. They will also be avoiding some speaking situations. Moreover, their feelings and attitudes, as revealed in questionnaires and interviews with them and with their parents and teachers, will suggest some negative speech attitudes but they won't be deeply ingrained.

Advanced Stuttering

Individuals who fit into the advanced developmental/treatment level are well into their teens and sufficiently mature to handle the assignments used in advanced treatment. Their stuttering pattern is similar to intermediate stuttering, but their patterns of avoidance and escape may be more habituated (ie, patterns appear to be highly automatized and rapidly performed). They will probably avoid difficult speaking situations whenever possible, and I often find strong negative self-concepts and negative anticipations of listener reactions as well. An individual with advanced stuttering may feel, for example, "I must be awfully incompetent if I can't even talk," or "People think I'm dumb because I stutter."

Closing Interview

Before the closing interview, I ask the adolescent if they are ok with having both them and their parents in the conversation. Also, before meeting with the parents and adolescent at the end of the evaluation, I take some time to write a summary of my findings and some very tentative ideas for where to go from here. This may be hand-written or printed, but it is important for the family to have something to refer to as we talk, as well as to take home and talk about among themselves or with relatives, if appropriate. Once they have had a chance to look it over, I ask them what questions they have.

Then, I verbally summarize my impressions of the teen's stuttering with plenty of positive comments about the teen and their realistic potential for learning to stutter more easily. I give my suggestions for treatment (or no treatment)—ideally integrating the teen's ideas for change that they shared earlier in the interview. I emphasize that treatment usually takes many months, because the stuttering has developed over many years and much is learned behavior which needs to be unlearned. I may add that not only behavior needs to be changed, but feelings and attitudes about oneself and one's stuttering must change too if easier talking is to last. Being at peace with one's speech, whether fluent or not, is the lifetime goal.

If the trial therapy has gone particularly well, I also ask the adolescent if they would be willing to show their parents how they can make stutters easier with some concentrated work. This is tricky because I don't want the parents to expect the teen to do this at home whenever they stutter. I explain—if we show easier stuttering to the parents—that this will only be practiced in therapy at first, not outside yet, until the teen feels they have mastered stuttering more easily and we have done lots of work on generalizing it to more and more real-world situations. I also suggest that the teen will use easier stuttering a little at home if and when they feel like it and having the parents accept it as normal speech will foster its growth.

If the teen is computer savvy and uses the internet (what teen doesn't?), I recommend the websites for teens who stutter. For example, on the Stuttering Foundation (www.stutteringhelp.org), there is a link to resources specifically for teens that can be found on the home page (you may need to scroll down). The "teens" link leads them to streaming videos for teens as well as a good deal of written material for free and links to other internet sites with resources for teens. These items will help them learn about therapy and develop realistic and motivating expectations about its potential outcome.

Another source of information for teens who stutter is the National Stuttering Association (www.westutter.org). On their home page, you can hover your mouse over "Who We Help" and choose "Teens" and find many interesting links. The National Stuttering Association also hosts national conferences, giving individuals of all ages an opportunity to share their experiences and receive long-term support.

Sometimes, it helps to have the teen you are assessing talk with a former or current teenage client who also stutters. This can provide substantial hope. This can be arranged for a future meeting and perhaps the current or former client's parents would be willing to talk to the parents of the teen you are evaluating.

As you talk with the teen and their parents about therapy (if it's called for), remember that some adolescent clients are reluctant to participate in therapy, rather than being highly motivated, because of their desire to close ranks with their peers and distance themselves from adults. If they are at all interested in help, I try to strike a bargain with them to try at least four sessions of therapy before they make a decision about treatment. As with all therapy for younger individuals, I strive to make the sessions a lot of fun so they will want to come back and they feel their stuttering is accepted in our clinic.

We end the closing interview by asking the adolescent and their parents if there is anything they've left out that they want to tell us or if they have any questions. Following that, we express our appreciation of the parents and the teen, and reaffirm plans for the future.

ADULT

The assessment of an adult who stutters can be more straightforward than for younger clients. Adults are usually seeing you because they want to get help. Although some clients may be discouraged because they have been stuttering for years and are understandably skeptical that you can really help them, many are highly motivated to work on their speech and ready to begin this work during the evaluation. Your challenge is to take advantage of this motivation, get them working immediately, and give them realistic hope that hard work and determination can change their speech and maybe their lives. Many aspects of my recommendations for assessment of an adult are adopted from Van Riper. Some of these I learned from his book, *The Treatment of Stuttering* (1973a). But other components came from my experience of being assessed by Van Riper himself, when I had just turned 20 years old.

Preassessment

Case History Form

This is the same form used for adolescents who stutter (Fig. 11.4), and it can be sent to the client and returned to you prior to the actual assessment.

Attitudes and Feelings Questionnaires

I assess clients' communication attitudes through observations, interview questions, and questionnaires. Typically, I use the adult version of the Overall Assessment of the Speaker's Experience of Stuttering (OASES-A, Fig. 11.5) and the Modified Erickson Scale of Communication Attitudes (S-24, Fig. 11.6) questionnaires. Because I want to be able to analyze completed questionnaires before the diagnostic interview, I prefer to send them to clients and ask them to complete and return the questionnaires before the interview. If this is not possible, clients can complete them when they arrive for an evaluation before the initial interview or, as a less desirable alternative, after the initial interview. Prior to the interview, follow-up questions based on information from the case history and questionnaires, which are described in the section on feelings and attitudes, can be prepared to further explore a client's attitudes.

Audio/Video Recording

It is important to sample a client's speech in several situations to get an adequate picture of their stuttering. I ask clients to video or audio record themselves talking in one or two different situations outside the clinic and get the recording to me prior to the evaluation. It is usually easy for clients to record themselves talking to someone on the phone, recording only their own voices and not the person on the other end of the line, therefore, not violating the other person's privacy. Some clients can also video record themselves talking face-to-face with a friend or family member, obtaining their permission to record. If I study the recording(s) before an evaluation, I am better prepared to understand the client's stuttering and to plan various trial-therapy strategies.

Assessment

Interview/Conversation

I begin by welcoming the client and reviewing the procedures I will use to evaluate their stuttering, such as interviewing them about their stuttering and their feelings and attitudes, video recording their speaking and reading, examining what they do when they stutter, and trying to determine if they can change it. I let them know that after I've interviewed them, I will ask them to wait while I analyze the information I've obtained before a meeting with them to share my findings and recommendations. If there are any forms or questionnaires that I haven't already obtained from them, I'll have them complete those while I analyze the other data. I video record the interview, and even though I have indicated that video recording will be part of the evaluation, I ask the client again, just prior to turning on a video recorder, whether they mind if I record our conversation.

I begin our interview with an open-ended question such as "Tell me about the problem that brings you here today," or "Why don't you tell me about your stuttering?" The first question might be used if I don't know what is motivating the client to come for an evaluation at this time; the second question I use when I already know from prior information why the client has come right now.

Once a client has had a chance to describe their speech problem, I ask further questions to try to get a deeper understanding. The following are typical questions that I ask with a brief commentary about why I'm asking them. Sometimes, I group several questions together (eg, a question to start the client talking about a particular topic and follow-up questions that I ask if the first question doesn't elicit all of the desired information). I ask only one question at a time, listen carefully to the client's response, and try to understand the client's underlying feelings.

1. **Tell me about the beginning of your stuttering and how it has changed over the years.**
   I realize that in answering the first part of this question, a client may just be reporting what parents told them about their stuttering. The accuracy of their response may be questionable, but at least I'll learn their perception of the onset. The second part of the question—about changes over the years—may reveal what kinds of things affect the way the client stutters. Do they stutter more severely because of a recent job change or a threat to their self-esteem, such as a divorce or loss of employment? Less frequently, I may find out that a client began to stutter in late adolescence or as an adult. If so, I would want to consider the possibility of neurogenic or psychogenic stuttering, which is discussed briefly in the upcoming section on "Diagnosis" and more fully in Chapters 8 and 18, on atypical disfluency.
2. **What do you believe caused you to stutter?**
   This may give some insights about a client's motivation. For example, a woman whose speech I once evaluated reported that her mother and several brothers stuttered and that her stuttering was, therefore, a genetic problem that could not be helped. This led us to confront the issue of whether or not she was likely to change. (Yes, change is quite possible no matter what a client's genetic history.)

   In addition, I sometimes find that clients have misinformation about possible causes of their stuttering. If I can give them more appropriate information, their attitudes about the problem may change, and their motivation may increase. I have met individuals who come to the evaluation believing that their problem is entirely psychological. After I discuss current views of stuttering, they are relieved to know that they *can* modify their speech and their attitudes about speaking, even with stuttering, without long-term psychotherapy.
3. **Does anyone else in your family stutter?**
   I might find that a parent stutters, which can be significant because a parent's attitudes about their own stuttering may have had a profound effect on the client. Moreover, knowing about other family members who stutter and how they have responded to it may provide a better understanding of the factors related to this client's stuttering, which may be useful in treatment. For example, someone I am interviewing may have had a parent who stuttered but who never talked about it. I might then want to explore whether the individual I am working with feels especially ashamed of their stuttering or, on the other hand, whether it gives them an important bond with the parent, or both.
4. **Have you ever had therapy for your stuttering? What did the therapy consist of? How effective do you think it was?**
   This information is important in planning therapy. For example, if a client had received a type of therapy that they felt did not help, it would be unwise to use that type of therapy with this client. But, if a client has had success with therapy but has regressed slightly or moved away before treatment was finished, using this type of therapy again may be most appropriate. It is important that clinicians be familiar with various types of therapy that clients may have undergone. Most current therapies emphasize either modifying stuttering behaviors and attitudes (**stuttering modification**) or learning to talk in ways that eliminate stuttering (**fluency shaping**). A third option is learning to talk openly with stuttering, with an attitude that it is a perfectly acceptable way to talk.
5. **Has your stuttering changed or caused you more problems recently? Why did you come in for help at the present time?**
   Responses to these questions allow clinicians to see the current problems faced by the client and also get a sense of the client's motivation. For example, a client may have been offered a promotion if they can improve their speech or may have recently learned of the clinic's treatment program and is hoping for some relief from a long-standing problem. The following four questions about the client's pattern of stuttering are closely related to one another:
6. **Are there times or situations when you stutter more? Less? What are they?**
7. **Do you avoid certain speaking situations in which you expect to stutter? If so, which ones?**
8. **Do you avoid certain words on which you expect to stutter? Do you substitute one word for another if you expect to stutter? Do you talk around words or topics so you won't stutter?**
9. **Do you use any special movements or extra sounds to get words out? Escape behaviors?**
   These four questions will provide information that is useful in planning therapy because they tell us something about the client's most difficult situations, how they feel about them, and how they deal with them. This information may also corroborate what has been learned from the questionnaires that the client completed and will also reveal how aware they are of their stuttering behaviors. Neutral (rather than negative) questions about escape and avoidance behaviors let the clinician show they accept these behaviors as they explain why escape and avoidance behaviors are used and strongly learned.

10. **Have your academic or vocational choices or performance been affected because you stutter? How?**
The client's answers can be used to help plan later stages of treatment in which new behaviors and new challenges are attempted. They may also prompt the clinician to refer clients in later stages of treatment to an academic or vocational counselor to help them make more appropriate choices for themselves.

11. **Have your relationships with people been affected because you stutter? How?**
As with Question 10, I can use this information to plan a client's hierarchy of generalization, moving from easy to difficult social situations gradually if the client finds social interactions difficult. I also need to know how much a client blames their stuttering for any of the difficulties they have in social interactions. A client may be socially inhibited because they are sensitive and vulnerable to expected listener reactions. Such sensitivity can be assessed by observing their facial expressions and body movements while stuttering as indicators of affect. If they appear to be relatively unaffected emotionally by their stuttering but professes to have difficulty relating to people, they may benefit from counseling or psychotherapy that focuses on resolving this interpersonal difficulty.

The decision to refer an individual for psychotherapy as an adjunct to stuttering therapy can seldom be made in an evaluation session. It may be that a few therapy sessions are needed to learn more about a person and to develop the client's trust before a successful referral can be made. If psychotherapy is recommended too hastily, a client may believe that I think his stuttering is too great a problem for me to handle, perhaps an insurmountable problem or one that I secretly believe is due to a psychological disorder. However, if I work with them and they start making some progress before I refer, they will likely feel supported and may be more likely to benefit from psychotherapy.

12. **What are your feelings or attitudes toward your stuttering? What do you think other people think about your stuttering?**
A client's responses will be used to help determine some of the foci of treatment, such as desensitization procedures to decrease fear as well as shame or guilt about stuttering. Perceptions about others' views of his stuttering may need to be confronted with various "reality-testing" tasks to find out what people really think.

13. **What are your family's (spouse's, children's) feelings, attitudes, and reactions toward your stuttering and toward the prospect of your being in therapy?**
This information can identify sources that may positively or negatively affect a client's motivation and may be an important consideration in planning therapy.

14. **Is there anything else that you think we ought to know about your stuttering?**
This gives the client a chance to get anything off their chest that they may be holding back or an opportunity to discuss issues that occurred to them only after other questions were asked.

15. **Do you have any questions you'd like to ask me?**

Sometimes, a client has questions about stuttering that they have been reluctant to ask, and this may give the clinician an opportunity to answer them. On the other hand, a client may want to ask about the length and type of treatment or other issues that are best dealt with after his assessment is completed. In this case, the clinician explains why they need to delay responding but will keep the questions in mind to answer during the closing interview.

Speech Sample

In this part of the evaluation, the client's overt stuttering behaviors are assessed. Although I always video record the entire evaluation (if the client has given permission), I pay particular attention to the recording of this section because I will need to analyze it carefully afterward. In the first 5 or 10 minutes of the interview, I try to let the client talk as much as possible without my interrupting or asking too many questions. This is a conversation, but one in which the client does most of the talking—at first. Clinicians use a variety of procedures for assessing overt stuttering. Next, I shall describe in detail the tool I currently use and then note other available options.

Stuttering Severity

As indicated in Chapter 9, stuttering severity is usually measured using the Stuttering Severity Instrument (currently, SSI-4; Riley, 2009; Fig. 9.3), a moderately reliable tool that is commonly used to assess the severity of stuttering. To obtain appropriate samples, I have the client talk about a familiar topic, such as his work, school, hobbies, vacations, sports, or entertainment. It is important to get about at least 300 syllables of the client's talking, so 5 or 10 minutes is usually enough, depending on the client's fluency. Then, I provide the client material at an appropriate reading level, such as the passages in the SSI examiner's manual, and ask them to read aloud for about 3 minutes to get 200 or more syllables of reading.

As I noted earlier, we often gather more than one sample of spontaneous speech from adults and adolescents. A sample of speech during a telephone conversation in the clinic can be video recorded and scored using the SSI. In addition, I use samples the client has brought or sent in. If the sample from another environment is audio recorded rather than video recorded, I score it for both frequency of stuttering and speech rate, as described below.

In some instances, an adult client will ask for therapy that doesn't work directly on their stuttering, but instead focuses only on attitudes and feelings and works toward talking without concern about stuttering. Those individuals may prefer to only have attitudes and feelings assessed, rather than the severity of stuttering.

Other Measures of Stuttering

If I am assessing stuttering many times throughout the course of treatment or assessing samples that I cannot visually analyze, such as audio samples recorded by a client in his natural environment, I use a combination of frequency of stuttering (percentage of syllables stuttered) and speech rate (syllables spoken per minute). These measures, which were first described in Andrews and Ingham (1971), together require much less time than the SSI. Another possibility when speech is assessed frequently throughout treatment is to have yourself and the client independently rate samples using the Lidcombe Program's 9-point severity rating scale (Fig. 9.4).

Speech Rate

In addition to measuring stuttering severity using the SSI, I also assess a client's speech rate. I believe, as many other clinicians do, that speaking rate often reflects the severity of stuttering, as well as its effect on communication. If a client's speech rate is markedly slower than normal, communication may be difficult for them. A description of the procedure for measuring speech rate was given in Chapter 9, "Preliminaries to Assessment."

Normal speaking rates of adults range from around 115 to 165 words per minute, or about 162 to 230 syllables per minute, with a mean of 196 syllables per minute (Andrews & Ingham, 1971). Adults' normal rates for reading aloud are faster, ranging from about 150 to 190 words per minute (Darley & Spriestersbach, 1978), or about 210 to 265 syllables per minute (Andrews & Ingham, 1971).

Pattern of Disfluencies

Throughout my evaluation of adult or adolescent stutterers, I observe the client's patterns of stuttering. For example, I try to roughly determine the proportions of core behaviors that are repetitions, prolongations, or blocks and ask myself a number of questions about the client's stuttering. During blocks, where and how do they shut off airflow or voicing? What are their escape and avoidance behaviors? Do they end the stutters quickly with pushing and tension? Are they able to tolerate being in blocks, or do they speak in unusual or vague ways to avoid stuttering? More details on various escape and avoidance patterns can be found in Chapter 7 on the development of stuttering. My aim, as I study the client's stuttering, is to figure out how much fear of stuttering there is. If there are a lot of avoidances and urgent escape behaviors, I would hypothesize that the client has a fair bit of fear of stuttering, and I need to focus on that as I gain the client's trust, get to know them, and help them learn to stutter more easily.

As I explore the behaviors that constitute a client's stuttering, I comment on these behaviors, acceptingly, and question the client about how typical this sample of their stuttering is, and ask about the escape and avoidance behaviors we've observed. If a client doesn't seem too uncomfortable confronting their stuttering, I ask them to teach me how to stutter like they do, and we work together, with both the client and myself emulating their various types of stuttering. This does not need to be an exhaustive exploration, because I will do much more in treatment. Here, I am trying to accomplish three tasks: (1) begin to decrease fear a little, by modeling an "approach" rather than "avoidance" attitude toward stuttering, showing clear acceptance and objectivity about behaviors that the client may feel are shameful and perhaps even terrifying; (2) study the client's emotional reaction when the client comes face-to-face with their stuttering and perhaps reduce some of their fear; and (3) teach both of us about what the client does when they stutter so that they can begin to reduce their emotional response to it and eventually stutter in a way that is freer or closer to typical speech. My first steps in having the client approach their stutters are the beginning of trial therapy, described in more detail in the next section.

Trial Therapy

I try therapy techniques with clients during their assessment sessions for several reasons. First, I try to get an idea of how a client responds to different therapy approaches, which provides me with information I may use in talking with them about possible treatments. Second, trial therapy can help me to make a differential diagnosis between developmental stuttering and stuttering with a neurological or psychological etiology. Third, it gives clients a preview of things to come and provides them with motivation to follow through on treatment. There is a fourth reason: to give the client hope that they can change.

I begin by asking a client to modify their stuttering, which can be done easily in the context of studying their patterns of disfluency, as described in the preceding section. In fact, this exploration of stuttering with a client is a condensed version of the first stage of treatment that aims to change stuttering to an easier pattern. Once a client is able to emulate their stuttering to a small degree, I carry out trial therapy by coaching them through the following sequence:

1. First, I encourage them to stutter, telling him we must have a sample of the behavior we are trying to change. Then, I ask them to "freeze" during a moment of stuttering but maintain the level of physical tension and posture of their stuttering as I encourage them to stay in the moment of stuttering. In other words, I ask them to catch a stutter and prolong it. This may require a little or a lot of modeling of how to hold a moment of stuttering right on the sound that's being stuttered. This is easier with a continuant sound, like /m/, and will be harder and need more coaching for plosives, such as /b/. You will probably have to model for the client how to prolong the posture required for holding a stutter on a plosive. It is key that

you and they identify the exact posture that is associated with the moment of stuttering and hold onto it. When I model this for the client, after I demonstrate staying in the moment of stuttering, I always finish the word slowly and easily, which I will ask them to do, later. It is important that during this activity, the clinician praises the client enthusiastically for catching and holding onto a moment of stuttering. This helps the counterconditioning process—pairing a positive stimulus (praise) with a behavior about which the client feels negative (the moment of stuckness). Also, anything you can do to inject humor into this process will help the counterconditioning.

2. Have the client become aware of what they are doing at the moment when they get into the stutter. For example, where are they holding back sound or airflow? Lips? Tongue? Larynx? All three? As you are helping them explore what they are doing when they stutter, use plenty of praise for being able to stay in the stutter. This is an experience charged with fear and frustration for most adolescent and adults who stutter. Try to create something very different—a satisfying experience that you provide by rewarding their maintaining of this stuttering moment. It's similar to treatment for a phobia: staying in contact with a feared object (a spider or even, in some cases, a rabbit) reduces fear if there is reward provided by another person. It has been said that an individual's physical awareness of what they are doing with their body as they stutter can be an antidote to the fear they might otherwise be feeling (Zebrowski, personal communication, October 18, 2011, channeling the famous clinician Dr. Dean Williams). This may be related to the use of proprioceptive awareness, that is asking the client to focus on how movement feels, to manage stuttering (Van Riper, 1973a).
3. Have the client change their behaviors that are increasing the burden of stuttering by (1) releasing excess physical tension wherever they can feel it, (2) starting to move structures that are being rigidly held, (3) getting voicing or airflow going, and/or (4) allowing themselves to breathe. I may stop a client's trial therapy here if they are unable to release the physical tension or does it only with obvious difficulty and frustration.

If a client seems able to make these changes in trial therapy, I go one step further. I ask the client to hold onto the stutter, which will become more voluntary after my coaching reduces their fear. I coach the client to prolong the airflow or voicing for several seconds (while I tell them how great it is that they can do this!) and then produce the remainder of the word slowly. (Some of my clients call this "catch and release.") You can see an example of trial therapy in a video on Lippincott Connect—"Diagnostic Evaluation: Trial Therapy" with the Chapter 11 videos. If a client is able to do this with coaching, I ask them to do it while reading without my coaching. This is enough. No matter how much or how little our client is able to do, I want to stop when they are feeling successful.

Another approach to trial therapy—one that I would only use for a client who seems to have little or no fear of stuttering—is to change the client's habitual way of talking so that stuttering is decreased substantially or prevented. Adults who fear stuttering, especially those with avoidance behaviors, will probably continue to have fear even if they learn a new way of talking to (temporarily) replace stuttering. The fear will often create a relapse in the new fluency. However, with those few clients who are unafraid of stuttering, I experiment with a slow way of talking that produces fluency. I begin by reducing my own speech rate as I describe the aim of this exercise to the client, which is to produce words very, very slowly. I use a written sentence that begins with a vowel or a glide, going over it word by word, teaching the client to use gradual and gentle onsets of voicing and to stretch each sound, whether vowel or consonant. This is essentially the "prolonged speech" or "fluency-facilitating targets" used by some fluency-shaping approaches, such as the Camperdown Program (O'Brian et al., 2017) and the Fluency Plus Program (Kroll & Scott-Sulsky, 2010). The clinician needs to provide a good model for each word and to give feedback frequently. When words are produced slowly enough with each part of the speech production system (respiration, phonation, and articulation) moving in slow motion and without excess tension, then fluency results. After a client is able to produce each word of the sentence in this way, they are then coached to produce the entire sentence, linking each word to the next. Breath supply should be monitored closely, so that pauses for breath are taken whenever the client would take a breath naturally. Again, accurate modeling and frequent feedback are crucial at earlier stages of treatment.

As an example, the sentence, "Apples are a red fruit," should take from 15 to 20 seconds to produce, with a pause for a new breath after the word "a." The /p/ in "Apples," the /d/ in "red," and the /t/ in "fruit" each should be produced without stopping airflow, making these plosives sound like fricatives. If clients are particularly adept at this, they can be taken all the way to saying short sentences in conversational speech that are produced in this slow, fluent manner. However, clients who have difficulty should be coached only through the production of the short, written sentence, and care should be taken to stop this activity before they experience failure.

This therapeutic approach—fluency shaping or "controlled speaking"—I would *only* use with the rare client who shows little fear of stuttering and who appears to have a relatively robust (nonsensitive) temperament.

Feelings and Attitudes

A variety of questionnaires can be used to assess various aspects of a stutterer's feelings and attitudes about communication and stuttering, as mentioned earlier. These include the OASES (Yaruss & Quesal, 2006) (Fig. 11.5), the Modified Erickson Scale of Communication Attitudes (S-24) (Andrews & Cutler, 1974) (Fig. 11.6), the Stutterer's Self-Rating of

Reactions to Speech Situations (Johnson et al., 1952), the Perceptions of Stuttering Inventory (Woolf, 1967), the Locus of Control of Behavior Scale (Craig et al., 1984), and Self-efficacy Scaling by Adult Stutterers (Ornstein & Manning, 1985). Any of these (I most often use only the first two) can be sent to the client before the evaluation and returned so that the clinician can score them ahead of time and have a preliminary idea about the client's emotions related to his stuttering.

Much of the exploration of emotions, however, is done informally, as well as through the questionnaires cited in the last paragraph. This work goes throughout the treatment but is started in the initial evaluation interview. As feelings are being expressed and the clinician creates an atmosphere of calmness and tolerance, the client-clinician relationship is begun. As they converse, the clinician tries to understand the client's feelings, sometimes asking questions to elicit them and sometimes restating the expressed feelings in a way that demonstrates the clinician is interested in them and accepts them. This approach is therapeutic. It is described by Carl Rogers in his book *Counseling and Psychotherapy* (1942). In this book, Rogers not only describes how the clinician works but also provides a detailed transcript of his work with a client who stutters (and has other issues) in his chapter "The Case of Herbert Bryan." We will revisit the counseling relationship in the next chapter, but for now, I will make a few comments about eliciting feelings in the evaluation interview.

In the assessment interview, described earlier, I wait until I have recorded about 5 to 10 minutes of the client's relatively uninterrupted speech to use for assessment of stuttering, and then I begin to explore the client's stuttering and their feelings about it. As I suggested in the section on "The **Pattern of Disfluencies**," I often stop the client and ask about the stutters that they have and we study them together. As I do this, I also probe the client's feeling with such comments as "When you get stuck like that, how does it feel?" or "If you get in a block like that when you are talking to someone, what are the feelings that go with it?" Before the assessment interview begins, I try to read the client's intake questionnaires, such as the OASES or Erickson S-24, to get some ideas about what are some of the emotional issues related to his stuttering. I use that information to explore the client's feelings—both those about being a person who stutters (feelings such as shame) and those that rise up when the client is (1) anticipating a stutter, (2) is stuck in a stutter, and (3) has just stuttered. It may also help to have the client try to get in touch with sensations within their body that are associated with these feelings.

Other Speech and Language Behaviors

As I interact with a client during the interview, I informally assess their comprehension and production of language, their articulation, and their voice. I also screen their hearing. If I suspect that there may be an articulation, language, voice, or hearing problem, I follow up with further evaluations. Procedures for assessment of speech sound production can be found in Bernthal et al. (2022) and in Velleman (2015). I let a client's concern about other disorders guide us in treatment. If, as I have found occasionally, a stuttering client also produces distorted /s/ or /r/ sounds, I discuss it with them. If they are not concerned, I don't believe it is necessary to treat that disorder. However, if I believe that an articulation, language, or other problem handicaps a client communicatively, I advise treatment for that problem also. Sometimes, I deal with voice problems differently. I have found that some stutterers may be hoarse, but I suspect this may be the result of laryngeal tension related to stuttering. If stuttering treatment is successful, hoarseness may disappear. Again, I take my cue from the client. If the problem bothers them and isn't remediated by treatment, I address it. If hoarseness is of recent origin and not associated with a cold, I may refer them for an otolaryngological examination to rule out serious laryngeal pathology.

Diagnosis

After I gather the information just described, I need to determine whether the client stutters and, if so, what treatment level is appropriate.

In rare cases, adults who are typically but highly disfluent may be referred by spouses, employers, or friends. Most of these individuals have phrase repetitions, circumlocutions, revisions, and hesitations, which are the types of disfluencies described in Chapter 7 as typical. In addition to the differences in type and number of disfluencies, secondary behaviors and negative feelings and attitudes will be absent. Our role in such cases is to explain to the individual that this kind of speech is not related to stuttering but has been shown to be associated with developmental language disorders and attention deficit hyperactivity disorder. If the client or referring person feels strongly that the disfluent speech interferes with communication, a fluency-oriented treatment described in the chapters on treating advanced stuttering may be offered to the client.

Another need for differential diagnosis, in addition to identifying cases of typical disfluency, is ensuring that cluttering, neurogenic disfluency, and psychogenic disfluency be identified and distinguished from "typical" or "developmental" stuttering.

Some of the salient features of cluttering in adults and adolescents are rapid and sometimes unintelligible speech; frequent repetitions of syllables, words, or phrases; lack of awareness or concern about their speech; disorganized thought processes; and language problems. Cluttering often coexists with stuttering, and both disorders may respond to a highly structured, fluency-shaping approach for treatment. Evaluation and treatment procedures for cluttering are described in Chapter 18.

Neurogenic disfluency in adults is usually the result of stroke, head trauma, or neurological disease. Symptoms are likely to be repetitive disfluencies but may include blocks as well. Because stuttering commonly begins in childhood, if a client reports onset of stuttering after age 12, a neurogenic-based disorder is a possibility. In almost all such cases, onsets of neurogenic-based fluency problems are clearly linked to a well-defined episode of neurological damage. A section of Chapter 18 is devoted to evaluation and treatment of neurogenic stuttering.

Disfluency that begins in adulthood can also result from psychological trauma. When late-onset disfluencies are seen that are associated with psychological stress and conflict or the onset of a psychiatric condition, psychogenic disfluency should be suspected. Traditional treatments, such as those described in Chapter 17 on treatment of advanced stuttering, may or may not be helpful. The patient should be referred for both psychological and neurological assessments, so that treatment needed in these areas will be identified and provided. See Chapter 18 for more information.

When a clinician determines that stuttering treatment would be appropriate for a client, whether the stuttering had a typical onset during early childhood or has another etiology, the focus turns to a consideration of what level of treatment to select for the client. As I indicated earlier, adults are most likely to be at advanced developmental and treatment levels. Signs of this level include the core behaviors of repetitions, prolongations, and blocks, all with tension; the secondary behaviors of escape and especially *avoidance*; and strong negative feelings and attitudes about communication in general and stuttering in particular.

Determining Developmental and Treatment Level

Because adults who stutter will usually have been doing so for years and will have repetitions, prolongations, blocks, escape behaviors, and avoidances, as well as entrenched negative feelings and attitudes, the most appropriate treatment is for advanced level stuttering, detailed in Chapter 17. For the rare adult who has little fear of stuttering the approach called "fluency shaping" or "speak more fluently" may be appropriate. That treatment protocol is also described in Chapter 17.

Closing Interview

I will assume here that the client is a person with developmental stuttering rather than another type of fluency disorder or with only typical disfluencies. By this point in the evaluation, I have a pretty good picture of their stuttering and how I will start therapy. I begin by summarizing my impression of their stuttering pattern (ie, core and secondary behaviors) and their attitudes and feelings. One of my aims is to let them know I have some understanding of their stuttering and why they do what they do when they stutter. I feel it is important to let them know that, given their level of stuttering, it is quite understandable that they would use the various secondary behaviors and avoidance tactics that they do. I accept these behaviors rather than criticize them and let them know that I feel I can work with them and help them discover other ways to respond. I try to ensure that they feel they will not be alone, that I will be working alongside them, and that I will gradually give them more and more responsibility to work on their own.

Then, I briefly describe some therapy options and discuss the possibilities with them. With my guidance, the client and I decide on a treatment approach. Afterward, I give them some written suggestions to begin the process of their taking responsibility for part of their treatment. This will also take advantage of the fact that, as indicated earlier, many clients are highly motivated to change at the very time they come for an evaluation.

If the client has few avoidances and relatively mild stuttering, I am likely to start treatment with fluency shaping. If the client's stuttering is moderate to severe and/or they relatively many avoidances and fears, I am likely to start with stuttering modification treatment. See the next chapter for an overview of both approaches. An exception that I may make is when a client has many fears and avoidances but seems unwilling to confront them. I may begin working with this client using fluency shaping. Some clients who are at first unwilling to "touch the hot stove" of stuttering will be able to confront and change their stuttering if they first get some fluency through fluency shaping.

Before I conclude the interview, I let the client know about the many helpful organizations that are dedicated to helping people who stutter. The National Stuttering Association, for example, holds in-person conferences and on-line events to bring together individuals who stutter and their families. StutterTalk provides hundreds of free podcasts about stuttering and their home page provides links to many other organizations that help stutterers. I make sure the client understands how to connect with this world of helpful contacts.

At the end of the closing interview, I ask a client if they have any questions about the evaluation. I also try to answer the questions asked in the initial interview that I postponed for response until after the evaluation. Clients sometimes ask how long treatment will take. This is a reasonable question, given that they need to budget time and money to undertake treatment, but I have no easy answer for this difficult question. With appropriate cautions about individual differences and unexpected issues, I reply that with hard work and a willingness to tackle difficult situations and to confront fears with my help, I believe that considerable progress can be made within a year of the onset of treatment.

A Video Recording of an Adult Diagnostic Evaluation

A video recording of an evaluation of an adult with advanced stuttering is available on the website. Although the recording omits discussion of the questionnaires usually given, it does capture the gathering of the speech sample, at the same time that the clinicians explore the onset and development of the client's stuttering. The client is questioned about their motivation for treatment, trial therapy is administered, and the client and clinicians develop an assignment for them to begin to work on immediately. At the end of the session, the client leaves with a positive feeling that they can change their stuttering and meet their goals. Aspects of the evaluation that you should pay particular attention to are described below.

On *Lippincott Connect*, you will find video clips (with others in Chapter 11 videos) of a young adult—Ben Barnet—that illustrate key aspects of an evaluation of an individual with advanced stuttering. The first clip is "Diagnostic Evaluation: Introduction." In this clip, the clinicians obtain a sample of Ben's speech when they ask him to tell them about the onset of his stuttering and his previous therapy. As you listen to his speech, notice his occasional repetitive stutters, a few blocks, and some avoidance behaviors (eg, starters). Compare his fluency when speaking to his fluency when reading.

In the second clip, "Exploring Ben's Stuttering," the graduate student clinicians find out about his motivation for therapy and explore with him what his stuttering is like. What do you observe about (1) the types of stutters he has, (2) his avoidances, and (3) how aware he is of what he's doing when he stutters?

The third clip, "Exploring Ben's Avoidance Behaviors," focuses again on his motivation for therapy. It is clear that Ben feels his stuttering holds him back from fully participating in life. Underlying this, I think, is his being unwilling to say exactly what he wants to say because he's reluctant to stutter.

The clinicians carry out some trial therapy (in the clip with that name) that helps Ben go ahead and get into his stutters, rather than avoiding them. They see if he can stay in his stutters and hold onto them and discover that when he doesn't fight them, the stutters gradually release themselves.

Because Ben understands what he must do to reduce his stuttering, the clinicians end the session in the "wrap-up" helping Ben develop an assignment to "get into the stutter." The clinicians help Ben understand that the more he confronts his fear of getting stuck, the more he will learn that the stutters will release themselves if he courageously stays in his moments of stuttering and accepts them. This will give him a feeling that he can control what he once feared.

Ben returned to our clinic 5 years later after carrying out this assignment day after day, month after month. In the video clips titled "Commentary," he reviews the recording of his initial evaluation and provides insights into what he was feeling and doing at that time as well as revealing how much his stuttering has changed. We will discuss the Commentary video clips later in the book when we discuss treatment of stuttering in adolescents and adults.

SUMMARY

- In evaluating a client who may stutter, your task is to decide the following:
  1. Whether their observed disfluencies or avoidances warrant treatment
  2. If they do, you should also find out more about the client's history, current environment, speech behaviors, and reactions.
  3. What treatment seems reasonable given these findings
- In assessing a school-age child, the important questions are as follows:
  1. How the stuttering is affecting the student's performance in school
  2. How the student feels about his stuttering
  3. How motivated they are to work on it
  4. How supportive the parents are of the student's problem
  5. How supportive the student's teachers are
- The assessment of the school-age child may proceed differently if they are being seen in a clinic versus at school. If seen at school, the IDEA affects the process and mandates how assessment is carried out. If seen in a clinic, the clinician will have more contact with the family but needs to reach out to the school setting.
- Key elements of the assessment for a school-age child are as follows:
  1. Initial contact and formal interview with the student's parents
  2. Interview with the student's teachers
  3. Interview with the child
  4. Analysis of speech
  5. Trial therapy
  6. Assessment of other factors, including academic adjustment
  7. Determination of appropriate treatment
- In assessing an adolescent or adult, the important questions are the client's level of motivation and ability to carry out assignments independently; the severity of stuttering and degree of avoidance; the client's feelings and attitudes about his stuttering; whether the problem is typical "developmental" stuttering or is cluttering, psychogenic, or neurogenic stuttering; and the appropriate type of treatment.
- Key elements of the assessment of an adolescent or adult are as follows:
  1. Obtaining preliminary case history, attitude questionnaires, and recordings made outside of the clinic
  2. Interviewing the client
  3. Analyzing the client's speech
  4. Conducting trial therapy

5. Interviewing parents if client is an adolescent
6. Determining appropriate treatment
7. Summarizing findings and making recommendations in closing interview with client

- Whether the person is to be treated as a normally disfluent speaker or as someone who stutters depends on your interpretation rather than a score. You must weigh what you see and hear to determine whether they indicate stuttering, normal disfluency, or even another disorder. From the flood of information you have gathered, you must extract the essential characteristics that support your choice of treatment.
- To hone your judgment, make evaluations a continuing process. The procedures I have suggested for assessment and diagnosis in this chapter will give you a good start, but stuttering is highly variable, and no individual can be completely evaluated in just an hour or two. Consequently, you will overlook an important element at times, and sometimes a vital clue will not be present in the samples of behavior you see during an initial evaluation. With good ongoing evaluation of a client, you will be able to change decisions and redirect therapy as additional information and understanding become available. You will also be able to evaluate the effectiveness of your treatment and improve it when needed.

STUDY QUESTIONS

1. What do you tell the parent of a school-age child who asks you what causes stuttering?
2. Compare the involvement of the parent and the teacher in the evaluation of a school-age child.
3. In what various ways do we assess the impact of the school environment on the school-age child who stutters?
4. What are the benefits of obtaining both a reading and a conversation sample with school children, adolescents, and adults?
5. In the sections on evaluation of the adult and adolescent, what different pieces of information that you may gather from the interview questions help you to assess the client's motivation?
6. What are two reasons we suggest continuing evaluation after the initial assessment of clients who stutter?
7. Compare the assessment of the feelings and attitudes of a school-age child with the assessment of feelings and attitudes of an adolescent. Compare them both with assessment of feelings and attitudes of an adult.
8. What are the stages of management (from less to more formal treatment by the SLP) for a school-age child who stutters?
9. What are the goals of trial therapy?
10. What are the major questions to be answered in the evaluation of an adult?

SUGGESTED PROJECTS

1. Role-play the part of a clinician in an interview with the parent of a school age child, having a friend or classmate play the part of a parent. Practice your listening skills by only listening and asking no questions as the "parent" describes in detail their student's stuttering problem. Switch roles, and then compare your impressions of the experience both as the parent and as the clinician.
2. Pair up with a friend or classmate who could pretend to stutter or with a person who stutters, and practice trial therapy (including exploring feelings) that is appropriate for a school-age child and then appropriate for an adolescent, and then appropriate for an adult. In what ways are these different? As you do trial therapy, try modifying stutters to make them less severe and modifying speech to produce fluency.
3. Pair up with a friend or classmate who doesn't stutter, and have them talk rapidly about a complex topic so they produce normal disfluencies. See if they are able to "catch" their normal disfluencies and hold onto them (eg, turn single repetitions into multiple repetitions or make prolongations longer). Can this be done with normal disfluencies? With only certain types of normal disfluencies?
4. Find websites on the internet that contain helpful information for (1) parents of school-age children who stutter, (2) teens who stutter, and (3) adults who stutter.
5. One of the challenges for clinicians is to get a good speech sample from a student who may be somewhat shy or reluctant to talk to someone they don't know well. Experiment with different ways of interacting with a school age child until you find a "best" method. For example, try asking lots of questions, try just playing quietly alongside a student, and try playing with a student and making comments about things you are playing with together.

SUGGESTED READINGS

Logan, K. (2020). *Fluency disorders* (2nd ed.). Plural Publishing.

Logan, who himself is a person who stutters, provides excellent guidance in doing clinical assessments, including how to obtain valid speech samples, make detailed analyses of them, and come up with treatment recommendations.

Manning, W., & DiLollo, A. (2018). *Clinical decision making in fluency disorders* (4th ed.). Plural Publishing.

These authors have had a great deal of experience in the field of stuttering and present excellent ideas about diagnosis and evaluation.

Shafir, R. Z. (2000). *The Zen of listening: Mindful communication in the age of distraction*. The Theosophical Publishing House.

This is an excellent introduction to the practice of careful listening. Shafir is a speech-language pathologist who has developed her ability to listen to clients and writes eloquently about the healing powers of mindful listening.

Shapiro, D. (2011). *Stuttering intervention: A collaborative journey to fluency freedom* (2nd ed.). Pro-Ed.

This is a very fine textbook on many aspects of stuttering—its nature, assessment, and treatment, written by someone who has coped successfully with his own stuttering for many years. The chapters on (1) preschool children; (2) school-age children; and (3) adolescents, adults, and seniors who stutter have insightful sections on assessment and diagnosis, as well as treatment.

Van Riper, C. (1973). *The treatment of stuttering*. Prentice-Hall, Inc.

In his text, on pages 215 to 219, Van Riper gives a step-by-step description of his process of assessing an adult's stuttering. Not surprisingly, Van Riper's approach takes into consideration that each client will be unique and his individual needs for therapy must be understood.

Yaruss, S. (2002). Facing the challenge of treating stuttering in the schools: Part 1. Selecting goals and strategies for success. *Seminars in Speech and Language*, *23*, 153–159.

This volume of "Seminars" is a rich source of information for school clinicians. Experienced clinicians, many of whom work in the schools, have written chapters on a wide variety of topics, including interpreting IDEA 1997, doing an evaluation in a school setting, and planning therapy for school-age children.

Zebrowski, P., Anderson, J., & Conture, E. (2022). *Stuttering and related disorders of fluency* (4th ed.). Thieme.

This fourth edition of a classic text originally edited by Richard Curlee in 1999 is replete with detailed chapters on the nature, diagnosis, and treatment of stuttering. More than 40 experts from all over the world have written a total 17 chapters with the latest information on stuttering, cluttering, as well as both acquired neurogenic stuttering and acquired functional (formerly called "psychogenic") stuttering. Students, clinicians, and clinical scientists will benefit from studying this all-encompassing volume of new information and recent perspectives on stuttering.

RECOMMENDED WEBSITES

www.westutter.com

This is a wonderful national organization that works with stutterers of all ages and their families via on-line and in-person conferences so individuals and families can meet and share their common experiences.

www.stutteringhelp.org

This website contains many resources helpful to individuals who stutter, their families, teachers, and speech-language pathologists. They constantly update everything so that the latest helpful information is available in the form of videos, lectures, classes, and many other resources.

www.stuttertalk.com

This website contains hundreds of podcasts related to stuttering. There are always new and interesting interviews and conversations, as well as an archive with more than 700 earlier podcasts.

III

Treatment of Stuttering

12

Preliminaries to Treatment

Chapter Outline

Chapter Objectives

After studying this chapter, readers should be able to:

- Understand the most important attributes of an effective stuttering clinician
- Understand how clinicians' beliefs about the nature and development of stuttering affect their choices about treatment goals and procedures at different ages
- Understand how counseling is a vital part of stuttering therapy and how the clinician implements counseling for clients of all ages and parents of children who stutter.

- Understand what important goals are for stuttering therapy and how they may vary depending on the client's age
- Understand the therapy procedures used to meet identified treatment goals

Key Terms

Clinician's beliefs: The perspective a clinician takes on the nature and development of stuttering that leads to their choices of assessment and treatment goals and strategies

Cognitive-behavior therapy (CBT): Treatment based on the notion that persons' perceptions of and thoughts about situations and about themselves determine their feelings and behavior. CBT aims to help the persons see situations and themselves more realistically and more compassionately

Counseling: The relationship that the clinician builds with the client and/or parents that is so vital in supporting well-being and change. This is a process initiated by the clinician so that everyone involved feels that they are part of a team working together with common goals and mutual respect to help the client

Critical thinking: An attitude of mind that encourages questioning; in the current context, the questioning is about whether a treatment will be effective for a particular client

Empathy: Ability to put oneself in another's place and to identify with the feelings that the other person has

Evidence-based practice: A commitment to use research evidence, client goals, and clinician expertise when choosing assessment and treatment goals and tools

Fluency-facilitating environment: A climate in one or more situations that makes it easier for an individual who stutters to speak more fluently. One example might be when parents speak more slowly than usual and increase pausing. Another example would be when family members are accepting of stuttering

Genuineness: Honesty about life, oneself, and other people; a sense that the clinician is comfortable with themselves, speaks straightforwardly, and takes actions that are congruent with their thoughts, beliefs, and attitudes

Therapy protocol: A detailed plan for carrying out treatment

Warmth: A feeling of positive regard for another person, often conveyed by tone of voice and body language

Before presenting the details of treatment in the next six chapters, I want to give you background information to use as you help your clients and their families accept and then manage stuttering. I'll begin by describing key attributes of clinicians who work effectively with people who stutter and how a clinician's beliefs about the nature of stuttering influence treatment decisions. Then, I will discuss **counseling**—the framework you will use as you build relationships with your clients and, when appropriate, their families, as a basis for problem solving. The clinician's attributes—described in the next section—provide the electricity that sparks motivation and contributes to progress as treatment takes place. Following this, I will provide explanations for the **therapy protocols** you can use, as well as how and why you use them. Then, I'll discuss common goals for stuttering therapy and finally the procedures to meet them.

CLINICIAN'S ATTRIBUTES

The clinician is probably the most important ingredient in stuttering therapy, other than the client. A clinician's knowledge, skills, and personality have a major influence on outcome. This is true whether therapy's major focus is to change behaviors, thoughts, feelings, outside variables, or some combination of these. In this section, I discuss some of the attributes that I think make a clinician effective, and I suggest how these can be developed. Unfortunately, there are no data that I'm aware of to support the importance of these attributes for stuttering therapy. In the field of psychotherapy, Rogers (1961) and others have spent a considerable amount of time and effort measuring the effects of some of these clinician attributes on treatment success. In the field of stuttering treatment, Manning and DiLillo (2018), Shapiro (2011), and Zebrowski (2007) have excellent chapters on the role of the clinician and the importance of the clinical relationship.

Much of my thinking about the treatment process has been influenced by my experiences as a client and later as a student of Charles Van Riper. He was a master clinician of stuttering therapy. Let us begin then with Van Riper's (1975a) description of three important clinician characteristics: empathy, warmth, and genuineness.

Empathy

Empathy, in stuttering therapy, is the ability to understand the feelings, thoughts, and behaviors of someone who stutters. Some clinicians prefer the term "compassion" instead of "empathy" because it implies being of service to your client (Holland & Nelson, 2020). You might think that empathy is much easier for clinicians who themselves stutter. However, Van Riper's own clinician, Bryng Bryngleson, was a fluent speaker who showed an impressive understanding of individuals who stutter. Once, Bryngleson assigned Van Riper the task of voluntarily stuttering to 10 strangers, but Van Riper was unable to carry it out. Exhausted from trying again and again and failing over and over, Van Riper sought out Bryngleson in his office. Bryng, as he was called, jumped up from his chair and headed for the door, saying, "It's OK, Van, just follow me and watch." Bryng then went into a nearby tobacco store, walked up to the clerk, and pretended to stutter—with the longest, loudest stutter that Van Riper had ever heard, causing the clerk to cower behind the counter. Van Riper was astounded. That single demonstration by his clinician had a huge impact on Van Riper. He felt deeply supported by Bryngleson's acceptance of Van's failure and Bryngleson's willingness to risk ridicule to help him. Remember this when you wonder how to show your clients empathy for their stuttering.

You can also get some idea of what clients experience by going out in public like Bryngleson did and stuttering voluntarily, though you don't have to stutter as long or as loud as Bryng did. My students are required, over the course of the semester, to carry out 15 pseudostutters—to friends, family, and especially to strangers—and to keep a journal of their own emotions about their experience. Every year they tell me that this assignment—which they hated at the time—opened their eyes to the challenges of stuttering. They find out not only how embarrassing it is to stutter but also how listener reactions can make them feel—both good, if a listener is accepting, and bad, if the listener is rude. It also quickly reveals how dread of specific speaking situations can build rapidly when the prospect of stuttering looms large—even when it's voluntary stuttering.

You can also develop empathy with all your clients by working on your ability to listen deeply and acceptingly. Listening should be filled with curiosity—about the person who stutters and the person's experience of stuttering, including pain and frustration and sense of failure in many stutterers. The clinician's sense of curiosity when listening will radiate to the client that you are sincerely interested in their thoughts, feelings, and their observations of their stuttering behaviors. In addition to listening with your ears, empathy can be gained by observing your clients' body language, posture, and the words they use. Van Riper said that he could improve his understanding of a client's feelings if he assumed the same body posture that the client had (C.G. Van Riper, personal communication, April 1965). Levine (2010), a psychotherapist working with patients who have experienced emotional trauma, writes eloquently about how a client's posture will often convey their emotional state. Clinicians may detect those emotions because the clinicians' own bodies unconsciously imitate their client's postures and, because of that, the clinician senses what the client is feeling. Levine notes, "Therapists working with traumatized individuals frequently pick up and mirror the postures of their clients and hence their emotions of fear, terror, anger, rage and helplessness" (Levine, 2010, p. 46). Even if many of our clients who stutter cannot be described as traumatized by their stuttering, they will still have strong emotions relating to their speaking difficulty, even if they themselves do not recognize it. By noticing these, the clinician can, over the course of therapy, help the client to deal with them.

Another way in which clinicians who work with stuttering can increase their empathy and compassion is by reading stories written by people who stutter and by parents of children who stutter. These narratives will help you better understand the experiences that have shaped their feelings and thus you will be able to respond to your clients more genuinely because you more deeply understand them. Good examples of such writings are *Out with It—How Stuttering Helped Me Find My Voice* (Preston, 2013), *Stuttering Interrupted—The Comedian Who Almost Didn't Happen* (Nina, 2019), *Life on Delay: Making Peace with a Stutter* (Hendrickson, 2023), and *V-V-Voice: A Stutterer's Odyssey* (Damian, 2014). I will describe these books and others in the suggested readings at the end of this chapter.

Warmth

This attribute has also been referred to as "unconditional positive regard" (Rogers, 1957). Much of it is conveyed in the tone of voice, facial expression, and body language of the clinician. Genuine caring comes from the heart and is conveyed automatically when it is present in the clinician. Clients whose clinicians demonstrate **warmth** feel accepted, liked, and nurtured. Warmth creates an environment that supports learning and helps clients respond to the challenges involved in making difficult changes, such as being open about their stuttering. Warmth is also expressed in the comments the clinician makes when a client has done something well. This is sometimes harder than you think. It surprises me, when I watch a video recording of one of my therapy sessions, how many opportunities I miss when I could be reinforcing the client with a "Good!" or "Well done!" said with sincerity. Therefore, I try to watch videos of myself working with a client to discover things that I need to work on. Although it is initially painful for all of us to watch video recordings of ourselves, this is one of the best ways we can improve. Clinicians should become aware of how much or how little enthusiasm they show and how much warm encouragement they give to their clients. These are important tools of therapy.

Genuineness

Van Riper (1975a) described a third characteristic of good clinicians: "**genuineness**," which he equated with Rogers' (1961) "congruence." Both terms refer to a clinician's honesty and self-acceptance. The clinician just tries to be who they are, "roughness, pimples, warts, and everything" as Oliver Cromwell said on having his portrait painted (http://www.thehistoryblog.com/archives/1773). Genuineness allows clinicians to be honest with their clients, not sugarcoating the hard lumps of reality that must be swallowed if real progress is to be made.

In his video "Therapy in Action," Van Riper said to his client with his characteristic bluntness, "Why do you have to have all that junk in your speech? Can't you just go ahead and say the word, starting with the first sound and working your way through it slowly, syllable by syllable?" (Van Riper, 1975b). My students often thought this side of Van Riper was cruel and couldn't understand why he would be so blunt. But I think Van Riper is just doing something vital in his therapy. He is showing the client that he can be tough. This means that the client would feel that Van Riper is tough enough for the client to be angry with him, to hate him, even to be able to express his rage toward him at times. All these things—as well as the opposite—feelings of love and caring between the client and the clinician are components of deep and effective therapy, especially when we work with older children, adolescents, and adults. When a client senses the clinician's genuineness, they gain trust and begin to believe that their clinician means it when they ask the client about their thoughts and feelings so that the client can let go and honestly express those feelings, convinced that the clinician will understand and accept them and their feelings, and be strong enough to be unhurt by them. Clinicians can cultivate their genuineness and strength by being open about their abilities and their limitations and learning self-acceptance through psychotherapy, meditation, spiritual practice, or other experiences that help them accept both their weaknesses and their strengths. This "groundedness" in the clinician will allow them to feel frustration and anger toward the client (and not have to express it) when the client shows resistance in treatment.

Ability to Push for Growth

This attribute is related to genuineness and is seen in clinicians' challenging their clients—particularly school-age and older—to change their ideas and regular ways of thinking, to take risks, to give up old patterns. This is likely to cause discomfort and resistance in clients, but when the challenges smell of hope and are made with the clear belief that the client can change, they can be powerful sources of motivation for the client to get to work and take on hard things.

Ability to Identify Positive Aspects of Clients and Families and Help Them Realize Those Strengths

Some years ago, psychology and counseling began to turn away from a focus on what was wrong with a person, moving toward seeing a person's strengths, talents, and potential for growth. In his description of "A Newer Psychotherapy," Rogers (1942) advocated for a growth-oriented approach to counseling by suggesting, "the aim is not to solve one particular problem, but to assist the individual to *grow*, so that he can cope with the present problem and with later problems in a better-integrated fashion." (p. 28, italics are Rogers'). He goes on to say, "For the first time, this approach lays stress upon the therapeutic relationship itself as a growth experience" (p. 30). This same prizing of client growth rather than clinician magic is also evident in newer approaches to counseling individuals with communication disorders (Holland & Nelson, 2020) as we'll see later on in this chapter. In fact, one sub-part of newer approaches is termed "Post-Traumatic Growth." Although we don't usually think of stuttering as the result of trauma (although sometimes it may be), it may be traumatic for families to realize that their child is stuttering and understand that it may affect all of them for some time. With a supportive clinician, as well as on their own, families may grow in their abilities to champion the child, radiating appreciation for the child's talents and aptitudes, as well as accepting the child's stuttering for now. For older clients, positively oriented clinicians can emphasize the client's skills and abilities, as well as successes in working toward their shared goals. Accepting failures as a natural part of progress is also a component of a strengths-based approach.

A Preference for Evidence-Based Practice

There are more traits than those listed above that characterize good clinicians. One is a clinician's desire and ability to base their clinical practice on evidence of its effectiveness. This is **evidence-based practice**. In choosing tools and approaches for evaluating and treating someone who stutters, clinicians who wish to grow look for evidence of the effectiveness and appropriateness of treatment approaches that they are using or considering. They work together with the client or family in the diagnostic evaluation to determine which treatment approach is likely to meet the client's or family's goals most effectively. The clinician measures the client's progress during treatment to assess whether this approach is working with this person. The clinician is flexible, creative, and insightful enough to find ways of altering treatment if it is not working.

Many treatments, including some described in this text, have relatively little published data that support their effectiveness. For example, my approaches to school-age children and adolescents/adults have been derived from years of experimenting in a more casual way, and only now have I developed enough consistency to start collecting data to be disseminated. This does not preclude my approaches being used. However, when my or any other treatment not supported by strong research evidence is used, clinicians should be particularly careful to assess how well particular treatment procedures work for *their* clients with measures made before, during, and after treatment. In addition, for those clinicians who find particular treatment protocols very effective, obtaining research evidence on them to share with others would represent a valuable contribution to the field. Ideas and information on evidence-based practice can be found in Bernstein Ratner (2005), Bothe (2004), Frattali (1998), Guitar (2004), Guitar and McCauley (2010b), Pietranton (2012), Sackett et al. (2000), and Yairi and Seery (2023). The American Speech-Language-Hearing Association (ASHA) has provided member access to useful tutorials on evidence-based practice at http://www.asha.org/Members/ebp/web-tutorial/.

An interesting example of an early attempt at evidence-based practice is the data that Van Riper (1958) kept as he experimented with different forms of treatment for stuttering. He attempted to write down in detail what variations he made with his treatment protocols each year and reassessed his clients 5 years after they had finished therapy. Although he admits his methods are not perfect, the chapter in which he presents 20 years of experiments in stuttering treatment is a fine example of evidence-based clinical practice for its time, more than 65 years ago (Van Riper, 1958). In this spirit, in the treatment chapters that follow, I suggest ways in which clinicians today can measure client progress.

A Commitment to Continuing Education

Another important attribute for clinicians is the habit of continually updating knowledge first gained in graduate school. New methods of evaluation and treatment are developed every year, and new data on treatment effectiveness become available. Continuing education is particularly important to be able to meet the treatment goals that clients and their families choose. Keeping up to date with the latest and best practices can be done by reading appropriate journals. Recent editions of books that review diagnostic and treatment methods for stuttering can also be helpful. Books might provide more background information than journal articles. Books may help you think about how well the method will fit with your and your client's goals and your current level of expertise. A good example of such a book is the 4th edition of *Stuttering and Related Disorders of Fluency* (Zebrowski et al., 2022).

New approaches to treatment often require training. Short courses at the annual ASHA convention and workshops offered through schools, hospitals, state associations, and other institutions are excellent sources of such training. However, before adopting a new approach, a clinician should critically analyze the quality of evidence that supports its claim to effectiveness.

Critical Thinking and Creativity

Clinicians should become discriminating consumers and ask, "Which new diagnostic tools and treatment approaches are effective, and which clients are they appropriate for?" This demonstrates **critical thinking**. Some new approaches are not all they are cracked up to be. For example, many years ago, a well-known psychologist and his colleague (Azrin & Nunn, 1974) suggested that teaching clients simply to take a breath and relax before speaking was an effective treatment for stuttering. Researchers at another clinic tested the approach and found it to be far less effective in their clinic than its developers had suggested (Andrews & Tanner, 1982). Nevertheless, there may be some aspects of relaxation and breathing that are useful for some clients in the hands of a clinician who becomes skilled at integrating these tools into a broader approach.

Another critical question is "Will this approach work for my clients in my environment?" Often a treatment that works under laboratory conditions with carefully selected participants does not work as well in the real world of a public school, for example. But clinicians may be able to adapt an approach to suit their situations. For instance, an approach developed for very young children in tightly controlled clinical studies with total fluency as its goal may need to be altered so that some degree of easy and open stuttering is an acceptable outcome when used with older children.

CLINICIAN'S BELIEFS

It is important for clinicians to weigh their beliefs about the nature of stuttering against the available data and then develop clinical procedures compatible with the **clinician's beliefs**—procedures supported by data, ideally data collected by others as well as the clinician. My own beliefs about the etiology and development of stuttering that were presented in the first few chapters are reviewed here only in enough detail to illustrate the relationship between beliefs and treatment procedures. My beliefs are that predisposing physiological factors interact with developmental and environmental influences to produce or exacerbate core behaviors that often (but not always) begin as repetitions. When children experience these early disfluencies as feeling out of control or as causing listeners to show alarm, they nonconsciously increase the amount of physical tension, trying to stop the runaway stutters, and they may speed up their attempts to say the word. The increase in tension makes the disfluencies even more distressing to them, compounding the problem. They then may add escape and avoidance behaviors to their behavioral repertoire as well as negative feelings and attitudes to their range of emotional reactions. They learn escape behaviors through instrumental conditioning, they learn speech fears and other negative emotions through classical conditioning, and they learn word and situation avoidances through avoidance conditioning. All of these factors and how they contribute to stuttering are reflected in the details of how learning influences the development of stuttering in Chapter 5 and in the description of the stages of stuttering development I described in Chapter 7.

How does this point of view about the etiology and development of stuttering affect treatment? Let's use the management of school-age children who stutter to illustrate this point. In my view, a child's treatment plan is determined by their developmental level of stuttering—which reflects the likely behaviors and emotions they have added to their speech and feelings about their speech. Each advance in level requires new components in treatment. A first grader with borderline stuttering who is not embarrassed or afraid to talk and who doesn't avoid talking requires a different treatment than a fifth grader with intermediate-level stuttering who has developed fears and avoidances in response to their stuttering. In my view, the first grader with borderline stuttering may be treated with an approach that focuses on increasing fluency and deals only minimally with negative feelings and avoidance behaviors. On the other hand, the fifth grader needs help to reduce the tension and struggle *and* the fears and avoidances. In contrast to these ideas about treatment, a clinician who doesn't believe that fears and avoidances are crucial in understanding and managing stuttering might treat both children with the same approach.

Another way in which clinicians' beliefs can affect management is in the assessment procedures they use. Assessment tools should provide clinicians with information that is essential for planning treatment and measuring progress. In evaluating the first- and fifth-grade children described above, I would evaluate each child's feelings and attitudes about their speech, as well as their use of word and situation avoidances, to accurately determine each child's developmental/treatment level and decide which aspects of the problem to focus on first. Another clinician—for example, one who is atheoretical or unconcerned about the etiology and development of stuttering—might simply want to measure each child's frequency and severity of stuttering.

A third way in which clinicians' beliefs about the nature, development, and treatment of stuttering can affect clinical behavior relates to how they counsel the parents of children who stutter. In counseling the parents of these two school-age children mentioned in the preceding paragraph, my beliefs would guide me to describe the etiology of stuttering as being related to the way a child's brain processes speech and language. Using terminology appropriate to the parents, I would talk about brain organization and development that may predispose a child to stutter, and I would emphasize that this suggests that parents don't cause stuttering. I would also explain that the child's way of producing speech and language can become more effective, which means that parents can be vital in helping a child overcome or manage their stuttering. I would also discuss with parents the importance of factors in the environment that might be contributing to the child's stuttering problem and discuss ways of modifying these factors. Lastly, I would use my understanding of the development and nature of stuttering to give parents a general idea of the course of therapy and possible outcome. Clinicians with other beliefs might not go into the nature of stuttering because they feel it is not well understood and would instead just counsel the parents about their role in the child's treatment.

In closing this section, I would like to quote Williams (1968) on the subject of the clinician's beliefs. The following paragraph was quoted by Van Riper (1975a) in his chapter on "The Stutterer's Clinician."

> *Before a clinician can do stuttering therapy meaningfully, he must assess his own beliefs about the nature of stuttering. Once he does this, he formulates a retraining program that is related to the basic concepts he holds about the nature of the problem. He adopts a language in talking about the problem. He devises procedures that he believes will achieve his goals of therapy (p. 441).*

Although in these words Williams suggests that the clinician chooses the goals of therapy—a common practice in 1968, it is likely that today's clinicians will have beliefs that the client and clinician choose goals together.

TREATMENT GOALS

Clients and their families have an important role to play in choosing goals that are paramount for them. Ongoing discussions between clinician and client about treatment goals strengthen a client's motivation to achieve them and enhance the relationship between clients and clinicians. The following statement by Baer (1990), an eminent behavioral psychologist, expresses this philosophy.

> *It seems only reasonable to learn that when stutterers are given control of the therapeutic consequences that presumably can change their output, some of them choose*

different targets than would their therapists or, probably, other stutterers, and some of them target not so much their speech output as they do a private response that they describe as sense of 'imminent loss of control' (p. 35).

Baer's comment about a client's subjective feeling of a loss of control is quite important and we will return to considerations of stutterers' own experience of stuttering (in contrast to a listener's experience) later.

Changes in Treatment Goals

Treatment goals for stuttering therapy change over the years as ideas about best priorities for people who stutter change. Therefore, in the current edition of this textbook, I will describe more recent goals for clients and clinicians. In Chapter 1, I described a change in attitude that has emerged from stuttering support groups and from some members of the National Stuttering Association (NSA). Paralleling changes in self-image in the Deaf and hard of hearing communities, many stutterers are starting to feel that they needn't be ashamed of their stuttering, but, instead, can be proud of how they have dealt with it and how they can help others in their environment become more patient listeners—a goal that will benefit all of the listener's conversational partners. They have reduced avoidances and aim to be typically talkative. They reject therapies that focus solely on talking more fluently at any cost. The goals of stutterers who have this new attitude range from not seeking any therapy to learning to stutter more easily, being open with listeners about their stuttering, and saying whatever they want to say without worry.

In this section on treatment goals, I advocate for the importance of client choice, with the client being the family for younger children and the individual themselves for older individuals who stutter. At the same time, those of us who are practicing clinicians probably have particular therapy approaches that we are good at and typically use with our clients. When we have listened to our clients' descriptions of what their goals are, we can discuss with them our own philosophy and areas of competence. Then, we work to reach mutual agreement about whether we should try to work together. Usually, we are able to meet client goals without changing our fundamental approaches to stuttering. If not, we can refer them to other stuttering specialists whose expertise more closely matches these clients' goals. And, when appropriate, we can update our own therapy approaches through continuing education.

Reduce Negative Feelings and Attitudes About Stuttering and Speaking

In the chapter on the development of stuttering, I described how people who stutter may acquire negative self-concepts through repeated experiences of stuttering and perceiving—sometimes correctly and sometimes incorrectly—that listeners are impatient or disapproving. Over time, a person's negative expectations in speaking situations become more engrained. This can lead to more stuttering. If a person who stutters expects rejection or disapproval, he may try very hard not to let the stuttering occur—not to let the stutter out—by adopting fixed, tense articulatory postures that trigger blocks. These are often devastating to the individual who stutters and make them feel helpless and out of control. This increasing tension due to strengthening negative expectations then "snowballs" downhill, gathering speed, from negative thoughts to more stuttering to more negative thoughts, on and on. This avalanche of events is at the heart of much chronic stuttering.

Good treatment can unroll the giant snowball. Clients can be toughened up (desensitized) to the experience of stuttering, decreasing their fears and negative expectations. They can also be shown how to say their feared words without as much struggle. As a result, they will approach speaking opportunities with more relaxed speech muscles and find themselves stuttering more easily or not stuttering at all. This in turn will lead to more positive expectations, which can lead to easier or less stuttering; thus, a positive cycle begins to replace the negative cycle that got them to a place of more severe stuttering and very negative feelings about themselves in the first place.

A different approach besides unrolling the snowball and gradually decreasing fear of the experience of stuttering is to give the client repeated experiences of being fluent with one of several approaches—in many situations, with increasing linguistic and social demands over a relatively long period of time and with much success and little failure. The aim is to replace expectations of stuttering with expectations of fluency. This seems to work best, in my experience, with children and with adults who have few avoidance behaviors. For those with much avoidance and struggle, the strategies described below can help.

No matter which approach is taken, the clinician's relationship with the client will be an important factor in the success of treatment. Figure 12.1 shows a clinician showing warmth and curiosity about a client's severe stuttering block. When the person who is stuttering encounters someone who is interested in their stuttering and does not reject it, they feel a little less negative.

Before we leave this section, I would like to describe a negative feeling we can label "loss of control." In Chapters 5 and 6, I talked about a nonconscious response to feelings of stuckness and loss of control: increased tension. This tension seems to me to be a defensive response to relatively loose disfluencies that are often the first sign of stuttering in a preschool child. This experience—the child's feeling stuck and feeling that their mouth is out of control—soon becomes conscious and remains an important part of stuttering as a child grows up. Key components of treatment, such as staying in the stutter, accepting it, and letting it relax are intended to reduce the negative feeling that an individual has that their speech—his stuttering—is out of control.

A
Wow, you are really having to work to get some of your stutters out. It must be exhausting.
B
It sure is!
C

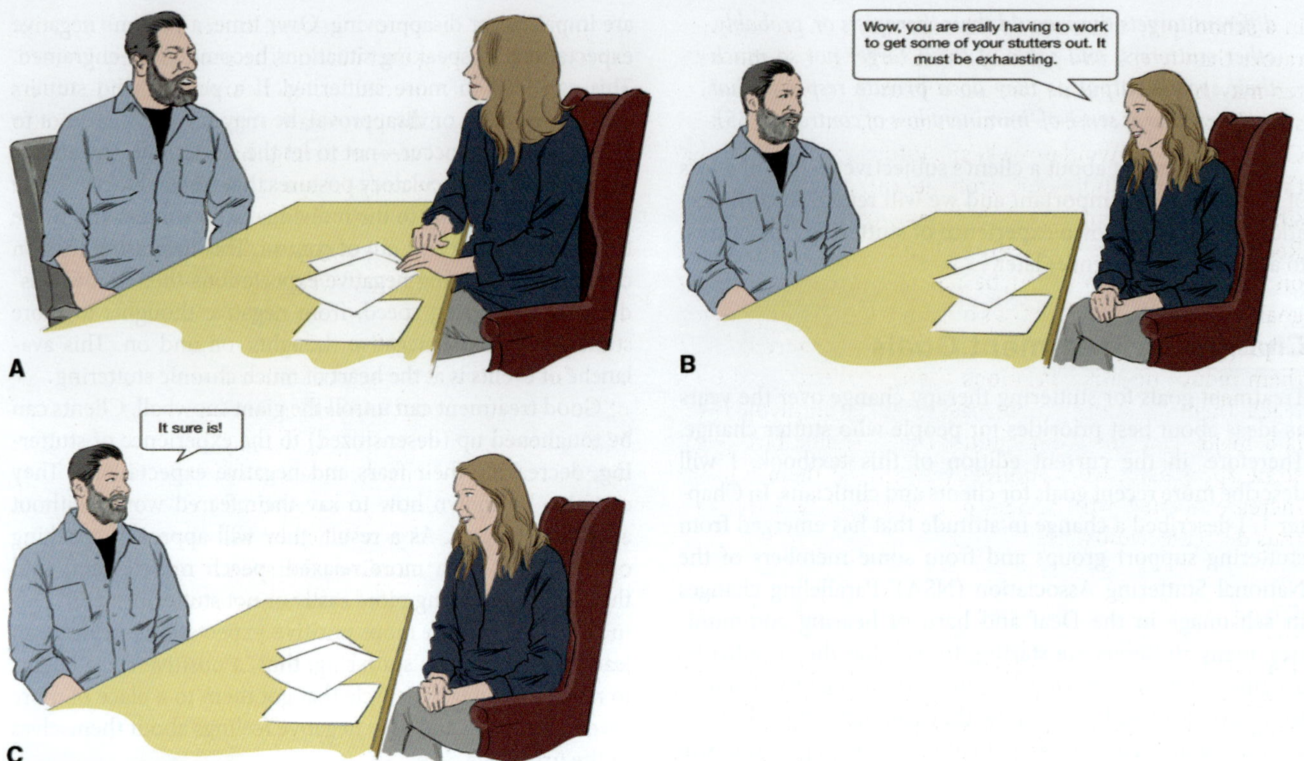

Figure 12.1 A clinician showing empathy in response to a client's stuttering. **A.** When the client is having a severe block, the clinician is calm and patient and shows real interest in what the client is saying. **B.** When the client finishes his stuttered word, the clinician makes an empathic response. **C.** The client, upon hearing the clinician's empathic response, relaxes a little and responds appreciatively.

Perkins et al. (1991) described the feeling of loss of control by the speaker as a key element in stuttering, perhaps the heart of it. Tichenor and Yaruss (2018, 2019) have added to this concept, noting that a client's subjective feeling of loss of control should be considered not only as part of the definition of stuttering important for its focus on the experience of the person stuttering rather than the experience of observers but also as a consideration for treatment.

Reduce the Abnormality of Stuttering

I think much of the abnormality of stuttering comes from the conditioned tension and struggle behaviors that occur during moments of stuttering. It shows up as squeezing of facial muscles and other speech muscles that may not be visible (such as laryngeal muscles) as the person is trying to say a word that feels blocked. Reducing this tension and struggle is an important goal for school-age, adolescent, and adult clients. In addition, behaviors that occur before the stutter (avoidance) and behaviors that are deployed to terminate the stutter (escape) should be eliminated or at least greatly diminished. These include (1) avoidance behaviors, such as the repetition of the sound "uh" before saying a word, and (2) escape behaviors, such as eyeblinks and head nods used to terminate a block. For some school-age children and older clients, it may not be possible to eliminate their stuttering. Instead, the stuttering can be changed so that it is easier and more comfortable for the speaker, interferes less with communication, and strikes the listener as something less noticeable or concerning. Van Riper and other experienced stuttering clinicians have suggested that a person who stutters may not always have a choice *whether* they stutter but they do have a choice about *how* they stutters. This choice includes stuttering in a way that is easier and briefer than their old habitual pattern. This new way of stuttering reduces fear because it feels and sounds more like normal speech and is often unnoticed by the listener. Once the person has confidence in his ability to stutter this easily, they are less likely to increase muscle tension in response to an actual or anticipated stutter.

Reduce Avoidance

Avoidance behaviors, as you will remember, are evasive maneuvers taken by individuals to keep from stuttering. Sometimes they may occur very close in time to the expected stutter, such as saying "um" or "well" just before attempting to say a feared word (as illustrated in the video of Ben in the Chapter 12 adult diagnosis clips on Lippincott Connect). Other times they may be quite separated in time from the expected stuttering, such as *not* volunteering to be in a school play or by driving 20 miles to talk to someone rather than telephoning them. Some individuals who stutter may have an innate predisposition to avoid negative stimuli because of their temperaments, as described in Chapters 2 to 6. Avoidances keep stuttering "hot," because they prevent an individual from learning that it is possible to stutter in an easy fashion and communicate well. Reducing avoidance is usually not the first treatment goal on the list, although it may be one of the most important goals for more advanced levels of stuttering. Usually, before helping clients reduce avoidances, clinicians need to help them reduce negative emotions about stuttering and then teach them to stutter more easily. Reducing avoidances is a major goal for older children and adults, but again, some approaches work indirectly by giving them tools to increase fluency, which then, one hopes, reduce fear and thus decrease avoidances.

Reduce the Frequency of Stuttering

This can be achieved in a variety of ways, but it is important to reduce the frequency of stuttering without creating other behaviors, such as taking deep breaths before speaking that may be distracting to the listener (and speaker) and may therefore hamper communication. Reducing the frequency of stuttering is a common goal for young preschool children whose stuttering is often more frequent repetitions and prolongations than typical children of their age. As children grow older and become adolescents and adults, their stuttering may become more severe and more complex—including blocks, escape, and avoidance behaviors. With these individuals, reducing the severity of stuttering becomes more important than reducing the frequency. An exception may be those older preschool children, adolescent, and adults who may have little negative attitudinal and emotional components to their stuttering. If they are really not bothered about their stuttering but still want to reduce it, procedures that reduce their stuttering frequency may be appropriate.

Increase Overall Communication Abilities

The ability to communicate easily and well varies a great deal from client to client. It may be affected by severity of stuttering, temperament, avoidances, and communication models in the family. For many of us who work with individuals who stutter, effective communication is a very important treatment goal. Some clients will become good communicators once the frequency and severity of their stuttering, along with their negative feelings and attitudes about speaking and stuttering, have been reduced. For other clients, guided practice and structured experiences in communication are essential. Once clients feel they can communicate easily, they often begin to seek out talking experiences, their avoidances drop away, and they become comfortable and open about any remaining stuttering that occurs. The goal of effective communication is most needed for older children and adults who have developed avoidances. Many of these clients, especially those with more severe stuttering, have been preoccupied with their stuttering and not spent much time learning to communicate effectively (Curlee, personal communication, March 3, 2004). They may still have hesitancies and a herky-jerky style of speaking that lacks the fluidity of normally fluent speech.

A good example of how stuttering—especially the fear of stuttering—can affect communication is shown in the video of Ben Barnet's initial evaluation on Lippincott Connect.[1] When asked why he is seeking therapy, he says, in essence, that he doesn't say what he wants to say. His talking is hard for listeners to understand because he has so many avoidances and "work-arounds" when he fears he will stutter that his narrative is hard to follow. Compare his style of talking in the evaluation video with his new way of expressing himself that is evident in the "Commentary" video clips made 5 years later.[2]

Create an Environment That Facilitates Fluency

This goal is paramount for working with young children who can often be treated by helping the family reduce pressures on the child's speech and increase positive aspects of the child's speaking environment in order to create a **fluency-facilitating environment**. For example, family members can spend one-on-one time with the child, using a slow speech rate and careful listening skills, thereby increasing the child's daily opportunities to experience fluency. The child's environment may be made more positive through praise and appreciation of their fluent speech and/or their other accomplishments. This goal of improving the child's speaking environment may also be important for school-age children. However, teachers and aides, as well as family members, need to be enlisted in facilitating the child's fluency. Older clients can make their environments facilitating to both fluency and stuttering by being open about their stuttering and sharing with others how listeners can be most helpful to them.

Increase Freedom to Speak

This goal is similar to what Shapiro is referring to in the title of his book *Stuttering Intervention: A Collaborative Journey to Fluency Freedom* (2011). For me, freedom to speak means being able to say what you want to say, when you want to say it. There may be some stuttering, but the

---

[1]See "Diagnostic Evaluation."

[2]See "Commentary" videos.

individual doesn't hold back from speaking because of it. Moreover, the individual's own reaction to their stuttering is not strong and therefore they are able to maintain natural eye contact and connect with the listener and communicate effectively. When the person feels free to speak, their struggle may be minimized with little negative emotion about their stuttering and far less tension and holding back as they speak.

The following observation by President Barak Obama captures the positive effect on listeners that a speech problem may have when the speaker is free to speak despite their difficulty:

> *[The President] had been moved by the images of Gabby Giffords (U.S. House of Representative member wounded in a mass shooting in 2011) testifying in front of the Judiciary Committee, her brave words somehow more stirring because of her labored speech. You could feel the impact of all the energy she had invested in her rehabilitation and speech therapy. (Leahy, p. 361).*

THERAPY PROCEDURES

The aim of this section is to outline the tools and strategies that clinicians can use to work on the treatment goals described above. By understanding which procedures are most likely to be useful in achieving each goal, clinicians can select those procedures that best suit each client and are in accord with their own beliefs. The procedures outlined here are more fully described in the therapy chapters on each developmental/treatment level.

Counseling

In some ways, "counseling" is the psychological background in which a clinician helps a client meet their goals for easier speech and more effective communication. In doing this, the clinician exhibits many of the attributes described in the first few sections of this chapter (eg, empathy, warmth, and others) and the stuttering client and their family are affected by them. The clinician's empathy, warmth, genuineness, ability to push for change, and optimism can deepen the client-clinician relationship. This relationship can be the energizer that motivates clients to take risks, to accept their stuttering for now, but, if they wish, to change their stuttering. This bond between stutterer and clinician can increase clients' self-confidence, give them satisfaction with changes they make and give them comfort when they fail.

Counseling wears different clothes and takes on different shapes in different phases of treatment. As I describe these features of counseling, I will depend in part on the book *Counseling in Communication Disorders—A Wellness Perspective* (Holland & Nelson, 2020). I will also call on my own experiences working with stutterers of all ages and their families.

Counseling With Parents of Children Who Stutter

Parents who have just realized their child is stuttering need information and support. For the information, the clinician can describe—using easy to understand terminology—what is known about the many factors that combine to bring about stuttering. These factors include the way the brain is organized slightly differently in many individuals who begin to stutter as well as aspects of the child's genetic temperament and personality that may make them respond to disfluencies in ways that can help prevent chronic stuttering, or, instead, may trigger different responses that may affect the frequency and severity of stuttering. For support, the clinician can suggest that treatment can help the child overcome the stuttering or help it become a minor issue that doesn't affect the child's success in school and enjoyment in being with other children and other adults.

As part of supportive counseling, it is vital that the clinician listen attentively to what the parents are thinking and feeling. Recently, I discovered in my files a mimeographed handout by Carl Rogers titled "Communication: Its Blocking and Its Facilitation" (undated). The handout conveyed the idea that the communication is fostered if you can understand another person's point of view without evaluating it. As you listen to parents talk about their experiences and concerns, can you understand their point of view without judging it? Even if parents blame themselves for the child's stuttering, can you simply try to express back to them what you think their thoughts and feelings are, to see if you've got it right? Don't try to correct what might be misperceptions on their part. Just convey that you are trying to understand where they're coming from. Their feeling of being understood will help them feel their thoughts and feelings are accepted and will allow them to take in new information when they are ready. This feeling of being understood by the clinician will foster the interpersonal relationship between clinician and parents. This relationship is the dynamo that allows the parents to become more effective in supporting their child as the child copes with their present stuttering and flourishes, learning to handle it effectively.

Throughout therapy, it is vital that the clinician listen, understand, and verbalize acceptance of the parents' point of view, even if that view is different from the clinician's. For example, parents may need to express their frustrations with the hard work of therapy, especially if they are doing some of the treatment at home. If the family is from a different culture than the clinician's, it is important that the clinician elicit parents' accounts of how the child's stuttering is responded to by peers, neighbors, and other relatives. Then, the clinician can acknowledge what the family is experiencing and adapt treatment to cope with this culture's responses. Another important setting in which the parents may need information and support is with the child's teachers if the child is in school. A meeting of the clinician, parent, and teachers may help the parents feel supported and help the teacher(s) understand how to respond to the child's stuttering.

Another school-related issue that cries out for the clinician's support of parents is the child's Individualized Education Program (or Plan) (IEP). IEPs are support systems for children with disabilities in public schools; they involve professionals in the school as well as the child's parent(s). For a child who stutters, the Speech-Language Pathologist (SLP) is involved and is thus given an opportunity to help develop a plan for the child and, also important, assist the parent(s) in contributing substantially to the process.

Holland and Nelson (2020) have an excellent description of the clinician's role in a chapter (by Damico and Damico) about counseling with parents. This same chapter also details ways in which the SLP can guide parents and teachers in recognizing and communicating the child's talents and strengths. Moreover, Damico and Damico emphasized the many ways in which the clinician can help the parents find other parents of children with similar issues, such as parent support groups, both in person and on the internet. In the case of stuttering, the NSA website (www.westutter.org) has links that allow parents (perhaps with the clinician's help) to find NSA chapters near where they live; many chapters have parent support groups. For example, using the NSA website, you can link to information on the chapter in Burlington, VT, that allows parents to find support groups, not only for themselves but also for their child who stutters. Informational and supportive videos for parents of children who stutter are available on the Stuttering Foundation website (www.stutteringhelp.org) and on the Friends website (https://friendswhostutter.org/kids). On this website, parents can click on links labeled "Parents of Preschoolers" and "Parents of school-age children." Watching these videos with parents and/or discussing them with parents can be supportive and helpful and continue to create the bond between parents and clinician that is so essential for successful treatment.

Counseling With Children Who Stutter

Working with children who stutter is often a delightful and satisfying experience. Much of the gratification comes from getting to know the child and building a trusting relationship so that the child is comfortable talking about their experiences and feelings, both about stuttering and about other aspects of their lives. That relationship depends in part upon the counseling that the clinician engages in throughout therapy. A major dynamic for building that relationship is *listening* to the child. This is not merely asking the child questions and attending to their answers. It is creating a connection with the child, making it so they are comfortable in telling you about their experiences and feelings. When you are able to do that and the child is comfortable sharing, it is critical that you respond both by silent attention as well as occasional comments and questions showing them that you want to understand what they are feeling and thinking. An example of a child sharing experiences and emotions is depicted on Lippincott Connect in the Chapter 12 videos. In this clip, titled "David Self-Rewarding & Emotions," we see David rewarding himself with candy for using a "slideout" as he calls them (they are loose and easy stutters) and then keeping track of how many he has done on a pad of paper, so he can get a reward of getting to play a game with me after he hits his goal. After he is well on his way to his target, I then bring up the topic of bad feelings about stuttering and David shares his experiences with stuttering and older kids. He is pretty open about being scared of stuttering. Note that he stutters on the word "scared" several times, turning each stutter into a smooth slideout. Because he's getting a steady supply of candies for slideouts, he re-uses the word "scared" repeatedly. At the end, we play a game of vertical checkers (as a break from the hard work of catching and changing stutters) and he gives me a tip about how to improve my game. David's openness about his stuttering did not come easily. At first, at age 6, he was reluctant to talk about stuttering at all, much less make changes in his stuttering. But with patience and lots of fun, games, and candies, David was willing to imitate my easy stutters and then he used "slideouts" on his own and gradually became quite fluent with only a few stutters. He is now in his 30s with a wife and child, working for a nationally known investment management company as a financial advisor.

One of the hallmarks of wellness counseling is focusing on the client's strengths rather than only dwelling on their stuttering. With David, it was easy to let him show off his prowess playing games and shooting hoops in a net hung from the back of my office door. Many children I have worked with have artistic talent that I incorporate into therapy, such as the drawing by Marcel displayed in Figure 7.6 in the chapter on typical disfluency and the development of stuttering. We used his drawing to talk about his feelings about the stuttering he had at the beginning of therapy, as well as plan the next steps in our work together. Another child, Isaiah, was very bright and talented at building things. When we finished some hard work on stuttering modification, he and I went to a room with many tools and together we built a handsome power strip that looked beautiful, even on the table in the treatment room. With every child, you can find talents and strengths to celebrate, so the negative feelings that come up as you confront stuttering will be lessened by the positive glow that accompanies recognition of the child's accomplishments.

The child's school is a vital place where the clinician can intervene if needed. Most teachers understand stuttering to some extent, but a meeting with the teacher can help fill their gaps in knowledge. A meeting between the child, the teacher, and the clinician can be really helpful, especially if the there are ways to improve the teacher's response to the child's stuttering. In a video on Lippincott Connect, titled "Classroom Teacher, Student, and Clinician," the child explains to her teacher that sometimes she has silent blocks when she's called on and the teacher mistakenly thinks she doesn't know the answer and calls on someone else. This brings new understanding to the teacher who becomes much more receptive to the student's stuttering in class.[3] With meetings like these, students feel supported and understood and the relationship with the student is deepened.

The book by Holland and Nelson (2020) gives many further examples and describes many ways in which the clinician can build a strong relationship with the child to foster acceptance and management of stuttering and the feelings that accompany stuttering. I recommend it.

Counseling With Adults Who Stutter

This section is highly shaped by my experience as a client of Charles Van Riper, as well as my own work with adults who stutter. Counseling begins as the clinician helps the client determine what their goals are for therapy. Sometimes the client wants to be 100% fluent with no trace of stuttering; sometimes the client wants to continue stuttering as they are now but without being concerned or bothered by it. The clinician needs to accept what the client says they want at this point, although the goals may change as they work together. Most clients, by the end of therapy, are content with some stuttering left in their speech, as long as it feels comfortable and easy and doesn't interfere with their communication. As Van Riper (1973a) discusses the counseling he employs with clients, he notes that it is not deep psychotherapy[4] but a highly supportive relationship. He suggests that the relationship really begins as he guides the client in confronting their stuttering when they work together to identify and understand what the stutterer is doing when they stutter. As this confrontation takes place, Van Riper works to reduce the client's fear by his own comfort with the client's stuttering. He says, "the analytic examination of the displayed behavior in the context of the therapist's genuine interest and freedom from punitiveness reduces anxiety" (p. 247). As the clinician guides the stutterer into more and more confrontation of stuttering behaviors and exploration of feelings before, during, and after moments of stuttering, the client may turn their strong negative feelings toward the clinician. Van Riper suggests that the clinician needs to tolerate displays of anger and hostility toward the clinician, suggesting that "good therapists are self-flushing." More resentment and resistance may be expressed by the client as the focus of therapy moves from *identifying* stuttering behaviors and feelings into *desensitization*—decreasing negative emotions that have been associated with stuttering. Despite that, the clinician must continue to show faith that the client will be able to become more at peace with their stuttering and then be able to change it. Van Riper says, "Faith is said to move mountains, but it is the therapist's dedicated care and concern, if not love, that moves stutterers" (p. 243).

In my own work with adults who stutter, I try to build a therapeutic relationship with a client by focusing attention on what the client is saying about their stuttering as we are working on it together and on the verbal and written reports the client gives me after working on assignments between sessions. I try never to ask a client to do something with their stuttering on their own that we haven't worked on together outside the treatment room. If we go to a shopping mall to practice staying in the stutter until tension is reduced and ending the word slowly, I always go into a store with a client and demonstrate what I'm asking the client to do. My students who don't stutter learn gradually to become comfortable with pseudostuttering in public that approximates what the client does when they stutter. They resent this assignment at first, but soon understand how important it is to learn to overcome their own fears of public stuttering in order to be truly empathetic and able to act as a model for their clients who need it.

I remember a young man named Ed who had particular trouble with words beginning with /s/. The student clinician and I went into many stores with Ed and practiced stuttering on /s/ words, but despite an hour of doing this, Ed was never able to get his /s/ words to become relaxed and easy. We complimented Ed on his courage and hard work and planned to work on it with him the next week. In debriefing after the session, the student and I were frustrated and saddened by Ed's failure. However, when Ed came to the next session, he announced that his fear of /s/ words was practically gone. Months later, he told us in a letter he wrote us later from his home far away, that the exercise in those stores was a game-changer for him and for his stuttering. I think the support we gave him as he confronted his fear was what made the difference.

Sometimes there are failures that don't turn around and become successes. These are events that you can learn from. Early in my practice, a graduate student and I worked with an undergraduate from a prestigious college in another town, requiring him to make a long drive to attend sessions. This undergraduate had a notable stutter but seemed unable to confront it and often mentioned he didn't want his parents to know that he was attending therapy or even that he stuttered severely when he was away from his home. After a semester, he dropped out of therapy and I struggled at that time to understand what we might have done differently that would have helped him. Now, nearly 40 years later, I think that we could have spent more time building trust and helping him express his fears and frustrations in a warm, accepting environment. Maybe that would have made a difference.

I think of counseling being used primarily in therapies that focus—at least in large part—on changing both feelings and

[3]The clinician in this video (myself) has a pony tail because he refrained from getting a haircut until he'd finished the 3rd edition of this textbook.

[4]However, Van Riper says the psychotherapy that he received as a student (who still stuttered at that time) at the University of Iowa was helpful in giving him insights about himself and making him "a happy stutterer."

behaviors related to stuttering. However, sometimes strict behavior shaping therapies, sometimes called "Fluency Shaping," have an opportunity for attentive listening to a client. Many years ago, I worked with a young woman who stuttered moderately and obviously but was relatively comfortable with herself and wanted a very brief treatment. My graduate students and I used a prolonged speech therapy that began with hours of speaking while under delayed auditory feedback that forced her to speak very slowly. We treated her for only 2 days, but many hours of each day were spent talking (with very slow, prolonged speech that was gradually speeded up) with two graduate students and myself. She recovered completely after those 2 days and was still fluent when I met her for lunch last summer, about 35 years after her treatment. I think the hours of talking about her stuttering and her life and being listened to attentively by the graduate students and myself may have been a contributing factor in her success.

Another female client I worked with, a charming middle-aged woman named Francesca, benefitted immensely from working with my entire stuttering class, weekly. A graduate student and I had started her off in individual therapy that focused on stuttering modification. Francesca was a quick learner and did not have extensive fear and avoidance. She was very comfortable in our adult stuttering support group and expressed interest in more frequent group activities, so I invited her to become a client that my whole stuttering class could learn from. When I was working on my master's degree, I had taken a stuttering class from Van Riper and he had a young man who stuttered come to that class to have Van Riper work with him in front of the class and then go on assignments with various class members in the afternoons. Why couldn't I try that? Francesca was warm and friendly with my entire class and thus it seemed natural to have various class members work with her. She came to every other class (thus, one day a week), and in that class, she seemed to have a relationship with each student. At the beginning of each class meeting, she would report on the assignments that she, class members, and I had come up with to work on with one or two class members outside of class and also on her own. As she was telling us how the assignments went, class members would make supportive comments and ask questions. When she was having trouble with a particular challenge, such as starting feared words with a slow and relaxed movement, a class member would volunteer to come to the front of the room and, with my input, help Francesca practice the desired way to attack feared words. Then, they worked out an assignment to do together outside of class, such as going to a nearby store to practice carry-over to the real world. The relationship with the class, the discussion of emotions, and all of our mutual support and appreciation were, in essence, the counseling that is so vital in working with adults who stutter. Further, her active participation in this learning environment made her stuttering of service to someone else, an experience that might be empowering in and of itself.

Procedures to Reduce Negative Feelings and Attitudes About Stuttering and Speaking

A number of therapy procedures can help clients become more realistic about how listeners perceive them and what this may mean to them. Cognitive therapy, for example, can be an excellent technique for helping clients think and feel more positively about their speech, listeners, and the situations that have elicited negative emotions in the past. Clients can learn to examine their thought processes and understand how what they *think* influences what they *feel* and how they *act*, particularly in regard to such maladaptive behavior as muscular tensing that leads to more stuttering. Some clinicians use **cognitive-behavior therapy (CBT)** as their sole treatment and others as a supplement to techniques for learning to speak fluently or to stutter in an easier way. The book, *Cognitive Therapy: Basics and Beyond* (Beck, 1995), is a good source for learning this approach, and I discuss cognitive therapy in the chapter on advanced stuttering. An excellent introduction to this approach with stuttering are two Stuttering Foundation DVDs: (1) *Tools for Success: A Cognitive Behavior Therapy Taster* and (2) *Implementing Cognitive Behavior Therapy with School-Age Children* (www.stutteringhelp.org).

A client I worked with some 30 years ago changed his attitude about his negative thoughts and attitudes about stuttering in general through confronting his fear of individual words. In a recent e-mail he said, as he looked back on his therapy all those years ago, "I eventually realized, through your therapy methods, that by breaking down my fear of stuttering, I reached the point that I really didn't care if I stuttered. Once I stopped being ashamed of stuttering, my fluency made a marked improvement. The last part took a long time, but I finally reached the point where not only could I talk about my stuttering, but I accepted it as part of who I am. I then incorporated my stuttering story and history into my business, 'Speaking of Success', where I coach others—mostly fluent speakers—in overcoming their fear of public speaking, as well as teach them public speaking skills."

Procedures to Reduce the Abnormality of Stuttering

These procedures are appropriate for clients who have developed struggle, tension, escape, and avoidance behaviors that make their stuttering obvious and sometimes alarming to the listener and the client himself. Therapies that target the abnormality of stuttering often use reward and mild punishment to change long, tense stutters into increasingly briefer and more relaxed ones and to diminish clients' use of escape and avoidance behaviors. To meet this goal, reward and punishment are often accompanied by a systematic program for reducing negative emotions. Such programs are founded on the belief that negative emotions elicit increased tension, escape, and avoidance behaviors and that these behaviors are maintained by the fact that they are rewarded when the stutterer finally gets the word out by squeezing and pushing on it. These approaches are often referred to as "stuttering modification."

A classic stuttering modification approach is that of Van Riper (1958, 1973a, 1975b), which begins first by reducing negative emotions through (1) objective study of the stuttering and then focuses on (2) desensitization to the frustration and embarrassment of it. Next, the clinician teaches the client to self-correct their stuttering after a stutter, where the self-correction is an easier form of stuttering, not a fluent utterance. Then, the clinician helps the client change to an easier form of stuttering while it is happening, ending the stutter in an easier way that is rewarded by its release. Gradually the client starts to begin their stutters in this easier fashion, in a way that makes the stutter much more like typical speech. Stuttering modification often results in a modified style of speaking that contains brief disfluencies produced in a slightly slower than normal way of talking. In an early description of this therapy, Van Riper (1957) sketched out how his therapy combines psychotherapy with behavior modification to help the client accept their stuttering as well as accept themselves as they learn to stutter easily in more and more challenging situations.

Some therapy approaches—both fluency-shaping approaches for older preschool children and adults as well as therapy approaches for preschoolers—don't aim to reduce the abnormality of the stuttering behavior directly, but instead focus on increasing fluency with the assumption that as fluency increases, stuttering diminishes to negligible levels.

Procedures to Reduce Avoidance

Some clients have very little avoidance, and once they learn to speak fluently, they enter speaking situations freely without expectation of difficulty. Others, however, because of temperament, learning, or both, have a strong tendency for avoidance that may be almost "hard-wired" because it is learned so well. Avoidance behaviors are usually serious issues that must be addressed in individuals who are school age (intermediate stuttering) or older (advanced stuttering). Treatment to reduce avoidance should begin by reducing negative emotions, particularly fears of stuttering and of listeners' reactions. Fear of stuttering can be tackled by a systematic program of rewarding clients with praise, support, or tangible reinforcement for "catching" a stutter, holding onto it and accepting it, and releasing it slowly and loosely. Fear of listeners' reactions can be lessened by the client and clinician alternatively pretending to have a bad listener reaction to the other's pretend (or real) stutters. This should be done in a way that's fun and gets rewards. This fear can also be reduced by clients' voluntarily stuttering to acquaintances and strangers. When a person who stutters can deliberately imitate their typical stuttering pattern and pretend to stutter, they finally feel in control during a stutter; this and the feeling of "stuttering" while also feeling in control is highly rewarding. Perhaps even more important than voluntary stuttering is the success and reward an individual feels if they are able to drop avoidance behaviors and go right into a feared word, stay in the stutter (showing it "who is boss"), then release it in a slow, controlled fashion. Figure 12.2 illustrates employing these strategies.

Reducing fear is not enough, however. Studies of animal behavior have shown that, even when avoidance symptoms disappear after fear is reduced, fear eventually returns and so do its symptoms—conditioned avoidance behaviors (Ayres, 1998; Bouton, 2016). Thus, new responses to the old stimuli must be taught. In stuttering therapy, an example of learning a new response to an old stimulus is for a stutterer to slow their speech rate as they say a word they expect to stutter on. This is an aspect of the "preparatory set" used in many stuttering modification approaches, as well as what I call "downshifting" to a slower speaking rate before attempting a difficult word, taught in fluency-shaping programs.

Avoidances are not confined to the moment just before a difficult word. Individuals who stutter may also avoid opportunities to speak by pretending to be busy when the telephone rings or by waiting for someone else to make introductions of new acquaintances. These avoidances can be treated by helping a client construct a hierarchy of easy-to-difficult speaking situations, in which they can use newly learned stuttering modification or fluency-shaping techniques. Clinicians can also motivate clients to continue seeking out new situations in which they can be open about their stuttering and can use their new strategies to manage stuttering. At meetings of the SpeakEasy Associations of Australia and the United States and conventions of the NSA (https://westutter.org/), there are always impressive testimonials by clients who have sought out public speaking opportunities, joined Toastmasters (an international organization of people who want to practice public speaking), or found other ways of increasing their approach behaviors and decreasing their tendency to avoid stuttering and speaking.

Procedures to Increase Overall Communication Abilities

For many children, adolescents, and adults, communication blossoms when fears of stuttering and listeners' reactions are reduced, and ease of speaking is increased. For others, long-standing habits of avoiding speaking situations and the accompanying lack of social experience have stunted the growth of their communication skills. For still others, concomitant problems, such as attention deficit or extreme shyness, may have prevented them from learning how to communicate well. Communication skills should be addressed in treatment whenever it appears that they are not appropriately developed. Observations of a client's communication and reports from a school-age child's teachers will indicate

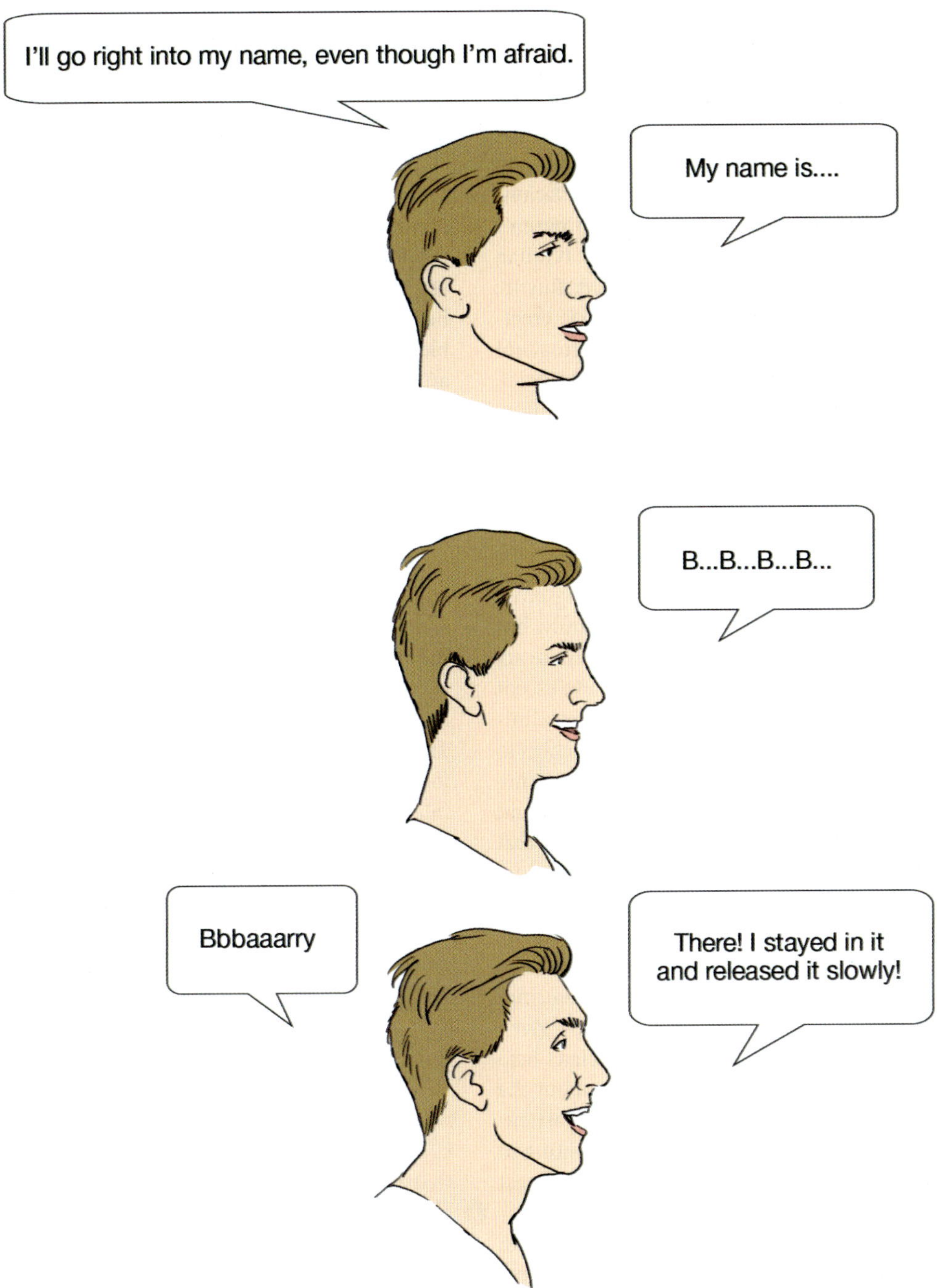

Figure 12.2 "Going into feared word, staying in the stutter, and releasing it slowly and loosely."

the areas that may need to be addressed. Specific skills that can be worked on include eye contact, turn taking, maintaining a topic, making relevant contributions to conversation, speaking intelligibly, clarifying and repairing what was said, and developing a willingness to initiate and maintain communicative interactions with others (Kent, 1993; Smith et al., 2000). Although these skills can be worked on individually, group therapy provides excellent opportunities for clients to practice them. Direct instruction, modeling, role-playing, and video-recorded feedback with discussion can be used to teach and refine communication skills.

Procedures to Create an Environment That Facilitates Fluency

Preschool-age children, especially those whose difficulties fall on the borderline between normal disfluency and stuttering, may need only a little change in their environments for their stuttering to disappear permanently (Starkweather et al., 1990). Treatment focuses on parents: counseling them in a way that reduces their anxieties, modeling for them, and continuing to support the changes they make. Parent-child interactions are usually the key element of the environment that can be changed to facilitate fluency. Video recordings and playback of these interactions in the clinic or observations at home, coupled with parent counseling, can help parents improve how they communicate with their child (Guitar, 1978; Guitar et al., 1992; Kelman & Nicholas, 2008; Rustin, 1991; Zebrowski et al., 2022). Parents usually work on creating a facilitating environment (slower speaking rate, frequent pausing, and increased attention to the child) during brief, one-on-one daily sessions with the child. In some families, other aspects of the environment may need to be changed, such as a home's hurried pace of life, stressful life events, and the communication styles of other family members. Older preschoolers may also benefit from a direct approach, involving contingencies for fluent speech and stuttering.

For school-age children, the creation of facilitating environments may include working with the child's family, but the school setting may be equally important, if not more so. Clinicians often work in partnership with a child or adolescent to make school a "fluency-friendly" environment. The clinician may arrange meetings with the child and their teachers to improve the teachers' understanding of the child's stuttering and to open lines of communication between the child and teachers. A child's peers can be invited to treatment so that they can improve their understanding of the child's stuttering, while the process of the child's openness about their stuttering with other children is begun. Freely discussing their stuttering with other students is one of the most powerful ways for a school-age child to make their environment more stuttering-friendly. For some children, a powerful boost can be given to therapy's progress if they are able, with the clinician's help and support, to make a presentation to their class about the nature of stuttering in general and their stuttering in particular. A good example of a child and her clinician presenting to the child's class is shown in a video on Lippincott Connect titled "A Child Talks to Her Class About Stuttering."

For adults, openness about stuttering is also a major way in which they can create a supportive environment. By commenting on their stuttering, by showing a sense of humor about it, and by sharing what techniques they're working on, adults who stutter can create environments in which their listeners are quite comfortable with the adults' stuttering. This helps them feel free to use various fluency-enhancing techniques.

My own treatment (and others' treatments) for each age are presented in the next five chapters. Descriptions of the other clinicians' approaches include their beliefs about the nature and development of stuttering as well as rationales for their choice of goals and procedures to treat each level. Both my own approaches and those of other clinicians have been developed and refined, usually over several years of trial and error. When possible, supporting data are provided for each treatment, but in many cases, where such data are not available, I suggest what data would be appropriate to gather.

Procedures to Reduce the Frequency of Stuttering

Operant conditioning procedures are often part of treatment approaches for achieving this goal and typically involve reinforcement for fluency and, occasionally, tactfully calling attention to stuttering and allowing a "do-over." Rewards may be verbal, such as the clinician's praise or approval, or tangible, such as tokens that can be redeemed for snacks, prizes, or an opportunity to take a turn in a game. Rewards for fluency and gently highlighting stuttering can be the primary tools used for treating beginning stuttering and are sometimes coupled with a hierarchy based on the complexity and length of utterances. In this case, clients move from producing one or two words fluently, moving on to longer phrases and then to spontaneous speech. Rewarding and highlighting stuttering may also be used as "shaping" tools for intermediate- or advanced-level stuttering, in which clients begin by speaking in a way that produces instant fluency, such as speaking very slowly, and then progressing to more and more normal-sounding speech in more and more difficult situations. This approach—sometimes called "prolonged speech"—was foreshadowed in remarks by Francis Bacon in the late 1700s (Siegel, 2007). Here are Bacon's words cited in Boswell's *The Life of Samual Johnson*, 1791:

> *In all kinds of speech, either pleasant, grave, severe, or ordinary, it is convenient to speak leisurely, and rather drawlingly than hastily: because hasty speech confounds the memory, and oftentimes, besides the unseemliness, drives a man either to stammering, a non-plus, or harping on that which should follow; whereas a slow speech confirmeth the memory, addeth a conceit of wisdom to the hearers, besides a seemliness of speech and confidence.*

The general term for treatments such as prolonged speech that focus on increasing fluency rather than decreasing the abnormality of stuttering is "fluency shaping."

SUMMARY

- The clinician's attributes are a vital ingredient in treatment success.
- Empathy, genuineness, and warmth are three clinician attributes that are widely acknowledged as important to the clinician's success.
- A clinician should be able to help clients grow and flourish in therapy and in their lives.
- Good clinicians seek to identify the strengths and talents of clients and promote them.

- An important component of best clinical practice is choosing evaluation procedures and tools that have been shown to be valid and reliable for the purposes for which they are being used. Thus, a quite valid and reliable measure for assessing the frequency of stuttering may not be valid and reliable if used to look at overall effect of stuttering on the quality of the client's speaking experience.
- Best clinical practice dictates becoming aware of evidence of effectiveness for treatment procedures that you use and adapting treatment procedures to fit clients' needs, as well as continuous assessment of improvement in attributes that have been chosen as goals for treatment.
- Continuing education is vital to keep abreast of new approaches and new evidence of effectiveness of current approaches.
- Clinicians should develop an informed set of beliefs about the nature of stuttering and fit assessment and treatment procedures to those beliefs.
- Goals for treatment and for continuing assessment should come not only from the clinician's beliefs but also from the client's (or family's) informed choices.
- Treatment procedures for meeting these goals must include counseling and can include methods of reducing frequency and severity of stuttering and secondary behaviors, reducing negative emotions and thoughts that interfere with fluency, increasing communication abilities, and developing environments that facilitate fluency.

STUDY QUESTIONS

1. What are the three important characteristics of a clinician described by Van Riper?
2. How might each of these characteristics facilitate progress in treatment?
3. What are the characteristics of evidence-based practice?
4. How might two clinicians' beliefs about the nature of stuttering result in two *very different* treatment approaches? How might these beliefs result in two *similar* treatment approaches?
5. How is counseling used with all ages of clients and all types of treatment?
6. Which of the treatment goals described in this chapter are appropriate for borderline stuttering?
7. Which are appropriate for beginning stuttering?
8. Which are appropriate for intermediate stuttering?
9. Which are appropriate for advanced stuttering?
10. Describe the differences between "fluency-shaping" and "stuttering-modification" approaches to treatment.
11. How might reducing negative emotions reduce stuttering frequency?
12. How might reducing stuttering frequency reduce negative emotion?
13. Which goal would you start with for a preschool child with borderline stuttering and why?

SUGGESTED PROJECTS

1. Video record yourself and a client during an evaluation or a treatment session. The first time you watch it, note only the things you think you do well. The second time you watch it, note one thing you would like to improve. Meet with a colleague or supervisor and discuss how to improve what you would like to and then work on that in another session and videotape yourself again. Watch this new tape for improvements in the behavior(s) you have chosen to work on.
2. Choose a treatment procedure you use and then search the literature to see if you can locate any information about its effectiveness.
3. Find a stuttering treatment approach that is described in detail and determine what the goals of treatment are, what the procedures are to reach these goals, and whether there is a description of how to measure progress on these goals. Examples are (1) Acceptance and Commitment Therapy for Adults who Stutter (Beilby & Yaruss, 2018; Beilby et al., 2012), (2) Avoidance Reduction Therapy for Adults who Stutter (Sisskin, 2018), (3) The Lidcombe Program (Onslow et al., 2017), and (4) Stuttering Prevention and Early Intervention (Gottwald, 2010).
4. Describe in detail your own beliefs about the nature of stuttering applied to children with intermediate stuttering. Given these beliefs, what therapy goals do you have for a child with intermediate stuttering?

SUGGESTED READINGS

Lieberman, A. (2018). Counseling issues: Addressing behavioral and emotional considerations in the treatment of communication disorders. *American Journal of Speech-Language Pathology, 27*, 13–23.

In describing counseling in our field, Lieberman notes that the helping relationship—in which the clinician creates a safe and supportive environment—is paramount for a client's making progress. At the heart of this relationship is a therapeutic alliance that is gradually formed between the client and clinician. This alliance helps clients feel that they are not doing the work of therapy alone. They feel supported and accepted as they are, whether they are leaning forward in progress or slumped in self-pity.

Manning, W., & DiLollo, A. (2018). *Clinical decision making in fluency disorders* (3rd ed.). Singular.

The first chapter describes many aspects of the clinician as well as of the clinical interaction in stuttering therapy. Also relevant to the topics in the current chapter is Chapter 7: Counseling and People Who Stutter and Their Families. This chapter contains an excellent description of the clinical relationship and other aspects of helping the person who stutters change their behaviors, thoughts, and feelings. The section titled "Basic Counseling Skills" is a good distillation of the key behaviors and attitudes needed for effective counseling. In Chapter 8, Therapeutic Process: Facilitating a Journey of Change, Manning and DiLollo describe goals for treatment and subtleties of how and when to work toward them. One of many excellent sections in this chapter is titled "Co-Drivers on the Journey: The Therapeutic Alliance."

Shapiro, D. (2011). The clinician: A paragon of change. In *Stuttering intervention: A collaborative journey to fluency freedom*. Pro-Ed.

This textbook contains two excellent chapters on clinician characteristics. One deals with the "magic" of the client-clinician relationship and touches on many of the attributes needed by effective clinicians. Another discusses the processes of students becoming qualified clinicians. The author talks about many aspects of supervision and analysis of clinical interactions.

Van Riper, C. (1957). Symptomatic therapy for stuttering. In L. E. Travis (Ed.), *Handbook of speech* (pp. 878–896). Appleton-Century-Crofts, Inc.

Although this is a very old chapter, it is an excellent description of how Van Riper combined psychotherapy with behavior therapy to create what we now call "stuttering modification" therapy. It is unparalleled in its explication of how his therapy motivates the client to confront his stutter and his "self" at the same time. Because of the emotional support and acceptance Van Riper provided, his clients were often able to reduce the abnormality of their symptoms and develop a "fluent stuttering" that passed for typical fluent speech.

Van Riper, C. (1958). Experiments in stuttering therapy. In J. Eisenson (Ed.), *Stuttering: A symposium* (pp. 273–290). Harper & Row.

This chapter describes the stuttering treatments that Van Riper experimented with in his first 20 years after leaving University of Iowa and setting up a speech clinic at what became Western Michigan University. Of particular interest are the systematic changes he made in treatment protocols year by year to develop the most effective methods and the 5-year follow-ups he made to measure long-term progress.

Van Riper, C. (1975a). The stutterer's clinician. In J. Eisenson (Ed.), *Stuttering: A second symposium* (pp. 453–492). Harper & Row.

This chapter is still a useful description of the attributes that may be important in clinicians who treat people who stutter. It also contains excellent sections on clinicians' roles in motivating clients and discusses the subject of whether clinicians who themselves stutter should treat clients who stutter.

Zebrowski, P. (2007). Treatment factors that influence therapy outcomes of children who stutter. In E. Conture, & R. Curlee (Eds.), *Stuttering and related disorders of fluency* (3rd ed., pp. 23–38). Thieme.

This chapter has excellent summaries of research relating to variables that can affect therapy outcome, including information about the relationship between the client and clinician.

Zebrowski, P., Anderson, J., & Conture, E. (2022). *Stuttering and related disorders of fluency* (4th ed.). Thieme.

This edited book contains the latest thinking on the nature of stutter, its evaluation, and its treatment. A multitude of experts from all over the world have contributed superb chapters that will help clinicians learn and employ the best techniques to work with stuttering.

SUGGESTED VIEWING

Hendrickson, J. (2022). I Stutter, But I Need You to Listen. Opinion, *New York Times*. On YouTube at https://www.youtube.com/watch?v=m0E_wMIwfSI

This impressively animated video presents John Hendrickson, a senior editor at Atlantic Magazine, describing his lifelong stutter and his decision to be open about it. Hendrickson happily reports that he is now saying what he wants to say when he wants to say it, without avoidance. He also addresses the important contributions made by listeners to improving communication.

Van Riper, C. (1975b). Therapy in Action—Dr. Charles Van Riper. Stuttering Foundation video #1080. Memphis, Foundation.

This classic video shows Van Riper working with a college-age student who stutters. It begins with a foreshortened evaluation and then the treatment stages of Identification, Desensitization, Modification, and Stabilization. A 20-year follow-up with the stutterer explores what, to him, were crucial elements in the therapy that made it so successful.

13

Treatment of Younger Preschool Children: Borderline Stuttering

Chapter Outline

Chapter Objectives

After studying this chapter, readers should be able to:

- Understand the difference between indirect and direct treatment
- Be able to plan and carry out indirect and—if needed—direct treatment of a younger preschool child
- Learn about data collection in the clinic by the clinician and at home by the parents, both of which can be used to guide treatment
- Learn the basics of treatment approaches advocated by others for preschool children

Key Terms

Direct treatment: Therapy that works directly on the child's speech by having them speak more fluently, stutter more easily, or both

Indirect treatment: Therapy that involves alleviating stresses that the child might be experiencing in communication at home and in other situations. It specifically does not have the child working on how they speak or how they stutter

Maintenance: The process of fading treatment while continuing to support the child and family so that fluency achieved in treatment does not diminish

One-on-one time: A period of about 15 minutes each day during which one parent is alone with the child and follows the child's lead in play and conversation. In this time, parents can practice new behaviors such as attentive listening to the child, making positive statements to the child after they speak, using a slower speech rate with pauses. Children can experience their parent's full attention in this interaction

Percent syllables stuttered (%SS): This is one measure of stuttering frequency that is often used as data to determine how much a child is stuttering at a particular time. We suggest using %SS along with SRs as an indication of whether treatment is working

Severity rating (SR): Numbers on a 0 to 9 scale given daily by parents to describe their child's fluency. The SR scale is shown in Figure 9.4 and described in detail in Chapter 9

Spontaneous fluency: A child's natural fluency that occurs without work or thought on his part

Younger preschool children: Children approximately between 2 and 3.5 years old. In this chapter, I will describe a number of different approaches to treatment of younger preschool children. I will begin by describing the approach I have been taking with this age group for more than 40 years.

AN INTEGRATED APPROACH

I would describe the stuttering in **younger preschool children** (2-3.5 years) to be usually at the "borderline" level with loose and relaxed repetitions. Treatment for them should be indirect, aimed at changing the environment, particularly parent-child interactions. The presumption is that an indirect approach will decrease environmental stress on the child and increase the bond between parent and child, create a positive atmosphere for the child when they are speaking, and, at the same time, will not call too much attention to their stuttering and will thereby not interfere with natural recovery.

A small number of young preschool children are a little more severe. They are starting to add tension to their stuttering and may be aware of and frustrated by it. I use reinforcement for fluent speech for these children. I aim at having them learn to stutter more easily and then gradually become fluent. Paramount in my approach is to make sure they feel good about talking and increasingly confident that they are in control of their speech.

In this chapter, I use the terms "family" and "parent" or "parents" interchangeably to indicate the important adult(s) with whom the child commonly interacts. Cultures and families differ in who should be involved in the child's treatment. When I imply that one parent is the major player in the interaction patterns I describe, the reader should freely adapt the treatment to suit each situation—one parent or two, older children or cousins, nannies, grandparents, or other caregivers.

Most treatment of stuttering at this age is indirect because it involves working with the family environment to increase fluency, rather than working directly on the child's speech. The initial focus is on helping parents feel less apprehensive and, therefore, more positive about their interactions with the child and helping them decide on what to do more of and what to change. I also attend to and try to understand their feelings of concern. If a child's family can discover new ways to facilitate the child's fluency and do more of what's already facilitating, they become confident in their ability to effect change in child's fluency. Taking a cue from attachment theory (Troutman, 2022), a parent can be guided to let the child take the lead in play, to verbalize what the child has just said ("Yes, you're right, the dolly is soft."), and to give the child specific praise ("I like the way you are putting the dolly in the car."). The parent's verbalizations are best spoken relatively slowly, with appropriate pauses. This speaking style may influence the child to talk in a relaxed way. Figure 13.1 shows a clinician listening carefully to the family's concerns and then guiding the mother to practice child-directed play in the clinic and at home. If indirect therapy by itself is not effective, then slightly more direct work on the child's speech by the clinician, with some help from the family, is appropriate.

I illustrate our approach to treatment with the case example of Ashley, the 2.5-year-old preschool child whom I introduced in Chapter 1.

"I like the way you are putting Dolly in the wagon".
"Dolly is soft"
"Yes, Dolly is soft!"

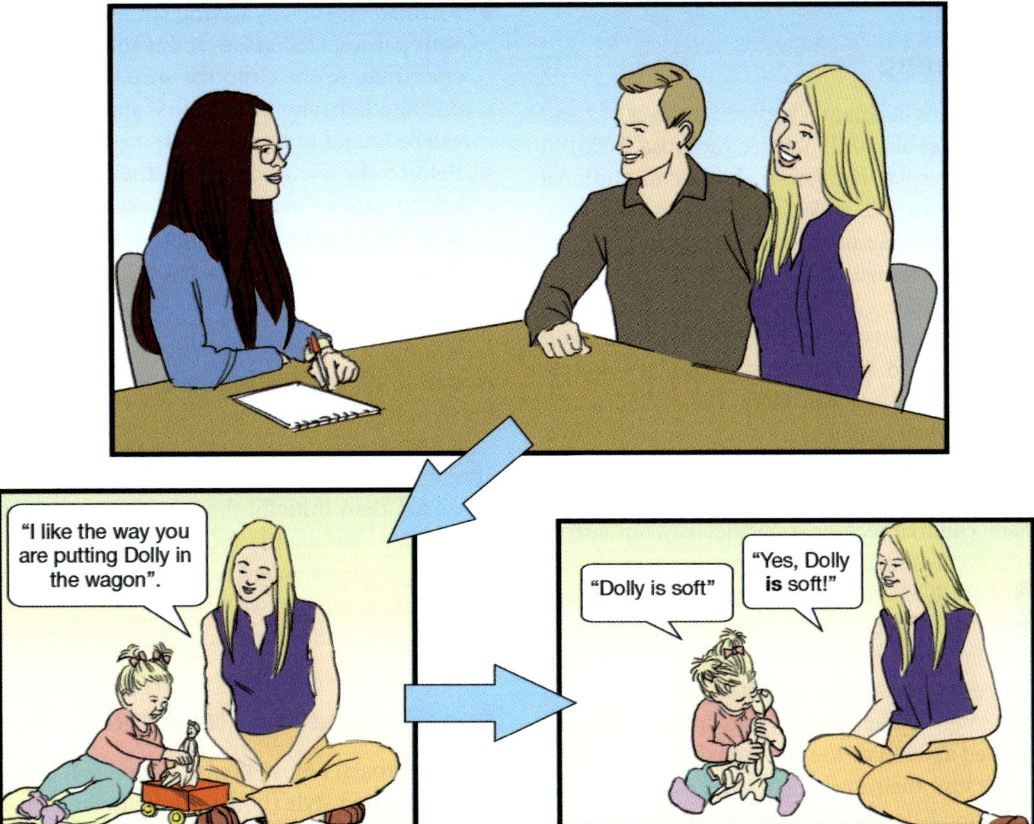

Figure 13.1 Clinician listens carefully to parents' concerns and guides mother to engage in child-directed play in clinic and at home.

Case Example

Ashley

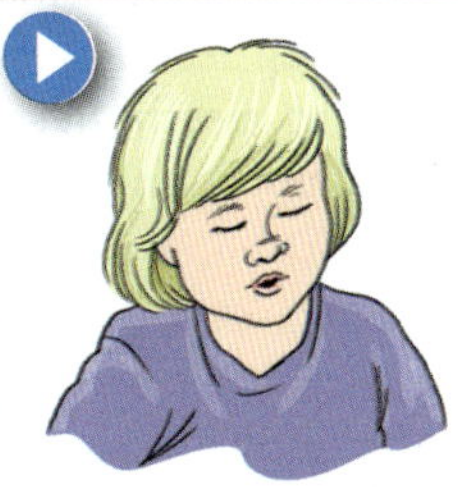

Ashley's stuttering, as you will remember from the video clip in Chapter 1, was characterized by multiple part-word and single-syllable whole-word repetitions. Two-and-a-half-year-old Ashley gave little indication that she was aware of her stuttering. Because her stuttering was quite frequent and gradually worsening, Ashley underwent treatment despite her young age.

Indirect treatment was carried out via once-weekly home visits by a clinician with experience in stuttering. The clinician began by playing with Ashley on the floor with a variety of toys including dolls and a dollhouse. The clinician used a slow rate of speech with many pauses, as we describe in this chapter. She did not ask Ashley to change her own rate but only modeled the rate for Ashley and her mother, who observed. Gradually, the mother took a greater and greater part, but the clinician continued to be part of play so she could observe the mother's own use of slower speech rate with more pauses.

After each session, the clinician and mother talked about how the mother was doing. The clinician was careful to praise the mother for what she was doing well before suggesting ways she could improve. In addition to slowing her speech rate and pausing more frequently, Ashley's mother also learned to turn most of her questions into comments. The clinician took data on the child's stuttering in each session.

This play therapy continued for about 8 weeks. Ashley's stuttering in the sessions disappeared, and her mother reported that she was more and more fluent in situations outside of the sessions. Five and a half years later, we video recorded an interview with Ashley at age 8. She was completely fluent, with no recollection of ever having stuttered.

Author's Beliefs

Nature of Stuttering

Stuttering usually begins in children between the ages of 2 and 3½ years (Bloodstein et al., 2021; Yairi & Ambrose, 2005). It emerges from the interplay between a child's constitutional predispositions (summarized in Walsh, Christ, and Weber, 2021), stresses in the environment, and the competition for resources as speech, language, and other capacities develop rapidly (eg, Smith & Weber, 2017). In these young children, stuttering behaviors are often characterized by a lack of tension in speech musculature and an absence of secondary characteristics—escape and avoidance behaviors. These children are often barely aware of their disfluencies. And even in children who show some signs of muscle tension early in their stuttering development, their stuttering and their awareness come and go. Because many children recover spontaneously, our aim in treatment is to prevent stuttering from becoming more severe and to maximize the likelihood that recovery will take place before the factors that influence persistence can do their work.

As I described in Chapters 5 and 6, my view of how stuttering becomes more severe is that children become distressed about their stuttering—either because they notice that their parents are alarmed about it or the children themselves react more strongly because their disfluencies feel out of control, or both. Their immediate response—often not consciously done—is to tense and push harder to get the word out. I liken this to the harder effort we use when a door is stuck and won't easily open. Soon after children try harder to get the word out, and are unsuccessful, they may develop escape and avoidance behaviors. If this escalation can be prevented, the plasticity of normal neural maturation will allow most of these children to develop neural networks like those of fluent children or to compensate for constitutional anomalies that create stuttering. To promote such flexibility in development to blossom into normal fluency, however, the clinician and family must provide an environment that fosters fluency and diminishes negative experiences with speaking.

In view of the presumed causes of borderline stuttering, our treatment focuses on these goals:

- Reduce the parents' anxiety about their child's stuttering, by listening carefully to their concerns, by helping them understand something about the nature of stuttering, by describing the path to recovery or to making any remaining stuttering a minor inconvenience, and by sharing videos designed for parents of children who stutter (such as Stuttering Foundation's [SF's] free videos "Stuttering and Your Child: Help for Parents" and "For Kids by Kids"). These experiences will lessen the likelihood that parents will convey distress about their child's stuttering to the child.
- Help the child feel good about speaking by having parents listen to the child attentively and make positive comments in response to what the child says.
- Facilitate fluency by having family members speak slowly with pauses, change questions into comments, and listen attentively to the child (be sure parents are just learning one new behavior at a time). If appropriate, older children can be taught to interact with the child using these skills.
- Reduce the child's alarm at their stuttering, in part by asking parents to comment acceptingly if the child seems at all frustrated when stuttering occurs.
- Reduce general stresses felt by the child in the family household.

The clinician should sequence these goals carefully so that parents don't feel overwhelmed if they are asked to do too much in too-brief a time.

If indirect therapy is not effective in reducing stuttering after 6 weeks, or if the child's stuttering proves to be more advanced than initially thought, I add slightly more direct procedures. My slightly more direct approach for stuttering in younger preschoolers consists of a hierarchy of activities that focus on playing with stuttering while reducing tension to result in a milder form and then gradually into fluency.

Speech Behaviors Targeted for Therapy

In the approach I most often use—indirect therapy—the family's interaction style (both speech and nonspeech behaviors) is the target of therapy. Thus, the child's speech behaviors are not a focus of the treatment but are, of course, periodically assessed. In those rare instances when this approach doesn't soon decrease stuttering, the child's stuttering behaviors and their emotions are targeted for change.

Fluency Goals

I believe that children who stutter at the borderline level who have no serious concomitant problems can achieve **spontaneous fluency**. With effective early intervention, this goal is readily achievable because the child's maturing nervous system gradually increases their capacity for fluent speech. In some cases, very mild stuttering may remain but not be an issue.

Feelings and Attitudes

Although the main focus of treatment is on the behaviors of family members and others who interact frequently with the child, a parent can do a great deal to reduce the child's negative feelings about stuttering when the child shows signs of frustration or dismay with their speech. This will be described in detail in the Procedures section, but I will make a few brief comments here. Usually, family members can tell if a child is showing signs of frustration or other distress about their disfluencies. Parents need to observe facial expressions, pitch increases, or whether the child stops in the middle of a stutter and changes what they are trying to say. When these or other signs of distress occur, a parent can make a comment, in a relaxed and accepting manner to reassure the child. It could be something like "I know it's hard when words get stuck, but it's ok. You're doing fine."

Maintenance Procedures

Many younger preschool children achieve fluent speech soon after their families have made some environmental modifications, and most maintain fluency without further treatment. However, it is important for the clinician to keep in contact with the family, even after formal treatment has stopped, to check on whether the child is reverting to older stuttering patterns. This support for **maintenance**, through telephone calls or e-mail, is gradually faded, unless the child begins to stutter again, calling for a return to treatment.

Clinical Methods

Working with stuttering at this level involves a variety of therapy procedures. I educate families by providing them with videos and reading material (such as resources available from the Stuttering Foundation (SF), and giving them opportunities to talk with other parents whose children have stuttered and have recovered) to help them understand something about the nature of stuttering and the ways in which they can help the child become more fluent. The clinician should be familiar with the written or video material before giving it to the family so that the clinician and the family can discuss it after the family has read or viewed it. I counsel families by listening to their concerns and by trying to understand their hopes, desires, fears, and frustrations. I brainstorm and problem-solve with families when I help them choose aspects of their interaction patterns to modify. I collect data on the child's speech and on the family's perceptions of their child's stuttering and fluency. And finally, I provide support as the child's stuttering decreases and the family strives to maintain their new styles of interaction.

Clinical Procedures: Indirect Treatment

This section describes the stages of indirect treatment, including continuing assessment of the child's speech at home and in the clinic, introduction of (1) positive comments to the child about what they've said, (2) a slower speech rate with pauses, and (3) introduction of other changes that the clinician and the family choose.

Severity Ratings

As I explained in Chapter 9 on assessment, during the closing interview the family is given a copy of the **Severity Rating (SR)** Scale (Fig. 9.4), and its use is explained to them. Although the scale was originally designed for use with the Lidcombe Program (LP) (see Chapter 14 for details), it is excellent for use with families of younger children who will be receiving indirect treatment. As you will remember, it is a 10-point scale that the family completes at the end of every day. Ratings range from 0 = no stuttering and 2 = extremely mild stuttering all the way to 9 = extremely severe stuttering (which may never be seen in a particular child). At each clinic session, after a baseline of the child's speech is collected in the first 10 minutes, the clinician and parent compare their SRs for the child's speech during the baseline measure. Agreement is defined as the parent and clinician's SR for that sample not differing by more than one point. If the difference between the ratings is greater than a single point, the clinician's rating is assumed to be accurate, and they discusses their rating with the parent to help the parent better understand the rating system and become "calibrated." The parent uses the scale to make a daily rating of the child's speech at the end of every day and brings or e-mails the week's SR chart to the clinician for discussion in each clinic meeting.

Baseline Speech Measures

At the beginning of each clinic visit, the clinician video records and observes the first 10 to 15 minutes of parent-child play. Attending to both the child's speech and the parent's interaction style, the clinician's first task is to decide on an SR for the child's speech in this parent-child play period. As noted, this will be compared with the parent's SR for the same sample. The clinician also notes aspects of the parent-child interaction, especially those on which the parent and clinician have agreed the parent will work on.

Family Interaction Patterns

As described in Chapter 10, in the section on assessment of the younger preschool child, my approach to treatment involves helping parents develop the most beneficial patterns of interacting with their child who stutters. After we have discussed our mutual SRs for the child during play and SRs for the past week, we watch the video recording we made at the beginning of the session of the parents' play with their child. As we watch the video, we share ideas on what might be the most facilitating interaction patterns for their child, including those that the parents are already using. That's important, because parents will be more receptive to change if they learn that they are doing many things well, but need to do more of them or need to tweak them somewhat. Together, we work out how they may expand on these patterns or continue them. In the following sections, I will describe some of the interaction patterns that I find to be most fluency facilitating for most children. You may find, however, that you and a family choose other facilitating patterns and you may want to begin with those. Examples of facilitating patterns are given in Table 13.1. Some of the key patterns include careful listening to their child, using a slower speech rate with plenty of pauses, and positive comments to child. As mentioned earlier, appropriate other family members besides parents can be taught these patterns.

TABLE 13.1 Family Interaction Patterns That May Facilitate Fluency

Listening time	All children benefit from feeling that what they have to say is important. This is especially true for the child who is beginning to stutter. Set aside some time each day as "listening time" with your child. Make it at least 5-10 min (or longer if you can) at about the same time each day, so your child can depend on it. Try to have it be a time when you can be alone with your child, free from distractions. During that time, refrain from making suggestions or giving instructions. Merely "be there" for the child, listening attentively to what they say or quietly playing alongside the child if they choose not to talk. The book on listening by Shafir (2000) is an excellent resource for improving listening skills.
Slow rate	It will benefit the child if family members reduce their conversational rate of speech to a slow, soothing style. Speech should sound relaxed and calm, with comfortable pauses throughout. An example of slow rate with pauses can be found in the YouTube video "Fred Rogers' 2002 Dartmouth College Commencement Address."
Pauses	The pace of conversation can be kept appropriately slow if the speaker pauses 1-2 seconds before starting to talk. This also helps to keep the speaker from interrupting another speaker.
Positive comments	Make many specific, positive, and accepting comments about what your child is saying and doing. Limit corrections or criticisms to important issues. Changes for the better usually happen more quickly when someone feels they are OK as they are. The child who feels good about themselves will be better able to use "listening time," "slow rate," and "pauses" to gain more fluency.
Fewer questions	It is natural to ask a child many questions in order to encourage them to learn new things and to display that knowledge. However, this makes some children feel "under the gun." So it may be a good idea to decrease demanding questions and instructions. If you are worried that your child won't learn enough if you are too laid-back, keep in mind that learning comes naturally to children. They learn best from your interest in things, especially from your interest and positive comments about the things they do and say.
Taking turns in family conversations	All children find it easier to talk if family members take turns rather than interrupting and talking over each other. A student and I published an article about how effective this approach was for her son who stuttered (Winslow & Guitar, 1994). She found that having family members hold a "talking stick" (an object like a salt shaker) when they took their turn was a helpful reminder not to interrupt each other.

As I work with the parents, watching their videos and discussing ideas for helping the child, I have the child play with another clinician—if available—or have the child play on the floor as the parents and I are sitting at a table.

Careful Listening to the Child and Making Positive Comments

I typically begin with this facilitating interaction because children who feel that their parents are listening to them and that their parents like what they are saying will feel positive about speaking and are less likely to increase tension and struggle when they stutter. When I watch the videos by myself at another time, I look for examples of listening and positive comments in video recordings I have made of the parents I am working with. In the next session, as we watch the video of these parents and their child, I point out these examples and compliment the parents. Once we have identified one or two examples of this, I ask them to find other examples of listening and positive comments. Once I think the parents understand what I'm asking them to do more of, the parents and I play together on the floor with the child (Fig. 13.2). I use careful listening and positive comments with the child myself, modelling for them.

For example, I can listen carefully to what the child says and if they say something about a car they are playing with—that they like it—after appropriate pause time, I may say something like "Yes, you sure are right about that car—it is a cool one! No wonder you like it." After I give the parents a few models, I ask them to try it.

Following the joint play, we explore the parents' thoughts and feelings about this activity and I make sure to listen attentively to what they say and acknowledge their feelings. If parents are comfortable with attentive listening and positive comments, I encourage them to practice them at home, ideally each day for 15 to 20 minutes. We also talk about the SRs that we've asked them to tally every day.

After several weeks—or less in some cases—parents will probably see a decrease in the child's SRs. If parents are

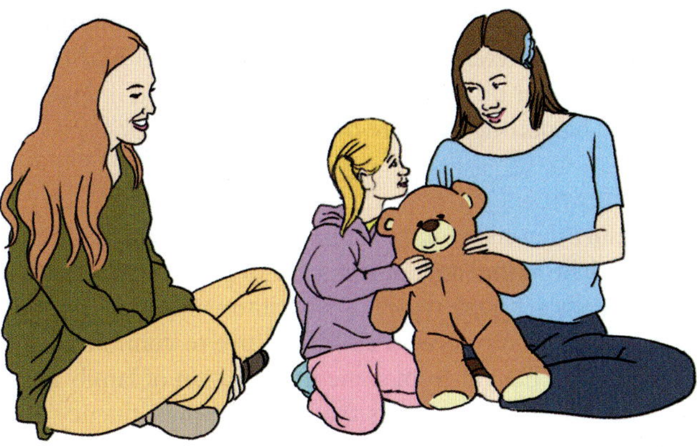

Figure 13.2 With clinician's help, mother learns to let child lead in play.

feeling that the stuttering is no longer an issue, it might be time to taper off the frequency of their meetings with me. Weekly contact with the parents is still vital, to encourage the parents to continue their careful listening and positive comments. If things continue to go well, and SRs are very low and stable, meetings can be made less and less frequent and when parents are ready, treatment can be ended. However, in most cases, some stuttering remains and it is appropriate to begin the next phase of treatment.

Slower Speech Rate With Pauses

For most families, the clinician starts by helping the parents reduce their speech rate and increase their pause time when talking with their child. The evidence reviewed in Chapters 2 and 3 suggests that individuals who stutter have constitutional deficits that make it challenging for them to produce speech at rapid rates. If parents provide a model of slower speech with plentiful pauses, this model alone will probably influence children to speak more slowly (Guitar & Marchinkowski, 2001). More importantly, a model of slower speech with adequate pauses has been shown to reduce children's stuttering (eg, Guitar et al., 1992; Stephanson-Opsal & Bernstein Ratner, 1988; Zebrowski et al., 1996). The clinician emphasizes that parents should not instruct the child to slow his speech rate; such direct instruction tends to be ineffective and annoying to the child. Mr. Rogers, whose children's television show aired from the late 1960s through the early 2000s, provides an excellent speaker for parents to emulate. A sample of his speech can be viewed on a 2002 YouTube recording Mr. Rogers' delivery of a commencement speech at Dartmouth College.

Teaching Slower Speaking Rate With Pauses

After rehearsing a slower speech rate with pauses, you can meet with the parents, model this style of speaking, and ask them to try it. Sometimes, beginning with a reading passage is easier than having a conversation. Most parents find it slightly embarrassing to speak this way at first, but your modeling this style will make it easier for them. Strongly reinforce them for the things they are doing well. Once they have a pretty good style, you can video or audio record their speech and play it back to them, and their experience of hearing and watching themselves speak this way will help them remember it. If you have a laptop with a camera, you can record a clip of them speaking this way and e-mail it to them so they will have it at home to refresh their memories from time to time. It is key that this type of speaking more slowly should not be one...word....at...a...time. This is often the way people speak when they are angry and I've had a least one preschool child tell his mother to stop talking this way. Our type of slower speech is smooth, with words linked together smoothly. Listen to Mr. Rogers' speaking style on the YouTube video mentioned earlier.

Trying Slower Rate With Pauses in the Clinic

After the parents feel comfortable using the new speaking style, the clinician and a parent can play with the child and use the slower rate with pauses. If the child asks the parent why they are talking in a funny, slow way, the clinician or parent may explain to the child that the parent talks too fast and needs to learn to slow down. With some children, we enlist them to remind the parent to slow down if they think the parent is talking too quickly. Children delight in correcting adults, especially their parents.

Using the Slower Rate With Pauses at Home

If the clinician is not satisfied with the parents' ability to speak with the child using this new speaking style, home practice should be delayed until the parents have mastered it. However, most parents pick up the new style quickly, and they can begin using it at home immediately. One parent should try to spend 15 minutes a day playing alone with the child and using the new speaking style. *The best time is in the morning because it may influence the child for the rest of the day.* Many families are too busy at this time, feeding and dressing their children and themselves. For them, one-on-one slow speech practice in the morning may be possible only on weekends. In this case, *any* 15 minutes per day of **one-on-one time** with the child is acceptable. Most important is that the parents do it on as many days as they can. If one parent does most of the one-on-one play with slow speech, the other parent should also use the slower speech rate when talking with the child whenever they can.

Monitoring Parents' Practice of Slower Rate With Pauses

Most parents benefit from consistent support for any changes they are making in their interactions with their child. I often keep in touch with them between clinic visits via e-mail or telephone, but I always suggest that they keep a brief journal of their experience with the new speaking style by making notes on the SR chart they are completing every evening. If parents are willing and able to video record themselves at home using the new speaking style during their 15-minute daily interactions, the recording is a fine motivation for them to practice and a good way for me to monitor their progress. In any case, their interaction with their child at the beginning of each session allows me to be sure they are using an effective speaking style and allows me to collect data on the child's percentage syllables stuttered during this interaction. When I'm observing this, I can also read the SR chart with the parents' notes about their daily work between clinic visits. In the discussion that follows the parent-child interaction, I am careful to reinforce the parents for everything they are doing well. In all discussions, the clinician's role is first and foremost to be an empathetic listener, allowing the parents to take the lead in assessing their progress and formulating plans to work on change.

Commenting on the Child's Speech When They Stutter

If the child is showing signs of frustration or other distress during their stutters, I ask parents to begin commenting by first letting the child know when they are talking well. I demonstrate this for them by saying something like "That's really good talking!" after the child has had a string of fluent sentences. I don't make a big deal of it but do say it with enthusiasm so that the child hears it and is pleased. Don't do this very often to avoid having the child become self-conscious. Once the child's fluency has been occasionally praised, then they are ready for the parent to comment when the child shows signs of frustration or is nonplussed during a moment of stuttering. Watch the video of Ashley on Lippincott Connect (Chapter 1, A Young Preschool Child: Borderline Stuttering, Segment 1). Notice that when she is trying to say the cat's name "Cookie," she repeats "Co-" many times and eventually you can hear a pitch increase and some breathlessness. She is also looking around, slightly baffled at what is happening to her. After she gives up and has finished her utterance, a clinician or parent *could* then say "Oh, that word 'Cookie' was hard to say. Sometimes words just get stuck and that's ok." A parent or clinician shouldn't do this very often or else the child may resent it or be embarrassed. Observe how the child reacts. If they seem even more distressed than before, back off of the commenting for a while and try again with a briefer reassurance, like "mmm-hmmm" after the stutter and then a comment letting the child know she's been heard and understood even though there was a stutter. If all goes well, the child may have a look of slight relief after she hears that everything is all right, even though the word got stuck.

Working With Other Aspects of the Parent-Child Interaction

As the clinician works with the parents or other family members on their positive comments, reducing speech rate, and pausing, the clinician continues to assess the child's progress toward typical fluency, as indicated by **percent syllables stuttered (%SS)** in the treatment setting, SRs at home, and discussions with the family. If these indicators of fluency do not portray a steady downward progression of stuttering in the first 3 or 4 weeks of treatment, the clinician and family should consider other aspects of the parent-child interaction that may be putting pressure on the child's fluency.

Modifications of Family Communication Style

Remember that most of the interaction patterns in families of children who stutter are not abnormal or particularly negative. They usually are quite typical of the culture in which the child is being raised. However, a child sensitive to communicative pressure may benefit from some modification of family communication patterns in ways that facilitate their fluency. It is vital that the clinician help the family understand that they are not causing the child to stutter because of inappropriate communication patterns. Instead, their communication is typical, but they can help their child by changing a few aspects of their communication to facilitate fluency.

One of the first things I do if I sense some aspect of the family communicative style might need a little modification is to have the parents watch again with me the video recording of their interaction with their child. As we watch together, I praise many things that the parents are doing well. Praise is vital in helping develop the parents' confidence and encouraging them to keep doing things they are doing well. As I praise the parents, I listen acceptingly to their comments even if they comment negatively about something they see themselves do. We watch together for things that the parents and I both feel might be putting pressure on the child. The best situation is when parents notice something to change—something that I also feel may be pressuring the child's fluency. Then together, we plan to change that aspect of the interaction and observe the results.

For example, in the 3rd week of treatment, a parent was doing a great job using a slower speech rate with pauses. However, the child's fluency—which had increased somewhat—had now plateaued. The parent and I watched the most recent video recording, and as we watched, I praised her slow speech with pauses. After a few minutes, the parent commented that she was surprised to see that she asked her child so many questions, rat-a-tat-tat, one right after the other. I agreed with her and we discussed alternatives, such as making comments instead of asking questions, and she tried this out during the week. The following week, the child's SRs showed further increases in fluency, and the parent's interaction with the child at the beginning of the session revealed an impressive decrease in questions. This change, accompanied by the slower speech rate with pausing, was enough to increase the child's fluency to normal levels, which was maintained long term.

Changes in Family Routine

In addition to changing conversational interaction patterns, a family may identify other stresses on the child that need to be changed, such as the amount of individual attention the child receives and the "busyness" of the family's schedule. My main function in helping families work on such stresses is to give them information about changes that others have found helpful and to be a sounding board for their plans for changing. I encourage them to assess, informally, the effects of these changes on the child's fluency and their overall adjustment. Although my praise and appreciation may help, a significant change in the child's stuttering is the real motivator. Notes the parent makes on the chart of daily SRs will help you and the family identify factors that may facilitate fluency or cause upward spikes in a child's stuttering. A parent, for example, noted on her SR chart that her child's stuttering flared up if she left the room while he was playing. She alleviated this stress by being careful to let the child know ahead of time if she were about to leave the room and that she would be right back. This example is a reminder of the importance of parents' attention for a child's self-esteem. When a child senses that their mother or father understands them and genuinely cares about them (cares about what the child likes to do, what the child thinks about things, and how the child feels), the child feels more comfortable with themselves, are less anxious, and are better able to speak easily.

To emphasize what I've said earlier, for many younger preschool children who stutter, a little more one-on-one time spent with a parent every day, preferably in the morning, can boost fluency tremendously. Although the morning can be the most difficult time for parents who work outside the home, one-on-one "fluency time" in the morning can have a positive effect on the child's speech for the rest of the day. If mornings are too difficult, some one-on-one time in the afternoon can also be very helpful. The time does not need to be long, just 15 to 20 minutes, but the parent needs to be with the child in a place where, ideally, they won't be interrupted.

The child should choose what to play or talk about, and the parent should follow the child's lead, participating as the child directs. As a parent becomes more and more comfortable with this nondirective play, they may want to explore ways of helping the child feel really understood. One of the parents we worked with, for example, learned to "mirror" her child's momentary emotions as they built a tower of blocks together. When the child placed a block on the tower and it fell off, the parent would quietly murmur a sound of disappointment, echoing the child's facial expression. This child made impressive gains in fluency in only a few weeks, and I believe that this parent's deep attention to the child may have contributed significantly to this change. Although parents may vary in the level of empathetic response they can achieve, increased caring attention is probably a realistic goal for most families. Attentive play can become child-directed conversations as a child grows older, and such conversations can continue the process of helping the child develop a sense of being loved, understood, and appreciated (eg, Troutman, 2022).

Course of Treatment

Sometimes families report that their attempts to make changes have been fairly successful. For example, they may have been able to make more positive comments, slow their speaking rates and to simplify their language, and may have seen improvement in their child. I let them know that their changes have been key factors in the child's improvement and stress the importance of continuing them. It is easy to resume old patterns after some improvement occurs, whether it's the challenge of losing weight or helping a child become more fluent.

Each child and each family are unique in how they respond to treatment, but it is possible to note some common trends. For example, some children become much more fluent soon after the family makes one or two changes in their environment. Occasionally, a child may become fluent immediately after an initial session, possibly because the family is less anxious about the child's disfluencies after sharing their concerns with a professional. Whatever the cause, early and immediate fluency gains should be viewed with cautious optimism. I share the family's pleasure at such dramatic change but suggest that their child's fluency may be fragile and will need to be nurtured by our continued efforts to create a facilitative environment.

Sometimes the path toward fluency is rough and irregular. The child may make little or no progress or may improve for a while and then return to their old pattern of disfluency. When this happens and the family or clinician feels frustrated by slow progress, further exploration of the family's feelings about the child's stuttering is called for. Many times, family members worry about the child's future, afraid that stuttering will be a serious handicap for the child. Sometimes there is lingering guilt about having caused the child's stuttering. Often it is hard for parents to accept the blemish they feel that stuttering creates on the family image.

Whatever the source of a family's anxieties, their concern about stuttering may easily radiate to the child in their reactions to the child's stutters. Unwittingly, family members may show their anxiety or disappointment through facial expressions or body language, which may make the child "hesitate to hesitate" and thus stutter more severely. Open and frank discussions with the family about their feelings and concerns are likely to be more helpful at this point than trying to change their reactions. In such discussions, the clinician's role is to make it easier for the family to talk about their concerns, so I listen carefully, try my best to understand them, and convey my understanding with acceptance and respect. When family members feel understood and accepted, it is easier for them to share their feelings and accept them. When this occurs, some feelings may change, and in turn, the child's stuttering may decrease, possibly because their stuttering no longer seems so terrible to the family.

Another barrier to changing a family's interaction patterns is the fact that some styles of interaction reflect important cultural values. For example, in the urban eastern United States, family members sometimes finish each other's sentences as a means of conveying a closeness and solidarity within the family that is highly valued. If they are asked to speak more slowly and pause between speakers' turn takings, such changes could conflict with one of the family's implicit cultural values. Another example might be parents who frequently teach, correct, and criticize their children's behavior. This "instructional" mode of interaction may reflect the importance that the family's culture places on education.

I believe that it is important to explore how the family feels about changes they are considering. Often, they can find ways to change other variables that will be as effective, thereby leaving unchanged those interactions that are of value to the family. Some years ago, I worked with a parent who spoke very rapidly to her 4-year-old child who was beginning to stutter. She resisted changing her speech rate because "it isn't the way we talk." In addition, she was frequently critical of her child's behavior. Consequently, I encouraged her to use positive reinforcement for fluency, as described in the LP approach to treatment of beginning stuttering in Chapter 14. At that time, I had just read the article by Onslow et al. (1994) and, borrowing just the positive reinforcement for fluency from that, asked this mother to let her child know with upbeat statements of praise that she liked their smooth fluency. The child's stuttering diminished almost immediately, and she was delighted with her ability to help her child.

Sometimes a family may resist change and doesn't fully participate in treatment. There may be psychological issues that need to be resolved through referral to a family counselor, or the family may have other, more serious problems with which to cope. In such cases, I talk with the family directly about my concerns. This usually leads to an open discussion of their situation, a referral to a family counselor, or, in rare cases, their decision to withdraw the child from stuttering therapy for the time being. If this happens, I let the family know that I remain available to them, and I try to stay in contact by occasional phone calls or e-mails to make it easier for them to resume the child's therapy if they wish to.

Maintenance

Indirect treatment of a younger preschool child is often effective within five or six sessions, over a period of 1 or 2 months. The child's speech becomes markedly less disfluent. Part-word repetitions become whole-word or phrase repetitions, which are more like typical children's disfluencies, and the family's concerns about the child's speech diminish. When this happens, I review with them the changes the family has made and the changes in their child's stuttering that reflect the child's improvement. Using this information, I help the family develop a plan to deal with periods of increased stress that may prompt stuttering to reappear. Most families feel that they have a handle on how to reduce stress on their child at this stage of therapy and their experiences in observing and changing their behaviors have given them confidence. If their child's stuttering suddenly increases, they know how to examine their speech rates or attentiveness when talking to the child and how to examine other aspects of their interactions and implement needed changes.

Effective maintenance for stuttering in younger preschool children is the result of two things: (1) helping the family to view the child's stuttering more objectively with less anxiety, guilt, or panic and (2) building the family's confidence in their own ability to implement problem-solving skills they've learned to use when the child's disfluencies increase. Sometimes, however, despite a family's best efforts to respond constructively, stuttering returns. This may occur after an increase in stress from some trauma or from typical life events, such as moving to a new house, or it may accompany a growth spurt in the child's language. On the other hand, it may be inexplicable. Whatever the cause, the family should feel comfortable getting back in contact with the clinician. I let each family know at the end of therapy that relapse is possible, not abnormal, and that I would look forward to seeing the child again if help is needed.

Supporting Data

Many years ago, my colleagues and I published two papers that evaluated the effect of changing parent-child interactions with a 5-year-old child who stuttered (Guitar, 1978; Guitar et al., 1992). Although this child was an older preschooler, the principles of working with the family on their interaction style were similar to those described for the younger preschool child. Our focus was twofold: (1) we guided the parents in making supportive statements to their daughter and (2) we taught the parents to slow their speech rates and increase pausing as they talked with her. We wondered what effect each different strategy would have on their daughter's stuttering. Our approach to treatment was to video record parent-child interactions over five treatment sessions and then view the videos with each parent. When viewing the videos, we let the parent decide what to work on in the intervening week and then recorded a new parent-child interaction after a week of work on changing the behavior they had selected. After six sessions, the child's stuttering had diminished to the level of normal disfluency; we followed the child for 10 years, and the stuttering never reappeared. In an analysis of the parents' behavior and the child's stuttering, we broke the child's stuttering down into primary stuttering (multiple repetitions without excess tension) and secondary stuttering (prolongations and blocks that showed muscular tension). Then, we analyzed the child's speech that immediately followed the chosen parent behavior. We found that the reductions in the daughter's stuttering were related only to changes in the mother's behavior, not the father's. Strikingly, the reductions in primary stuttering were significantly related only to the mother's slower rate. The slowed rate didn't reduce secondary stuttering. Conversely, the increase in the mother's accepting and approving comments to her daughter were significantly related only to their secondary stuttering and not their primary stuttering. This small study suggests the possibility that primary and secondary stuttering may be independent and related to different parent behaviors. Thus, the parent-child interactions for each family may contain different but important variables to manipulate if a client has both types of stuttering.

A variety of other studies have shown that changes in parent's communicative interactions affect their children's stuttering. Stephanson-Opsal and Bernstein Ratner (1988) demonstrated that when the mothers of stuttering children slowed their speech rates, the children's stuttering decreased. Starkweather et al. (1990) reported on 29 children they treated for an average of 12 sessions (some required as many as 40 sessions), all of whom completely recovered. Their approach involved primarily modification of the parents' behavior, including reduction of speech rate, having special speech time, matching parent language to child language, and reducing parents' negative reactions to stuttering. Zebrowski et al. (1996) showed that decreases in mother's speaking rate and pause time were associated with decreases in stuttering in some children. Were these children who showed mostly primary stuttering?

Further supporting data on this approach are presented in the outcome measures of the Michael Palin Center's treatment of preschool children, described later in this chapter. Data on 55 children treated with Palin PCI (Parent-Child Interaction) treatment indicated long-term improvement on stuttering frequency, attitudes about speaking, and parent perception of child's stuttering, assessed a year after the start of treatment. Moreover, yet more supporting data come from reports by Franken et al. (2005) and by de Sonnerville-Koedoot et al. (2015) that provide evidence of the effectiveness of parent-child interaction therapy (the RESTART Program, which is described in the next section). The study by de Sonneville-Koedoot et al. reported that 65 out of 91 children treated with this approach were no longer stuttering 18 months after treatment. In the next chapter on treatment of older preschoolers, the treatment approach described by Gottwald (2010) uses a great deal of indirect treatment but supplements it with **direct treatment** when needed. She reports that 26 of 27 children who were stuttering notably before treatment were speaking normally a year or more after treatment ended.

Clinical Procedures: Slightly More Direct Treatment

I don't use more direct treatment with every child who is a borderline stutterer, but it is a good alternative to combine with indirect treatment when indirect treatment alone does not decrease the child's stuttering significantly after 6 weeks. The causes of failure with an indirect approach are often unknown. Sometimes, a family seems unable to modify the child's environment as planned, or they do, but the child's stuttering persists unchanged or increases. In these few cases, I try a slightly more direct approach, as described in the next section.

Most younger preschool children with borderline stuttering are often minimally aware of their disfluencies. Their repetitions appear relaxed, and they show no signs of defensive reactions to their stuttering or using extra effort to "fight" their stutters. They also are normally fluent a great deal of the time, and I think they have the capacity to develop entirely normal fluency. Consequently, when borderline stuttering is a little more severe, I add slightly more direct treatment. I focus on the child's fluency, assuming that they will easily be able to increase the amount of fluency they have and "outgrow" their stuttering with our help.

However, I begin by training the child's parents to use praise for the *content* of what a child says, whether fluent or not. For example, if a child says, "Fido barking" the parent might say "Oh, you're right, he *is* barking at that doggie out the window." Then, gradually, the parent can also praise fluency, by saying something specific like, "Your speech was really smooth when you said you wanted a cookie." The clinician and parent should decide how frequently to use positive reinforcement, but most children are annoyed by praise if the parent gives it too often. A few children are annoyed by any praise at all given by the parent. In this case, the parent and the clinician can talk with the child about using something besides typical praise. Some children prefer their own phrase. One child wanted his parent to say "That was good monkey talk!" Another child asked for a gesture (thumbs up) instead of words.

As in parent-child interaction therapy, parents continue to keep daily logs of the child's overall fluency for each day, using the 0 to 9 SRs described earlier. When the child has made substantial progress in decreasing severity, the clinician guides the parent in gradually replacing praise for fluency in the daily one-on-one sessions with praise used occasionally during other activities during the day. While the parent is carrying out this slightly more direct therapy, it is important for them to attend weekly meetings with the clinician to demonstrate using the procedure, to share SRs, and to discuss progress and problems. It is also important for the family to continue one-on-one sessions with the child and *to continue the changes made in their interactions and family lifestyle.* If needed, the clinician can use a little stuttering modification in addition to positive reinforcement for fluency. This approach is described in Chapter 14, under the heading Stuttering Modification Treatment.

OTHER APPROACHES

The approaches of two other clinicians and the resources of the SF are described here. They are appropriate not only for borderline stuttering in younger preschool children but for beginning stuttering in older preschool children as well. I have selected them because they all involve the child's family, which I consider of major importance when working with preschool children. The nature of intervention ranges from monitoring the child's stuttering to helping parents change their interaction patterns to direct work on the child's way of speaking, if needed.

Even though two of these approaches present data on their effectiveness, clinicians using any approach should collect their own data on progress and outcome. As suggested in Chapter 9, baseline measures of the child's stuttering at the beginning of treatment should be made in a valid and reliable way. Because the fluency of preschool children is highly variable, recordings of the child's speech should be made at home as well as in a clinical setting. The Stuttering Severity Instrument-4 (Riley, 2009) should be used to assess frequency and severity. When treatment begins, weekly measures of progress should be made; percentage of syllables stuttered in the clinic and daily SRs of speech at home made by a parent are effective and efficient. When the child has achieved fluent speech (SRs at home of 0 [normal fluency] and less than 1%SS in the clinic), a maintenance program should be started, involving continued measurement at home and during gradually faded clinic visits. Children with borderline stuttering can be expected to achieve stable, normally fluent speech within 6 months. Clinicians should assess how long a child is in treatment before fluency is achieved and how well the child maintained that fluency a year after treatment ends.

Palin Center Parent-Child Interaction

Treatment

The team at the Michael Palin Center for Stammering has developed a therapy approach for children under the age of seven. The approach is based on the understanding that stuttering is a heterogenous condition, influenced by physiological, linguistic, cognitive/affective, and environmental factors (Kelman & Nicholas, 2020). Children are born with the genetic predisposition to stutter, and this increased neurophysiological vulnerability to stuttering is influenced by these other factors (Starkweather, 2002). The approach has evolved over a number of years and is now heavily influenced by the principles of Solution Focused Brief Therapy (briefly described in Chapter 11), meaning that the therapist works with the parents to identify the child's strengths, as well as areas for support. The parents are encouraged to identify what they are already doing that supports the child's confidence, fluency, and communication skills, to reinforce and increase these helpful behaviors. The therapy also seeks to reduce the impact of stuttering on the parents, so that they are less worried about it now and for the future, as well as increase their knowledge and confidence in how they can support their child.

A detailed description of the Palin Parent-Child Interaction therapy program (Palin PCI) has been published in Kelman and Nicholas (2008, 2020), and illustrative video clips can be found in Botterill and Kelman (2010). The approach begins with a thorough evaluation of a child's strengths and needs. The child's receptive and expressive language, phonology, speech rate, social communication skills, and temperament are evaluated. This gives an indication of any factors that may be contributing to the stuttering and the impact that it is having. A detailed parent interview elicits information about the child and their communication in the context of the family, and the parents' ideas are sought about what facilitates the child's fluency, communication, and confidence. The parents may have observed, for example, that the child stutters less when they have had plenty of rest and stutters more when they are competing for speaking time, such as at the dinner table. The parents' ideas are valued and incorporated into therapy, which consists of three strands: Interaction Strategies, Family Strategies, and Child Strategies. The Interaction and Family Strategies are introduced in the first six sessions of therapy, with Child Strategies introduced later, if necessary, and when these foundations are in place.

Palin PCI involves both parents (if they live with the child) attending a weekly clinic session for 6 weeks with their child. A video recording is made to establish which interaction styles are likely to be facilitating the child's communication, confidence, and fluency and which styles might be developed further. In the session, the therapist video records each parent playing with the child and this is watched together. The clinician invites them to comment on the helpful things they are already doing that they notice in the video. Examples of helpful interactions are (1) following the child's lead, in playing and in talking; (2) making sure the child has enough time to say what they want to say before the parent responds or interrupts; and (3) keeping good eye contact with the child while the child is speaking so the child really feels listened to.

Family strategies are also introduced. These might include turn taking turn in the family; confidence building through praise; or, managing behavior. Also, families are encouraged to talk openly with the child about stuttering, avoiding any taboo or "conspiracy of silence" about stuttering and focusing on the importance of confident communication, whether the child is stuttering or not. Parents are encouraged to consider their use of language around stuttering and the message that negatively loaded words and phrases, such as "having a bad day," can have.

After these discussions in the clinic meetings, each parent practices Interaction Strategies at home, playing with the child in special times lasting 5 minutes, between three and five times a week. The parents are also encouraged to generalize their Family Strategies into the home environment and include siblings where possible.

After the last of the 6 weekly clinic meetings, the clinician and the parents make plans for the next 6 weeks—a period called "consolidation"—during which the parents work independently of the clinician at home, continuing their special times and sending a log of these to the therapist each week. The clinician responds via e-mail or phone. At the end of this 6-week consolidation period, the family meets with the clinician for a review of progress. If the child and parent are pleased with progress and noticing signs that the impact of stuttering is reducing and the child is communicating more easily, the parents are asked to continue with the changes they are making, and another review is scheduled 6 weeks later. If the child is struggling to speak, becoming more concerned about the stuttering, showing signs of avoidance behaviors, and/or developing unhelpful strategies to reduce the stuttering, then more direct treatment is introduced. This may include activities to increase knowledge about stuttering, encourage openness, and desensitize to the stuttering, alongside more direct speech strategies such as increased pausing or speaking more slowly. If at all possible, the child's communication and stuttering are monitored for a minimum of 1 year.

Supporting Data

Data have been published for 13 children, showing short-term (5 weeks) (Matthews et al., 1997), medium-term (6 months) (Millard et al., 2009), and long-term (12 months) (Millard et al., 2008) efficacy. Using experimental single-subject methodologies, the clinician-researchers at the Michael Palin Center have demonstrated that the indirect components of this approach (Interaction and Family Strategies) can be effective in reducing the frequency of stuttering in children (Matthews et al., 1997; Millard et al., 2008, 2009). In addition, there is evidence that the approach can reduce the impact of stuttering for both the children and the parents and increase parents' ratings of knowledge and confidence in managing the stuttering (Millard et al., 2009). By including only children who had been stuttering for more than 12 months, collecting data over a baseline phase prior to therapy, and using statistical analysis that compared change against variability in the baseline phase, the researchers concluded that improvements were attributable to the therapy.

In an important larger study involving 55 children who were treated and followed for a year, Millard et al. (2018) showed that the children treated with Palin PCI showed significant reductions in frequency of stuttering and in the impact of stuttering on their lives. The authors also found that the children's perceptions of themselves as communicators improved and their parents were relieved of much of their worry about their child's stuttering and became more confident in how to support their child.

RESTART

The acronym RESTART comes from a study comparing this approach with the LP: "Rotterdam Evaluation Study of Stuttering Therapy—Randomized Trial." The RESTART program was developed in the Netherlands and is based on the Demands and Capacities (D&C) Model (Gottwald, 2010; Starkweather et al., 1990). In Chapter 6 on Theories of this textbook, I described the Demands and Capacities Model and explained relevant treatment procedures that derive from this theory. A good example of Demands and Capacities treatment is given in Chapter 14 in the section describing Sheryl Gottwald's approach to working with older preschool children. The RESTART program uses this approach but adds a highly structured effort to assess the demands placed on the child, especially in parent-child interactions, and to analyze the child's capacities.

In essence, RESTART therapy involves training parents to decrease demands on the child, including those in linguistic, cognitive, emotional, and motor domains. Parents set aside 15 minutes a day, 5 days a week as a "special time" for the child, focusing on what the child wants to talk about or do. During this time, a parent focuses on reducing the demands—especially those related to communication—and providing support. The manual for the RESTART treatment approach using the Demands and Capacities Model is available online at http://www.nedverstottertherapie.nl/wp-content/uploads/2016/07/RESTART-DCM.Method.-English.pdf/.

Treatment planning for RESTART begins with a thorough assessment of the child and parents. This assessment focuses not only on an analysis of the child's stuttering but also their cognitive, linguistic, and emotional strengths and weaknesses. In addition, the clinician makes a detailed assessment of accuracy, flow, and rate of speech motor movements to determine if there are deficits therein. Parent-child interactions are analyzed from video recordings made before an initial parent conference.

The parent conference begins with an exploration of the parents' feeling about their child's stuttering, especially their concerns that they might have caused the stuttering. Then parents are introduced to the Capacities and Demands model so that the parents and clinician can work as a team to develop a treatment plan.

In phase I of treatment, parents are guided in reducing demands on the child, such as by reducing speech rate, increasing pause time, and asking fewer questions. These changes first take place in the clinic, with clinician guidance, and then at home, during daily "special times" in which one parent plays with the child. Parents keep notes on their interactions at home and discuss their findings and questions in the once-weekly clinic meetings. This pattern may go on for many weeks and the child's stuttering is assessed by both the clinician and the parent to determine if the reduction of demands is reducing stuttering. If so, treatment is gradually faded and contact with the clinic is gradually lessened, until no longer needed.

Phase II of treatment—used only if the child's stuttering is not substantially reduced in phase I—focuses on increasing the child's capacities. Speech motor training ("speech gym") is undertaken, first in the clinic and then at home. If needed, the child's language and emotional resilience are treated. This continues until the child's fluency is typical or nearly so. If stuttering remains, phase III is undertaken, which involves direct treatment of stuttering, such as learning to stutter in an easier way. The child is also taught to be comfortable and unselfconscious about any remaining stuttering.

Supporting Data

In 2015, several investigators associated with the RESTART program published a study that demonstrated the effectiveness of RESTART (de Sonnerville-Koedoot et al., 2015) compared to the LP (see Chapter 14 for a description of LP). Results indicated that of the 199 children who participated (99 randomly assigned to LP, 100 to RESTART), approximately equal percentages had recovered completely when they were assessed 18 months after the beginning of treatment. Specifically, 70% of the children treated with RESTART and 76% of the children treated with LP were found to have less than 1.5% syllables stuttered at this follow-up measurement time. Although it may appear that the Lidcombe was slightly better than the RESTART program, given the variability of stuttering seen in each group, the 6% difference could have occurred by chance. Other measures of their recovery were also positive for both treatments at the final assessment. This study strongly suggests that both direct (LP) and indirect (RESTART) treatments are effective. Unfortunately, the effectiveness of these approaches could not be compared with natural recovery because ethical considerations prevented the use of an untreated control group. An economic analysis of both RESTART and LP indicated that LP was slightly more economical to treat children, but the costs were not greatly different.

Stuttering Foundation

The Stuttering Foundation (SF) provides a wonderful array of resources for stutterers of all ages and their families. The Foundation's publications and videos are especially helpful for families of young preschool children (borderline stuttering), but they also have many resources that are aimed at all levels of stuttering. To access resources for families of young preschool children who are stuttering, click on this link https://www.stutteringhelp.org and then at the bottom of the SF homepage you will see another link to click: "For Parents of Pre-Schoolers." Among the useful material that parents and clinicians can find on this link are "7 Tips for Talking with Your Child" (a 16-minute video), "Stuttering and Your Child: Help for Parents" (a 30-minute video), and "If You Think Your Child is Stuttering" (a brochure that is available as a down-loadable pdf).

Another important resource is Conture's *Stuttering and Your Child: Questions and Answers*, 5th edition (2015) published by SF, provides families, teachers, and others with information about stuttering and how children who stutter can be helped. It covers a wide range of issues, including stuttering versus normal disfluency, the possible causes of stuttering, changing the home environment, dealing with others' responses to the child's stuttering, and treatment. Although formal aspects of treatment are left to professionals, specific advice is given in highlighted pages about how parents, babysitters, day care centers, and teachers can help children who stutter. Parents are instructed how to be good listeners, how to increase the times when the child feels they are being heard, and how to reduce both conversational and lifestyle pressures on the child. Babysitters and day care centers are advised to react as normally as possible to the child and to treat the child like other children, while ensuring that the child has plenty of time to say what they want to say without feeling rushed. Teachers are encouraged to give the child support for oral recitations, allow the child the same speaking opportunities as other children, and help the entire class develop good speaking and listening practices.

One of the SF's most popular publications on the treatment of stuttering in young children is the video, mentioned previously, *Stuttering and Your Child: Help for Parents* (Guitar et al., 2010). It is available free as streaming video on the SF website, on YouTube, and as a DVD that can be purchased inexpensively. This 30-minute video, in both English and Spanish, was designed to be used by families working alone, as a preliminary tool, as well as by those who are in treatment with a clinician. The video teaches families to make changes in the child's environment, primarily in two areas: communicative interaction and family lifestyle. It also describes when to get help from a speech-language pathologist and what to expect in an evaluation and from treatment. The SF website quotes an American Speech-Language-Hearing Association book review that refers to this video as "perhaps the best buy in the nation for information on children and stuttering."

All of the SF's publications emphasize that families are not the cause of stuttering but that families can create an environment that facilitates the growth of fluency. The following suggestions for changes in families' conversational interactions are described in detail in both publications, and parents demonstrate them in the video:

- Talk more slowly.
- Use plenty of pauses in your speech after the child finishes talking.
- Ask the child fewer questions.
- Spend time physically close to the child, such as having them in your lap when you read to them.
- Allow silent time in conversations so that the child doesn't feel compelled to talk and isn't interrupted.
- Help the child learn to take turns talking.

The following suggestions are for families wishing to change some aspects of their lifestyle to facilitate their child's fluency:

- Try to find an opportunity each day, preferably in the morning, when special attention can be given to the child so that they are getting one-on-one time with a parent or another caregiver. During this time, the focus should be on listening to the child and letting them direct the play. The best interactions at these times are those when the parent is talking little and is primarily there for the child as they talk and play.

- Slow the pace of life, when possible. Give the family more time to do fewer things.
- Develop regular, consistent times for meals, naps, and bedtimes.
- Use reasonable and consistent discipline.
- Make sure the child gets plenty of rest.
- Provide plenty of time for the child to transition from one thing to another. For example, getting ready to go to a birthday party after playing quietly at home may require an extra 10 or 20 minutes because the two activities are so different. Parents might, for example, talk to the child about what the birthday party will be like, so the busy-ness of the party won't be so unexpected.

In addition to these ideas for changing a child's environment, the SF's publications suggest that parents should try to become aware of what events or situations are associated with the ups and downs of their child's fluency. Some children who stutter are more sensitive to common, everyday life stresses; things that may not bother most children may cause a child who stutters to become more disfluent. Some examples might be visits by strangers, holidays, a parent leaving for or coming home from work, or an argument between parents. If it can be predicted when more stressful events might occur, extra support can be provided to the child during such situations.

A family working with their child on their own is advised that if their child's stuttering does not show a gradual decrease after these changes have been in place for over a month, they should seek help from a speech-language clinician who specializes in treating childhood stuttering.

In addition to an extensive online bookstore with many low-cost publications and video material, the SF website also has a page with guidelines from ASHA for seeking insurance coverage for stuttering evaluation and treatment (www.stutteringhelp.org/insurance.htm).

SUMMARY

- Borderline stuttering in young preschoolers is characterized by an excess of typical disfluencies, particularly part-word repetitions and single-syllable whole-word repetitions. Although the child may have a high frequency of disfluencies and may repeat sounds many times, they are typically not frustrated or embarrassed by the disfluencies. If these emotional reactions do occur, they are usually transitory. Onset of stuttering is relatively recent (less than a year) in borderline stuttering.
- The occurrence of borderline stuttering in young preschoolers is thought to be the result of an interaction between a child's neurodevelopmental predisposition and typical developmental and environmental stresses. The family is not to blame for the stuttering but can be vital in creating a facilitating environment that increases fluency.
- Treatment is usually focused on helping families make changes in their conversational interactions and in family routines.
- Changes in the family's interaction patterns include helping family members: (1) make positive comments when the child has been speaking, to enhance the child's positive feelings about talking; (2) slow their speech rates; (3) pause for 2 or 3 seconds after the child finishes talking before they begin to speak and adding pauses in their own speech; (4) listen attentively to what the child is saying; (5) ensure appropriate turn taking by all members of the family, including the child; (6) ask fewer questions that require long answers; and (7) use vocabulary and sentence complexity that are close to the child's level when speaking to them.
- Changes in the family routine should include the following: arrange a time, preferably in the morning, when one parent or caregiver can have 10 to 15 minutes of uninterrupted time with the child. During this time, the parent should be primarily there for the child, listening and paying attention to what the child is saying and doing, and appropriately reflecting the child's feelings. This can be a time in which a parent or caregiver practices the interaction patterns suggested earlier.
- The family should be encouraged to carry out the following changes in their lifestyle: (1) create structures and predictable routines to increase the child's sense of security; (2) slow the pace of family life, so that there are calm transitions from one activity to another; (3) ensure that the child's life is not too busy or rushed; and (4) use consistent, reasonable discipline with the child to ensure that the child feels their family is in control.
- If a child's stuttering does not begin to decline within a month or 6 weeks after these changes have begun, slightly more direct treatment should be undertaken. In this approach, for mild borderline stuttering in young preschoolers, parents are taught to use occasional praise for fluency during one-on-one sessions with the child.
- Other clinicians' indirect approaches to stuttering in this age group include parent counseling coupled with changes in parent-child interaction patterns, enhancing the child's capacities in speech-motor control, language, and emotions. Also, families are encouraged to work on making the home environment and family life style more relaxed.
- One other more direct approach teaches children to use slow and smooth speech and to take turns in conversation. Another approach assesses the linguistic level at which a child is fluent and then moves the child through a hierarchy of longer and more complex responses while keeping them fluent for longer periods of time.

STUDY QUESTIONS

1. What are some aspects of family conversational interactions that may put pressure on the young preschool child vulnerable to stuttering?
2. What changes can a family make in their home to relieve speech and language pressures?
3. Discuss how the clinician can facilitate changes in family routines that may help the child's fluency.
4. What are some of the barriers to change that are found in some families? How can the clinician help the family overcome these barriers?
5. Compare one of the other clinician's more indirect therapies with one of the more direct therapies.

SUGGESTED PROJECTS

1. Conduct an informal ABAB study (called a "reversal design") of the effect of slowing your speech rate on a conversational partner who is not aware of the purpose of your study. You will need to record your conversation so that you can analyze the data afterward.[1] In the first A condition, conduct several minutes of conversation at a normal rate; in the first B condition, conduct the same amount of conversation at a slower rate. Then repeat the two rates in two subsequent A and B conditions. Was your speaking partner affected by your speaking rate?
2. Pretend that you are the parent of a child who is beginning to stutter. Search the library and the internet for advice about how to help your child, and determine whether there is consistency in the advice or whether conflicting information is given.
3. Examine the materials presented in this chapter that describe the therapies of other clinicians and determine whether the approaches are designed just for stuttering in young preschoolers or whether the authors intend them for older children as well.

SUGGESTED VIEWING

7 Tips for Talking With the Child Who Stutters (Stuttering Foundation; www.stutteringhelp.org).

This free 16-minute video provides excellent suggestions for both clinicians and parents, appropriate for helping preschool children who stutter when an indirect approach is used or is combined with a direct approach.

Stuttering and Your Child: Help for Parents (Stuttering Foundation; www.stutteringhelp.org).

This 30-minute video, available free from the Foundation, will help parents whose child is beginning to stutter. It is appropriate both for parents who are working without the help of a clinician and for parents who are beginning therapy with a stuttering expert. It describes how parents can help their child by making changes in their interactions with their child and in their lifestyle at home.

Chmela, K. (2004). *Working with preschoolers who stutter: Successful intervention strategies.* (Video) Stuttering Foundation.

This is a video of a convention presentation designed to teach clinicians how to work with preschool children who stutter, using modeling of easy, relaxed speech when talking to children and counseling parents to develop a fluency-friendly environment. It is available for continuing education for a reasonable price.

SUGGESTED READINGS

Gottwald, S. (2010). Stuttering prevention and early intervention: A multidimensional approach. In B. Guitar, & R. McCauley (Eds.), *Treatment of stuttering: Established and emerging interventions.* Lippincott Williams & Wilkins.

This is a very useful detailed description illustrated by video clips of the direct and indirect treatment for preschoolers who stutter developed by Gottwald and Starkweather over the past 25 years.

Guitar, B., & Conture, E. (2015). *The child who stutters: To the pediatrician* (5th ed.). Stuttering Foundation.

This free booklet provides information about the nature of stuttering and signs to look for in deciding which children should be referred for treatment. Handouts with suggestions for parents are also provided.

Guitar, B., Kopff-Schaefer, H. K., Donahue-Kilburg, G., & Bond, L. (1992). Parent verbal interaction and speech rate. *Journal of Speech and Hearing Research, 35,* 742–754.

This article describes therapy with parents of a young child who stutters and the analysis of parent-child interactions. The analysis of parent variables affecting the child's stuttering demonstrates that her stuttering can be categorized as either easy repetitions (tension-free) or blocks (tense). These two different types of stutters are affected by different parent behaviors (speaking rate or nonaccepting comments).

Kelman, E. & Whyte, A. (2012). *Understanding stammering or stuttering: A guide for parents, teachers and other professionals.* Jessica Kingsley Publishers.

This book's title comes from the fact that both "stammering" and "stuttering" are used in the United Kingdom for what is called "stuttering" in the United States. It provides an explanation of the nature of stuttering as well as guidelines to help the child and to find professional treatment.

Richels, C., & Conture, E. (2010). Indirect treatment of childhood stuttering: Diagnostic predictors of treatment outcome. In B. Guitar, & R. McCauley (Eds.), *Treatment of stuttering: Established and emerging interventions* (pp. 18–55). Lippincott Williams & Wilkins.

[1]You should ask your conversational partner's permission to record them, but without explaining the purpose of your "experiment." Perhaps you could tell them—before you start—that you are studying your own speech characteristics. Then, after you have analyzed the data, you could share it with them, explaining your true purpose.

A very thoughtful description of the use of diagnostic data to predict short- and long-term outcomes. Interestingly, successful short-term outcomes appear to be related to less severe stuttering at the beginning of treatment, but successful long-term outcomes are more related to diagnostic indicators of expressive (rather than inhibited) temperament and to lower language scores at the beginning of treatment.

Starkweather, C. W., Gottwald, S. R., & Halfond, M. H. (1990). *Stuttering prevention: A clinical method.* Prentice-Hall.

This book details a program of assessment and treatment for children who stutter and for their parents. It is the basis for treatments based on the Demands and Capacities model.

14

Treatment of Older Preschool Children: Beginning Stuttering

Chapter Outline

Chapter Objectives

After studying this chapter, readers should be able to:

- Describe the characteristics of a child who has beginning stuttering
- Describe the author's beliefs about stuttering, targets in treatment, goals for treatment, how much to involve feelings and attitudes in treatment, and maintenance procedures
- Delineate the procedures involved in the Lidcombe Program, the stages of therapy, and the criteria to complete each stage
- Describe the procedures for Stuttering Modification Treatment
- Explain how formal training may be obtained for using the Lidcombe Program
- Outline the components of Sheryl Gottwald's "multidimensional approach"
- Describe a number of different approaches to working on stuttering co-occurring concomitant speech or language problems

Key Terms

Concomitant speech and language problems: Difficulties with articulation/phonology and/or difficulties with language that sometimes accompany stuttering. When this occurs in some children who stutter, it poses the problem of which disorder to work on first. Several approaches have been used by experienced clinician-researchers

Demands and capacities: The perspective that the factors associated with the onset and persistence of stuttering are the demands placed on the child by her environments, balanced (or not) by the child's innate capacity for fluent speech

Lidcombe Program (LP): An operant conditioning-based approach to stuttering treatment, delivered in the home by a parent or other caregiver and guided via weekly meetings with the clinician

Older preschool children: Children between 3.5 and 6 years of age

Operant conditioning: A type of behavior modification that uses rewards and punishments to increase or decrease the frequency of a behavior

Severity Rating (SR) Scale: A scale from 0 to 10 used daily by parents to assess a child's stuttering. May be used by clinician as well during weekly clinic sessions

Stage 1 of the Lidcombe Program (LP): The initial step of LP in which the child becomes normally fluent. Criteria for completing Stage 1 are 3 consecutive weeks in which (1) the parent's weekly SRs are 0 to 1 during the week before the clinic visit and 4 of the 7 SRs are 0 and (2) the clinician's SR for the entire session is 0 to 1

Stage 2 of the Lidcombe Program: When the child meets the fluency criteria to complete Stage 1, this maintenance stage is begun. Weekly clinic meetings are faded systematically so that the parent and child meet with the clinician in this sequence: 2, 2, 4, 4, 8, 8, and finally 16 weeks apart. The child must continue to meet fluency criteria

Stuttering modification: A treatment approach that helps the client to decrease negative attitudes and feelings about their stuttering and guides them to stutter more easily. It may result in the elimination of stuttering as a problem or, at least, a reduction in the effort needed to talk

Unambiguous stutter: A moment of stuttering that is so clear that the parent or the clinician has no doubt that it should be categorized as a stutter

Verbal contingencies: Comments to the child made immediately after an event (eg, fluent utterance; stutter) that are intended to change the frequency of that event

AN INTEGRATED APPROACH

Children with beginning stuttering are usually between 3.5 and 6 years of age. To distinguish them from children with milder, borderline stuttering, I refer to them as **older preschool children**. They have probably been stuttering for at least several months, and their parents may well be concerned that it is not a transient problem that will disappear on its own. What follows are some details on the core and secondary behaviors of their stuttering, as well as feelings and attitudes that often characterize stuttering in this age group.

These children's most common core stuttering behaviors are part-word repetitions that are produced rapidly, usually with irregular rhythm. Prolongations may also be present. Both the repetitions and prolongations may contain excessive tension, which can be heard as abrupt endings to the repetitions and/or as increases in vocal pitch in repetitions and prolongations. Blocks may also be present, with evidence of tension and struggle. Secondary behaviors are typically escape devices, such as eyeblinks, head nods, and increases in pitch as the child tenses their vocal cords trying to get the word out. A few avoidance maneuvers may be observed, such as starting sentences with extra sounds like "uh" or changing words when a stutter is anticipated. In many cases, when the frequency of stuttering becomes high, these children may put their hands to their mouths to push words out or may momentarily avoid talking. Children with beginning stuttering usually feel frustrated and sometimes panicked with their difficulty in talking but have not yet developed a strong anticipation of stuttering or learned to be ashamed of their speech.

I will illustrate our approach with a description of Katherine's treatment. She is the 3-year-old child I introduced in Chapter 1. The course of her treatment is depicted in Figure 14.1.

Case Example

Katherine

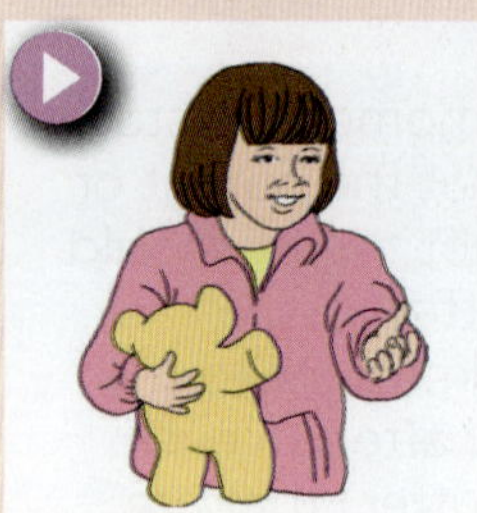

Katherine's therapy began when she was 3 years old and stuttering severely—on 21% of her spoken syllables. As you may remember from our description of her stuttering in Chapter 1, Katherine's pattern was characterized by repetitions, prolongations, and blocks, with a predominance of blocks with much struggle behavior. She had changed from bubbly and talkative to withdrawn and reluctant to engage in conversation.

At the time she came in for an evaluation, two other clinicians and I had recently been trained in the Lidcombe approach—a treatment described in this chapter. Several weeks after the evaluation, we began Katherine's therapy by training her mother in using **verbal contingencies** (praise) for Katherine's fluent speech during daily, 15-minute practice sessions at home. We also trained Katherine's mother in making daily ratings of the severity of Katherine's stuttering. During our weekly clinic meetings with Katherine and her mother, we measured the frequency of Katherine's stuttering in conversation at the beginning of each session. The rest of each session was spent on problem solving any issues that came up during practice sessions and training Katherine's mother in the next steps of treatment. These next steps included using verbal contingencies for stuttering and then using verbal contingencies for stuttering and for fluency during natural conversations throughout the day.

After several weeks went by, we saw notable improvement in Katherine's stuttering, shown by both our weekly measures of her stuttering frequency in the clinic and her mother's daily ratings of the severity (SRs) of Katherine's stuttering at home. The steady decline in Katherine's stuttering continued, interrupted by an occasional spike upward when a stressful event occurred, such as a visit by relatives or a family trip. At one point, Katherine's stuttering shot up for several days, and we worked with Katherine's mother to figure out the source of the problem. We discovered that Katherine's father, in his eagerness to help, began to use verbal contingencies without training when he was alone with Katherine and overdosed her with several hours of contingencies each day. Once that was resolved and Katherine's father was trained to use contingencies judiciously, her stuttering continued to decline steadily. Katherine became fluent after about 6 months of treatment. Over the following year, the clinicians continued to stay in touch, but Katherine and her mother came in to the clinic less and less frequently.

Seven years after therapy had been completed, we contacted Katherine and her parents to assess her status. She had been completely fluent ever since treatment ended and was highly verbal with only dim memories of ever having stuttered. Her parents have become a valuable resource for other parents of children who are beginning to stutter as they contemplate treatment.

Author's Beliefs

Nature of Stuttering

As I've described in chapters in the "Nature of Stuttering" part of this book, I believe that beginning stuttering arises when children's neurodevelopmental sensorimotor difficulties related to speech production interact with their temperament and other developmental and environmental influences to produce or exacerbate repetitions, prolongations, and blocks. This is essentially the position taken by C. S. Bluemel in his book *The Riddle of Stuttering* (1957). It was further articulated by Johnson and colleagues (1959), who suggested that the problem of stuttering arises as a result of interactions among (1) the amount of the child's disfluency, (2) the reaction of his listeners to the disfluency, and (3) the child's sensitivity to his own disfluency and to listeners' reactions. I would add to Johnson's list of interacting factors any pressures that a child may feel internally (eg, to speak quickly and in long, relatively complex sentences) and any anxieties the child may experience as the result of moving, the birth of a sibling, or other life events.

In some children, beginning stuttering emerges gradually after they have gone through a period of borderline stuttering as younger preschool children. As these children get older and if stuttering continues, they begin to respond to negative experiences of repetitive disfluencies with increased tension. However, in some children, beginning stuttering appears suddenly, close to the onset of stuttering. They may be easily frustrated or highly distressed when many of their speech attempts result in repetitions or prolongations that feel out of their control. As these children respond, at first nonconsciously, to these core behaviors, they increase tension and develop a variety of escape behaviors that are reinforced. Their eyeblinks, head nods, and pitch increases are rewarded because they often result in the release of stutters. Gradually, classical conditioning influences when and where the child's stuttering occurs. Specifically, negative emotional experiences that are associated

Mother and child in clinic session

Mother and child in practice session at home

Mother and child in natural conversation at home

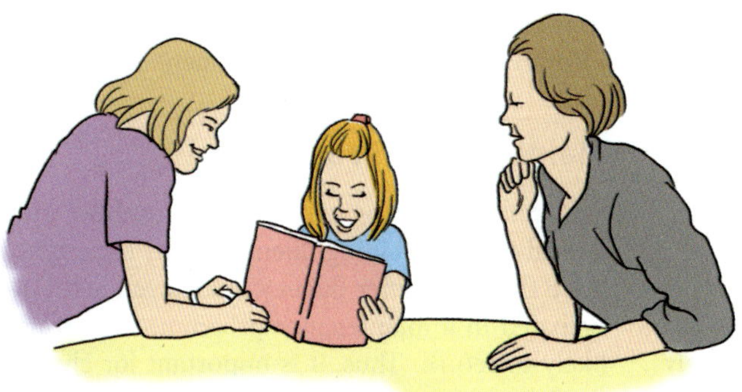

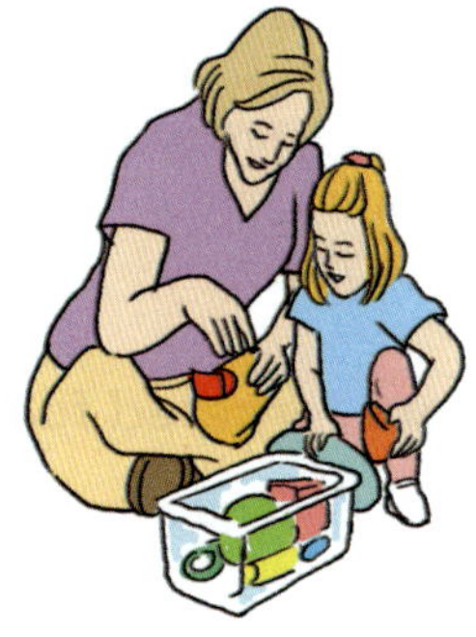

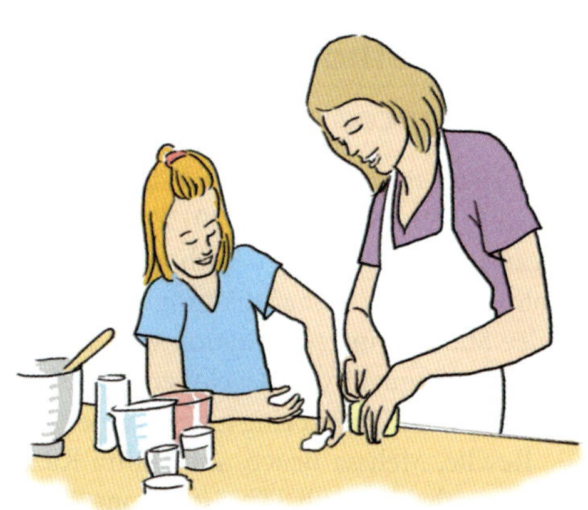

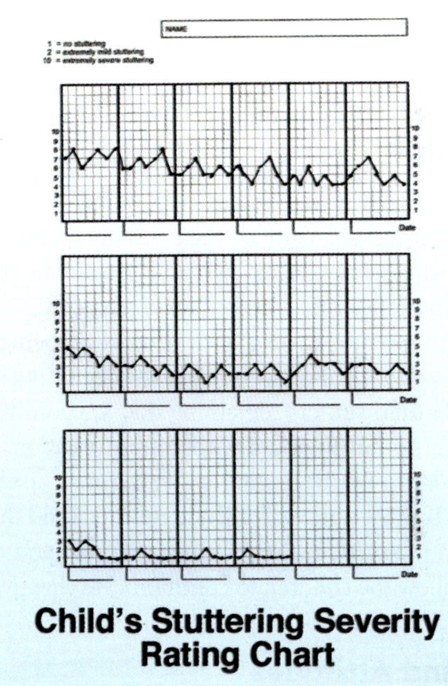

Figure 14.1 An overview of Katherine's treatment with Katherine's mother conducting most of the treatment at home.

with stuttering become etched into memory and associated with various contexts, such as the telephone, impatient listeners, or particular sounds and words. As stuttering spreads and becomes more pervasive and more consistently present, these children become aware of their stuttering, although at first, they may have little shame about it and do not dread speaking situations. Because of the plasticity of the brain at this age, some children with beginning stuttering develop better sensorimotor control of speech production, and their stuttering goes out the door it came in. Their stutters diminish in frequency and severity and disappear or become a minor nuisance. Other children, perhaps those with more widespread sensorimotor deficits, a more sensitive temperament, or larger doses of other developmental and environmental stresses, continue to stutter and often develop more advanced symptoms.

Like Bloodstein (1975), I believe that if we can provide a child who has beginning stuttering a sufficient number of positive, fluent speaking experiences during treatment, fluency will replace stuttering. Bloodstein, whose 50-year career was focused on the nature and management of childhood stuttering, strongly advised treatment that would ensure that "the child experiences daily successful, pleasant, and rewarding speech with a minimum of stuttering" and that these daily experiences be created by the parent at home (Bloodstein, 1975, pp. 61–62).

Echoing Bloodstein, I believe that this may happen best when treatment is administered by the parent at home, where it can be done many days a week. It also appears effective if natural fluency is elicited at first in highly structured situations, systematically reinforced, and then carefully transferred to more and more real-life situations in which stuttering has been occurring.

Speech Behaviors Targeted for Therapy

Usually, intervention for beginning stuttering focuses on fluency, with the expectation that children at this stage are likely to respond well to techniques with that focus. Sometimes, however, when the child is beginning to experience fewer repetitions and an increasing number of very effortful stutters, the focus may expand to include not just fluency but also methods of modifying disfluencies so that they are less effortful. Despite these goals as major targets for therapy, however, creating a context that is playful and therefore fun is also seen as crucial.

Fluency Goals

Almost all children who are treated with effective therapy for beginning stuttering will gain or regain spontaneous, typical fluency. In most cases, a year or two after treatment ends, the children will have little or no recollection of having stuttered and will not have to monitor their speech or work at being fluent. Some who are stuttering more severely at the beginning of treatment may have mild stutters remaining that are hardly noticeable and which do not interfere with communication. In rare instances, children with beginning stuttering may continue to stutter in ways that are noticeable. These children (and their parents) can learn to accept the remaining stuttering and develop attitudes that allow the children to communicate effectively.

Feelings and Attitudes

As noted earlier, a child with beginning stuttering has occasional frustration and intermittent concern about talking. They have only mildly conditioned fears or avoidances of stuttering. Thus, it is typically unnecessary to focus directly on feelings and attitudes in therapy—in most cases—for a child with beginning stuttering. I do, however, work on feelings if the child seems frustrated or ashamed of their stuttering, as you'll see in the later sections of this chapter where I talk about specific techniques.

The feelings and attitudes of these children are, however, influenced by the family. The clinician teaches the family member providing the at-home treatment to be matter-of-fact about the child's "smooth" and "bumpy" speech. The clinician and family member openly discuss the child's stuttering during their weekly meetings when the child is also present. These aspects of treatment are intended to reduce any embarrassment or shame that was associated with stuttering and foster the child's acceptance of stuttering as just a little slip-up, like bumping into a table or tipping over their tricycle. This is a far cry from the "conspiracy of silence" that formerly characterized the treatment of children who stutter.

Maintenance Procedures

Systematically fading contact with the child and their family is vital for maintaining fluency. In my experience, if families leave treatment after fluency is achieved without having participated in a maintenance program, stuttering seems more likely to return. Thus, it is important for clinicians to stress the importance of maintenance procedures at the outset of treatment. Moreover, the clinician and family should continue with careful data collection as contact is faded, so that the family can return to regular weekly meetings and discuss appropriate contingencies for fluency and stuttering if any relapse occurs.

Clinical Methods

Clinical Procedures: Lidcombe Program

For the past many years, I have been using the **Lidcombe Program (LP)** (Guitar et al., 2015; Onslow et al., 1990, 2003) to treat preschool children with beginning stuttering. I was initially trained in using this program in a workshop led by Rosalee Shenker in collaboration with the Montreal Fluency Centre. Subsequently, I developed more expertise through consultation and mentoring from Rosalee and my colleagues, Julie Reville, Melissa Bruce, and Danra Kazenski. Follow-up training with Elisabeth Harrison—one of the developers of LP—further sharpened my skills. For readers interested in using this approach, I urge you to obtain formal training at one of the many workshops offered around the world by the Lidcombe Program Consortium. More information on LP is available at http://www.lidcombeprogram.org. On this website, the link to "Lidcombe Program Trainers Consortium" provides a brief video "lptc-an introduction" in which the program is described in a way that both families and clinicians can get a clear overview of the program and its flexibility to adjust to different families and different children. On the website, there are also links to pages that provide information in the following categories: Families and Caregivers, Speech-Language Pathologists, and Teachers and Health Professionals. The information for Speech-Language Pathologists includes copies of materials needed for using the Lidcombe Program, including the treatment guide that can be found by clicking on the Research and Publications link. More information about stuttering treatment can be found by connecting with the Australian Stuttering Research Centre (ASRC), available through Google and other search engines. Moreover, an excellent chapter in Guitar and McCauley (2010), written by Harrison and Onslow, gives a detailed description of LP. Fourteen short video clips on *Lippincott Connect* (Chapter 14 videos) show Harrison (a master LP clinician) treating a preschool child using LP. Although LP is ever-evolving as its developers continue to identify improvements through their research, the essentials of the interventions have not changed significantly, making these resources of continuing value.

Overview

The Lidcombe Program uses **operant conditioning** procedures (ie, verbal response contingencies), which are administered by a parent in the home during brief one-on-one practice sessions and natural conversations each day and are guided by weekly meetings with the clinician. Treatment begins in structured conversations—practice sessions designed to elicit a maximum of fluent speech by the child so that the child receives mostly positive reinforcement. At the beginning of treatment, it is important to provide frequent praise, sufficient to let the child know that they are fluent (eg, "That was really smooth talking!"), *acknowledgment of fluency* (eg, a very low-key "That was smooth"), or *request for self-evaluation* (eg, "Was that smooth?"), which is used only after a fluent utterance. After the child becomes used to praise for fluency, the parent begins to comment infrequently on the child's stuttering. When the child stutters, the parent provides a gentle *acknowledgment of the stutter* ("That was a little bumpy") or *a gentle request for self-correction* (eg, "Say 'truck' again."). Although in an operant framework, these latter comments are seen as mild punishments, I think that many parents and children will experience them as pretty innocuous. Table 14.1 lists verbal contingencies for fluency and stuttering.

The ratio of verbal contingencies for fluency to verbal contingencies for stuttering is kept very high to make the program a positive experience for the child. In other words, the parent responds to the child's stuttering only after the parent has given an appropriate number of praises for fluency. The ratio is determined by the parent and clinician as they observe how the child responds to both kinds of contingencies. As the child's stuttering decreases during practice sessions, contingencies are also given during the natural conversations each day. The parent continues to provide verbal contingencies for fluency and stuttering, but in more casual way, in natural situations of daily life, such as when the parent is talking with the child in the car, in the kitchen, or at a store. Once the child meets the established criteria for fluent speech

TABLE 14.1 Verbal Contingencies for Fluent Speech and Unambiguous Stuttering

	Examples of Verbal Contingencies
Fluent speech	■ Comments should be specific to speech (ie, "nice" or "very good" is too general, but "that was nice, smooth talking" is right on). ■ Always give at least as many praises for fluency before a contingency for stuttering. ■ Adjust the types of praise to those that the child seems to enjoy. Here are some examples: ● "That was smooth." ● "Great, your words are smooth!" ● "Nice smooth talking!" ● "No bumps there, excellent." ● "I didn't hear any bumps." ● "Wow, that whole story was totally smooth." ● "Was that smooth?" (The answer should always be "yes" and followed up with another instance of praise.) ■ Also praise for spontaneous self-evaluation (ie, if the child says "I was really smooth today" or remarks on his own smooth or bumpy talking).
Unambiguous stuttering	■ Use low-key friendly delivery and move quickly to a praise. ■ Use one request for correction after several praises. ■ Some children become so smooth during a session they do not need any contingencies for stuttering. This is okay because the goal is practicing stutter-free speech. ■ In early responses to stutters, some Lidcombe clinicians merely comment acceptingly on stutters rather than asking the child to re-do them: ● "Oops, I heard a little bump." ● "That was a little bumpy." ● "There was a bump." ● "You got a little stuck there." ● "You only need to say ______ once." ● "Say ______ again." (Use if child is comfortable with repeating stuttered word.) ● Remember only to praise smooth speech; it's important not to praise bumps! However, praising the child's willingness to continue talking after a bumpy patch supports communication and therefore warrants consideration.

in all situations, the treatment is gradually faded in a systematic fashion during Stage 2, which is the maintenance stage of treatment. Throughout the program, the clinician and parent regularly assess the child's stuttering using the severity rating chart and use those measures to make treatment decisions and problem solve any barriers to progress.

Stage 1: The First Clinic Visit

Stage 1 of the Lidcombe Program begins with the first clinic visit when the clinician meets with the parent (or other caregiver) and child to accomplish three goals: (1) to explain severity ratings (SRs) to the parent, (2) to assess the child's stuttering and overall ease of speaking, and (3) to teach the parent to conduct daily practice sessions. Stage 1 clinic visits are typically 1 hour in duration.

Assessment of Stuttering Using the SR

Assessment of the child's stuttering is carried out primarily by using the **Severity Rating (SR) Scale** (see Chapter 9; Figure 9.4). This is a 0 to 10 scale that the clinician and parent use in each clinic meeting. In addition, the parent records SRs at the end of every day, reflecting their judgment of the child's stuttering severity that day. The daily SRs are crucial data used to assess the child's progress and make decisions about verbal contingencies. On the SR Scale, a 0 represents no stuttering, a 1 represents extremely mild stuttering that a casual observer would not notice, and a 10 represents extremely severe stuttering.[1]

In the first clinic meeting, after discussing the scale in detail with the parent, the parent and I play and talk with the child to obtain an adequate, representative sample of the child's stuttering. I then ask the parent to tell me what SR they would give the child's speech in that sample, which I compare with my own judgment of the child's SR. It is usually possible with only a little discussion to ensure that the parent is using the scale appropriately. On the rare occasion that the parent's rating differs from mine by more than 1 point plus or minus, I explain how I came up with my rating and then try to determine if the parent seems to understand my rationale and is likely to be accurate in their future ratings. I often say to a parent if there is any stuttering, the score can't be 0, and if you think about is the stuttering is mild, moderate, or severe, it will help you come up with a score that is in the lower, middle, or top part of the scale. If I have doubts, I use video clips of the child's speech to help teach the parent how to use the scale. I typically ask the parents to make videos of the child's speech at home during the first few weeks of treatment so that I can continue to "calibrate" the parent's ratings. Once I'm sure that the parent understands the scale, I ask them to rate the child's speech at the end of every day and to bring the ratings to our weekly meetings. The standard Lidcombe procedure has the parent bring in a chart that displays each day's SRs of the child. I encourage the parent to add comments to the chart if the child has gone through a period of increased stuttering, sickness, or other event that the parent feels may have an impact on severity or the child's response to treatment. If it would be helpful to the parent, there is an online scale available from ASRC downloads. This can be filled out online and e-mailed to the clinician.

Assessing the Child's Percentage of Syllables Stuttered (%SS)

The use of %SS to assess the child's stuttering is optional because it simply assesses the frequency of the child's stuttering, rather than characteristics of the severity of the stuttering. When I am conducting LP treatment, I usually assess the child's %SS at the beginning of treatment and at other important points in the program such as when the child moves from Stage 1 to Stage 2. For a formal assessment using %SS, I typically video record the clinic session and later score the child's stuttering from their speech in that sample, which should be at least 300 syllables.

Teaching the Parent to Conduct Daily Practice Sessions

A critical part of the first clinic visit is to show the parent how to conduct the daily practice sessions. It is most important to create situations that not only are fun but also stimulate and encourage a lot of fluent speech in the child. This enables the parent to begin treatment using a great deal of positive verbal contingencies for fluency. To demonstrate for the parent, I begin by using a picture book or picture cards with the child to elicit short, fluent words. To keep the child's interest, I talk with a lot of enthusiasm and move through the pictures quickly. I usually name a picture or two myself as a model for the child and then ask them to name some pictures. After the child is engaged in the task and is producing a good deal of fluent speech (because the task is designed to limit the length of the response and thus producing much fluency), I praise the child's fluency immediately by saying something specifically about their speech, such as "That was really smooth talking!" or "You said that really smoothly!" It is important to make the praise *directly relevant to the child's fluency*, rather than general praise (ie, not "You are doing well!" but "You said those words really smoothly"). After modeling for the parent, I ask them to work with the child, and I coach the parent if necessary.

With children who have more severe stuttering, I may need to begin with single-syllable words or have the child repeat the word after me. Children who have milder stuttering can progress quickly from single words to carrier phrases (such as "I like _____") and to short sentences of three or four words. Figure 14.2 shows a linguistic hierarchy that most children can quickly climb on the way to natural conversations in the beginning of Stage 1. It is important to keep in mind and share with the parent the idea that the point of the

[1]The Lidcombe Program changed the 0 to 9 scale to a 0 to 10 scale in 2023, to make it similar to many scales that are 0 to 10.

Conversation
Two to four sentences
Sentence
Carrier phrase and word
Single words

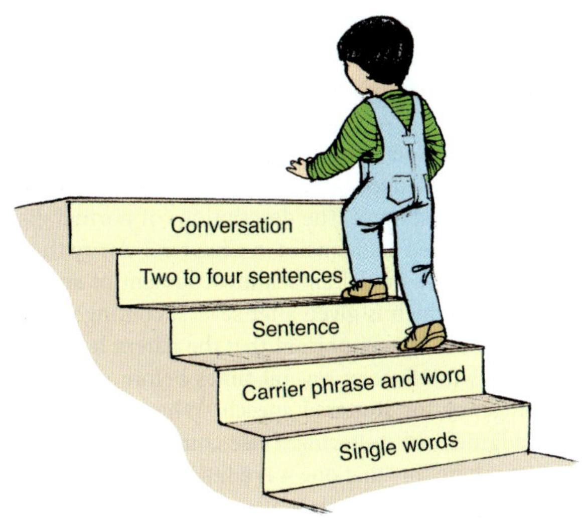

Figure 14.2 Linguistic hierarchy used for practice sessions at the beginning of Stage 1 in the Lidcombe Program.

linguistic hierarchy is only to ensure that the child is producing many fluent utterances and thus receiving frequent praise for fluency. There is no need to adhere to the linguistic hierarchy in obsessive way. As long as the child is producing plentiful fluency, the goal of therapy is being achieved.

One of the mistakes parents often make when they first begin is to use positive verbal contingencies for fluent speech that are too general. They might say, for example, "That's good" or "You're doing well." In this case, I simply restate the need for specific praise and observe the parents doing it.

Another common error is for parents to let the child make longer responses than are appropriate, thereby allowing more stuttered than fluent utterances to occur. Fortunately, a little discussion and lots of modeling will usually clear this up. For those children who need to start at the one- or two-word utterance stage, specifically praising their use of one or two words will help keep them at this level until it is appropriate for them to move to longer utterances.

As I mentioned earlier, it is crucial that the parent make the practice sessions fun for the child. It may be helpful to suggest games and activities for the sessions. Table 14.2 lists some of the activities that parents can use with the child in these practice sessions.

At the end of the first clinic visit, I review the activities and tasks the parent will be doing over the coming week and respond to any questions they have. Some parents benefit from taking notes or being given a written description of things they will be doing; others like to have a follow-up contact from me. In all cases, I encourage them to call or e-mail me if they have any questions or concerns during the week.

Stage 1: Subsequent Clinic Visits

Most subsequent clinic visits have three goals: (1) to assess the child's stuttering, (2) to discuss the current progress, and (3) to introduce new procedures when appropriate. Each session begins with the clinician and parent assessing the child's stuttering using the SRs. This assessment is made from the child's conversational speech when talking with the parent and the clinician with no verbal contingencies given, until a representative sample of the child's speech has been obtained (about 300 syllables or 10 minutes). The clinician determines in their own mind what SR rating to give the child's speech and then asks the parent for their rating of that sample. Once the parent has announced their SR rating, the clinician then shares with the parent what the clinician's rating is. If the parent and clinician ratings differ by more than 1 point, a discussion ensues that helps the parent align their ratings with those of the clinician, or, in some cases, influences the clinician to change their rating. In some instances, the parent may be initially rating the child's articulation or language instead of, or in addition to, their stuttering, so this must be clarified. Accurate parent SRs are essential to the integrity of the treatment program. These ratings, along with the clinician's ratings, determine whether treatment is progressing successfully and signal when to fade practice session conversations and transition to treatment in natural conversations. They

TABLE 14.2 Suggested Games and Activities for Structured Treatment Conversations

Grab bag	The parent puts interesting items into a large cloth bag or pillowcase, and the child guesses what each is by reaching into the bag and feeling the item.
Picture naming	Using picture books or picture cards, the child names each picture. At the one-word level, the child only names the pictured object. As longer utterances are permitted, the child can use a carrier phrase such as "That's a ______," or she can name the item and its color, such as "red rabbit."
Reading a story	Parent and child look at a familiar book while the parent reads or tells the story. To elicit a word or phrase, the parent asks the child to complete a sentence, such as "Then Goldilocks said, 'Somebody's been sleeping in my ______.'"
Rhyme closing	Parent makes up a rhyme and leaves the last word blank, like "Once there was a man—he cooked his eggs in a frying ______."

also indicate when to move from Stage 1 to **Stage 2 of the Lidcombe Program.**

After the clinician and parent complete their ratings of the child's speech, they discuss the week's SRs and the progress of the home treatment. As they talk, the child usually plays by themselves in the same room, with some interaction and encouragement from the parent and the clinician. The openness with which discussions of the week's progress take place is a hallmark of the Lidcombe Program. There is no attempt to keep the child from overhearing the parent and clinician discussion of the child's stuttering. The matter-of-fact manner in which the clinician and parent discuss the child's speech seems to make it more likely that both the parent and child will feel less anxious about the child's stuttering and may reduce any shame the child might feel about their difficulty. During the parent and clinician's discussion, some children often make noise to call attention to themselves. In my experience, this is not because the child objects to the discussion of their stuttering but is only an attempt to bring the focus back more obviously on themselves. At such times, it may be helpful if the clinician simply tells the child, "Right now, I want to talk to your mommy/daddy for just a minute; then we'll play again!" or the parent may take a minute to play with the child.

As the clinician looks over the parent's weekly SRs, the clinician may ask about the days in which ratings are higher or lower than average, or the clinician and parent may brainstorm solutions to problems that may be indicated by lack of change in the ratings. This is often a time when videos of the practice sessions from home are useful, so that the clinician can assess how they are being conducted. It is also essential that the parent demonstrate treatment during each clinic visit to show how they are conducting the treatment at home by doing a few minutes of a practice session with the child using the verbal contingencies (Fig. 14.3). When adequate progress is being made and home SRs and clinic assessments indicate that the child is becoming more fluent, new treatment procedures can be introduced.

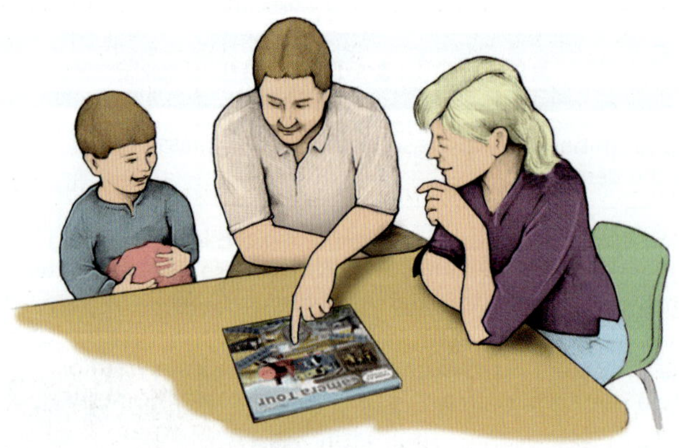

Figure 14.3 Clinician observing a father demonstrating a practice session with his child.

Once a parent is appropriately and accurately reinforcing fluency, they may be taught to use mildly negative verbal contingencies for stuttering in practice sessions. The mildest such contingency is verbally acknowledging the occurrence of an **unambiguous stutter**. Only unambiguous stutters should be acknowledged because normal disfluencies should not be treated as stutters. The descriptions of normal disfluencies and stuttered disfluencies in Chapter 7 clarify this difference. I typically model an acknowledgment of stuttering for the parent, which is given after several contingencies for fluent utterances. It is important that the parent learn to use contingencies for fluency several times before using a verbal contingency for stuttered speech. When I demonstrate acknowledgment of stuttering, I use comments like "a little bumpy one there" or "that one was a little bumpy." I make the statement quietly, immediately after the stutter and without any negative inflection in my voice. Acknowledgment does not require a response from the child, although some children will spontaneously repeat the word that was disfluent, and the parent should praise the attempt. After I have modeled how to acknowledge stutters, I ask the parent to try it, but only after they have praised several of the child's fluent utterances. Most children hardly seem to notice the acknowledgment, although some may stop momentarily and look at the parent when it is given. Typically, I ask parents to continue using contingencies for fluency and begin using acknowledgment of stuttering for a week before introducing further verbal contingencies for stuttering. What I have described is my way of using the LP treatment. However, there is flexibility in how verbal contingencies are delivered, and each clinician should decide on their own—after they receive training in LP—exactly how to teach parents to deliver contingencies.

In the following weekly meeting, I introduce requests for self-correction of unambiguous stuttering. This verbal contingency asks the child to say the stuttered word again with a phrase such as (if the child has stuttered on "I") "Can you say 'I' again?" *Such requests are made in a positive, supportive manner*, and it is important that the parent practice this contingency after the clinician demonstrates it. Some parents may be hesitant to request a self-correction and may convey their concern to the child. Others may inadvertently use a slightly negative or impatient tone when asking for a correction. However, a clinician's patient modeling and subsequent coaching can do wonders to shape parents' responses into helpful, supportive requests.

After the child has repeated the word fluently, the parent should praise the self-correction with comments like "Nice job of making that word smooth." If a child ignores a parent's request for self-correction or refuses to self-correct, the parent just moves on. If the child says the word again but stutters again, the parent may say something supportive like "That's OK; sometimes those words are hard."

In the subsequent weeks, the clinician monitors the child's progress and ensures that the parent is delivering verbal contingencies effectively. The clinician also checks to see that the child is enjoying the practice sessions and is responding well to the contingencies for both fluency and stuttering. Every child and every family are different, so the program must be individualized in each case. For example, some children may indicate they are uncomfortable with such praise as "That was really smooth talking." In this case, the parent can ask the child what they would like the parent to say when the child is talking smoothly. Alternatively, the parent can use one of the other verbal contingencies for fluency. Some children who don't react well to praise will happily respond to requests to self-evaluate their fluency. One child I worked with preferred that the parent put a penny in a jar, which made a nice "plink" sound, rather than verbally praise their fluency. Another child who loved the Boston Red Sox asked his mother to say "That's Red Sox talking!" after fluent speech. You can guess what the child asked the parent to say after the child stuttered. It had to do with a New York team.

Stage 1: Introducing Verbal Contingencies in Natural Conversations

When treatment has progressed well for 2 or 3 weeks, and SRs indicate an increase in stutter-free speech, a gradual transition can be made from practice sessions to natural conversations. Thus, verbal contingencies of praise, acknowledgment of stutters, and requests for correction can now be given in typical daily conversations, such as during meals, riding in the car, shopping, and playing. When treatment is first introduced in natural conversations, practice sessions usually continue for a time to make the transition easy. When contingencies in natural conversations have been going well for a week or two and stuttering continues to decrease, practice sessions can be faded gradually. For example, each week, one or two practice sessions may be dropped until they have all been discontinued and replaced with contingencies in natural conversations.

There are several reasons why practice sessions may subsequently be reinstated or even increased. The first reason is if SRs increase when natural conversations have largely replaced practice sessions, practice sessions should be reinstated until the child's SRs have returned to earlier levels. Another reason for continuing or reinstating practice sessions is if the child asks to continue practice sessions for a period of time as the transition to natural conversations is made. Sometimes parents feel that things are going so well in practice sessions that they believe the transition to natural conversations should be made slowly.

Several issues may warrant consideration when using contingencies in natural conversations is just getting underway. Parents may wish to begin with just praise for fluent utterances and then add acknowledgment for fluency and for stuttering, requests for self-evaluation, and, finally, requests for self-correction of stuttering. If problems appear in response to any of these verbal contingencies, they can be solved immediately. It is also important that verbal contingencies not be given relentlessly throughout each day but are used selectively at first, so that the parent can judge how the child is responding. If the child reacts well, which is usually the case, the parent can begin using verbal contingencies in more and more conversations, but at the same time, the parent should make sure that the child is not overwhelmed by too-frequent attention to their speech. The child needs to experience the normal flow of conversation for its own sake, rather than feel that everything they say is being evaluated. This is especially essential for sensitive children but is probably valuable for all children to avoid increasing the child's sense of being scrutinized for their speech.

Another issue that may arise relative to contingencies in natural conversations is who is giving the verbal contingencies. In general, only the person who has been meeting with the clinician should be conducting practice sessions and giving verbal contingencies in natural conversations. In some cases where it seems really needed, both parents, and even other family members, may be involved in the natural conversations. When this is done, it must be done very carefully and be individualized for each family. Any individual who is giving verbal contingencies must be meeting with the clinician to make sure that the contingencies are done properly. This will ensure that *many more instances of praise* for fluency be given than requests for self-correction of stuttering and that requests for self-correction be done in a supportive manner. Also, the focus on the content of the conversation rather than its fluency needs to remain a top priority.

Contingencies in natural conversations at home and weekly meetings in the clinic continue until the child is essentially fluent and can move to Stage 2. This point is reached when two criteria are met: (1) the parent's SRs for 3 weeks in a row are all 0s and 1s, with at least four of the ratings being 0 each week, and (2) the clinician's SRs *for the entire clinic visit* are 0s or 1s for these same 3 weeks. Meeting these criteria is vital if the child is to remain fluent after treatment. If the clinician has any doubts about the reliability and validity of the parent's SRs, they should request that the parent bring an audio or video recording of the child's speech at home to confirm that the criteria are met. The clinician can also check with others who have daily contact with the child to verify that the child has the level of fluency that the parent's SRs indicate.

Stage 2: Maintenance

One of the most important components of the Lidcombe Program is its maintenance procedure. Because relapse is common in stuttering treatment, parents are cautioned when they begin Stage 1 of the Lidcombe Program that it is essential that they continue to work with the clinician through the end of Stage 2. They are reminded of this throughout Stage 1 so that the procedures of the second stage are expected. Stage 2 consists of 30-minute clinic visits that are scheduled at gradually wider intervals. Typically, there are two visits at 2-week intervals, then two visits at 4-week intervals, then two visits at 8-week intervals, and, finally, one visit 16 weeks later. During this period, parents continue to provide verbal contingencies for fluency and stuttering just as they did during Stage 1 and continue to record SRs, but the clinician guides the parents in gradually decreasing their verbal contingencies until they are completely discontinued.

To progress through this schedule of visits, the child must maintain the same level of fluency achieved to begin Stage 2 (clinician SRs of 0 or 1 for the entire clinic visit and parent SRs beyond the clinic visit of 0s and 1s, with at least four ratings of 0 during any given week). When the parent and child come in for a scheduled clinic visit, the clinician has a natural conversation with the child without providing verbal contingencies, followed by a discussion of how the child's speech has been since the previous visit, using the severity ratings from the previous week that are provided by the parent. This discussion, as always, is focused on the parent's SRs and reports of how the child is responding to verbal contingencies. At each visit, the clinician and parent decide whether to continue decreasing the frequency of clinic visits or to make some changes, such as keeping to the current frequency of visits, resuming or increasing contingencies in natural conversations, or reinstating both practice sessions and contingencies in natural conversations. It is also possible that some aspect of the verbal contingencies may need to be adjusted. For example, sometimes a child becomes so fluent that when stutters do occur, parents or other family members apply contingencies to stuttering without concurrently giving more contingencies for stutter-free speech. Sometimes, making this adjustment of reinstating praise for stutter-free speech will solve a problem of stuttering re-emerging or increasing in frequency. In other cases, stuttering reappears because of momentary period of stress, such as the birth of a sibling, or the family moving to a new home. In such cases, reinstating weekly visits may help the parent and clinician get the child back on track.

Stage 2 takes about a year to complete for most children. Although minor relapses may occur, parents are usually able to accurately assess what changes need to be made to bring the child back to essentially stutter-free speech.

Extensive research has been done on the use of telehealth to deliver LP (eg, Wilson et al., 2004). There is strong evidence that telehealth delivery produces results as good as clinic delivery.

Problem-Solving

In general, the Lidcombe Program runs smoothly without much difficulty if clinicians carefully follow the manualized format that is described in the Treatment Guide. However, it is common for minor problems to arise during Stages 1 and 2. This section describes some common problems that may occur and their possible solutions. For more detailed descriptions of troubleshooting and special cases, see the Lidcombe Program Treatment Guide (March 2021), available as a download from the Lidcombe Program Trainers Consortium website (asrc@fhs.usyd.edu.au).

Sometimes, progress toward fluent speech is stalled for several weeks, or previous gains are momentarily lost. If so, I usually begin by talking to the parent about what they think might be occurring. Parents are often able to pinpoint something they have changed about the way they are doing treatment. Or it may be that a parent misunderstands some aspect of treatment. Thus, it is essential to have parents demonstrate how they conduct treatment, and it may be even more helpful to have them bring in a video of treatment at home. Examples of things that may go wrong include the following: (1) parents are less attentive to praising fluent speech regularly so that fewer positive reinforcements are made than requests for corrections; (2) parents become lax about the consistency of practice sessions so that many days are missed and treatment becomes inconsistent; (3) other family members, while trying to be helpful, make mistakes in providing verbal contingencies because they have not been trained; (4) the child is overly sensitive to verbal contingencies and asks parents to stop using them; and (5) some children who stutter severely at the beginning of treatment have trouble generating adequate fluency in structured sessions; (6) some children have co-existing deficits like phonology and/or language problems, and LP treatment take longer.

The problems that arise from misunderstanding the parameters of treatment can usually be resolved by supportive feedback and guidance of the parent and modeling of appropriate behavior. Other issues, such as conducting treatment inconsistently, may require brainstorming with the parent about how treatment can be conducted more regularly. If a child isn't enjoying conversations, progress will be stalled. But it is not difficult to coach parents in delivering treatment in ways that are enjoyable, effective, and fun for both parent and child. Clinicians who have worked with preschool-age children have usually learned how to keep a child interested and achieve therapy goals at the same time. It may be appropriate for other family members to become involved in practice sessions, but they must be trained by the clinician to deliver contingencies effectively. Practice sessions may be shared by both parents and other caregivers, but the clinician should ensure that whoever is delivering treatment is doing so accurately, and direct training is the best way to achieve this.

If a child objects to the parent's verbal contingencies after treatment has gone on for some months, it is usually helpful to ask the child how they would like the parent to respond to fluent speech and to stuttering. Some sensitive children prefer nonverbal contingencies such as a wink or a "thumbs up" after several fluent utterances and just a quick eye contact after a stutter.

With children who have moderate or severe stuttering, it is critical to structure their treatment conversations so that the child is largely stutter-free and only stutters occasionally. One way to do this is to ensure that in practice sessions, the child is, at first, using only short utterances (which are more likely to be fluent). Short fluent utterances should be reinforced but not longer ones. This "differential" reinforcement of shorter utterances will teach the child to make short, fluent utterances for the first part of the training. Then, after the child is reliably experiencing mostly fluent speech in the practice sessions, longer utterances can be stimulated. With the help of the clinician's instruction and modeling, the parent can learn how to move the child up a linguistic hierarchy of increasingly longer and more complex sentences while preserving fluency. It should be noted, however, that if the child remains stutter-free even when using longer sentences at the beginning of treatment, the parent should allow that.

The Lidcombe Program is an effective treatment approach, and its effectiveness is maximized if the clinician attends a training workshop conducted by the Lidcombe Program Trainers Consortium. Information about workshops, research articles on treatment outcome, and a treatment manual are available on the Lidcombe website (Lidcombeprogram.org). After training, the clinician can join an online Lidcombe discussion group, which provides a wealth of information about various challenges that may arise in treatment.

Outcome Research on the Lidcombe Program

A number of studies have reported that the Lidcombe Program is effective in eliminating stuttering in most preschoolers. A long-term outcome study of 42 children treated with the program showed that their stuttering was at near-zero levels 4 to 7 years after treatment (Lincoln & Onslow, 1997). Other research reported that the mean number of clinic visits needed to complete Stage 1 treatment in a sample of 29 children was 18 clinic visits (median = 16) (Rousseau et al., 2007). In response to concerns expressed by critics that the Lidcombe Program might produce negative psychological effects, Woods et al. (2002) compared pre- and posttreatment measures of the *Child Behavior Checklist*[2] (Achenbach, 1988) and the *Attachment Q-Set*[3] (Waters, 1995) and found no ill effects of treatment on the children's psychological health. In fact, the *Child Behavior Checklist* showed improvement in the children's behavior after treatment.

An important research tool for assessing treatment effectiveness is a randomized controlled trial. To use this procedure to test stuttering treatment, a group of children who stutter would be divided in half. One-half would be given a treatment, and the other half would be given no treatment (the untreated group would eventually be treated once the study data have been collected). Just such a study was carried out in New Zealand (Jones et al., 2005). When the Lidcombe-treated group (n = 29) was compared with the untreated group (n = 25), a significantly (P = .003) greater improvement was seen with the Lidcombe-treated group. The "effect size" was 2.3 %SS. This means that the difference between the treated group and the control group final levels of stuttering relative to their variability in stuttering was very large; in fact, the authors indicate that it was more than twice the minimally clinically significant difference stated in their treatment protocol before the study was done.

While the majority of research on the Lidcombe Program has been done in Australia, publications from researchers in the United Kingdom, Canada, and other countries have appeared. For example, Miller and Guitar (2009) showed that Lidcombe can be very successful when implemented by supervised graduate students with excellent outcomes for 15 preschool children. It was found that duration of treatment (number of sessions required to reach the end of Stage 1) was predicted by scores on the Stuttering Severity Instrument (Riley, 2009); children who stuttered more severely before treatment took longer to become fluent. This is important information for clinicians so they can let parents of children with more severe stuttering know that treatment may take 20 sessions or more. In a later study, Guitar et al. (2015) combined the data from these original 15 children and added 14 more children, all of whom were assessed pretreatment and 2 years after treatment. Long-term outcome indicated that most children showed near-zero stuttering, and for the few others, stuttering was substantially reduced. Stuttering severity before treatment was a strong predictor of outcome; such children who were more severe before treatment had slightly more residual stuttering at long-term assessment. In this study, girls did slightly better long term than boys when assessed 2 years after treatment. In other studies, Latterman et al. (2008) assessed the outcome of Lidcombe treatment in Germany, showing it to be quite effective, and Femrell et al. (2012) reported on its success in Sweden.

The Lidcombe group in Australia has also published data on conducting the Lidcombe treatment in a group setting (Arnott et al., 2014) as well as webcam delivery of Lidcombe to parents over the internet (O'Brian et al., 2014). In both of those treatment environments, the Lidcombe approach was found to be effective compared to traditional delivery procedures. Recent research has also explored the mechanism by which the Lidcombe Program works (Amato Maguire et al., 2022; Santayana et al., 2021).

In summary, the Lidcombe Program appears to be an effective treatment for older preschool children who stutter, with a vast number of studies supporting its use. There have been recent concerns about Lidcombe's emphasis on stutter-free speech—given the popularity of accepting stuttered speech as "normal" because of neurodiversity. However, in my experience, when Lidcombe is carried out by a trained clinician, children and parents feel great relief when stuttering is eliminated. The children I have treated with Lidcombe beam with pride when they announce, as treatment is ending, "I'm a good talker!" and their parents glow with the satisfaction that they have been a major factor in this change.

---

[2]The Child Behavior Checklist is a form filled out by parents to determine if a child has a behavior problem.

[3]The Attachment Q-Set is a tool to assess how securely a child feels attached to their parent/caregiver.

Stuttering Modification Treatment

More Direct Treatment on Stuttering for Beginning Stuttering

Some preschool children who stutter are beginning to have negative feelings about their disfluencies but are not showing the full-blown signs of struggle or escape behaviors that characterize most beginning stuttering. Still, they may occasionally express real frustration with their stuttering.

Typically, I work with these children using **stuttering modification** for about 45 minutes each week. I also continue to provide encouragement and support to the family in helping them make the child's environment as facilitating to fluency as possible. Our treatment activities are presented in a hierarchy that the clinician and child ascend as far as is necessary to bring the child's disfluencies into the "typical disfluency" range. Progressive steps are taken when the clinician senses that a child is feeling competent at the current step. Thus, improvement may be rapid or slow and sudden or gradual, depending on the child's feeling of comfort and mastery with the tasks at hand. There is no need to hurry this process. It should take place within the context of games and activities that make the focus on stuttering casual and are, above all, fun. The clinician needs to remain alert to the child's immediate sense of confidence and self-esteem in selecting the moment to move the child to the next step in the treatment hierarchy.

Modeling Easy Stutters

I begin this approach to stuttering modification rather indirectly by providing models of easy stuttering in my speech. If the child's repetitions are fast and abrupt, my models are slow with gradual endings. If the child has many repetitions or long prolongations, I repeat or prolong sounds briefly. These models are done casually during play with the child. I don't produce them immediately after the child stutters but insert them randomly, about once every two or three sentences, as if I were stuttering as I talked.

Once the child has become acclimated to the models of easy stuttering after 10 or 15 minutes of play, I begin to make, *occasionally*, accepting comments about them. I might say, for example, "Hmmmm, I used slidey speech on that word, didn't I?" or "That word stuck a little, but that's OK and I slid right out of it." Most children appear to be shyly interested in what I am talking about, and this approach can continue to develop. A few children, however, may react negatively and say such things as "Don't do that!" or "I don't like it when you do that." For them, this approach needs to proceed slowly to allow my acceptance of them as they are and my support during play activities to gradually counteract the child's anxiety.

If the child has begun to experience the first pangs of frustration from stuttering, which can be inferred from their questions or complaints about getting stuck on words, I will try to help them express this. Even though I am making comments that show acceptance of my own pretend and real stuttering (since that sometimes occurs), I occasionally may produce a longer than usual stutter and say, "Sometimes they go on for a long time. That makes me mad sometimes." I continue to try to sense what the child is feeling and to empathize as naturally as possible. I use this empathic focus not only when I am modeling easy stutters but throughout treatment.

For children who evidence periods of acute frustration with their stuttering, parents should be coached on how to make empathetic statements in a calm, soothing, slow style when the child is going through a difficult time. As I do therapy, I try to involve the parents in appropriate activities both at home and in the clinic. If their indirect treatment has not been effective, I need to be sure that the parents do not feel pushed aside by my direct therapy with the child. They need to remain active participants.

The Child Begins Active Participation: "Catch Me"

When I sense that a child is comfortable with my easy stuttering models, I see if the child will take part. I may say, for example, "Can you help me? Sometimes when I get stuck on a word, it goes on and on. Then, I try to make my stuck words real slow and loose, and it helps me get unstuck. But sometimes I forget. If you hear me go on and on like thi-thi-thi-thi-thi-this, just say, 'There's one,' and then I'll try to change it to make it slow and loose with slidey speech." When the child catches me, I will change a fast, tight repetition to a slow, loose one. As I model stuck words, I choose a style of stuttering similar to the child's.

Praise should flow liberally when the child catches one of my modeled stutters. This provides the child with a sense of accomplishment that is associated with something they previously felt to be out of control, even though now it is in my speech. For many children, tangible rewards, such as small snacks or turns at a game, are important motivators and should be used along with praise to establish the child's ability to catch the clinician's stutters. Figure 14.4 illustrates "Catch me."

The Child Begins Active Participation: Play

This stage can either follow or precede "Catch Me." It depends on the clinician's judgment about which activity would be more comfortable for the child. Sometimes you may start one of these stages but find the child is not ready and you switch to the other. The playing with stuttering stage engages a child in following the clinician's lead in playfully imitating disfluencies that are similar to their own, such as repeated or prolonged sounds. The purpose is to desensitize the child to the frustration that sometimes arises in more severe borderline stuttering. It is a process that may take place because play can give a child a sense of mastery without the risk of failure. The concept of play is quite interesting. Scientists speculate that children's play is an opportunity for them to practice and master skills that are needed in adulthood. Playing with stuttering may take advantage of children's natural tendency to play and provide them with the pleasure of mastery and

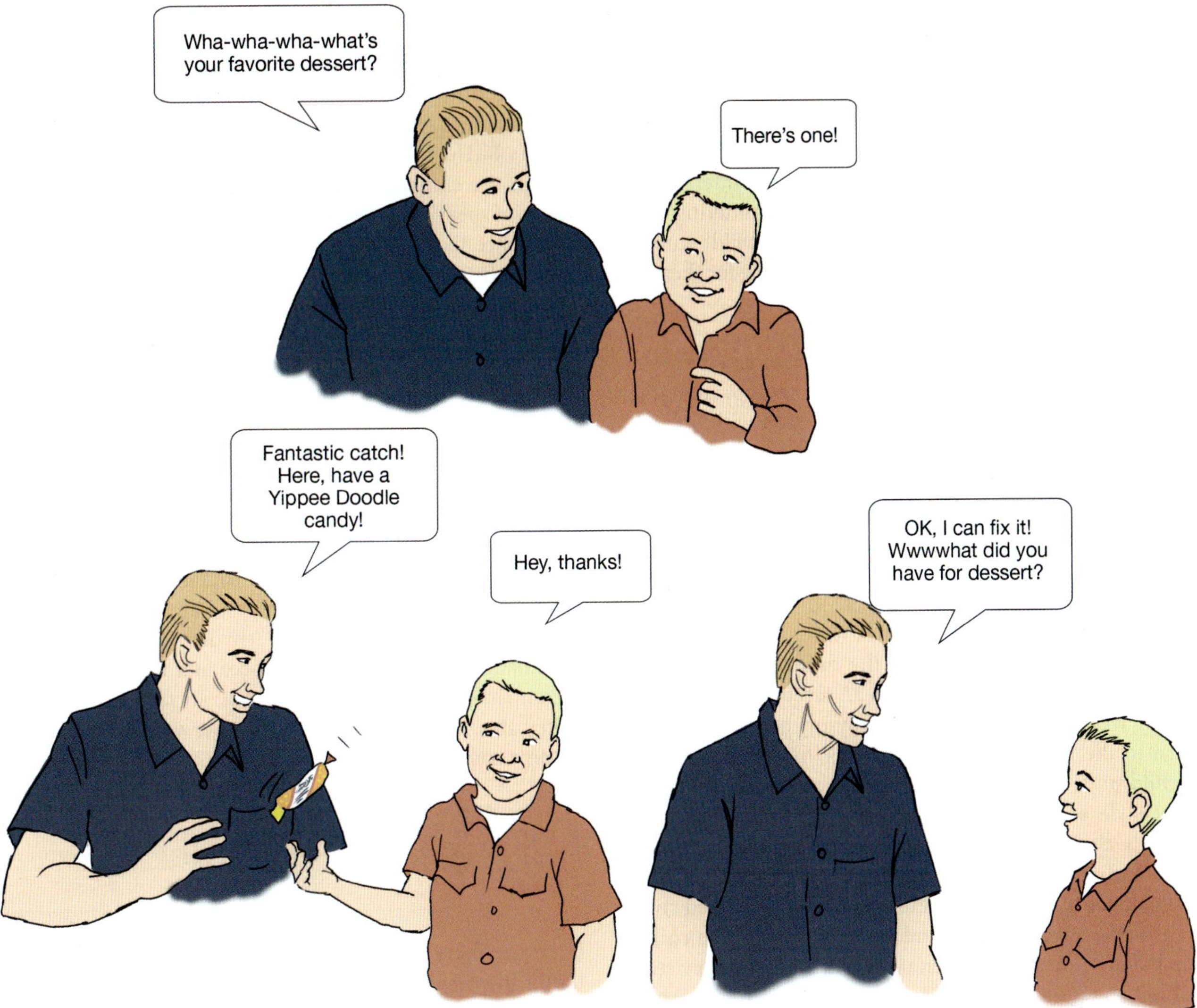

Figure 14.4 Child catches clinician's tense stutter, clinician rewards child, then clinician changes stutter to an easier one.

control over something that has been frustrating and sometimes even frightening.

Take, for example, the child who stutters primarily in a repetitive fashion. The clinician might say, "Let's play a game of saying some sounds over and over and see how many times we can say them. I bet I can say a whole bunch of times! Watch this. Ba-ba-ba-ba-ba! Can you do it that many times?" Or it can begin by making sounds for animals, puppets, or other toys: "Hey, this is a zebragella! It goes 'lllllla! llllla!' (using prolongations). Then, it jumps around like this (clinician jumps around) and chews the carpet" (clinician pretends to chew the carpet).

The clinician and child can keep incorporating such play into their routine as long as the child finds it fun and the clinician can free themselves to enjoy uninhibited play. From playing with repeated or prolonged sounds, the clinician can build a bridge to playing with repeated or prolonged sounds in conversation and, in time, to the child's actual stutters.

One of my former students read what I had written about this sort of play with stuttering in an early edition of this textbook and uses it very successfully with kids, to desensitize them to the fear of stuttering and help them change what they do when they stutter—going from tense to loose stutters. I describe her work and illustrate it in Chapter 15, on therapy for intermediate stuttering in school-age children.

The Child Produces Intentional Stutters

After the child is able to catch the clinician's stutters and appears comfortable doing it, the clinician should begin looking for opportunities to ask the child to produce a stutter intentionally. This can be done most easily by pretending to have trouble producing slow, loose stutters. For instance, the clinician might say, "I can't seem to make this one slow and loose. Can you show me how to do it?" Again, this should be done intermittently and casually mixed in with other activities that are fun for the child.

Praise and, if needed, tangible rewards are used to help the child build confidence. When the child is able to produce slow and loose stutters, the clinician can let the parents know, in the child's presence, about this accomplishment, focusing on the child's ability to teach the clinician. If the child seems proud of this accomplishment, the clinician can take advantage of this opportunity and have the child show intentional stutters to the parents. This not only desensitizes the child to stuttering with the parent, but it also desensitizes parents to the child's stuttering and models acceptance of the child's stuttering for them.

The Child Changes Their Own Real Stutters

For many young children whose stuttering fluctuates between mild and severe levels, these more direct therapy activities focused on stuttering modification, combined with a facilitating environment provided by parents, may be enough to advance their fluency into the typical range within a few months. For those whose stuttering persists, still another stage of stuttering modification may be necessary. In such cases, I look for opportunities when the child seems ready to modify their own stutters.

I begin by responding to a few of the child's real stutters with accepting comments to help the child feel comfortable with their stutters. I might say, with an accepting voice, "Oh, that one was a little bumpy on 'my-my-my car…,'" and then return to the business of playing. After further play, when the child stutters again, the clinician can model an easier and slower style of stuttering on the same word and comment positively about it. I then ask the child to imitate my easier stutter and praise them for doing so, using reinforcements and guidance to shape their stuttering to a slow, relaxed style.

I look for slightly slower and easier stutters in the child's speech and reward them. Even if the child intentionally stutters, but in an easier way than they stuttered previously, I reward them. From this point on, the clinician uses a combination of modeling and reinforcement to shape the child's stuttering. It is the deliberate slowness and "easiness" with which the child produces repetitions or prolongations, along with the sense of playing with stuttering, that make it possible for the child to begin *feeling a sense of control.* This in turn should reduce their frustration and fear, further diminish tension, and enable them to move through stutters with minimal effort.

After the child is able to make their stutters slower and easier in the clinic, generalization may occur away from the clinic without the need for formal transfer activities. Such "spontaneous" generalization may be a result of the child's increased self-esteem from gaining mastery over behavior they previously felt uncomfortable about and felt was out of their control. Consequently, emphasis should be placed on the stutters that a child handles successfully, rather than when they lose control.

If generalization is not occurring automatically, I work with family members to make the child's ability to play with and modify stutters a point of pride at home. Initially, the child can teach parents and siblings to stutter in the clinic under the clinician's guidance. Then, the clinician can work with the child at home and involve family members if possible and if needed, so that the parents learn to use positive reinforcement selectively to increase the child's slow and easy stutters and let the child know that they are appreciated. Even though the emphasis here is on slow and easy stutters, the effects of speech and language maturation and the increasing confidence that the child feels in their speech as a result of reduced frustration should result in typical fluency.

Sometimes a beginning stutterer may not be able to get to mastery over their tense stutters and turn them into easy ones. Then, the clinician and family need to be sure to help the child realize that stutters are OK and that they can go ahead and talk anyway and communicate effectively, using good eye contact with their listeners and openness about their stuttering.

One final note about direct therapy with young children who stutter: Van Riper once told me that one of his daughters began to stutter quite severely at a young age and he found a way to help her, using direct therapy. Van Riper and his wife used what now might be called "rhythm therapy." They had their daughter speak short sentences in a rhythmic manner, accompanied by clapping her hands. In fact, all the family talked this way for several weeks, after which his daughter became completely fluent, despite a minor relapse or two.[4]

ANOTHER CLINICIAN'S APPROACH: SHERYL GOTTWALD

I present Sheryl Gottwald's approach to working with stuttering in preschool children because it has good outcome data indicating that it is effective. This is not data from an isolated lab, but the findings of a clinician as she did therapy. It is a well-rounded "multidimensional" (to use her adjective) approach that helps parents change the home environment, helps the child change feelings and attitudes, and guides the child in changing the way they stutter, to an easier way of stuttering that typically leads to fluent speech.

Gottwald (2010) has refined an approach first developed at Temple University by Starkweather et al. (1990) and extended by Gottwald and Starkweather (1999). They designed it for children ages 2 to 6 who stutter. This treatment popularized their concept of **"demands and capacities,"** described in Chapter 6, that ascribed stuttering to a combination of the demands placed on a child by their environments (internal and external) interacting with their innate capacity for fluent speech. Because there are many factors maintaining the child's stuttering, Gottwald terms her approach "multidimensional." Among the dimensions are treatment focused on

[4]Compare this with the syllable-timed speech approach for preschool children who stutter, reported by Trajkovski et al. (2009).

the parents to reduce stresses in the child's environment and treatment focused on the child to strengthen the child's fluency. Gottwald carries out her assessment and treatment by working to understand the family's and child's needs, working with their strengths, and supporting them deeply as they deal with their challenges.

Modifying the Environment

Gottwald is very sensitive to each family's needs as she works with them to help them modify the child's environment. She describes her orientation this way: "Families bring their own individual needs for emotional support; until their feelings of sadness, guilt, frustration, and other emotions are addressed and acknowledged, it will be so much more difficult for them to make the changes necessary to support their child's fluency. We discover what families need by talking with them about their hopes, observations, feelings, and needs" (Gottwald, personal communication, July 2018).

The initial component of treatment—parent counseling—provides parents with a simplified version of what we currently know about the nature of stuttering. Figure 14.5 was drawn from a video clip of Gottwald counseling a mother and father whose child is stuttering. A series of video clips illustrating Gottwald's approach is available on *Lippincott Connect* for Chapter 14.

Some of the information that Gottwald shares is that stuttering is highly variable and that many factors may influence its ups and downs, including factors that the family may be able to change. The family is also introduced to an etiological (focusing on what the cause might be) model of stuttering, which explains stuttering as emerging from interactions between the child's capacities and the demands placed on the child. The clinician also helps the family find ways of talking about stuttering with their child. They learn to support the child by commenting sensitively when the child has difficulty getting a word out. Open acknowledgment of stuttering is intended to reduce the child's and the family's negative feelings about stuttering. For example, a parent might say to a child who has just stuttered and appears frustrated or ashamed, "Sometimes those words really get stuck. It's OK. I'm here to listen." This conveys to the child that the parent has the time and is focused on listening patiently.

During individual counseling, families are also taught to change other aspects of their behavior that may be affecting their child's fluency. For example, family members may learn to respond to the child's stuttering without interrupting, looking away, or otherwise conveying impatience. To decrease pressure from the family's speech and language environment on the child, family members may be taught to slow their speech rates, pause more frequently, and simplify their language when talking with the child. To increase the child's self-esteem, families may be urged to create times each day when the child has a parent's full attention. Sometimes, family members may be bombarding the child with questions or otherwise pressing them to speak. As a remedy, they are shown how to talk about what they are thinking and doing as they play with the child, thereby modeling the behavior they want to encourage. Table 14.3 lists some of the things that family members can do to facilitate fluency.

In addition to changing behavior directly related to speech, families are also counseled about other stresses in the home. For example, Starkweather et al. (1990) have noted that a hectic family lifestyle can exacerbate a child's stuttering. Once parents understand that a too-busy family schedule may be a factor in their child's stuttering, they are often able to reduce the hustle and bustle in the home and are gratified when their child's stuttering subsequently diminishes. In addition, a slower pace and more relaxed lifestyle can often provide increased satisfaction for all family members.

Gottwald sometimes supplements individual family counseling with group therapy in which two to four other couples whose child stutters are involved, when that can be arranged. This gives families an opportunity to share experiences and

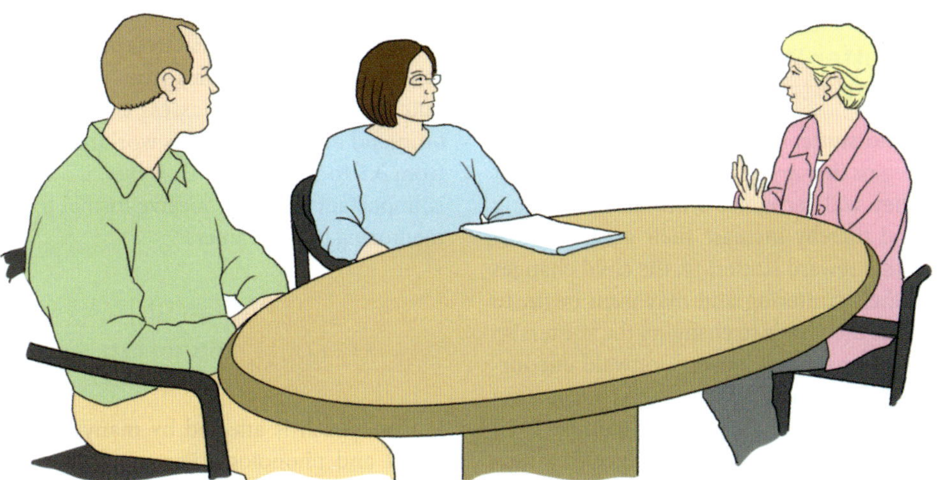

Figure 14.5 A clinician counseling a family about treatment for their child.

ideas and to support one another. As members of a group, parents receive support from one another and can share ideas for helping their children. The clinician's role is to help the group members develop a sense of mutual trust by modeling concern, acceptance, and respect for all group members and their ideas and feelings. Generally, the group talks about topics they select, although the clinician may also suggest topics that are often concerns of most members, such as regression during treatment and termination of treatment.

Modifying the Child's Speech

The other major component of Gottwald's therapy—besides working with the parents or caregivers to change the child's environment—is modification of the child's speech. This involves parent and clinician modeling and reinforcement, as well as the clinician's instruction when needed. Instruction in changing stuttering with older preschool-age children is a natural outgrowth of the parents and clinician talking openly about stuttering with the child. The procedures that the authors use to modify a child's speech are as follows.

Children Who Stutter With Minimal Struggle

First, the clinician talks and plays games with the child in a very fluency-enhancing setting. This situation includes the clinician talking slowly in a relaxed way with plenty of pauses and silences. Then, the clinician teaches the child to talk in a slow, relaxed way. This is done with very little linguistic demand on the child; for example, a game they play may require only simple short sentences. Gradually, as the child becomes more and more fluent in this situation, demands are gradually increased. This may entail games and conversation involving longer and more complex utterances, or the clinician may speed up their speech rate. For those children who continue to stutter in this low-pressure situation, Gottwald teaches them to stutter using "easy bounces" at the beginning of an utterance, li-like this.

Children Who Stutter With Moderate to Severe Struggle

For those children who stutter with noticeable tension and struggle, Gottwald begins therapy by talking with them about stuttering, so that they will recognize what they are doing when they stutter and thereby increase their acceptance of it. By playing games that reward stuttering, the child changes their feelings about their stuttering and may even begin to stutter on purpose. This then leads to changing the stutters so they become gradually looser and looser. Gottwald encourages these children to use bouncy speech (re-re-repeating sounds easily and loosely) or stretchy speech (lllllllllike this) in which easy, loose prolongations take the place of struggled stutters. As she works on helping the children change their stutters, Gottwald also works to help them express their feelings as a way of leading to improved attitudes about their stuttering and a better understanding of it.

Termination

Individual and group parent counseling and modification of the child's speech continue until the family environment and the child's speech have met the following two criteria. First, the environment has changed enough so that major stresses have diminished and the family seems to understand the dynamics that may exist between environmental stresses and the child's stuttering. Second, the child's stuttering has decreased to the point at which they are normally disfluent, with an occasional mild instance of stuttering.

Supporting Data on Gottwald's Multidimensional Approach

Starkweather et al. (1990) reported that most of the children they have treated have regained normal fluency. Of 39 children whom they treated using this approach, 7 dropped out, and of the remaining 32 children, 29 recovered completely, and 3 were still in treatment at the time of the report. The average child requires about 12 sessions of therapy using this approach, although some children require much more before therapy can be terminated.

Gottwald and Starkweather (1999) treated an additional 15 families with their approach. Although 1 family dropped out, the children of the remaining 14 families achieved normal fluency and reported maintaining it a year after the children were dismissed from treatment. Further data on her approach were provided by Gottwald (2010) involving the children of 27 families. Again, 1 family dropped out, but 26 families reported their children had normal fluency 1 year or more following dismissal from treatment.

Compared to LP, Gottwald's treatment based on the Demands and Capacities model appears to be equally effective and, on average, takes fewer sessions (12 in Gottwald's approach; 18 in LP). However, LP has generated many more outcome studies of their treatment program and has used randomized control trials (the "gold standard" of treatment outcome measures) to assess treatment effectiveness. I recommend both to clinicians working with preschool children from 3.5 to 5 years old. However, if a clinician chooses LP, it is important that they receive formal training and follow-up mentoring by LP trainers.

TREATMENT OF CONCOMITANT SPEECH AND LANGUAGE PROBLEMS

Fluent speech is affected by many variables, including language and phonology. For example, there is evidence that many children who stutter also have language and/or phonological problems (Bloodstein et al., 2021; Hall et al., 2022;

Ntourou et al., 2011). However, there is a tendency in graduate programs to focus students' training in fluency disorders on individuals whose only problem is stuttering. Once these newly trained clinicians graduate, they take positions in the real world and find that their caseloads are brimming with children who not only stutter but also have concomitant problems. I hope this section will help clinicians develop strategies to help these children. Treatment for stuttering plus other issues must be well-planned and flexible to be successful with both deficits. It is also important that evaluation of these children identifies concomitant problems because the co-occurrence of stuttering with language and/or phonological problems can suggest that natural recovery from stuttering without treatment is unlikely (Leech et al., 2017, 2019; Sasisekaran, 2014). The co-occurring deficits indicate that clinicians should treat these children as soon as possible rather than adopt a "wait and see" approach.

When concomitant problems are found, the challenge is to plan how best to work with these other problems along with treatment of stuttering. A very useful resource for working with both stuttering and two of these concomitant deficits is the chapter by Hall, Garbarino, and Bernstein Ratner titled "Language and Phonological Considerations" in Zebrowski et al. (2022). Many of the suggestions I give in this section come from this chapter. One of their principles is that treatment must ensure that the linguistic and phonological demands of the therapy activities do not stress speech production capabilities. For example, trying to teach a child to use easy onsets while speaking long and complex sentences may be too challenging. Similarly, asking a child to stay in a moment of stuttering while reading sentences with phonological elements that the child has not mastered may lead to failure.

Evaluation

A preschool child being considered for stuttering therapy should be assessed not only for stuttering but also for aspects of language and phonology as well. The article by Brundage et al. (2021) provided a detailed description of a thorough evaluation of a preschool child who stutters. Moreover, the aforementioned chapter by Hall et al. (2022) not only gives a rationale for an in-depth evaluation but also provides a case example of such an assessment, in Box 13.1. In addition, the reader should consult Chapter 10 in the textbook, *Assessment of Preschool Children who Stutter*, for the components of an evaluation. The latest editions of *Clinical Evaluation of Language Fundamentals Preschool*, 5th edition (Wiig et al., 2013), and *Goldman-Fristoe Test of Articulation*, 3rd edition (Goldman & Fristoe, 2015), should be used to assess aspects of language and phonology.

TABLE 14.3 Modifying the Speech and Language of Family Members

1. Use a speech rate that more closely matches the child's.
2. Pause between conversation turns.
3. Eliminate questions requiring long, complex answers.
4. Respond to the content of the child's message with positive comments regardless of fluency.
5. Acknowledge struggled stutters by using meaningful words, such as "That's okay."

Treatment

Treatment of children with stuttering and concomitant problems must focus both on stuttering as well as one or more concomitant issues. But how do you decide which to focus on? First one and then the other? Where do you start? The literature in this area suggests that there are three possible ways to organize treatment: sequential, concurrent, and cyclic.

Sequential Model

The sequential approach begins with identifying the child's most pressing problem and treating that until a certain degree of mastery has been achieved. Then, the next most prominent problem is dealt with. A weakness of the sequential approach is that if the first problem treated requires a long time to master, other problems may be neglected even though their prime time for treatment may be passing.

An example of a sequential approach is how clinicians using the Lidcombe Program usually deal with concomitant problems (Unicomb et al., 2013). When using Lidcombe, it is imperative that only stuttering be treated during Stage 1, during which the parent and child are highly involved in working on fluency. Typically, the Lidcombe Program from the beginning to the end of Stage 1 is conducted first, and then, any other speech or language problem is treated. In some cases, however, when another problem is particularly severe, such as when a phonological problem is so severe that most of what the child says cannot be understood, phonological treatment is conducted until the child's speech is intelligible. Then, Stage 1 of Lidcombe can be implemented, and treatment of the other problem(s) can be resumed when Stage 1 is finished. During treatment using the Lidcombe Program, it is crucial that parents understand that the focus is on fluency only, so that their SRs are not affected by the other disorder(s). Placing the priority on the treatment of stuttering is recommended because of its greater likelihood of chronicity and exacerbation as children grow older. This contrasts with most other developmental problems that tend to improve a little or at least not worsen appreciably if treatment for them is delayed.

Concurrent Model

Clinician-researchers using other approaches—not the Lidcombe Program—have recommended a variety of ways of responding to other **concomitant speech and language**

problems in beginning stutterers. One approach is to work on phonological and language problems *at the same time* as they work on fluency, if other problem(s) are severe enough to warrant intervention. Bernstein-Ratner (1995) provided a good overview of how these children can be identified and how therapy can be designed so that it considers the whole of these children's communication challenges. Guidelines are given for concurrent approaches for stuttering concomitant with phonological and language issues.

Ratner presented the example of such an approach with phonological problems as described by Conture et al. (1993). These authors used an indirect approach, avoiding the traditional "corrective" type of therapy and providing the child with plenty of models of target phonemes through extensive auditory stimulation and opportunities for improved production. This is done in an accepting environment rather than correcting the child when they are wrong and asking the child to try again with more attention and effort. Hill (2003) begins with receptive training and then follows with a sequence of working on phonological change, sound play, sound approximation, and rehearsal of correct sound production in a few target sounds. If language is an issue, the clinician again begins with receptive training, followed by integrating practice with proper syntactic forms into the fluency hierarchy of more and more complex language. For example, the clinician provides appropriate instructions and materials and has the child practice a specific syntactic structure while using easy, relaxed speech.

Another good example of the concurrent approach is given in chapter by Hall et al. (2022), describing therapy for a 3.6-year-old boy with stuttering and a severe phonological problem. This case example (Box 3.2 in their chapter) is particularly useful because of the details given about the assessment, the treatment of the phonological problem, and the involvement of parents in indirect stuttering therapy.

Cycles Model

This approach alternates fluency treatment with language or phonology therapy over the course of the year (Hodson & Paden, 1991; described in Bernstein-Ratner, 1995). Bernstein-Ratner points out that this provides children with initial periods of concentrated learning of new skills (for a specified amount of time irrespective of whether or not the client meets criteria for finishing the treatment), followed by opportunities for spontaneous generalization of these skills to other settings while the other treatment is cycled in. This alternation continues until one of the problems is resolved so that all attention can then be given to the remaining issue(s).

Again, the chapter by Hall et al. (2022) provided an excellent case example (Box 13.4). The child described here is 3.11 years old and has a receptive-expressive language disorder. After several months of language therapy, the child begins to stutter and treatment then uses a cyclic (and concurrent) approach to treating both issues. Both the child and his mother are involved in the treatment.

To recap, in schools and clinics, as well as in private practice, it is not uncommon to assess and treat children who stutter but also have other communication problems. Three approaches are described for planning and carrying out treatment that consider the interactions between stuttering and other issues such as phonological and language problems. Other concomitant problems, such as attention deficit hyperactivity disorder, will be discussed in Chapter 15 on Treatment of School-Age Children.

SUMMARY

- Beginning stuttering arises from an interaction between children's constitutional predispositions and developmental and environmental influences to produce primarily repetitive disfluencies with increased tension. These stutters may commonly become more severe, evolving into prolongations and blocks with tension. Escape and avoidance behaviors may sometimes appear as a component of the disorder, as children experience increasing frustration with their inability to complete a word.
- A key element of treatment for children of this age is to prevent them from having negative emotions associated with their stuttering, including experiences they may have as part of their therapy, such as learning that speaking can be fun and rewarding. When children have negative experiences, the danger is that they will react to stuttering (and anticipated stuttering) with tension and struggle that will begin a cycle of increasingly negative feelings and increasingly tense stuttering, coupled with escape and avoidance behaviors. Focusing treatment on increasing fluency and building the child's confidence in their fluency can help prevent this cycle.
- Children with beginning stuttering usually have a large amount of fluency that can be reinforced and generalized to situations that previously elicited stuttering.
- The Lidcombe Program is a parent-delivered, operant conditioning program for preschoolers in which the parent is guided to conduct daily treatment conversations and apply verbal contingencies to fluency and stuttering. Treatment begins in practice sessions and moves to natural conversations throughout the day, so that treatment is conducted in the child's natural speaking environment, promoting generalization to all aspects of the child's world. Once the child is fluent in all situations, the clinician manages a phased withdrawal of clinic contact with careful monitoring of progress so that the family can respond to any relapses by reinstating needed features of treatment and then return to the fading process.

- Some children may not be suited for the Lidcombe Program. A stuttering modification approach for these children includes helping the family create a fluency-supporting environment, having the clinician model easy stutters and, if needed, then gradually getting the child to identify easy stutters and then imitate them and gradually change their own harder stutters into easier ones.
- Another clinician, Sheryl Gottwald, uses an approach based on the "demands and capacities" concept and treats both the family and the child. Gottwald uses an individualized treatment in which the clinician gets to know each family and each child so that their needs can be met in a way that plays to their strengths and supports their challenges.
- It is important to help children who have concomitant problems (like phonological or language challenges) work on them in a way that takes into account the influence of stuttering on these issues and vice versa. Many clinician-researchers have described approaches that do just that; they include sequential, concurrent, and cyclic treatments.

STUDY QUESTIONS

1. Describe Stage 1 and Stage 2 of the Lidcombe Program for the beginning stutterer. What is the goal of each phase?
2. Describe practice sessions and natural conversations in the Lidcombe Program.
3. Describe the two major ways of collecting data on the child's progress in the Lidcombe Program.
4. Describe how data are used to guide the child's progress in the Lidcombe Program.
5. What is a major difference between the Lidcombe Program and Stuttering Modification?
6. Compare the Lidcombe Program and Stuttering Modification with Gottwald's approach. In what ways are they similar, and in what ways are they different?
7. Describe Gottwald's use of "easy bounces" and "bouncy speech" to change a child's more tense stutters.
8. Describe how the treatment of beginning stuttering and concomitant phonological and language disorders can be managed.

SUGGESTED PROJECTS

1. Develop a hierarchy based on length and complexity of utterances that could be used by a clinician who is working with beginning stuttering and wants to move from single words to conversational speech.
2. Develop a hierarchy, based on increasing social complexity, for a child with beginning stuttering. Design it for use by a typical, two-parent family with older and younger siblings and grandparents who visit frequently. In other words, design a series of interactions that a parent could take a child through that would have the child practice fluency in more and more challenging social situations with the family members listed.
3. Interview the family of a child with beginning stuttering who was treated successfully. Find out what they perceived to be the most helpful aspects of treatment and what advice they would give to other families just beginning treatment.

SUGGESTED READINGS

Bernstein-Ratner, N. (1995). Treating the child who stutters with concomitant language and phonological impairment. *Language, Speech, and Hearing Services in Schools, 26*, 180–186.

In this insightful overview of the treatment of children with concomitant disorders, Bernstein Ratner identifies several models that have evolved.

Guitar, B., & McCauley, R. (2010b). *Treatment of stuttering: Established and emerging interventions.* Lippincott Williams & Wilkins.

Several interventions described in this book are applicable to older preschool children, and each is accompanied by video clips illustrating treatment. Of particular importance to the current chapter is the chapter by Harrison and Onslow about the Lidcombe Program.

Packman, A., Onslow, M., Webber, M., Harrison, E., Arnott, S., Bridgman, K., …, Lloyd, W. (2016). *The Lidcombe Program treatment guide.* Available under Research and Publications using the link for Speech Language Pathologists at http://www.lidcombeprogram.org

This manual gives detailed information about the procedures that clinicians use in administering the Lidcombe Program. The manual is frequently updated as new information is obtained about how to make the program effective.

Shapiro, D. (2011). *Stuttering intervention: A collaborative journey to fluency freedom* (2nd ed.). Pro-Ed.

The section on direct intervention in the chapter on intervention with preschool children has many excellent suggestions for treatment, including ideas for building up resistance to fluency disruptors and encouraging expression of emotion. In addition, there is an excellent section on working with children who stutter and have concomitant disorders.

Zebrowski, P. M., & Kelly, E. (2002). *Manual of stuttering intervention.* Singular.

The chapter on treatment of the preschool child, particularly treatment of those children who are likely to persist in stuttering, contains many excellent ideas for direct work on stuttering. Many case examples are given. The authors are both world-renowned stuttering therapists.

Zebrowski, P, Anderson, J., & Conture, E. (2022). *Stuttering and related disorders of fluency*, (4th ed.). Thieme.

As I indicated when I cited this book in earlier chapters, this fourth edition of a classic text originally edited by Richard Curlee in 1999 is replete with detailed chapters on the nature, diagnosis, and treatment of stuttering. More than 40 experts from all over the world have written a total 17 chapters with the latest information on stuttering, cluttering, as well as both acquired neurogenic stuttering and acquired functional (formerly called "psychogenic") stuttering. Students, clinicians, and clinical scientists will benefit from studying this all-encompassing volume of new information and recent perspectives on stuttering.

15

Treatment of School-Age Children: Intermediate Stuttering

Chapter Outline

Chapter Objectives

After studying this chapter, readers should be able to:

- Describe the characteristics of a child who has intermediate stuttering
- Describe the author's beliefs about stuttering, targets in treatment, goals for treatment, how much to involve feelings and attitudes in treatment, and maintenance procedures
- Outline the goals and activities of these components of treatment: exploring goals, beliefs, and feelings, as well as changing stuttering behaviors, being open about stuttering and accepting it, performing voluntary stuttering, reducing fear and avoidance, coping with teasing, maintaining improvement, and learning and generalizing fluency skills
- Describe important aspects of working with parents and working with teachers to help the school-age child who stutters
- Describe the treatment procedures of (1) Yaruss, Pelczarski, and Quesal; (2) Walton; and (3) Harrison, Bruce, Shenker, Koushik, and Kazenski

Key Terms

Easier stuttering: Stuttering that involves less struggling and fear and makes the speaker feel able to "just talk"

Cognitive behavioral therapy: Working with thoughts and beliefs that may give rise to the negative emotions associated with stuttering

Desensitization: Helping the individual become less sensitive to negative experiences such as stuttering or negative listener reactions

Exploring: Approaching and getting to know something you may have been afraid of

Fluency disrupters: Stimuli that put pressure on someone's speech so that they stutter. Examples are interruptions and fast-talking conversational partners

Fluency skills: Skills that improve fluency, such as slow rate and easy onset of phonation

High-quality stutter: These are stutters that are held without any avoidance until fear and tension are reduced. The stutters are then released slowly and loosely. They are the results of learning to "stay in the stutter"

Proprioception: This is one of the "fluency skills," referred to above. It involves closely attending to sensory feedback associated with speech movement (such as the feeling of the jaw and tongue moving) to guide speech. This attention to proprioceptive feedback may reduce the impact of faulty auditory feedback that may hinder fluency

School-age children: Children between 6 and 14 years old

Staying in the stutter: Going right into the stutter, without any avoidance behavior, and prolonging the articulatory posture and sound associated with the moment of "stuckness," with the purpose of extinguishing the threat and fear associated with the experience of being stuck

Voluntary stuttering: Deliberately stuttering or pretending to stutter so that one loses some of the fear of stuttering

AN INTEGRATED APPROACH

The typical school-age child who stutters (intermediate stuttering) is usually an elementary or junior high school student between 6 and 12 years of age who has been stuttering for several years. I use the word "child" or "student" to refer to the client, but I am aware that when a youngster is 10 years or older, in many ways they are more like an adolescent than a child. The school-age student will probably exhibit tense part-word and monosyllabic whole-word repetitions, as well as tense prolongations. Blocks with tension and struggle are also common in these students. They are the most disruptive aspect of their stuttering, both to them and to listeners. The student may also use escape devices, such as body movements or brief verbalizations (eg, "uh"), to break free of stutters once they are stuck in them. If their stuttering has advanced further, they may use avoidance strategies such as starters, word substitutions, circumlocutions, and evasion of difficult speaking situations. The very same "uh" that began as an escape device *during* the moment of stuttering may suddenly appear *before* a moment of stuttering, as learning does its sinister work of teaching the students' behaviors that make speaking feel harder. What has happened is that the torment of being jammed in a stutter creates negative emotions that spread like a wildfire when the student anticipates a word or sound that they have had trouble on before. If they're like me, they will end up using a multitude of "uh's" until their feared word or sound finally feels like it can be said fluently.

Another notable feature of the student's disability is the shame and embarrassment they feel because they stutter. Humiliations have piled up, squashing the student's self-esteem. They are afraid of getting stuck in a stutter and afraid of real or imagined rejection because of it. Shame becomes a constant companion, dogging them when they must speak. Because they are in school and must talk in class as well as on the playground, they are constantly experiencing humiliation because they can't talk like other kids. They even may be teased and bullied by their peers because of their stuttering.

There are exceptions. A few **school-age children** who stutter are not humiliated by their difficulty. They may have grown up in unusually accepting and supportive homes. They may have compensating talents—like superb athleticism or a towering intellect. Or they may just have resilient temperaments that keep them from feeling bad for very long when bad things happen. These rare students will benefit from focusing on **fluency skills** at the start of their therapy. However, some who begin therapy with fluency skills may need to add stuttering modification to their toolbox if it turns out that they are not able to fully manage their stuttering focusing on fluency. In my opinion, all students who stutter benefit from aspects of stuttering modification that help them feel ok about stutters when they appear. This reduces the threat and fear that upcoming stutters can generate, and reduces that shame that stuttering can hammer into the student's self-image.

The treatment approach I will describe in the next section is for most of the school-age children who stutter. This approach aims to first reduce students' negative emotions and then teach them easier and easier ways to stutter that become closer and closer to spontaneous fluency. Some steps in this approach are depicted in Figure 15.1.

I illustrate our approach to treatment with the case example of David, the 6-year-old elementary school student whom we introduced in Chapter 1.

Author's Beliefs

Nature of Stuttering

In intermediate stuttering, anomalies in the neural pathways supporting speech production, combined with a child's vulnerable temperament, interact with developmental and environmental factors to prevent natural recovery and produce or exacerbate the core behaviors of repetitions, prolongations, and blocks. School-age children respond to these disfluencies with increased tension because of their fear of being stuck and out of control and their efforts to push words out that then makes stuttering worse. As students experience more and more of these increasingly severe core behaviors (tense blocks that stop forward movement), they become distressed because their speech has gone haywire and they can't fix it. In desperation, they blink their eyes or nod their heads to break out of a stutter. They feel embarrassed as their stuttering becomes more severe and noticeable, and they often realize they are the only kids doing it—they are unlike their peers or anyone else they know. And if they do happen to know others who stutter, for example, a father or cousin, they may have learned that these individuals are not open about it.

The more these students stutter when talking to family and friends, the more these students dread it happening again. These moments of anticipatory fear spread via classical conditioning—that is, through the repeated pairing of negative stuttering experiences (emotions) with various sounds, words, and speaking situations. As more of their talking is infiltrated with stuttering, they try to cope by avoiding—dodging feared words and difficult situations, saying "I don't know" when asked a question, or throwing in extra sounds to get a stuck word moving. Avoidance behaviors are reinforced when these tricks seem intermittently successful in preventing stuttering. Because longer and more abnormal stutters lead to more negative listener reactions, children with intermediate stuttering develop the belief that stuttering is bad and, therefore, they are bad when they stutter. Shame about their speech becomes a feature of their daily life. As speech-language clinicians, we want to keenly anticipate this negative emotion and redouble our efforts to help these students experience their own power to resist it.

Because the tension response plus escape and avoidance behaviors, and negative feelings and attitudes are all learned, they can be modified by new learning. The context for this change must be an accepting, supportive environment that focuses on the child as a person, rather than just on his or her stuttering. Many students with intermediate stuttering feel that they have failed in previous therapy, especially if their previous therapy has emphasized fluency above all, and thus have disappointed their parents and teachers by not becoming fluent. Thus, I try to help these children feel accepted with their current level of stuttering as well as help them experience mastery and success with their speech *and* with their communication.

If treatment can provide a student with a sufficient number of emotionally positive speaking experiences in therapy, such as experiences in which they feel "in control" of their speech and their listeners' reaction to it, the increased fluency and positive feelings associated with speaking will generalize to other environments. The clinician can use operant and classical conditioning principles to achieve this increased fluency and generalization, rewarding beneficial changes in stuttering and associating speaking with pleasurable experiences. Furthermore, because possibly long-term predisposing neurophysiological factors may contribute to the core behaviors in the speech of many students who stutter, it is

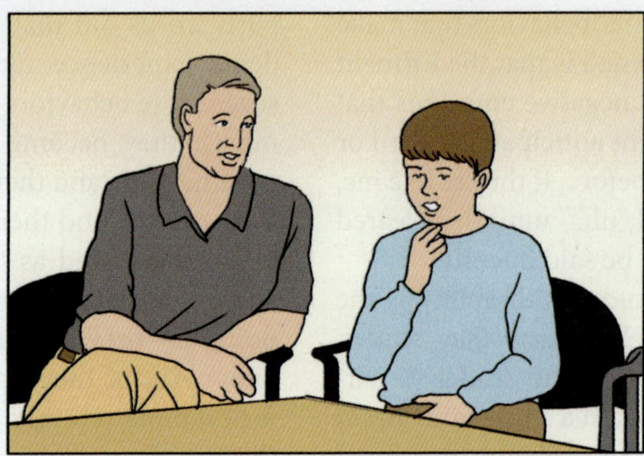

Student Explores His Stuttering

uh-uh-mmm-uh-uh-my
Not quite

Try it with me...mmmmmyyy
mmmmy
Nice job!

Mmmmmmyy stutters are easier now that I'm no longer afraid of them.

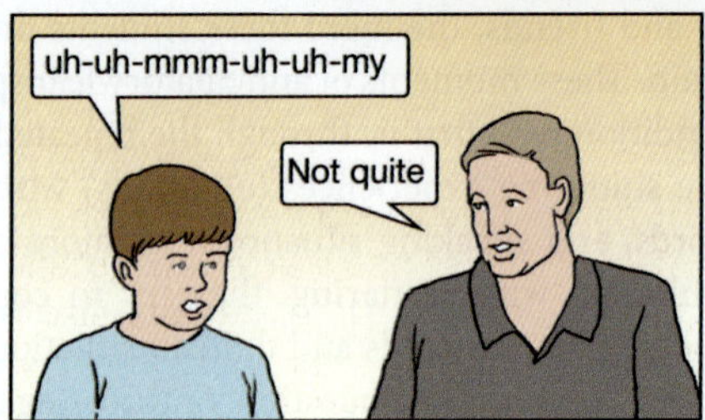

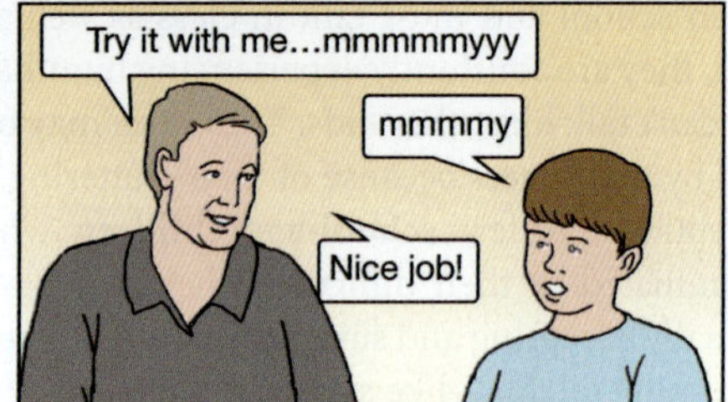

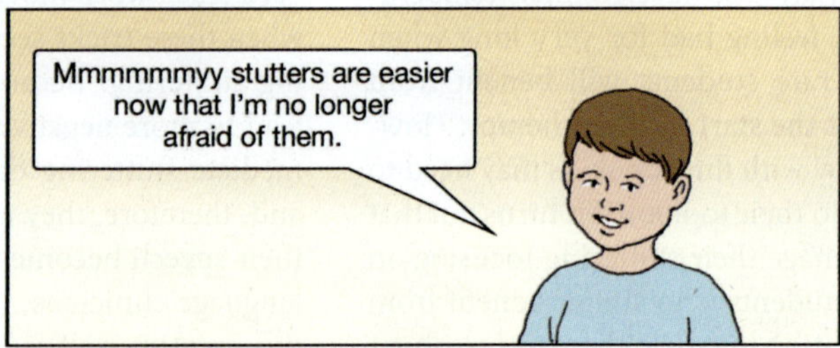

Student Learns to Make His Stutters Easier

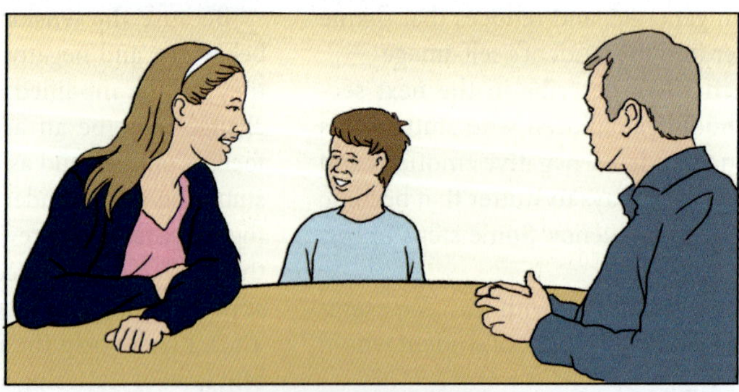

Student Generalizes His Fluency Skills to New Listener

Figure 15.1 Overview of integrated treatment for stuttering.

also important to help them cope effectively with any remaining disruptions in their speech. These twin goals of (1) coping with the remaining stuttering and (2) gaining positive speaking experiences can be achieved using a combination of reducing negative feelings associated with stuttering, increasing self-confidence through success in reducing tension and thus modifying stuttering, and teaching students to stutter more and more easily. In implementing these goals with a school-age child, I find that the child's age and maturity influence the selection of clinical procedures.

Finally, it is important to reduce developmental and environmental influences that may be contributing to the child's stuttering. I can do this by working with the student's parents, the student's classroom teachers, and the student's class, helping

Case Example

David

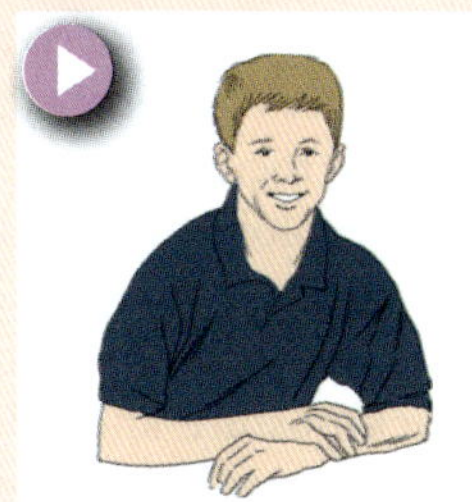

When David was 6, he began weekly treatment with me (and a graduate student), when I was using an early version of the treatment described in this chapter. In the first months of treatment, David was extremely sensitive about his stuttering and unwilling to work directly on it during the exploration stage of treatment. In fact, he wouldn't even discuss his stuttering and would often walk out of the therapy room when I brought it up. My response to his reluctance was to pepper my speech with easy stutters (slightly drawn-out onsets of words lllliiike this). I'd occasionally probe whether he was willing to talk about his stuttering (he wasn't). Our activities were confined to shooting hoops with a basketball net attached to the back of my office door and bowling with plastic pins and balls as I kept up a steady flow of easy stutters. I would sometimes comment that I needed to use easy stutters to control my stuttering (David later said he never believed I really stuttered but was just pretending). One day, David spotted a jar of candies on my desk and asked if he could have one. I traded him one in exchange for him trying an easy stutter. Thus began a steadily effective therapy strategy. Over the next year, he increasingly warmed to the idea of changing his stuttering from hard blocks to easy "slide-outs" (as he called them) while earning candies. The candies always went home in a bag that his mother put away in a drawer and then surreptitiously returned to me for recycling as rewards for easy stutters. David's slide-outs were simply his going into a feared word (or sometimes a word he expected to be fluent on) in a loose easy, slow manner and sliding through it without tension.

I tried to teach David fluency skills such as slowing and **proprioception** but he always favored slide-outs. We practiced slide-outs with many listeners in many different situations. At some point, David decided on his own to keep a score sheet of the number of slide-outs he used in the therapy room and outside. Perhaps because he received a reward for each slide-out, at first, David began to put in slide-outs even on words he wasn't stuttering on. In fact, he had begun using "**voluntary stuttering**" without being aware of that as a technique. Slide-outs became a fluency skill for him. Soon, David would give himself a check mark for each slide-out without my having to tell him; I intermittently praised him after he used a slide-out and he reinforced himself. I think this self-reinforcement of keeping a record of his successes was an important part of his therapy that he invented himself. See the video "David Self-Rewarding & Emotions" on Lippincott Connect that captures both David discussing being scared of stuttering and rewarding himself for slide-outs.

In addition to working on the ease and fluency of his speech, David improved his attitudes about speaking, largely through talking with his class about his stuttering. Always a bit of a ham, David was happy to make presentations to his classes in third, fourth, and fifth grades. He showed posters and video clips he had made, answered questions, and had other students come up and "learn how to stutter." During his elementary school years, the course of therapy was full of bumps and detours, as well as great gains in fluency. Once when his family sold their house and built a new one in a different neighborhood, he was thrown for a loss and started to stutter more severely again. During this time, he was also teased by another student who was having his own problems at home and school. A few months' work with David, his parents, his teachers, and his friends, as well as the child who teased him, brought him through this relapse stronger than ever, and he continued to gain confidence in his speech throughout junior high and high school without further therapy. When he graduated, he was essentially fluent with a few minor repetitions and prolongations.

I should add to this account that David's parents were a major help to his therapy. They were always willing to come to our clinic and talk over his progress (even in the early days when he wasn't making any), as well as promoting therapy activities at home (such as buying him a punching bag to release his frustrations during a relapse). At my suggestion, they tried to reinforce his fluency at home, particularly at the dinner table. This lasted all of 2 weeks and came to a screeching halt when David declared he just wanted to talk and not do therapy at home as well as at the clinic. What he wanted was just his parents' general support of him, which they gave unstintingly.

David's sister and brother were very sympathetic to him when he was going through a bad patch, and David was surprisingly open to talking with them about his stuttering. David was also open with many others about his stuttering, including my class and a local television program. I think another key aspect of his recovery was his participation when he was in high school as a mentor in group therapy for younger school-age children. He was a much-loved "older brother" to the group and helped them immensely by modeling his slide-outs as well as leading them into situations outside the clinic. He even threw in some voluntary stutters to give them courage to try it too.

Recently, David read the above description of his therapy and thought it was accurate, but he said this: "One thing you might want to add was that once I kind of 'owned it' as my thing that made me different, that changed my attitude a lot and helped me become more open about it."

them create an environment that accepts the student regardless of the student's progress with speech, thus helping the student to feel less shame and free to try different ways of handling their stuttering. In addition, I help the child communicate directly with their parents and teachers about how parents and teachers can best help the child deal with their stuttering.

Feelings and Attitudes

How much attention should be given to the student's feelings and attitudes about their speech? A lot. When a student is frustrated, embarrassed, and afraid of stuttering and of speaking, the clinician must help them feel okay about themselves and their speech. Furthermore, because these students are starting to avoid certain words and speaking situations, it is important to reduce these avoidances and fire up the "approach" neural systems in the brain. I discuss this in more detail later in this chapter, but the concept is that activating approach behaviors in students who stutter may stimulate emotions in the left hemisphere that would accompany more relaxed and forward-moving speech. If this is to happen—for the child to change from avoidance to approach emotions and actions—the child must feel the clinician's acceptance of him *as they are now*. This acceptance is conveyed, especially at the beginning of therapy, by the clinician's evident curiosity about what the student is doing when they stutter, why they do it, and whether that helps them. It is also conveyed by the clinician's genuine interest in the student, even apart from their stuttering and fluency. The clinician can discover many positive things to admire in the child and let them know how accomplished they are.

The client-clinician relationship is one of the most important things in therapy (eg, Wampold, 2015). Thus, if the child wants to talk about something other than his stuttering, this can be very healthy and the clinician should listen attentively. Many school-age children have told me, years after therapy, that one of the most helpful things I did was to let them talk about whatever they wanted, and I listened without stopping them to have them work on their stuttering. Your therapy room should be a place where a student can talk about personal issues and not worry about whether they stutter or not.

I have an additional thought about the importance of the clinical relationship. In Chapter 6—when I discuss my perspective on secondary stuttering—I suggested that the reaction that becomes the fear of stuttering starts out as a nonconscious perception of threat: the threat of being out of control and helpless to stop it. An accepting clinician may be a partial antidote to the perceived threat. As the school-age child repeatedly experiences the clinician as an interested and nonpunitive listener—an adult who is on the same team as the child—the child may then let go of some of his or her nonconscious defensive responses. Because there will be failures as well as successes, the clinician will benefit the child most by accepting the failures and really playing up the progress made by successes. The accepting clinician will find things to praise about the failures such as noting what the student did as they made an effort to approach the challenging situation.

Speech Behaviors Targeted for Therapy

The speech behaviors targeted for intermediate stuttering therapy are primarily moments of stuttering. Unlike treatment of beginning stuttering, which focuses on increasing fluent speech, this therapy begins with a focus on stuttering behaviors that are first approached, explored, gradually accepted more, then changed. The change is accomplished by helping the child be present in the moment of stuttering, being able to hold onto the stuck posture and relax and let it go slowly and loosely. This has a profound effect of reducing the fear that was causing the physical tension that has been creating the awful feeling of being out of control.

Fluency Goals

What are the fluency goals that are realistic for school-age children? A few intermediate school-age children who stutter can become typical or spontaneously fluent speakers. This is more likely for younger than for older school-age children. Those who don't become completely and effortlessly fluent will benefit enormously by developing tolerance and acceptance of their remaining stuttering—a truly significant challenge. This acceptance allows them to stuttering more easily as they learn to be present in the moment of stuttering and slowly and loosely finish the word they have been stuck on. The experience of many who have stuttered and have done this is that they are able to stutter in a looser, milder way because when fear which is decreased, tension with all its attendant escape and avoidance behaviors occurs less frequently. Essentially, we are asking the child to stutter in an honest, straightforward way without the ducking and dodging that so often interfere with communication, but instead remain calm as they momentarily accept the stuckness and let the tension diminish. In short, a realistic fluency goal for many intermediate school-age stutterers is acceptable stuttering, that is, fluency mixed with mild or very mild stuttering. For some, the ability to accept the stuttering and make it easier and easier gives them a sense of mastery over something that had previously terrorized them. In fact, many will feel absolutely triumphant when they get stuck in a stutter but are able to look their listener in the eye and dexterously finish the word they are stuck on.

Strategies to Help Maintain Positive Changes

As I described in Chapter 5 on Learning and Unlearning, our primary treatment approach to changing stuttering behavior in schoolchildren is to decouple the link between the conditioned stimulus (stuttering or anticipated stuttering) and the conditioned response (increased tension and struggle and accompanying escape and avoidance behaviors). We do this by helping the child tolerate and accept their stuttering as it is happening and then let them experience the release of tension that happens when they can tolerate and accept their moments of being stuck. Then they can have the triumph of being able to finish the word easily and feel in control. As this happens multiple times, the student's experience of threat and fear gradually decrease so that when they sense an approaching stutter, they now realize—even nonconsciously—that they may not have the conditioned response of increased tension and the expected stutter may be produced easily and loosely. In learning terms, we are "extinguishing" the threat/fear that was triggered by the stuttering. However, research reveals that behaviors that were eliminated by extinction can reappear (1) when some time has passed since the extinction treatment was delivered and (2) when the individual is in a context different from that in which they received the extinction treatment (Bouton, 2016). The effect of the passage of *time* can be seen when individuals are treated in an intensive therapy format and then discharged. Commonly, their stuttering returns, slowly or suddenly, several weeks after treatment ends. Hendrickson (2023) gives a vivid account of this happening in his chapter titled "The Fluency Factory." The effect of *context* is evident in Hendrickson's account: treatment is administered in a protected setting, but the individual needs to go home after therapy and cope with the slings and arrows of his home and work. It is also seen when a child is treated in a therapy room by an accepting clinician and becomes quite fluent but stutters when they go back to his classroom. Change of context had sudden effect on my own speech. When I received stuttering therapy from Van Riper, I left his treatment group prematurely (and against his advice) and started to hitchhike around the country to test my newly fluent speech. I stood on the edge of the highway going out of town with my thumb in the air. The driver of the first car that stopped to pick me up asked me "Where are you going?" I answered, "Chi-chi-chi......Chi-chi-chi......" My stuttering was back, for Round 2. It hadn't given up. But neither had I.

To maintain positive gains, treatment must include strategies designed to keep the extinction of the old fear active for the long term. Treatment should be tapered off gradually rather than end suddenly, and the clinician should maintain intermittent contact with the child for a time afterward. Some students who end therapy with improved fluency can be enlisted as mentors to younger children who stutter. This can help them remember what they did to achieve greater fluency as well as increase their self-esteem. It is probably also a good idea to prepare students for the likelihood that stuttering will bother them again in the future because of the reasons just given. Fear is a tricky foe that will lurk in the new scenery of their future life. Not the students' fault, but the nature of the beast that they are learning to repeatedly put down, and then do their best to exile for the long term.

Clinical Methods

In the first stages of therapy, to help the student reduce negative emotion, I use a combination of (1) listening acceptingly as we talk together about the student's stuttering, including their feelings about being seen as someone who stutters, and (2) joining the student in playing with stuttering—to make therapy fun, to reduce anxiety, to reward hard work, to approach the fear associated with stuttering, and to learn to reduce tension and struggle. When the student is less afraid and not so ashamed of their stuttering, I use modeling and coaching to teach them a different response to the anticipation and experience of stuttering.

I also work with the student's parents and teachers to create "stuttering-friendly" environments that increase the student's comfort using the techniques we learn together in treatment. The measures I use to assess progress are described in the section titled "Progress and Outcome Measures."

Clinical Procedures: Stuttering Modification

In this section, we get down to some of the nitty gritty of therapy—the methods that help us actually achieve the goals we want to our clients to achieve. My clinical methods for intermediate stuttering have been influenced by many people, but Charles Van Riper has been my prime inspiration. Many of the techniques and much of the philosophy in my approach come both from therapy with Van Riper (1973b) for my own stuttering and from the chapter in his treatment book entitled *Treatment of the Young Confirmed Stutterer*. I am also indebted to Julie Reville, who shared her intuitive clinical approaches with this age group. Many activities that she and I developed for treating children with intermediate stuttering are presented in our workbook, *Easy Talker* (Guitar & Reville, 1997). More recently, I have been influenced by Danra Kazenski, my former Ph.D. student and now a colleague in our department at the University of Vermont. She has an exceptional understanding of stuttering and of school-age children. She works with children individually, in small groups, and in large ones.[1] We share so many ideas and strategies that I never know which ones she came up with and which ones I did.

In the next many sections and subsections, I describe the steps of stuttering modification that I use when I work with students. As you read these sections, remember that every student you work with will be different. You should sequence the activities and goals to fit the needs and the readiness of

[1] Danra was recently selected by the National Stuttering Association (NSA) as Chapter Leader of the year. Check out the website she created, with help from NSA: www.burlingtonstutters.org.

each student and you should be flexible enough to change activities and goals if something isn't working. In the Case Example at the beginning of this chapter, you will remember that David resisted therapy for many months. With his family's blessing, I kept him in therapy despite lack of obvious progress and gradually coaxed him into imitating my pretend easy stutters. With rewards (many self-administered) for trying new ways of stuttering, he developed his own tools for speaking more easily that he called "slide-outs." Obviously, this was a luxury that would only be open to a handful of privileged students. Nonetheless, even continued brief contacts may help the child feel supported and be welcome to come back to work on stuttering when they were ready.

Beginning Therapy: Exploring and Changing Stuttering

I start treatment by getting to know the child—who they are, what they like to do after school and on weekends, and all about their family and their pets and their favorite snacks and drinks, and games they like to play, and anything else that comes up naturally in our conversation. I let my real interest in them reveal itself. Most of the time I'm paying attention just to what the student says and conveying that I'm appreciating them as we talk. Their daily life, their favorite activities, and their experiences all provide the metaphors and analogies that we will use as we work together. Some of the time I'm also quietly observing the child's stuttering, to the extent that it shows up in our conversation. As we talk, I convey my comfort with their stuttering by my relaxed attention during their moments of stuttering. At first, I just watch and listen carefully to learn what the child does when they stutter; eventually, when the student seems to be ready, I help them explore their stutters, as described in the following sections.

Exploring

Exploring is the opposite of avoiding; it is an "approach" behavior that can reduce negative emotions. When I proposed a theoretical background for persistent stuttering in Chapter 6, I speculated that the temperament of many children who have developed intermediate-level stuttering might be biased toward avoidance and withdrawal from threatening stimuli. To help them ignite their "approach" neural circuitry[2] (Gray, 1987; Kinsbourne & Bemporad, 1984), I use play to make stuttering approachable. This idea is put into practice by engaging such youngsters in appealing, enjoyable activities that counteract their natural tendency to avoid.

For some students, you may want to use the first "explorations" (eg, deciding about what should be goals of our therapy, and what are our beliefs about stuttering) to help them understand the nature of what you and they will be working together on. For others—those who seem tentative or impatient—you may want to dive right into exploring the core behaviors of their stuttering (see the section with that title further along in this chapter) and then show them how they can change these behaviors. Students who are unsure about being in therapy need an immediate taste of success if they are to buy into the process.

Exploring the Goals of Therapy

A student needs to know where they going in therapy. I begin by letting them know we will draw a map of where we're going together. Depending on the student's age, I will ask them about past therapy, what they learned, and what they'd like to get out of this therapy. Most school-age children will probably answer that they would like their stuttering to be totally gone. I might respond that we can work toward that goal, but then I would ask them if it would be okay if they had a little stuttering sometimes when they're excited or in a hurry. I let them know that at first, they and I will be working to get to know their stuttering and what makes it happen. Then we'll work on helping them make talking easier. I might tell them that this at the very beginning of therapy or after several sessions. It's often helpful to draw some pictures or diagrams to make the activities and sequence of therapy easier to grasp. Figure 15.2 illustrates the possible sequence of therapy for our approach. However, it may help to discuss with the student if this looks ok to them and then maybe the student can help redraw the sequence if they would like to make changes in what you are going to do together.

Exploring Beliefs About Stuttering

A student with intermediate stuttering must be given some explanation for his stuttering. He knows he stutters and has been stuttering probably for a number of years, and he needs to have an explanation for why he talks differently from his friends. So, what do I say to this youngster?

Choosing words that are appropriate for the child's age and comprehension level, I let him know that stuttering is not his fault and that much of it is stuff he couldn't help and you can help him learn a better way to handle his stuttering. I let him know that he must already be a good learner to have learned all the things he does when he stutters. This means he will be good at learning some new, easier ways to talk. To help him realize that stuttering is not his fault, I may say that just like some kids have trouble drawing pictures of things or other kids find it hard to play a musical instrument, he has a little more trouble getting words out smoothly if he is talking fast and has lots of ideas to get out. If he loves to do certain things and is pretty good at them, I will tell them that they are really good at some things, and, like most kids, he will have to practice to get good at speech. I let him know about famous people who also have the same problem, like Ed Sheeran, Bruce Willis, Elvis Presley, Marilyn Monroe, James Earl Jones (Darth Vader in the original *Star Wars* trilogy), Samuel L. Jackson, and Nicholas Brendon (star of the TV show "Buffy

---

[2]Whereas avoidance tendencies are part of right-hemisphere emotions, approach tendences are more likely located in the left hemisphere. Thus, the exploring and play may well kindle these left hemisphere emotions.

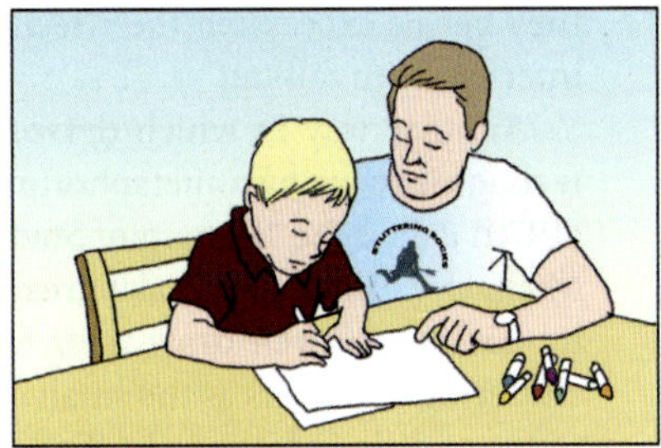

Exploring goals, beliefs, and feelings

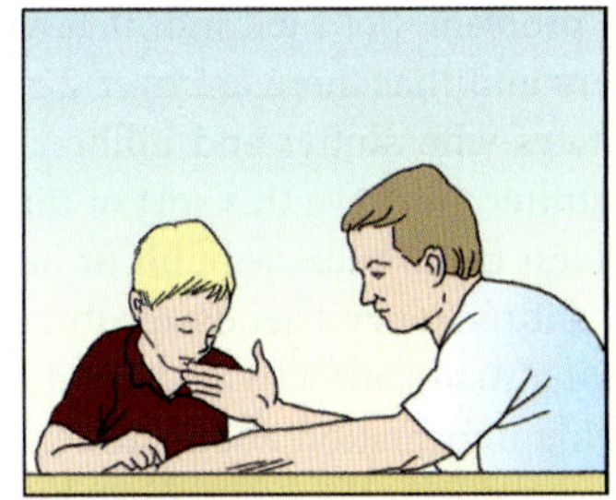

Exploring and changing core behavior

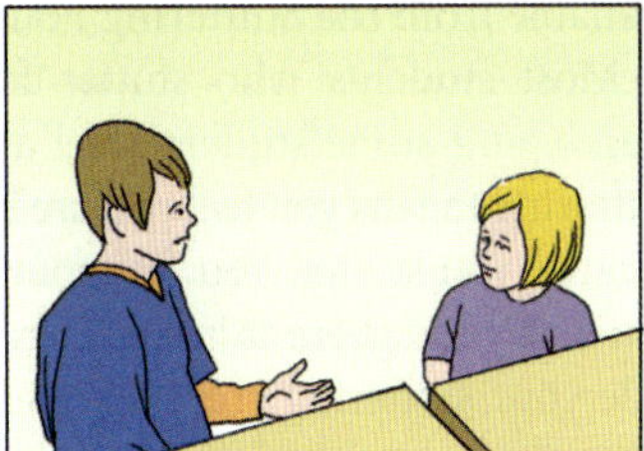

Openness

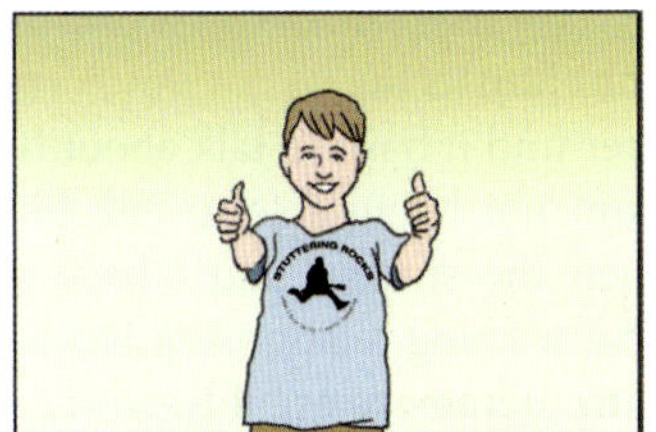

Acceptance

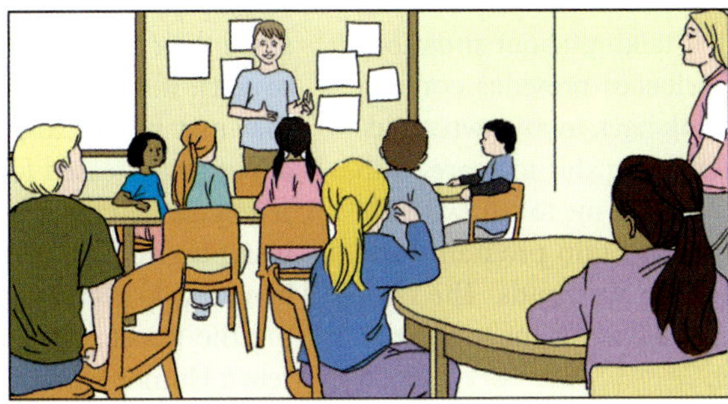

Transfer

Figure 15.2 The sequence of therapy.

the Vampire Slayer"). Jony Ive, the famous designer of the Apple iPhone, Apple Watch, and many other Apple products, stuttered as a young man and was bullied and teased about it, but eventually became typically fluent. Many sports stars also stutter (or used to), such as Shaquille O'Neal and Tiger Woods. Lots of famous people stutter, but they have learned to change their stuttering so it is hardly noticeable, and so can the student. The Stuttering Foundation home page (www.stutteringhelp.org) has a long list of famous people who have stuttered and have lived fulfilling lives, managing their stuttering so it is hardly noticeable.

I go on to explain that any tendency to stutter the student was born with accounts only for the fact that sometimes when he talks fast or is excited or tired, he finds that he stumbles over words. This is the part I call natural stuttering. Other parts, the most bothersome parts, like getting really tight when he stutters or putting in extra sounds or eye blinks, are learned, often when other people are surprised by our stuttering and react in a way that makes us feel weird. If these behaviors are learned, he can change them. One tool I sometimes use to help teach intermediate stutterers about stuttering is the video, *Stuttering: For Kids by Kids*, which is available from the Stuttering Foundation (Scott & Guitar, 2004). This DVD has great examples of kids who stutter talking about the difficulties they face and how they have worked on their speech. One of the videos on Lippincott Connect shows a child describing how useful the *For Kids by Kids* video was to him. In the videos on Lippincott Connect for Chapter 15, Cam's father talks about how helpful the *For Kids by Kids* video was to Cam, during the parent interview (on the video titled "CM: Introduction") and Cam himself talks about how much hope he got by watching the *For Kids by Kids* video when I am talking with him about how his stuttering has been for the past several years, in the Chapter 15 video "CM: Trial Therapy."

In helping a student to better understand their stuttering, I think it is beneficial for them to know that a lot of children stutter and that they are not the only person in the world who stutters. Often, a student may not know any other students who stutter and may believe that he is one of only a very few who have this problem. So, I tell him that about 1 in every 100 kids stutters and that there are over 2 million people in the United States who stutter and millions more around the world who stutter. I believe this sort of information helps a child to feel less alone because of his or her stuttering. Both Friends (https://www.friendswhostutter.org) and the National Stuttering Association (www.westutter.org) have websites that provide information about stuttering for kids and parents and also have annual meetings in which kids who stutter meet other kids who stutter. These meetings are often life-transforming experiences.

Exploring Feelings About Stuttering

Most students who stutter find it hard to talk about the hurt and shame they feel from not being able to talk like their peers. This changes when the student and I have worked together for a while and a trusting relationship has built up. Nonetheless, I try, early in therapy, to see if they will share a little of what they have experienced as they try to navigate a very verbal world with broken words. Van Riper (1973b) suggested that school-age children who stutter are able to talk about difficult situations even if they can't identify difficult sounds and words. He believes that talking about situations in which they have had bad experiences provides comfort and even inspires hope. When I think back to my own childhood, I can imagine feeling relief in being able to share, with an accepting clinician, how hard it was for me to talk with the class about my favorite TV shows and radio programs and what I liked to do after school and on weekends. The class sharing time was mostly a time of dead air for me and probably for most children who stutter.

I ask kids about the times that are hard for them because they stutter. If they are willing to share, I listen attentively and praise them for talking about hard times. I often comment on the experiences and feelings that other children have when they stutter, such as the angry and sad feelings that result from being teased, being told by adults to slow down, having words finished for them, and being interrupted. Together, we go onto the internet and find places where other kids have shared their stuttering experiences, like the "Just for Kids" link on the Stuttering Home Page (http://www.mnsu.edu/comdis/kuster/stutter.html).

I find that some children express their feelings more freely through drawings. Thus, I may ask them to draw pictures of what stuttering is like. I begin by telling the student that some stutters are like a stuck door (or whatever is most relevant to his type of stutters), and I draw something that represents the feeling. I usually make jagged lines to represent frustration and talk to the child about how stutters like that might feel. Then, I ask the child to draw a picture showing how it feels when he gets stuck on a word. In explaining his drawing, the child is often able to express how he feels. Therefore, I use drawing throughout therapy to help the child deal with old feelings of hurt and new feelings that are encountered during various stages of therapy. My experience has been that children's feelings often affect their fluency. The more practice they get in expressing their feelings, the less those feelings interfere with talking.

Another way in which drawings can be used to explore feelings is by using a metaphor proposed by Joseph Sheehan (1970) called the "Iceberg of Stuttering." Clinicians from the Michael Palin Centre make great use of the iceberg analogy by having children draw their own icebergs showing their stuttering behaviors as the small top part of the iceberg above water and their feelings in the large underwater portion. A good depiction of this can be seen in the video mentioned earlier, *Stuttering: Basic Clinical Skills* (Guitar & Fraser, 2007), available from the Stuttering Foundation.

Most students who stutter feel at least a smattering of shame, and some students feel a lot of it. Being ashamed of stuttering means you feel you are bad or stupid or incompetent because you stutter. You feel your parents are disappointed in you and your peers think you are not very cool. You want to hide your stuttering and hide yourself in a closet until it goes away. As you can imagine, the burning urge to hide your stuttering does not help you work on it to change it and make it go away (or at least to decrease it). Because shame wants you to keep your stuttering under wraps, it is hard for students to share their feelings of shame with anyone. But there is a place to start. If the student is able to talk about difficult situations, they may be able to talk about teasing. And how they may feel about being teased for stuttering is one of the faces of shame. If you can tell the child about what other kids have said about being teased, this may get the flow started. Sometimes, I have been able to get a child to draw a picture of being teased. Drawing the teaser as particularly ugly can provide a little comic relief. Humor is often a balm to hurt. There are some links to a section on teasing in the Just for Kids section of the Stuttering Home Page. By looking at them, a child who stutters may realize how most kids who stutter get teased, and they can see what other kids have said to teasers.

Another key to relieving hurt feelings and shame is for a student to let the world (or at least a few friends) know about their stuttering. Being able to tell his class about their stuttering, with the clinician's help, is immensely helpful. It can relieve shame and reduce teasing. If you go to Lippincott Connect, you can watch a video titled "A Child Talks to Her Class About Stuttering showing a class presentation that a child did with her therapist. Also, especially for children in a support group, wearing a shirt that proclaims "Stuttering Is OK!" can be fun. In fact, as I write these words, I'm wearing my T-shirt that shows a leaping guitar player and says in big words "Stuttering Rocks!" Given my last name, this t-shirt's inscription has special meaning to me, but there are lots of similar t-shirts out there.[3]

By now, the student has shared with me their moments of stuttering and their feelings about them. Moreover, the

[3]T-shirts that say "Stuttering Is OK Because What I Say Is Worth Repeating" are available from the Stuttering Foundation www.stutteringhelp.org for $10. Another source of cool things that advertise stuttering is https://www.etsy.com/shop/VTStutteringTherapy.

student has found me to be an understanding and accepting listener. Some deconditioning of speech fears has already occurred. Thus, some basic groundwork has been laid in preparation for the following stages of treatment.

Exploring and Changing the Core Behaviors of Stuttering

I guide a child to approach and explore the core behaviors of their stuttering using three principles taken from treatment research on anxieties and phobias in animals and humans (Mineka, 1985). I believe these are relevant to stuttering because Mineka and her colleagues (eg, Mineka & Oehlberg, 2008) suggest that the uncontrollability of aversive events is an important aspect of the threat they pose to the subjects. You can see the parallel with stuttering. These principles of treatment, adapted for stuttering, are (1) the clinician must be unafraid of stuttering; (2) the student must explore and study their stuttering; and (3) the longer the student is able to remain in contact with moments of stuttering, the more their or her fear will be reduced.

First Principle: The Clinician Must Be Unafraid of Stuttering

Taking the first principle and applying it to stuttering, the clinician can demonstrate their lack of fear of stuttering by showing their curiosity about the student's stuttering. The clinician can listen carefully to what the student is saying but at the same time be noticeably attentive to what the student is doing when they stutter. After getting to know the student and with introductory remarks about wanting to learn about the student's stuttering, the clinician can comment on the student's stuttering. The clinician might tell the student that the clinician needs to learn as much as possible about the student's stuttering in order to help them. Then the clinician would ask the student if it's okay if they make comments on the student's stutters as the clinician tries to study them. Most kids will give at least a reluctant assent. If one particular stutter is more tense or longer than others, the clinician can say "Oh, there was a good stutter. Seems like you really squeezed your tongue when you said that word." This comment has the effect of letting the student know the clinician is more than okay with the student's stutters and even curious about them. Later on in therapy, the clinician can ask the student to teach the clinician how to pretend stutter like the student does, having the student coach the clinician to improve the clinician's stutters so they are more like the student's. The clinician can also show the student the clinician is unafraid of stuttering by taking the lead in practicing in all situations (unless the child wants to take the lead). When I worked in a school system in Washington, DC, I often asked a student to stutter on purpose or make changes to their stuttering when we went into the administrative assistant's office. I always went first, modeling for the student some pretend stutters in my own speech. The clinician should cultivate and renew their own lack of fear of stuttering. The clinician should be able to pseudo-stutter comfortably when talking with the student alone as well as in public to acquaintances and strangers.

Second Principle: The Student Must Explore Their Stuttering

Exploring is the beginning of accepting and potentially changing. In this stage of treatment, the clinician helps the student get in touch with what they are doing when they stutter, and that is the doorway to being able to modify it. Depending on the sensitivity and reluctance of the student, I might begin to discuss the student's stuttering with them when we are drawing pictures, playing a game, or doing something else the student enjoys. Thus, I can alternate between helping the student explore their stuttering and moving back to an activity that is fun. To start, I simply comment on the student's stuttering in an accepting manner. I take note of how they respond and whether they appear uncomfortable or whether they acknowledge their stuttering even subtly and nonverbally when I comment on it. This first approach to stuttering may go quite easily if I have won the student's trust and they are not excessively embarrassed by their stuttering. Those who are very sensitive can be helped to face their stuttering by proceeding slowly.

For an especially sensitive child, I begin by providing them with a feeling of mastery over something else, such as a board game, drawing, or "shooting hoops" in the therapy room. I then alternate between exploring their stuttering and giving them relief through other activities of their choice. See the case example of David at the beginning of this chapter.

As I explore a student's stuttering with them, I not only comment on it but also ask them to describe what they're doing when they stutter. For example, I might say, "Okay, there was an interesting one. What did you do when you stuttered on that word? Where did you feel that stutter?" Then, I help them feel and identify what they actually do when they stutter. For many students, this focus on stuttering behavior—especially if they are rewarded for it—creates an openness about stuttering that can begin to change their emotions from shame and helpless confusion to a more hopeful and objective outlook. For many students, this might be the first time anyone has openly talked with them about their stuttering.

Let me pause for a moment here to say more about rewards. Most students, especially those under the age of 10 or so, are delighted to have frequent rewards for their work. Therapy must be fun, and rewards help make that so. Therefore, when I first begin to work with a student, I ask them about their favorite candies or sodas or other things they'd like as little rewards for their hard work. I also check with the student's parents to make sure they are okay with soda or candy as rewards. As they get older, some students are not as motivated by candy or soda rewards. Some students can work out with their parents a credit system in which a student gets points in treatment as reinforcements for accomplishments. Points are later cashed in for something the parents agree to buy for the child. One example of a point system was developed by a student named Cameron (who agreed to have his name used). When therapy began, when he was 7 or 8, he was happy to get candy rewards; then, when he was older, he said let's drop the candy. He and his parents agreed to a point system that eventually netted him (after many, many points) an electric guitar. Both reward systems (and the electric guitar) can be seen or heard in the videos of his evaluation (see video clips of a diagnostic evaluation of a school-age child on *Lippincott Connect*) and videos of his treatment (see "Cam's Popcorn Video" on *Lippincott Connect*). In high school, Cameron formed a band and they still play together as he works his way through college.

Going back to the early exploration of a student's stuttering, I teach them about "speech helpers," which are the lungs, larynx, and articulators, and their involvement in speech production. A cardboard or plywood cutout of a head, neck, and chest with speech helpers drawn on it may help. For examples, see Exercise 1-1 in *Easy Talker*, our workbook that is listed in Suggested Readings at the end of the chapter; also watch the "Exploring Talking and Stuttering" part of *Stuttering: Basic Clinical Skills*, a DVD available from Stuttering Foundation (Guitar & Fraser, 2007). This part of the video includes having the student get to know their stuttering (and therefore being less afraid) as well as learn to change it.

For a more sensitive student, I start with instructions about how speech helpers work during *fluent* speech and wait a bit before I explore what the student does with their speech helpers when they stutter. For children who are a bit less emotional about their stuttering, I go right into exploring with the student what their speech helpers are doing as the student is stuttering. In this part of treatment, the student learns the parts of their speech mechanism, what they do when they talk, and what they do when they stutter. The student is also learning that stuttering is not a scary monster that attacks them but simply things the student does that hold back their speech as they try *not* to stutter.

As the student and I talk about their speech helpers for younger students or articulators for older ones, I ask them to *feel* what they are doing when they stutter. I ask them to pretend to stutter and make the pretend stutter as tight as a real stutter would be. This is an important moment in therapy. If they can stutter voluntarily (pretend stutters) and be rewarded for it, their fear of stuttering will diminish a little.

If the student is able to do some pretend stutters, we then try to make stuttering fun, crazy, and weird. We have contests to see who can have the longest stutter, the loudest stutter, or the craziest stutter. My colleague Danra Kazenski takes kids through exercises in "silly stuttering" where they play with stuttering and reduce the fear and shame associated with it by having fun with stuttering.

Figure 15.3 shows an example: Danra is having a child show how a monkey might stutter. They are both enjoying this play, and it is loosening up the child so that he can experiment with changes in his stuttering, going from tense and struggled stutters to looser and easier ones that feel in control.

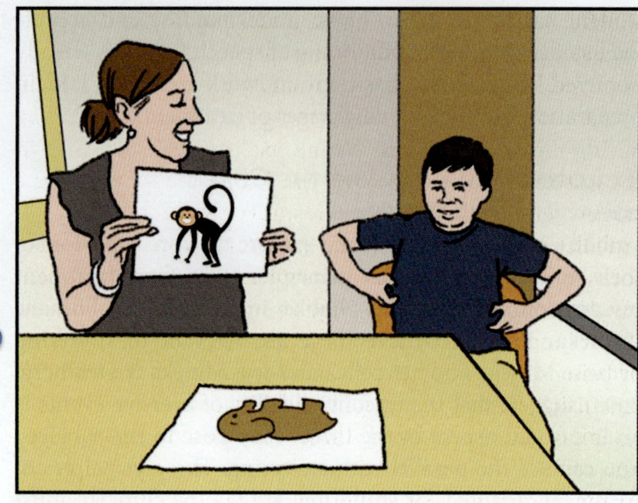

Figure 15.3 Danra and her client Aden Gagne doing "silly stuttering."

Once a child is comfortable with discussing his stuttering and even playing with stuttering, I move to having them reduce their fear of being stuck in a stutter—this is the heart of changing the behavior. I begin by having the child try to "catch me" stuttering. See how I describe it in Chapter 14. The "catch me" game can be played earlier in the flow of therapy, but whenever it is done, it should be adapted to how sensitive the student is. Some children don't immediately like the idea of catching my pretend stutters right at the beginning of therapy, so I may delay this work until after we've explored their stuttering. To start, I throw in a few pretend easy stutters and ask them to let me know, by signaling (pointing at me or saying "there's one"), whenever they notice a stutter in my speech. Easy stutters can be repetitions, prolongations, or blocks, but they are produced slowly and without much tension. In these pretend (or, for me, sometimes real) stutters, I try to stay in (prolong) the actual moment of stuttering (holding onto the posture of the articulators when the stutter is "stuck"), even if it means slightly distorting a stuttered plosive or two. I reward the student when they successfully catch my easy stutters, and I sometimes talk about what I did when I pretended to get stuck. This lets them know that I am not afraid of stuttering and in turn provides a model of talking objectively about stuttering. Clinicians can do this "legitimately" even if they don't stutter. For an older child, it might be useful for them to explain that the clinician doesn't stutter and ask the student if they mind if the clinician does some pretend stutters. Most children know that the clinician's stutters are voluntary and are okay with it. This is especially true if the child has previously coached the clinician to pretend stutter in a way similar to their real stutters.

After several minutes of putting easy stutters in my speech (where I stay in the moment of stuttering) and having them catch me, I ask the child if it's okay if I try to catch their stutters.

As I prepare to describe catching the child's stutters and having them stay in them, let me spell out what "**staying in the stutter**" means and why I use it. The phrase "staying in the stutter" refers to holding onto the stuckness of the stutter—the articulatory posture when the stutter is tense—and letting sound or airflow continue as tension decreases and then ending the word loosely and slowly. The aim is to extinguish the threat (nonconscious) and fear (conscious) that are triggered by being stuck in a stutter. See LeDoux (2015) for an important distinction between threat and fear. These negative emotions can only be damped down if the clinician praises and rewards the student as they continue to stay in the stutter. As the student is more and more successful at this, they will find it easier to do. I also use the phrase "**easier stuttering**" to mean the same thing. With apologies to the reader for excessive terminology, when I refer to a "**high-quality stutter**," I mean one that hits all the targets of "staying in the stutter."

Back to helping the student have a positive experience when I, with the student's permission, catch their stutters: I try to make this as positive an experience as possible for the student, by being pleased with their stutters and sometimes rewarding their stutters when I catch them, helping the student feel good about themselves and their work. As I suggested in Chapter 12: Preliminaries to Treatment, I think the relationship that the clinician has with the student can be a powerful force in helping the student reduce negative emotions (both nonconscious and conscious). The overall goal here is to change how the student feels about the stutters *as they are having them*. Thus, when I catch one of the student's stutters, I use coaching and modeling to help them *stay in the actual moment of stuttering*—the core behavior. Stutters go by very quickly and the student won't particularly enjoy staying in the heart of the stuckness, so it may take a considerable amount of modeling, persuading, and rewarding to have them stay in the stutter and tolerate it. Also, some sounds don't make it easy to stay in the stutter. For example, on a stuttered plosive, it is hard to stay in it and keep some sound or airflow going. On a stuttered /b/ in "Barry," you need to keep your lips together, vibrating, while the /b/ sound is steadily coming out. Yes, this distorts the typically exploded /b/, but it achieves the goal of learning to tolerate and transcend the fear that initially permeates the heart of the stuckness. The sound /p/ can be even more challenging because only the sound of airflow is heard as the posture is held and the lungs continue to expel air. Also particularly difficult are laryngeal blocks that shut off all sound and airflow. You must help the student stay in the posture and gradually get sound or airflow going. For voiced sounds, the laryngeal block can be released and eased out of by using vocal fry. Once the student learns to tolerate the discomfort of staying in the stutter, *in an environment that accepts and even rewards their staying in the stutter*, the fear begins to diminish. And because it's the fear that triggers the tension, the stutters themselves become easier and looser.[4] This experience—of being able to tolerate being in the stuckness of the stutter—done over and over and rewarded by the clinician tends to lead to easier stutters. Then, the child anticipates easier stutters—*stutters that feel in control*. So begins the happy spiral of easier stutters begetting anticipation of easier stutters, leading to more and more and more easy stutters and increased freedom to talk. Once "staying in the stutter" (and having the tension melt away) has been learned fairly well in the therapy room, generalization can begin. Or it may begin to happen spontaneously as the child feels success.

Before I talk in detail about generalization, I thought it would be good to share an example of a school-age child learning to stay in the stutter, keep good eye contact, and release the word slowly once the tension has melted. Recently, when I was looking through old folders for examples of students' work on staying in the stutter, I came across my notes from a session in 1993, when working with a student about 9 years old I'll call "Charlie." Here they are:

> *A good session on Thursday. We began with a chat. He didn't mention stuttering. He asked to have candy. Yes, two pieces. I said I needed help on my book; he described what was going on when he stuttered and moved through it easily. After a little of this, he reiterated how it made him worse to focus on stuttering too much. He asked to play bowling and I said okay if we can make it a reward for holding a stutter and looking at me and then moving through it slowly. We bowled and I rewarded him verbally and with candy when he stuttered. This really took off. He really got a kick out of getting candy so easily and piling it up; he got 10 pieces of candy, had great "managed" stutters with good eye contact, and good easy releases. He even rewarded me when I had some easy ones. At the same time, he was teaching me about bowling and I did really well and he accepted being beaten by me. At the end of the session, as we said goodbye, his mom tried to ask a lot of questions about what he had worked on. When he said bowling and candy, she said she hoped he'd worked on his speech as well; he kind of ignored this, and went on about something else. I must find a tactful way of talking to her about this—I think she'll bring it up.*

In addition to making notes after each session, I sometimes video record parts of therapy, with the child's permission. After he does some particularly good work, I ask him if he'd like to see the video clip of it. Video playback works particularly well if the child can be put in charge of recording and playback. Some students will get a kick out of learning to

[4]In the video clips for evaluation of school-age children, one clip called "Trial Therapy" demonstrates how a clinician can coach a child (Cameron) into staying in the stutter and letting it go easily.

edit their videos so they look and sound pretty good. Lippincott Connect contains a video called "Cam's Popcorn Video" in videos for Chapter 15 that shows what a school-age client and his graduate clinician can put together to show his family and his friends what he's doing in therapy. When we finished the video, he asked if we could send it to India to help children there. Recently, I let him know that his video is being seen around the world.

Third Principle: The Longer the Student Is Able to Remain Calm in Contact With Moments of Stuttering, the More His Fear Will Be Reduced

The third principle taken from the phobia treatment literature (Mineka, 1985) suggests that extended amounts of time in contact with feared object (stuttering) will help reduce fear of it. The idea of being "in contact" with stuttering behavior may have an important meaning in the context of speech motor control. A student who has been stuttering persistently for several years may have lost easy access to proprioceptive awareness (nonconscious physical feeling) of their speech or may never have had it to an appropriate degree. This may make it difficult for them to use proprioceptive information to coordinate speech movements. Therefore, as a child explores their stuttering, I help them increase their conscious awareness of what they're doing when they stutter, particularly for more severe moments of stuttering. If I can guide them to stay in the moment of stuttering until it's likely that they *can* release the block, they can feel what they're doing and then will realize that they can control the tension and movement of their speech structures. *The shift that they will feel as they hold on to stutters for an extended period of time will seem like a change from being out of control to being in control.* It is, as we say to our kids, "Showing the Stutter Who's Boss." The feeling of being in control may indeed result from a change in the activity of brain areas that control speech movements. It may be a shift from a motor area of the brain that is not well supplied with sensory feedback to a motor area with better sensory information that controls movement. This shift in brain areas has been shown to be a correlate of motor movement that is changed to become under the subject's control (Guitar et al., 1988; Humphrey & Reed, 1983). For a good example of a student staying in contact with a moment of stuttering, see the video of Dean Williams on *Lippincott Connect*.

Another interesting video of staying in the stutter and showing the stutter who's boss is titled "Allison's Video," which is in the Chapter 15 videos on Lippincott Connect. It shows a 9-year old girl playing with her stuttering with the help of a clinician who is making the whole enterprise lots of fun.

Openness, Acceptance, and the Beginning of Mastery

At this point in therapy, the student is starting to feel less embarrassed and ashamed about stuttering. They are not so terrified when their articulators seize up and their listener looks down. Now, they are on their way toward mastering what was once, to them, a fatal flaw. For a student with intermediate-level stuttering, working for this mastery is a lifelong process. At first, it takes immense effort and attention—his stuttering has been Darth Vader, Voldemort, and Goliath, all rolled into one. But when teaming up with a strong clinician, supportive parents, empathetic peers, and caring teachers, stuttering can be sent packing or at least cut down to size. Gradually, success is no longer measured in fluency but in little moments of manageable stuttering.

Being Open About Stuttering

A major milestone for the child traveling along the road toward mastery of easier stuttering is becoming more open about stuttering. The clinician, by their own models of voluntary stuttering in public places, can inspire the student to talk about stuttering casually with friends, to refer to it in humorous ways when it happens, and to educate people about it. Children differ widely in their readiness to be open about their stuttering. However, once most of them feel some sense of mastery over immobilizing fear that has made them feel helpless in the past, they are much more able to let people know about it. If a student stutters in class, I rehearse casual comments that they can make about their stuttering when, for example, they are giving an oral report or answering a question in class. The student might say, for example, "My report is about how maple syrup is produced. Before I begin, I just want to say that I'll probably stutter sometimes while I'm talking, but don't let it bother you. I might take a little longer than most reports but I assure you it will be over!" Or the student might say, "I'll probably stutter, but it's no big deal." Basically, it is not so much the content that is important as the fact that the student acknowledges their stuttering and that they're coping with it. They feel good that they have acknowledged it, and their audience is more comfortable than if they stutter and try to hide it. One vehicle a student can use to be open about their stuttering with family and friends is a zany video about stuttering that they make with their clinician. Take a look at the music video clip of Allison and her clinician dancing with stuttering. It's on *Lippincott Connect* and is titled "Allison's Video."

A student may also benefit from developing a repertoire of casual comments to make about their stuttering if they get particularly hung up on a word while talking to friends, relatives, or strangers. They might learn to say, "Wow! I really got hung up there," or "I'm really running into a lot of blocks, but let's get on with it." In my experience, the most effective comments are those that the student comes up with spontaneously when they feel comfortable with their stuttering. These are unforced, often funny remarks that put the child and his listeners at ease, like saying "Who burped?" after you have an unexpected burp.

Teaching other children and teachers about stuttering can be a powerful tool in combating the shame and embarrassment that often accompany a student's stuttering. Although this can be done with small groups of students brought into the therapy room or in meetings with the child and their teachers, our experience has been that eventually sharing information about stuttering in front of the entire class is extremely effective for many children. When and if a student is ready to do this, we work together to prepare, rehearse, and then give a presentation that informs the class about stuttering in general and the student's own stuttering in particular. A question-and-answer period is a crucial part of the presentation because it gives the student's classmates a chance to express their curiosity about stuttering. It also gives the student an opportunity to demonstrate their expertise in the very behavior that previously made them feel so helpless. We usually bring along some item of interest to share with the class, such as a YouTube video of a famous person who stutters or a cell phone app with a Delayed Auditory Feedback so the child can let his peers experience the kind of stuttering that results from trying to talk with the delay.

Here is an example of how this can work. A second grader who was very sensitive about their stuttering was also rather proud of a brief segment on a local television station that showed him working on his stuttering. He was willing to show a video of this segment in class and answer questions about his stuttering. The following year, I accompanied him to class for a full-scale presentation about stuttering. This presentation included posters he had made, demonstrations of therapy techniques, and a question-and-answer segment. A year after this program, the child had a particularly rocky beginning to the school year because his stuttering had returned full force after his family moved to a new house in a new neighborhood. However, he was still willing to do another presentation with me. This time, he used more video clips of himself talking, because he was more reluctant to talk at length; however, he talked to the class about some of the "ups and downs" in his progress with stuttering.

Another example of openness is the experience of is a second-grade student, Nejla, who came to therapy in our clinic, accompanied by her public school clinician. Together, they produced a brief video with jazzy music to show to her class as the centerpiece of a live presentation she made with both the school clinician and the graduate student she worked with in our clinic. The presentation to her teachers and peers can be seen in the video clips on *Lippincott Connect* for Chapter 15 titled "A Child Talks to Her Class About stuttering."

Accepting Stuttering

The therapy, up to this point, has usually made the student a tiny bit more accepting of their stuttering, but the road to real acceptance is often long. In fact, true mastery of managing stuttering includes being able to accept failure some of the time. As you have gotten to know the student, you and they will probably be able to come up with some helpful analogies for acceptance of failure in the world of performance. What does the student admire? Ballet? Soccer? Baseball? Music? Farming? Car racing? Cooking? In any performance—in any endeavor that humans try to master—there is some failure. Mastery comes not from intolerant perfectionism but from being able to miss the target at times and keep on trying. As LeBron James (four-time most valuable player in the National Basketball Association) has said, "You have to be able to accept failure to get better." (https://www.quotezine.com/lebron-james-quotes/).

When the California State Fullerton baseball team started out with a losing season in 2004, a professor of kinesiology at the university got the team together and gave them advice to forget any bad plays or poor at-bats they'd had in the past, "flush them down the toilet," and concentrate on now. To keep them from forgetting his advice, he gave the team a miniature toilet that they put at the top of the dugout during each game. When they won the College World Series at the end of that season, their championship rings were engraved with the words "Next Pitch" (Witz, 2018). A child who stutters can be taught to forget past bad experiences and just concentrate on what he is doing now. Even if he fails, he can focus on the things he did right.

The clinician can be vital in helping the student accept his failures and find the little successes. This will come up frequently as the student is trying to master staying in the stutter, letting the tension release itself as threat and fear go down, and ending the word slowly. When the clinician provides a model that the student isn't able to match, they can find some things about the student's try that the clinician can praise. For most people, feeling good about a try helps them use feedback about what they need to adjust their aim. So, when a student stays in a stutter for only a brief moment and then ends the word quickly, let him know enthusiastically that he made a good try. Then give them another model and have them produce the stutter *along with you*. Having them stutter along with you will help them come closer to the target and will deserve some enthusiastic praise.

I'll return later in this chapter to the idea of accepting stuttering and missed targets, especially when we talk about transferring new skills to the world beyond the therapy room. For now, I'll recommend some very informative reading relevant to this topic. In the book *More Than Fluency* (Amster & Klein, 2018), there are two chapters that will give you many ideas about helping students deal with stuttering that happens even when they are trying not to. "Avoidance Reduction Therapy for Stuttering" is one chapter and "Acceptance and Commitment Therapy for Stuttering" is another.

Another idea about accepting stuttering came from a poem about stuttering that started us helping children develop positive responses to their stuttering. Several years ago, a graduate student and I were helping a 10-year-old girl learn to stop fighting her stutters and learn to handle them with grace and ease. One of the steps in her exploring her stutters was to get to know her stutters and "make friends with them." The graduate student, Charles Barasch, wrote a poem for the girl to help her accomplish this:

Getting Unstuck (Reprinted from the book *Home Movie* (2022, Finishing Line Press) with permission of the author.)

for a young girl who stutters
When breath hides in your stomach
like a fish under stone,
and when it's hooked thrashes
and teases, dive down and follow,
let it think it's pulled you in
while you swim past swaying weeds,
through the shadow and light
inside yourself. And when it thinks
it owns you, sing to it like a mermaid,
it will fall in love with you
and do whatever you want.
It will follow you home
and be your liveliest companion,
it will dance for you
and do tricks for your friends,
you will think you've never met anyone
so intelligent or funny.
The house you set up together
will be happy until the end of your days.

We have found that if students can have a creative response to their stuttering, by making their own poems about stuttering, drawing pictures of their stuttering, or making models of what stuttering is like using Play-Doh, the hurt is somewhat healed. One of the school-age children we worked with recently sent a letter and drawing to the Stuttering Foundation website to have it displayed for other children to see. If you have a student who would like to have his or her creative endeavor displayed on the website, go to this page: https://www.stutteringhelp.org/drawings-and-letters-kids/.

Transferring New Skills to the Real World

If you have taught your student who stutters to go right into the stutter and hold onto it (with intermittent praise and rewards from you) until the tension is reduced, ending it slowly, and if they can do it reliably in the treatment room, it's time for transfer. Your student may be already transferring their skills to their speech with their family, especially if their parents have been supporting and reinforcing his practice. Now is the time to prepare for transfer by planning hierarchies and engaging in voluntary stuttering and **desensitization.**

Voluntary Stuttering

Voluntary stuttering has been around for a long time, at least since Van Riper's own therapist (Bryng Bryngleson) taught him to use it in the 1930s. Bloodstein et al. (2021) have a good description of the origins and evolution of voluntary stuttering. When I work with students, I often ask them to voluntarily put in their speech the target we started shooting for during the exploration phase of treatment: staying in the stutter. We begin doing this in the therapy room. Once the student has been able to emulate my model of holding onto the stuttered sound, letting the tension release, and ending it slowly, I ask them to put in pretend stutters using that technique of stuttering. In fact, many of the students I work with will spontaneously use voluntary high-quality stutters to earn rewards. When I dole out rewards, I don't discriminate between real and voluntary/pretend stutters, in part because I often can't tell the difference. And the student may not be able to discriminate either. Getting rewarded for these voluntary high-quality stutters makes them feel like little victories. As we transfer these skills, the positive feelings associated with these stutters help to counteract the discomfort of being perceived as a kid who stutters in real-world situations, like when talking with friends.

Eye Contact

Although in some cultures, eye contact between speaker and listener is not always appropriate, improving culturally appropriate eye contact has long been a consideration in stuttering therapy. As clients become more open with listeners about their stuttering and work on easier stuttering in public, improved eye contact is often a target of treatment. In her fascinating book on dog behavior, Horowitz (2009) describes how eye contact in dogs and wolves can be an assertion of authority and it may sometimes work that way for humans. However, Senju and Johnson (2009), researchers studying eye contact suggest that "In humans…eye contact provides a foundation of communication and social interaction" (p. 127). Just what we want as we work with stutterers learning to be comfortable talking in public. To me, another benefit of working on eye contact in our therapy is that increased eye contact is an element of approach behavior, which is accompanied by left-hemisphere emotional activation increasing not only approach behavior but also exploration and release of ongoing behavior, as I described in Chapters 3 and 6 and is discussed in detail in Davidson (1984), Kinsbourne (1989), and Kinsbourne and Bemporad (1984). Thus, in my view, increasing culturally appropriate eye contact, as stutterers transfer their modified stuttering and fluency skills into the public, decreases inhibitions generated from right hemisphere emotions, reducing physical tension and allowing freer and easier speech. In addition, normal eye contact with listeners enhances communication and helps meet the goal of not only easier speech but improved communication. At the same time, it's important to be real. If you've ever engaged in a casual conversation in which eye contact is mentioned, you've probably found that you experience a marked feeling of awkwardness, wondering if your own eye contact is overly intense, too fleeting, or otherwise out of whack with what is "normal." It's important to share this observation with children working on this issue. Further, if the child has a coexisting diagnosis of autism spectrum disorder (ASD), the issue of eye contact becomes even trickier, an idea I will return to in a later section of this chapter.

Desensitizing Students to Difficult Situations and Challenging Words

Most students who stutter have some bugaboo situations in their daily lives that trigger stuttering. For me, it was reading Bible verses aloud in Senior Boys' Sunday School as we went around a room reading aloud, in an old barn that was heated only by a woodstove. Sometimes we read the New Testament and so the sound /ʤ/ in the word "Jesus" was often a challenge because it came at the beginning of so many verses. For kids I've worked with, difficult situations often included being called on in class, being asked to say their name, and telling a joke or a story about something that happened to them. We begin desensitization by developing a hierarchy of situations in which we will practice high-quality stutters.

Planning a Transfer Hierarchy

I think it would be too daunting for most children to plan a hierarchy filled with all the situations that are hard for them, so we just begin with a few not-too-hard ones. Desensitization means simply working on high-quality stutters in situations that are challenging. Thus, you and the student think of a situation that is slightly hard, plan what the student might say in this situation, and then start by role-playing the situation in the therapy room. For example, the transfer hierarchy might begin with a situation called "Someone asks you your name" (if that's a challenging situation for the child). At first, the clinician asks the student his name in the therapy room and the child has a high-quality stutter, either real or voluntary (ie, pretend). Then they might go into the hallway outside the room and repeat the situation with me. At some point, the child might feel comfortable enough to do this with another adult, such as a parent or a school staff member, along with me. Once the work is being done outside the therapy room, like in the administrative assistant's office, rewards and praise might be saved until the child and clinician get back to the therapy room and are alone together, unless the child is happy getting praise or a tangible reward in public.

An example of a hierarchy involving some of the steps in therapy that we have described in this chapter is shown in Figure 15.4.

Transfer Activities

Reducing Fears Related to the Classroom

Let's consider the situation of a student being afraid to speak aloud in the classroom. In this case, I would invite, with the

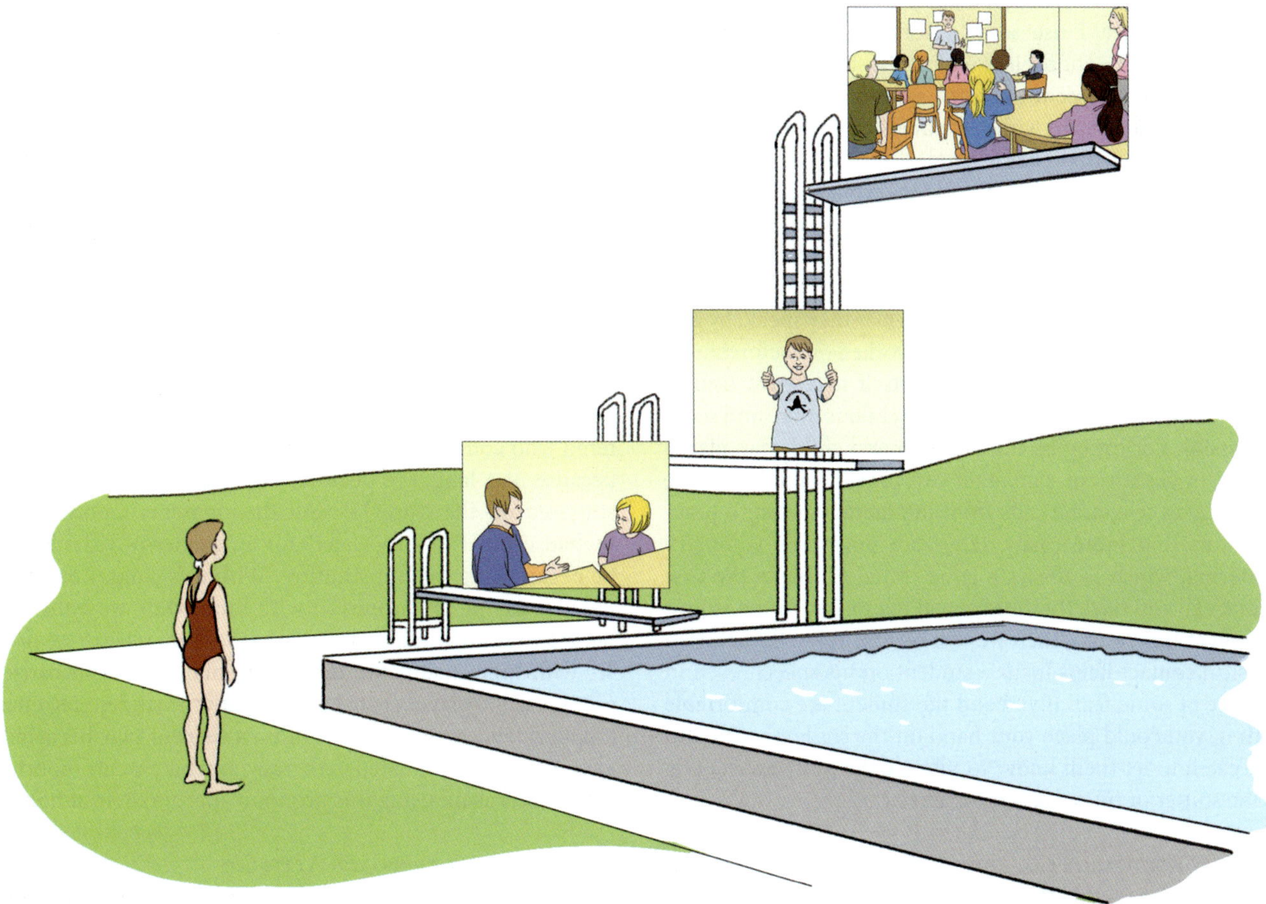

Figure 15.4 Using an easy-to-hard hierarchy to overcome fear and avoidance.

student's consent, one or two of their classmates into therapy. I would play the role of the classroom teacher and have this small group of two or three children ask and answer questions. When the child begins to feel comfortable doing this, I would expand the group to three or four classmates. Next, it might be helpful for the student and the rest of us to go to their classroom during the noon hour or at recess. After explaining our goal and therapy procedures to the classroom teacher, I would have the student sit at their desk and have the teacher ask questions about their lessons. These activities are about as far as I can go in simulating a student's fear of this situation. The student needs to take the last step of these therapy procedures by themselves. They have been successful in a series of situations that successively approximate their feared situation, and their classroom teacher is now sensitized to the student's problem and understands the student's therapy. The chances are that after some initial ambivalence, the student will overcome their reluctance to talk in class. But of course, that will not be all the time; it will probably vary from day to day and week to week.

Scaffolding

I have found it useful with some children to "scaffold" their staying in the stutter during transfer activities by creating a stuttering-friendly environment, letting the listener(s) know that *we* are working on *our* speech. If the clinician doesn't stutter, the child is probably happy with listeners thinking they both stutter. I use some voluntary (pretend) stuttering, staying in the stutter and ending loosely, as a model and encouraging the student to do the same. I am always careful to plan this beforehand with the student and ensure that they are comfortable with it. For example, I may tell a stranger in a mall that the student and I are working on our speech and we'd like to ask them some questions. Depending on the student's readiness, I may ask the first question or the child may. If the situation has been difficult in the past, I may coach the student in their use of staying in the stutter, as they speak, by giving them subtle signals that we have worked out beforehand.

Transfer on the telephone lends itself to a great deal of scaffolding, which can be faded as the child is more and more successful. For example, the clinician and child may plan a variety of gestures or signs that can provide support as the child makes telephone calls from the therapy room to practice stuttering more easily. If we are practicing voluntary stuttering, which is always a good thing, I'll make the first phone call and have the child signal me to stay in the stutter whenever they want. Then we will reverse roles. Sometimes, physical contact helps focus a student on his speech even in the face of some fear. If you and the student are comfortable with it, you could place your hand on the student's arm and squeeze it to let them know you notice that they are staying in the stutter or offer a fist-bump afterward.

More on Reducing Fear and Avoidance

Some children take a little longer than others to transfer their ability to stay in the stutter and let the tension melt before finishing the word slowly. Their learned fears and avoidances may be particularly strong and may require a concerted effort to overcome. The right analogies or comparison can help many children in this situation to deal with their fears. I get them to think about other fears they have overcome or about people they know, such as family members, who are afraid of such things as the dark, bugs, snakes, spiders, or swimming in deep water, and I enlist the student's help in listing ways they might overcome their fears. I also look for examples in pop culture of fearless leaders or those who overcame obstacles, like Batman Harry Potter, Spiderman, or Ninjago. By analyzing how people get over their fears and describing the rewards of facing fears and conquering them, I am often able to motivate students to tackle their fears of difficult words and situations.

Sometimes, we forget that fears are very natural, and perhaps some fears—like a fear of crocodiles—are important to help us survive. Let students know that it's natural to be worried about words or situations that have given them trouble in the past. But they should also know that the fear of these things itself causes them to tense up and likely plays a role in their stuttering. Here are some steps to help them to reduce their fears: (1) be okay with having some fear; (2) study the words or situations so they can learn about them; (3) practice staying in the stutter over and over before going into real-life challenging situations; and (4) get rewarded for going ahead and trying something despite their fear, even if they're not completely in control of their stuttering. In fact, if the student can just shoot for making their stuttering gradually less and less tense, it will be an easier target to hit, and they will succeed more and more.

Reducing Word Fears

It is usually easier to help students overcome their fear and avoidance of particular words than of particular situations. This is because the clinician can provide students with more support in confronting word fears in the therapy room than they can provide them when students confront their situational fears in daily life. The clinician can also use feared words over and over again within the therapy situation. For example, I worked with a young school-age student who stuttered who consistently substituted "me" for "I." This was not because of a language disorder but because he consistently stuttered on the word "I," and their parents reported that he had used "I" appropriately for a number of years before he began using this substitution. With this child, I began to practice saying "I" in unison with him, while we both pretended to stutter on it and stayed in the stutter. Next, we used "I" with high-quality stutters many, many times in carrier phrases while playing games. Gradually, the student regained his confidence in saying "I." Within a week or two, his avoidance of "I" was eliminated in therapy, and his parents reported that he was again using this pronoun appropriately at home.

Developing an Approach Attitude

In working on their fears and avoidances, students must understand (as we've suggested before) that they don't have to be completely successful in using high-quality stutters in all situations all of the time. In fact, as they first tackle feared words and situations, they may stutter in their old ways many times, and even a long time later, that same stuttering can come back. Even so, students should be rewarded for trying. The "approach attitude," which we sometimes refer to as "seeking out" (Guitar & Reville, 1997), may reduce fear and tension so that high-quality stutters are more obtainable. Repeated exposure to these feared words or situations, when supported by the clinician, will make a big difference in applying new skills to feared words and situations. The student-clinician relationship is paramount here. With a clinician who is highly supportive of the student and who models approach behavior, the student can override an avoidance-prone temperament and gradually develop approach attitudes and behaviors. My own therapy with Van Riper was successful in part because he was alive with a "Damn the torpedoes, full speed ahead!" persona and I have carried his image around in my imagination ever afterward.

Coping With Teasing

It is important to minimize teasing that a student is receiving because of their stuttering. The clinician can deal with this at any time, but it may be helpful to address teasing after the student has mastered some fluency skills and is transferring them. (I address this issue in more detail when I discuss counseling parents and classroom teachers.) Regardless of how hard parents, teachers, clinicians, and friends may try to eliminate teasing, I doubt that it is possible to eliminate all of it. Thus, I try to give a child some defenses against the teasing that he is likely to receive.

I agree with Van Riper (1973a) that the best defense against teasing is acceptance if a child is emotionally mature enough to feel and express acceptance. For example, if a child can say, "I know I stutter, but that doesn't give you the right to make me feel bad about it," or some similar statement, this will disarm most teasers. Nobody likes to tease someone who does not appear to be bothered. Running away, on the other hand, just reinforces teasing. Nevertheless, I have found that it is difficult for a school-age child to calmly accept and admit their stuttering when they talk to their tormentors. When I have been successful, I have done the following things.

First, I discuss the importance of calmly and openly admitting stuttering to teasers, rather than saying nothing. I explain how this type of response usually discourages teasers. I then explore with the student the sorts of statements they can imagine themselves making. The words they use must be words with which they feel comfortable. Next, I initiate role-playing with the student. As I play the role of the teaser, the student's task is to respond calmly to my heckling. They practice saying the types of statements they have chosen to use to counteract the teasing. I role-play this many times until the child feels comfortable with their response and can see themselves doing this in a real-life situation. Finally, the day comes when they try out this new behavior. I hope it works, but if it does not, I will be available to give the child support and encouragement in our next meeting.

I have also found that if I have two or more students who stutter or if I can form a group of several children who have speech or language problems, we can write and perform a play together about a child who stutters who triumphs over teasing.

Some children are especially sensitive to teasing and need patience and understanding as they work to develop effective responses. These children may have more inhibited temperaments, and their first reaction to a threatening situation is to withdraw or avoid. Hence, these children need practice in asserting themselves. In our role-playing, I experiment with a variety of ways in which the child can feel that they confronted the teaser. For some children, it might be teasing back; for others, it might be reporting the teaser to a teacher or the principal. A tactic taught by Bill Murphy, an experienced speech pathologist who also stutters, is to have children say "So?" back to the teaser after every taunt. Because it's a short utterance, children who stutter can often say it fluently and with gusto. Other excellent advice is contained in publications by Hughes (2014); Murphy et al. (2013); and Yaruss et al. (2018). A good list of resources related to teasing of children who stutter can be found at http://www.mnsu.edu/comdis/kuster/infoaboutstuttering.html#teasing/.

Maintaining Improvement

By this point in therapy, a student is usually speaking well in most situations. They are having a great deal of natural fluency in many situations and high-quality stuttering in others. Their speech fears and avoidances have been eliminated or significantly reduced. I do not dismiss the student from therapy at this point but gradually phase them out of therapy. I typically see a student for therapy once a week, even after major changes have been made and stabilized, then and decrease frequency to a twice-monthly basis for another month or so. If all continues to go well, I see them for a series of "checkups" over the next 2 years, first monthly, then bimonthly, and finally once a semester.

During these checkups, I obtain samples of the student's speech and oral reading and discuss with the student how they have been talking in everyday speaking situations. I also interview the student's parents and classroom teacher about the student's speech at home and school. If I find that the student's fluency has regressed or that they have begun to use avoidance behaviors again, I re-enroll the student in therapy. My experience is that some students may have one or two mild regressions before their fluency stabilizes. Such regressions are often associated with the beginning of a school year or with transfers from one school to another or with other disrupting factors.

When I return a student to therapy, it is usually for only a month or two. During these "booster" sessions, the student may need to have their stuttering management skills "tuned up." They may need a brief refresher course on the importance of not avoiding, or they may just need an opportunity to talk to an understanding listener about their stuttering. In time, these regressions and our reevaluations become further apart until finally the day arrives when the student, their family, and I decide to dismiss the student from treatment. My hope is that even though "dismissal" sounds rather final, the student realizes that they have an ally in me and in other Speech-Language Pathologists (SLPs) who know about stuttering. That attitude could help the student return to treatment if they think they need some additional help—in a month, a year, or a decade.

Clinical Procedures: Teaching Fluency Skills

A focus on fluency in students has a long tradition. In his chapter *Treatment of the Young Confirmed Stutterer*, Van Riper (1973a) advocates building up a student's fluency: "We always try to increase the amount of fluency in these children, and we want them to feel it and recognize it when it does occur rather than to focus their attention only on the stuttering" (p. 434).

One use of fluency skills is for the rare school-age students who are more like borderline stutterers in their relative lack of fear toward stuttering. They don't need the procedures described at the beginning of this chapter: exploring stuttering, staying in the stutter, and other stuttering modification strategies aimed at extinguishing fear. Instead, these rare "low-fear" students may need only a small amount of desensitization, and they can begin therapy by learning fluency skills to ease stuttering. Fluency skills are ways of producing speech that are likely to reduce stuttering. However, one must be cautious in teaching fluency skills, because they have been misused when they are taught as the only way to reduce stuttering. Remember: stuttering is acceptable. But there is no need for students to struggle and sweat when they are stuck. Fluency skills can make stuttering easier and reduce the Herculean efforts some stutterers make to get words out.

Another use for fluency skills is to help students who do fear stuttering but seem to be unable to make progress in desensitization until they have increased their fluency—seeing some hope for their speech and motivating them to stay in therapy. They may benefit from work on fluency skills training and then work on desensitization. Still other students may have benefitted from stuttering modification but feel they need to learn more to really solidify their increased fluency and may benefit from a period of focusing on fluency. By contrast, some students who have done well with stuttering modification therapy are just burdened by learning fluency skills. David, who is featured in the case example at the beginning of this chapter, decided that fluency skills were not helpful after he had made great gains using stuttering modification. Thus, we didn't spend a lot of time having him work on fluency skills.

Clinical Procedures: Working With Parents

I have five goals in mind when working with parents of an intermediate stutterer: (1) explaining the treatment program and the parents' role in it, (2) discussing the possible causes of stuttering, (3) identifying and reducing **fluency disrupters**, (4) identifying and increasing fluency-enhancing situations, and (5) eliminating teasing. I will discuss each of these goals in turn.

Explaining the Treatment Program and the Parents' Role in It

First, I discuss the stages of our therapy program with the student's parents, letting them know how I hope to take the mystery out of stuttering for their child by exploring with their child what they do when they stutter. I also tell the parents about our goal of teaching their child to hold onto stutters and learn to tolerate the previously feared stuckness of stuttering in order to release the tension. To the parents, it may even sound like their child is stuttering more when they use staying in the stutter to reduce the tension. It's important that I not only demonstrate this strategy for the parent but also have them try it and get good at it so they will know what to be pleased with in their child's speech. Second, I tell the parents that therapy may take time, perhaps 1 to 3 years and in some cases even longer. Third, I inform them that communicating with their child about their stuttering is important and that they should express their acceptance of their child's stuttering and acknowledge their understanding that it is often difficult for him to work on it.

Explaining the Possible Causes of Stuttering

I believe it is important for the parents of a school-age student who stutters to be given an explanation of the possible causes of stuttering. I explain current thinking about the nature of stuttering. In some cases, parents have no information about the causes of stuttering. Since I want them to participate in their child's treatment, they need to understand the rationale for our treatment program. Many parents feel guilty about their child's stuttering because of some outdated or inaccurate information they may have. They may have been exposed to an explanation that is no longer considered valid, or they may have been given some erroneous information by a well-meaning but misinformed friend or relative. Such parents then blame themselves for some supposed misdeed on their part. They need good, current information about the nature of stuttering. Often, just supplying this information relieves them of their guilt. The following materials have been helpful supplements to parent counseling:

1. On the "Stuttering Home Page" website (http://www.mnsu.edu/comdis/kuster/stutter.html), there is a link titled "Information About Stuttering," which leads to another link for parents of children who stutter. Articles, essays, books, and other materials for parents are provided directly there or are described so that parents can find them elsewhere.
2. On the National Stuttering Association website (http://www.westutter.org/whoWeHelp/NSA-Family-Programs/parents/School-Age.htm), there is a wealth of information for parents of school-age children who stutter.
3. On the Stuttering Foundation website (http://www.stutteringhelp.org/), a link titled "For Parents of School Age Children" leads to many useful items including "If You Think Your Child is Stuttering: 7 Ways to Help"—a video that provides useful information to parents. The Foundation also has other videos, *Stuttering: Straight Talk for Teens* and *Stuttering: Straight Talk for Teachers*, that can be helpful for parents.

Using language that is appropriate to the parents' level of understanding, I provide the type of information that I presented in the early chapters of this book. I describe how developmental and environmental influences may interact with predisposing physiological and constitutional factors to produce or exacerbate a child's initial repetitions and prolongations. The student responds to these disfluencies with increased tension in their effort to inhibit them. In time, the child also learns a variety of escape and possibly starting behaviors to cope with their repetitions and prolongations. I go on to suggest that predisposing physiological factors are most likely neurological in nature and are related to a student's deficits in speech production. I suggest that the student may have problems in timing the fine motor movements required for fluent speech. I add that students who stutter may also have a more sensitive temperament, and that could compound the stuttering by making the student more likely to have learned emotional reactions to their speech difficulties. I also note that in many cases, the predisposing physiological factors may be genetic in origin. Thus, there are many possible sources for the student's speech difficulty. I also suggest that because of the way the brain may be organized—with perhaps a very active right hemisphere—the student may have special talents in the areas of drawing, music, engineering, and other visual and creative endeavors. The Apple designer of the iPhone, the iPad, and many other Apple products, Jony Ive, stuttered as a child, perhaps because of a very active right hemisphere, but gained fame and fortune in part because of the way his brain is organized.

I explore, with the parents' assistance, the developmental and environmental influences that may be interacting with the student's predisposing factors to affect the student's stuttering. These are reviewed in Chapter 4. In some cases, I may not identify any developmental or environmental factors that seem to be contributing to the problem; however, when I do identify one or more possible factors, I attempt to lessen their influence. My experience suggests that in most cases, the solution to reducing the impact of developmental and environmental influences is fairly straightforward. In a few cases, when it may be more difficult, I have suggested that counseling by a family therapist may be helpful.

I also talk with parents of a student who stutters about avoidance behaviors. I describe these behaviors to them and explain how their child's word and situation avoidances are behaviors the child has learned to use in coping with the embarrassment and fear of talking. I also explain how, in therapy, I will be helping their child eliminate their use of these avoidance behaviors. I will also point out that avoidance learning is unfortunately a rather tenacious form of learning so that they will need to model patience as the child "unlearns" avoidances.

Some parents feel responsible for their child's stuttering and may feel they need to find a cure for it. While I'm discussing the possible causes of stuttering and after I've mentioned the possible neurological differences in students who stutter, I often bring up the possibility that their child will always stutter but that it needn't make the child's life any less full and rewarding. Because this can be such an important issue for parents, I try to judge whether this moment is the right time to discuss it. For example, if this is an initial phone conversation, I might not bring it up at that time. But if this is a face-to-face meeting and we have some time to talk about their concerns, I find it helpful to let parents know that a student who is still stuttering after age 9 or 10 years will probably continue to have at least a little stuttering throughout their life. In saying this, I am sure to indicate that most individuals who stutter into adulthood don't let their stuttering get in the way of their goals, and I will cite some examples of famous people who have achieved success even though they stuttered. At this point, I am careful to let them respond to this information. Parents sometimes envision difficulties in academic, social, and career areas for their child who stutters, and it is important for them to express these concerns and for me to listen deeply to them.

Identifying and Reducing Fluency Disrupters

As I explained in other chapters, environmental influences are often critical factors for managing beginning and borderline levels of stuttering in preschool children. Intermediate-level stuttering in students who stutter is more complex and requires direct treatment of a student's behaviors and attitudes, but environmental factors are important for this level of stuttering as well. The home environment of a school-age child who stutters may involve stresses and fluency disrupters that can be substantially alleviated if the clinician can join forces with an interested, motivated family. I begin by asking family members to observe when the child stutters most and when they stutter least. With this information, I brainstorm with them various ways to reduce potential stresses and to observe the effects on the child's stuttering. For example, some children stutter a lot when there is competition for attention at the dinner table or when several children arrive home from school at the same time, all wanting to talk to their parents. In other cases, changes in a family routine—like during holidays or when a crowd of relatives descends on the family—may spark an increase in a child's stuttering. Whatever the sources of stress, I encourage the parents and other family members to take the lead in identifying them and in planning ways of reducing such stress. Talking with the child about upcoming events can help. Even in cases in which stress may result from relatively abstract sources, such as a family's attitude that stuttering is shameful, the family is unlikely to change unless they feel that they and their points of view are respected and understood by the clinician. In an accepting environment, a trusting relationship can be developed, and a family may be open to seeing the child and his stuttering in new ways.

Increasing Fluency-Enhancing Situations

During the process of identifying the times when a child stutters more frequently, families also discover there are times when a child is extremely fluent. These may be specific situations or just days or weeks when the child is particularly fluent. Whatever the case, families can find ways of increasing factors that promote fluency and giving a child plenty of opportunities to talk when they are fluent. For example, a child may be especially fluent when they are talking to a parent at bedtime, when they are sleepy and relaxed. This provides a parent an opportunity to comment on the child's "easier speech" and to let the child know that they can imagine how good it must feel to talk easily. The clinician can help parents find ways of increasing fluency-enhancing situations and of reinforcing their child's fluency without implying that the times when they stutter are bad. Often the child and parent just talking, one-on-one, can produce lots of fluency as well as good vibes for the child. Encourage the family to empathize with the child about fluency being great but that stuttering just can't be helped sometimes.

For those children who are willing to work on their fluency with members of their family, a program of home therapy can be developed cooperatively by the child, parent(s), and clinician. Regular contact between the clinician and family members is important to facilitate and guide this component of treatment. Face-to-face meetings are ideal, but phone calls, journals, or e-mail will also suffice. A typical home program would include severity ratings made by both parents of the child's speech at home and by the child of their speech at home and at school. The specific behaviors to be rated and an effective reward system are negotiated by the child, parents, and clinician.

Parents' Involvement in Eliminating Teasing

If any of an intermediate stutterer's siblings are teasing the student about the student's stuttering, his parents need to stop it. I have found the best way to do this is to have parents have a serious talk with the teaser. They need to explain that teasing makes stuttering worse and must be discontinued. Usually, this is sufficient. If it is not, I have found it effective for me as the child's clinician to talk to the sibling about the importance of not teasing their brother or sister. In fact, the teaser can be taught what behaviors on their part can be really helpful to the student who stutters. Having an adult other than a parent talk seriously about this matter sometimes carries more weight with teasers.

Another important issue for parents is their reactions to teasing by other children at school. Although this is a serious matter, parents may do more harm than good if they are overly upset by classmates or others at school teasing their child. The student who is teased will take their cue from their parents. If parents are openly distraught about their child's being teased at school, the child will be more deeply affected by it. Parents, of course, need to respond if the child tells them that other kids are teasing them at school. They can listen to everything the child wants to tell them and also to find out if the teacher or principal know about it and are taking action to stop it. If parents let the school take care of the incident and convey to the student that they have faith in their ability to handle it but are also empathetic to the student's concerns, they will help the child maintain a good perspective on it. However, if the teasing continues without further reaction from the school or the school is not sympathetic to begin with, the clinician can offer to talk with the principal or classroom teacher, depending on where the teasing is occurring and being dealt with.

Clinical Procedures: Working With Teachers

I believe it is very important to have an intermediate stutterer's classroom teacher(s) involved in the student's treatment program (Fig. 15.5). After all, the child spends as much, if not more, time with the teacher than any other adult. In the remainder of this section, I'll use "teacher" to mean both one of the child's teachers and many of them. I have four goals in mind when I am working with a classroom teacher: (1) to explain the treatment program and the teacher's role in it, (2) to facilitate the teacher talking with the student about their stuttering, (3) to help the student and teacher work out the student's class participation, and (4) to help the teacher eliminate teasing.

The students in the University of Vermont 2017 summer camp program for school-age children who stutter created a "survival guide" for both students and teachers. It would be useful to share this both with the student's teacher and their

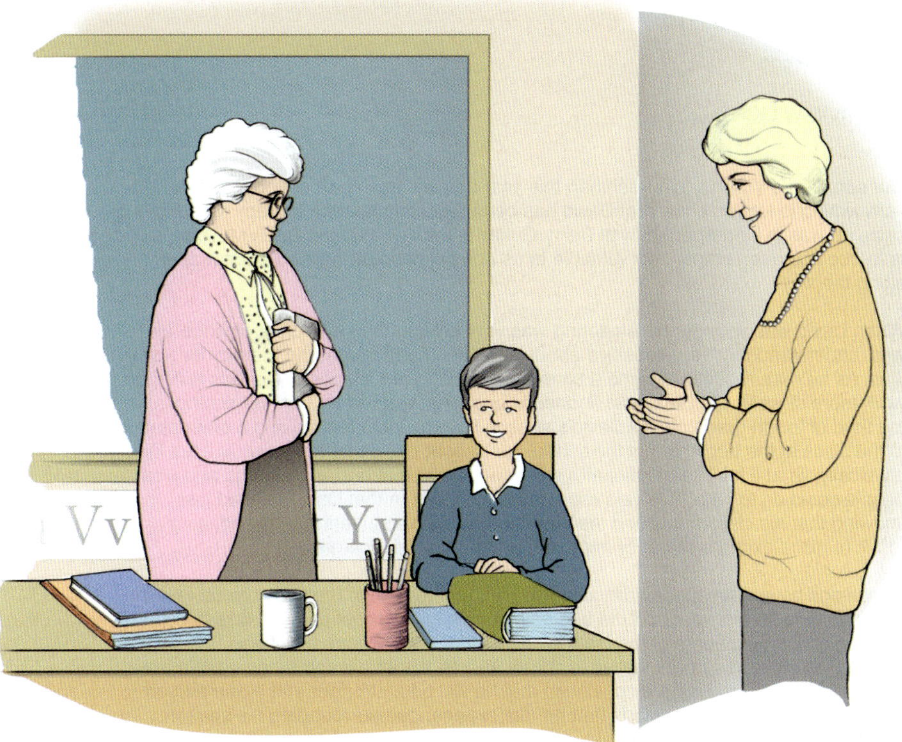

Figure 15.5 It is important to have the classroom teacher involved in the child's treatment.

parents as well as the child themselves. It's available via this link: http://westutter.org/wp-content/uploads/2017/08/BTS-Survival-Guide.pdf/.

Explaining the Treatment Program and the Teachers' Role in It

Involving the student's classroom teacher(s) in treatment works best if the student gives their permission for this to take place. Even the most reluctant students usually agree to let me make a contact with the teacher. If the student has several teachers, I always ask which teacher(s) the student would like me to talk to. Sometimes, a meeting with several teachers at once is efficient. When I worked as a speech-language pathologist in junior high and elementary schools, I gave in-services about stuttering to teachers at the beginning of the school year. If such in-services can be arranged, the Stuttering Foundation DVD *Stuttering: Straight Talk for Teachers* (Scott & Guitar, 2012) makes a powerful addition to a presentation on the problems faced by school children who stutter and how teachers can help them. Or consider showing another of the Foundation's DVDs: *Stuttering: For Kids, by Kids* (Scott & Guitar, 2004).

Another helpful way for the teacher to learn about the student's stuttering and their need for support is for the student's parent to write a letter to the teacher, with the student's consent. David's mother (David is the Case Example at the beginning of this chapter) wrote a wonderful letter to his teacher. This is shown in Figure 15.6. When you read about Patty Walton's therapy program further along in this chapter, you will see that she works with each student to help them write a letter to their teacher, explaining that they stutter and may have some trouble speaking in class. The student also lets the teacher know what they can do to help the student with their stuttering.

When I work with a student, I am sure to meet with the student's teacher(s) to give them an overview of the student's treatment program. I discuss how I am helping the student increase their fluency, eliminate their avoidance behaviors, and improve their overall communication ability. I want the teacher to understand the rationale behind these procedures. Therefore, I am careful to answer any questions the teacher may have, believing that helping the teacher understand our goals will have at least three benefits: (1) the teacher will have a better understanding of how to interact with the student, (2) the teacher will be better able to give me feedback regarding the student's fluency in the classroom, and (3) the teacher will have tools to work in the future with other students who stutter. I use the Teacher's Assessment of Students' Communicative Competence (TASCC) (Smith et al., 2000) described in Chapter 11 (see Fig. 11.1) to measure the student's baseline levels and progress. I also explain the teacher's role in the student's therapy and discuss why and how I would like the teacher to implement the three goals of (1) how to talk with the student about their stuttering, (2) how to help the student cope with oral participation, and (3) how to eliminate any teasing the student may be receiving. I discuss each of these in the following paragraphs. It is important for the clinician

August 30, 1999

RE: DAVID WILKINS

Our son, David Wilkins, is a freshman this year and will be in one of your classes. I am writing to let you know that David has been receiving speech therapy for stuttering since he was in kindergarten, with Barry Guitar at the Luce Center at UVM. This resource has been immensely valuable to us and we have all learned a great deal along the way.

When David was younger his stuttering was very pronounced and quite obvious. He was, understandably, very sensitive about his speech and fought the therapy for some time. As he matured and became a bit more accepting of his speech, he was willing to work more closely with Barry and find techniques that worked for him. Beginning in the third of fourth grade part of David's speech therapy included making a presentation to the class at the beginning of the school year about this stuttering — what it felt like physically, what it felt like emotionally, what people did that hurt his feelings and what people could do to help. This was especially significant in that David relaxed just knowing that his classmates and teacher understood his stuttering a bit and, as a result of his relaxing, his fluency improved and his confidence grew.

Transitions have always been difficult for David, but he seems pretty comfortable with the upcoming school year and the beginning of his high school career. He is familiar with the school and some of the teachers and students because his sister, Tina, is a senior. He is a solid student, active in sports and he is friendly and outgoing. We are very proud of him and we are convinced that he will be a stronger and better person for the struggles and frustrations that he has experienced surrounding his speech.

David is very fluent at the moment, and has been for some time now, but he will always have to live with some residual stuttering, along with its ups and downs, for the rest of his life. It may be awhile before you are aware of any dysfluency on David's part, and if you notice anything, it would be helpful to him if you are simply patient and a good listener, and if you don't try to finish his sentences for him.

David is aware that I have written to you and this alone will help him get off to a more relaxed start to the school year. Thank you for taking the time to read this and for being aware of what could be a sensitive situation.

If you have any questions please do not hesitate to call me at 202-555-0179 or Barry Guitar at 202-555-0183.

Ellen Wilkins

Ellen W. Wilkins
CC: Phyllis Cole and Barry Guitar

Figure 15.6 Letter to teacher by mother of a student who stutters.

to express their appreciation for the teacher's important work and to acknowledge how busy the teacher is just carrying out their work with the entire class.

Teachers Talking With the Child About Child's Stuttering

A friend of mine recalled going all the way through school from kindergarten through high school without any teacher ever mentioning their stuttering. They stuttered severely year after year, and everyone knew they stuttered, but nobody ever acknowledged it. This silence, they said, was very painful. I believe that it is better for classroom teachers to sit down with students who stutter and talk calmly with them about their stuttering, letting them know that the teacher is aware of their stuttering and would like to help them. The teacher should tell students that she will not interrupt or hurry them when they are talking. Just this sort of acknowledgment and acceptance of a student's stuttering by a teacher will make them feel more comfortable in the classroom.

Coping With Oral Participation

The teacher should also talk with the student about the student's oral participation in class. I believe it is important for a student who stutters to participate orally in class, even though it may take some courage for them to do it. If the clinician has built a strong empathetic relationship with the student, the clinician can inspire and support the student's efforts. It is also important for the student to eventually feel comfortable participating, and the teacher should seek the student's input on this matter. Possibly, some classroom procedure, such as calling on students in alphabetical order, is creating apprehension for the student who stutters and could be modified. For example, the student may prefer to be called on early, before their apprehension builds up. Or the teacher can ask the student questions in class that, at first, require minimal answers. If it goes well, more complicated and longer answers can be required. Perhaps the teacher and student can plan ahead for what questions the teacher will ask. With an understanding of the student's feelings and flexibility in procedures, most teachers can help a student who stutters become much more comfortable in their oral classroom participation.

Managing Teasing in School

It is not unusual for elementary or junior high school students who stutter to be teased about stuttering at school. If a classroom teacher becomes aware of teasing, they should attempt to stop it. As I indicated during my previous discussion of teasing in the home, I believe the best way to do this is to have a serious talk with the teaser. The teacher needs to explain that the child's teasing is making the stutterer's speech worse and that the teaser needs to discontinue it immediately. The teacher should make it clear that this behavior will not be tolerated. Some teasers are themselves troubled children and will need help from the school counselor to change their behaviors.

Progress and Outcome Measures

Measures of progress and outcome, as described in Chapters 9 and 11, need to be taken to assess the effectiveness of treatment. Data on stuttering and fluency (%SS–percentage syllables stuttered), Stuttering Severity Instrument [SSI-4], measures of attitudes [CAT and A-19], and assessment of communicative competence [TASCC]) can be used to measure progress during treatment and outcomes after maintenance.

This concludes the description of my approach to treatment of a school-age child with intermediate stuttering. I now describe the clinical procedures of some other clinicians. As you have seen, the major focus of my approach is to reduce the negative emotions associated with stuttering and combine that with a strategy to manage stuttering. Teaching fluency skills is reserved for later in therapy or is to be used for those few students who have few negative emotions.

APPROACHES OF OTHER CLINICIANS

Walton: Helping School-Age Students Speak More Easily While Changing the Way They Stutter

Walton has been working with school-age students who stutter for almost 40 years; her therapy reflects many lessons learned during her long experience with school-age students as well as preschoolers and adults. Her well-organized approach begins with a careful assessment that includes measures of stuttering severity, analysis of the child's stuttering pattern, assessment of the student's reaction to their stuttering, and their attitudes and emotions. She also assesses the parents' attitudes and behaviors toward their child's stuttering.

Walton's treatment plan varies for each student, but the following components are the core of her approach. She begins by exploring with the student what they want help with. She also touches on acceptance of stuttering. Walton's years of experience with stuttering have taught her that for students to begin accepting their stuttering, they need to experience some sort of change—an inkling that they can minimize and ultimately manage their stuttering.

To begin the process of change, Walton focuses on "fluency skills" in the sense that students learn what they do when they talk fluently—they become aware of their speech articulators and feel them move; she teaches them proprioception, the feel of easy onsets, light contacts, other tools that help them feel their fluency. Then she helps them become aware of what they do with their speech articulators, their voice box, and their airflow when they stutter. Figure 15.7 depicts a clinician guiding a child to feel what a stuttering moment feels like and, at the same time, reduce the feeling of panic and the urge to finish the word quickly. This experience is crucial and Walton works with the student extensively on being present during the moment of stuttering, not rushing, becoming aware of the physical tension they are creating.

Then the student is coached to gradually let the word out. In this way, Walton helps the student feel a sense of control, learning that they have choices in how they stutter. She lets the student know that the tension they employ when a word feels stuck is fighting the stutter and "the more you fight your stutter, the more your stutter fights back." Walton teaches them to use a loose, almost tension-free "bounce" when they stutter, beginning with the bounce as a voluntary stutter and then helping them use that with a real stutter. She begins with words and short phrases and works into using these stutters in conversations. Walton works with the student over many weeks, to give them repeated experiences of anticipating a stutter and going right into it, staying with it, holding it,

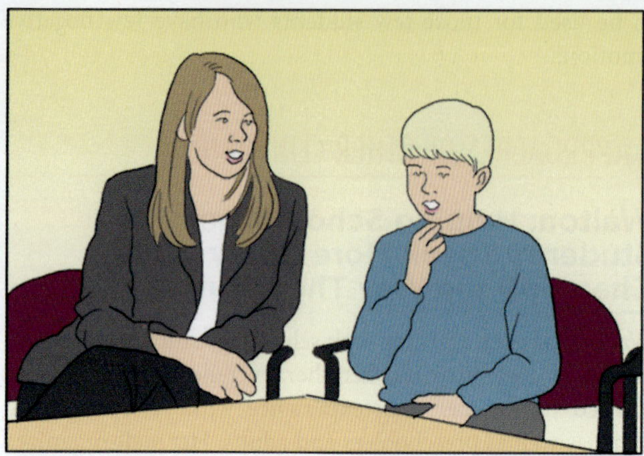

Figure 15.7 Clinician guiding a student to stay in the moment of stuttering and reduce the tension.

not responding to triggers of tension, and finishing the word slowly and loosely. The student gains a sense of empowerment with repeated experiences like this in many situations, moving from easy challenges to harder ones. As the student shares with Walton their thoughts and feelings about learning to manage their stuttering, she is vigilant to make sure she is carefully listening to everything the student shares with her, whether it is positive or not, to validate what the student says, what they think, and how they feel.

Walton has developed an exercise for students that helps them focus on feeling calm and able to make changes their stuttering despite their fears of listener reactions. Walton has students try to carry a full glass of water while walking down a hallway having to bat away paper balls that she is throwing at them. After they discover that they spill much water with the distraction of batting away paper balls (representing the feared listener reactions), they are then asked to walk down the hallway and ignore the paper balls she throws at them. They succeed wonderfully in keeping the water in the glass when they ignore the paper balls. Walton then helps them understand that they can ignore their thoughts and worries about listener reactions and focus attention on relaxing and managing their stutters.[5]

As Walton works with students on changing how they respond to anticipated and actual stutters, she also helps them deal with emotional responses. Incorporating some of the elements of the psychotherapy titled "Acceptance and Commitment Therapy," Walton talks with the student about how they think and feel about their stuttering. The student is encouraged to accept the fact that being unable to say words smoothly is indeed frustrating and may make you feel ashamed. But those feelings are normal and can be accepted and changed as the student makes a commitment to making their stuttering easier and feeling ok about it. Walton also uses **cognitive behavioral therapy** to help students realize that they may be "overthinking" the negativity of stuttering. For example, the student may imagine that listeners are bothered by the student's stuttering, whereas they might be surprised by it sometimes, but mostly they just accept it. The clinician and student can go out in public and survey people about what they think of stuttering and learn that most people aren't bothered by it. The clinician can go to a store with the student and deliberately stutter to a clerk and ask the student to observe the clerk's response—do they laugh? Do they turn away? In a conversation over an ice cream afterward, the student will hopefully see that the listener is actually quite patient. The student can do other exercises like this, some with and some without the clinician. The student will gradually learn that stuttering really isn't as bad as they thought. Walton uses a lot of these tools to move the student toward being much more comfortable talking, whether they stutter or not. She also helps the student use easy voluntary stuttering so the student can stutter (or seem to stutter) and feel in control, as well as calmly observe that listeners actually are accepting of stuttering.

Walton believes strongly in parent counseling, which involves educating parents about stuttering and about treatment, teaching strategies that the parents can be involved in to help the child at home, openness about stuttering at home so that stuttering is okay to talk about, making home a "safe house" for stuttering, helping parents have realistic expectations about treatment, and encouraging them to reduce criticism of the child and their speech. She also emphasizes working with teachers, including finding out from teachers about the child's speech in the classroom, educating teachers about stuttering (particularly this student's), and enlisting teachers' support to facilitate transfer of therapy techniques into the classroom. She works with the student to help them write a letter to their teacher(s), talking about the student's stuttering, and letting the teacher know what would help the student in class. Some students may request that the teacher not call on them unless they raise their hand. Or the student may want the teacher to realize that when the student tries to answer a question but appears to be silent, this may just be because they are having a silent block (not because they don't know the answer) and will soon get speech going again.[6]

Yaruss, Coleman, Beilby, and Herring: Treating the Experience of Stuttering

Much of my description of this approach comes from a recent chapter by this group on treating school-age students in *Stuttering and Related Disorders of Fluency* (Zebrowski et al., 2022). This chapter has many helpful tables detailing

[5]Walton gives credit to Jane Harley of the Michael Palin Centre for the ball-throwing, water-carrying exercise.

[6]This is the case in the video clip of a student named Cristy and I talking with one of Cristy's teachers about Cristy's silent blocks that the teacher misinterprets. The video on Lippincott Connect is titled "Classroom Teacher, Student, and Clinician."

treatment activities and insightful subsections describing their approach to challenging issues. If you wish to read a much more detailed depiction of their treatment, I recommend *School-age stuttering therapy: A practical guide* (Reardon-Reeves & Yaruss, 2013). The authors of the current chapter on treating the experience of stuttering have always had a wide focus, encompassing the child's and the family's whole experience when the child has a serious issue with stuttering. Of particular importance is the child's communication in the various social interactions in school, in the family, and with friends. This view of stuttering is also reflected in the assessment tool developed by Yaruss and Quesal (2006, 2016): *Overall Assessment of the Speaker's Experience of Stuttering.*

Activities within this model given in the chapter in Zebrowski et al. (2022) include (1) helping the child learn to manage their moments of stuttering by reducing their feelings of being out of control by lessening physical tension in stuttering (see Fig. 15.7); (2) helping children reduce their negative emotional and cognitive reactions to both the moment of stuttering and to the experience of having an obvious difference in the way they speak; (3) helping children deal with others' reactions to their stuttering—those of classmates, friends, and their family. As children are working with the clinician on these goals, they also work toward greater comfort, participation, and enhanced communication in social situations. For example, practice of activities in 1 to 3 are done in more and more challenging social situations.

The clinician is also working with the child to educate family members, teachers, and classmates so that they show more understanding and acceptance of the child's speech. For example, the clinician may support the child to give a presentation to their class to explain stuttering and make it OK to them. In my experience, such a presentation can make a major difference in how the child's teacher, their classmates, and the child themselves feel about and react to their stuttering in school. For an example of such a presentation, see the video titled "A Child Talks to Her Class About Stuttering" available on *Lippincott Connect*. In the current chapter, the authors emphasize the child and clinician working together to help the child learn how to feel comfortable with voluntary stuttering and how to use it to give the child the feeling of mastery, when the stuttering is done deliberately and feels like it is being controlled by the child. Another issue discussed in Yaruss et al.'s chapter is teasing and bullying. These are insightfully addressed in Murphy et al. (2007b, 2013).

The clinician always monitors how comfortable the child is as clinician and child work together to move up a hierarchy toward more openness about the child's stuttering in more and more situations. The clinician strives to be empathetic when the child wants to avoid situations or feels they aren't ready to take on harder tasks. These new challenges can wait until the child is ready. As the child and clinician work together on these endeavors, the therapeutic alliance between them is a key factor in successful therapy and needs to be deepened as therapy progresses.

TREATMENT OF STUTTERING ACCOMPANIED BY ATTENTION-DEFICIT/HYPERACTIVITY DISORDER (ADHD)

Many students have occasional difficulty focusing for long periods of time or sitting absolutely still in class or church, but only a small percentage—around 5% to 8%—have the neurodevelopmental disorder of attention-deficit/hyperactivity disorder (ADHD). The combination of stuttering accompanied by ADHD has been suggested to be between 4% and 26% of children who stutter (the result of different studies with widely different findings). A more precise report on ADHD and stuttering in children indicated that among 62,450 children studied in the National Health Interview Survey, 30.3% of male children who stuttered and 15.8% of female children who stuttered also had ADHD (Briley et al., 2021). There are two components to ADHD—inattention and hyperactivity—which may co-occur in some students, whereas other students may have only one of these manifestations.

Signs of inattention are

a. difficulty paying attention, even when spoken to;
b. being easily side-tracked while working on a task;
c. being very disorganized and messy; and frequently losing things.

Signs of hyperactivity include

a. fidgeting in seat and often leaving seat inappropriately;
b. talking incessantly and interrupting others;
c. running around like the "energizer bunny."

Treatment recommendations for students who stutter and have one or more signs of ADHD suggest both traditional stuttering therapy combined with medication by an appropriate physician for the ADHD. When stuttering therapy is carried out, my preference is to use stuttering modification for the stuttering issues, but with some added structures to help a student with ADHD compensate for attention-related problems. A number of clinician-researchers have suggested organizational features that will help. I'll describe them (while adding in my own tweeks). Donaher, Healey, and Soffer, (n.d.) recommend:

1. Begin by getting to know the student—their favorite activities, most and least favorite classes in school, TV shows they like, games they are good at, treats they like to snack on. The student should feel your real interest in them. All this information can be helpful in developing ways to explain stuttering to the student and to explore their ADHD issues.

2. Work with the student to create a structure for each therapy session, and post a timeline for components of therapy for you both to share. Each therapy session should include some activities that the child really likes and can beat the clinician at, such as throwing tennis balls at empty soda cans. Sports and games that the child likes can be brought into the therapy room and can be used as metaphors for things you work on in therapy. Examples are basketball played with a hoop that can be hung from a door and a bowling set that can be set up in the treatment room with plastic balls and pins.
3. Give the student clear and concise instructions and guidance about what you want them to try. Have the student tell you about what you are working on together. The repetition of it back to you will help them understand and let you know how well they understand it.
4. Draw pictures and act out behaviors you would like the student to learn. Watch the video on *Lippincott Connect* titled "Cam's Popcorn Video" to see how I had Cam act out two ways to handle stuttering: blasting through stuttering versus easing through stutters smoothly.

In a highly informative video presentation at an Oxford Dysfluency Conference, Donaher (2011) indicated that many clinicians have students who stutter on their caseload with "subclinical" ADHD. These students may not have strong or obvious enough symptoms to qualify as having true ADHD but may have some signs of short and inconsistent attention spans, hyperactivity, and/or impulsivity at home, in school, or in the therapy room. Those who do have true ADHD may be helped with a combination of stimulant medication (eg, Concerta, Ritalin, or Adderall) and behavior management. However, stimulant medications may make stuttering worse while improving ADHD. Consequently, nonstimulant meditations (eg, Strattera) along with social skills training and cognitive behavior therapy may be tried for students who stutter. Little research has been done on this combination for stuttering. Donaher cited relevant studies by Riley and Riley (1979, 2000) that showed that the presence of ADHD in students predicted poorer outcome after stuttering therapy. Importantly, the Rileys found that if inattention is treated *prior* to stuttering therapy, outcomes are more positive. In the video from the Oxford Dysfluency Conference, Donaher describes the treatment for students in his clinic (Children's Hospital of Philadelphia) who stutter and also have some ADHD traits, especially inattention. Donaher's approach is to choose "target behaviors" such as those associated with inadequate attention and focus on those with the help of the family and teachers. Examples of target behaviors include fast speech rate, and inability to focus on a task for a period of time.

My own approach to these particular deficits would include

1. Fast speech rate:
   a. Play games that include pushing a cart around the room with obstacles at fast speed, then pushing cart around obstacles at slow speed. Reward when obstacles are not disturbed when using slow speed.
   b. Have student walk slowly through obstacle course or around room. Reward when student can walk slowly around obstacle course.
   c. As above, but have student talk slowly (as you walk slowly) about favorite foods and snacks while walking slowly. Reward for keeping speech slow.
   d. As above, but clinician tries to hurry student to make them talk fast. Reward student for keeping speech slow as they walk slow.
   e. Have student talk slowly about a fun topic (like favorite sports, favorite teams, favorite TV shows, favorite video games) and reward student intermittently as they talk, if speech rate is kept slow.
2. Inability to focus on a task for a period of time.
   a. Together with student, decide on an enjoyable task (like reading silently from a favorite book or drawing a picture of playing a favorite sport) and decide together how long to focus on it for (start with an easy target of how long to focus on task). Reward student if they can keep focus for target time.
   b. If the above worked well, set a slightly longer time and see if the student can meet that and receive a reward.

In summary, your caseload may contain students who stutter who also have ADHD; some may have subclinical ADHD, particularly inattention and possibly hyperactivity. Both of these traits may interfere with therapy as well as with performance in the classroom and at home. It is important to identify particular deficits and help students remedy these before, or along with, therapy for their stuttering. A number of articles and videos related to stuttering with ADHD are cited in the recommended reading and viewing sections of this chapter.

TREATMENT OF STUTTERING ACCOMPANIED BY AUTISM

Treating stuttering accompanied by ASD in one individual can be challenging, especially for clinicians who have not previously worked with either. Therapists can benefit by reading the few case studies about treatment of stuttering in individuals with ASD and by reading the even smaller number of studies of small groups of individuals with both disorders, as well as viewing tutorial videos on this topic. This section is intended to provide readers with some foundational pieces of information to help them in these tasks.

In 2013 with the publication of the Diagnostic and Statical Manual of Mental Disorder, Fifth Edition (American Psychiatric Association), the dominant definition characterizes ASD as a spectrum that no longer includes subvariants such as Asperger syndrome. Where formerly three components had been as central to the diagnosis, now only two diagnostic characteristics are included: (1) difficulties in social communication and social interaction and (2) restricted, repetitive, and stereotyped patterns of behavior. *Difficulties in social communication and interaction* are considered present when three types of symptoms are noted: (1) difficulties in social-emotional reciprocity, such as failures to respond or initiate social interaction; (2) difficulties in nonverbal social interactions, such as those related to eye contact, use of gestures, and other forms of nonverbal communication; and (3) difficulties in developing and maintaining relationships, such as a lack of interest in peers. *Restricted, repetitive patterns of behavior, interests, and activities* are considered present when at least two of the following symptoms are noted: (1) stereotyped or repetitive actions on objects, movements (eg, frequent rocking back and forth), or speech; (2) insistence on routines; (3) very restricted interests that are intense or extremely focused (eg, a seeming obsession with a cartoon character); and (4) over or under reactivity to sensory experiences (eg, extreme positive or negative reaction to particular auditory, visual, tactile, or other sensations). Additionally, each of the two main diagnostic features need to have been present since early development and to undermine on the individual's ability to function in their families or communities. Whereas challenges in cognition and language were previously included as part of the definition, those are now viewed as potential co-occurring diagnoses. Determining the severity of autism overall is based on the degree of support required given the prominence and ubiquity of symptoms seen in the areas of social interaction and restrictive repetitive behaviors.

You may be wondering how often stuttering and ASD co-occur. A survey by Blood et al. (2003) of 2,628 children who stuttered found that 21 children who stuttered (0.8%) were also diagnosed with ASD. In a later study, Scaler Scott et al. (2014) reported on a group of children with ASD, a group of children who stuttered, and a control group. They found that 4 of the 11 children with ASD (36%) also had a diagnosis of stuttering. It should be noted, however, that the behaviors of the ASD group that were labeled stuttering were a variety of types of disfluency, some not stuttering-like disfluencies. As has been reported by others (eg, Sisskin, 2012) disfluencies in ASD include (1) stuttering-like disfluencies (part-word repetitions, single-syllable word repetitions, prolongations, and blocks); (2) other disfluencies (interjections, revisions, phrase repetitions, and multi-syllable word repetitions); (3) atypical disfluencies (final part-word repetitions, mid-word breaks, final-sound prolongations, and final phrase repetitions).

Three characteristics of ASD are important to be aware of when you are developing treatment strategies for the co-occuring disorders. *Social Impairment* is a key characteristic. Individuals with ASD have problems with the pragmatics of social interaction, such as responding to comments by the conversational partner and turn-taking in conversations. They may be over- or underreactive to stimuli such as loud noise or bright lights or prompts from the clinician to "remember you're supposed to be speaking slowly." *Difficulty With Communication* (both verbal and nonverbal) is manifest in these students being unable to read facial expressions, unable to understand metaphorical use of speech, and lack of awareness if the student isn't being understood by a listener. *Restricted Interests and Compulsivity*—being obsessed with a video game or a cartoon character, like Barney and his dinosaur friends. Individuals with ASD also may display self-stimulating behavior like hand flapping and rocking back and forth.

When students with ASD also stutter, they usually don't show the shame and embarrassment that is seen in typical students who stutter. The disfluencies of ASD students are sometimes referred to as "speaker-oriented disfluencies" because they seem to serve a purpose for the speaker, like holding the floor while speaking, to prevent interruption.

As we now get into details of treatment, we will begin with *Considerations for Design of Treatment.* Much of the ideas that follow are taken from a compelling video of a presentation on ASD and stuttering given by Vivian Sisskin (2012). Sisskin herself raised a child with ASD so she speaks from the experience of a parent, as well as a clinician who has worked with ASD for many years. Her ideas for planning include (1) consider the importance of the particular deficit to overall improved communication. For example, if stuttering is a minor issue, not bothering the family or other listeners, or the individual themselves, then don't treat it; (2) sessions should be designed to hold the student's attention. For example, use activities that student is captured by, such as social stories (Gray, 2010) and comic strips (Gray, 1994); (3) many students with ASD are more responsive to visual stimuli versus auditory stimuli. They also benefit from knowing the sequence of events that will occur in a session. Therefore, it may benefit students with ASD if clinicians post visual schedules of what will happen and when it will happen, for each session. (4) Develop individualized teaching strategies. Model the behavior change, elicit the change from the student, then give the student a favorite reward (reinforcements are critical); use mini-steps to make progress; scaffold heavily to help them learn (eg, to have a student identify a stutter, have them identify something simple like a cough or the word "I," then model the type of stutter you want them to identify in their own speech, by asking them to identify it in your speech, then in their own speech).

Now I'll talk about specific *Programming Considerations.* The best evidence from studies of treatment of ASD and stuttering suggests that a behavioral approach is most effective—eliciting changes in stuttering and rewarding changes with something the student really likes, coupled with praise. Gradually, praise can be used alone, but you can also use counters that can be cashed in for time the student can use as they choose. Remember that students with ASD are concrete thinkers so choose activities that can be explained and modeled in simple, concrete terms. Do more showing than telling. Help them understand the uses of communication, like getting just what they want, without too much delay. Because you will be focusing on changes in stuttering, help them to learn to communicate about stuttering. It may help to let them choose their terms to indicate different aspects of stuttering, like repeating words or sounds.

The *Fluency Goals* for students with ASD and stuttering include the following: (1) increased awareness of what is the target for change (best if you can help student discover for themselves what is to be changed); (2) investment in change—help student see why it might be useful to them to make the change; (3) concrete strategies—like Runyan & Runyan's Fluency Rules Program (1986) or another set of rules that the student can follow; and (4) use familiar concepts as you work with students for change. For example, show the student a visual depiction of word said with repetition (for example) as you say it with him doing it also. Then in small steps work up to having him say a phrase with the word not repeated. The Stuttering Foundation presentation by Vivian Sisskin (2012) has a powerful case example illustrated with videos of a child learning to eliminate word-final repetitions. This child also reduced stuttering-like behaviors and was shown to maintain these gains for a long period of time.

To summarize, students with ASD and stuttering can benefit from stuttering therapy, particularly if the clinician understands the student's learning style and limitations. Both the family and the school can become a part of the therapy team and generalization can take place with lasting effect.

SUMMARY

- My approach to stuttering in school-age children is primarily what we often call stuttering modification because it is aimed not at eliminating stuttering but modifying it to be easier and comfortable for effective and enjoyable communication. It involves work on both emotional and attitudinal aspects as well as how stutters themselves are managed.
- My treatment for the typical school-age child who stutters begins with an exploration of stuttering with the clinician clearly demonstrating acceptance of the student's stuttering. This will begin to decrease some of the negative emotions associated with it. After considerable therapy aimed at reducing fear and shame of stuttering, the clinician should demonstrate and guide the student in catching the "stuck" part of a stutter and staying in the stutter until the rush to blurt out the word subsides. This will help the student decrease the threat and fear of the moment of "stuckness" in stutters and thereby reduce the tension. After tension is reduced, the child then finishes the "stuck" word (which is now "unstuck") slowly and easily. As the child masters this strategy, they begin to have easier stutters that feel in control.
- In the approach for most children, after learning to stay in the stutter (strongly reinforced by the clinician), reducing fear and tension, and learning to end the stutter slowly and loosely, the young client then works on continuing to reduce their fear and avoidance by (1) being open about stuttering, (2) accepting their stuttering, (3) learning to use voluntary stuttering, and (4) becoming desensitized to stuttering in a variety of situations. Following this, transfer activities take place.
- Other clinicians, whose therapies are described in this chapter, use many of these same techniques. Most of them foster a change in attitudes about speech and stuttering, not only to provide positive expectations for fluency but also to help clients accept any residual stuttering so that they will deal with it rather than avoid it. Many also prepare the student to deal with teasing. I've included two different approaches to help readers see how they too may consider adding different elements to their treatment.

STUDY QUESTIONS

1. What is the "approach" attitude that I recommend for school-age children who stutter? What are some reasons why an "approach" attitude might help a child with intermediate stuttering?
2. What is the theoretical rational for "Staying in the Stutter?" In other words, why would staying in the stuckness of the stutter cause stuttering to become easier?
3. What is a "stuttering-friendly" environment, and how could you create one in a child's home and school?
4. Describe what the "exploration" phase of my treatment approach is designed to accomplish and how it meets that goal.
5. Suggest three ways in which you might assess to what extent the goals of the exploration phase of treatment have been met with a particular child.
6. When you are working on a transfer hierarchy and the child seems unable to transfer improved fluency to a particular situation, such as giving a book report, what can you do to achieve success on this step?

SUGGESTED PROJECTS

1. Avoidance reduction is an important component of the major treatment described in this chapter. Experiment with your own fears and avoidances to see if you can decrease them by using a "seeking out" attitude. For example, if you dislike making phone calls, devote a week to making extra phone calls and seeking out opportunities to make phone calls you usually wouldn't make. After the week is over, assess whether this experience decreased your dislike of making phone calls.
2. Watch the Stuttering Foundation video *For Kids by Kids* (available free at www.stutteringhelp.org) and plan how you might use various clips from it to help a child explore their own and others' stuttering.
3. Draw a "road map" with pictures that you could use to help a student at the beginning of therapy learn about what they will be doing over the course of therapy.
4. Develop new ways, new metaphors, and new activities to help a child learn to "Stay in the Stutter," let tension subside, and finish the word loosely and slowly.

SUGGESTED READINGS

Donaher, J., Healey, C., & Soffer, S. (n.d.). ADHD and stuttering. Available as free downloadable brochure from Stuttering Foundation.

This is a brief pamphlet that describes the symptoms of ADHD, discusses stuttering and ADHD, and provides ideas for treatment of children with ADHD. The pamphlet includes many references for learning more about ADHD.

Guitar, B., & Reville, J. (1997). *Easy talker: A fluency workbook for school-age children.* Pro-Ed Publishers. Available used on Amazon.

This is a workbook for elementary school children that tells the story of several children at a camp working on their stuttering. Along with the story, sequenced concepts and techniques are presented, with workbook activities for children to complete. This book integrates stuttering modification and fluency shaping.

Manning, W., & DiLollo, A. (2018). *Clinical decision making in fluency disorders* (4th ed.). Delmar Publishers.

The chapter called "Treatment of Young Children" contains excellent information on approaches with children between 2 and 12 years old. The first author is an individual who stuttered throughout childhood and young adulthood but essentially no longer stutters.

Ramig, P., & Dodge, D. (2005). *The child and adolescent stuttering treatment and activity resource guide.* Thomson Delmar Learning.

Goals of treatment, ideas for Individualized Education Programs (IEPs), steps in treatment, activities to teach elements of therapy, tips for involving parents and teachers, and a multitude of handouts (in Spanish and English) are some of the valuable contents of this book. Cluttering evaluation and treatment are also covered.

Reardon-Reeves, N., & Yaruss, J. S. *School-age stuttering therapy: A practical guide.* Stuttering Therapy Resources, Inc.

This book is an accessible guide for clinicians to use for school-age children and adolescents who stutter. It provides goals and activities, worksheets and forms to use for initial and continuous evaluation of students, and treatment plans.

Van Riper, C. (1973). Treatment of the young confirmed stutterer. In *The treatment of stuttering* (pp. 426–451). Prentice-Hall.

In this chapter, Van Riper provides a comprehensive discussion of a classic stuttering modification approach to the treatment of the intermediate stutterer.

Walton, P. (2012). *Fun with fluency: For the school-age child.* Pro-Ed.

This is a well-organized approach that combines stuttering modification and fluency shaping for the school-age child who stutters. This book provides a great deal of material that can be copied and used for each individual child.

Yaruss, J. S. (Ed.) (2003). Facing the challenge of treating stuttering in the schools. Part 2: Selecting goals and strategies for success. *Seminars in Speech and Language, 24*(1), February issue.

This journal issue is full of relevant and practical ideas for working with intermediate stuttering in a school setting.

Yaruss, J. S., Murphy, B., Quesal, R., Reardon-Reeves, N., & Flores, T. (2004). *Bullying and teasing: Helping children who stutter.* National Stuttering Association.

The philosophy behind this book is to empower children who stutter to take charge of teasing situations themselves. However, it also provides excellent suggestions for parents, teachers, SLPs, and school administrators.

Yaruss, J. S., Pelczarski, K., & Quesal, R. (2010). Comprehensive treatment for school-age children who stutter: Treating the entire disorder. In B. Guitar, & R. McCauley (Eds.), *Treatment of stuttering: Established and emerging interventions* (pp. 215–244). Lippincott Williams & Wilkins.

This chapter and accompanying video provide an excellent illustration of a broad-spectrum approach to treatment that targets affective, behavioral, and cognitive aspects of stuttering.

SUGGESTED VIEWING

Donaher, J. (2011). ADHD and children who stutter. In *Presentation at Oxford Dysfluency Conference.* Stuttering Foundation.

This hour-long video captures a presentation by Joseph Donaher who works with children who stutter and also have ADHD. Donaher explains in detail the signs of ADHD and cites many research publications that discuss the combination of the disorders and their treatment.

Sisskin, V. (2012). *Autism spectrum disorders and stuttering.* Presentation at Stuttering Foundation's Mid-Atlantic Workshop, Children's Hospital of Philadelphia. Available on Stuttering Foundation website: stuttering help.org.

This is a very informative 2-hour presentation by a master clinician who works with both stuttering and ASD. Sisskin is also the parent of a child who has ASD and this informs her work. The case studies presented here are vivid and help viewers understand the challenges of working with children who stutter and also have autism.

16

Treatment of Adolescents: Advanced Stuttering

Naomi H. Rodgers, Ph. D., CCC-SLP

Chapter Outline

Chapter Objectives

After studying this chapter, readers should be able to:

- Summarize the unique challenges and opportunities associated with stuttering in adolescence
- Describe how to establish a trusting **therapeutic alliance** with adolescents who stutter
- Summarize the steps to help adolescents stutter more easily
- Explain methods for addressing difficult thoughts and feelings about stuttering

Key Terms

Acceptance: Letting internal experiences just be there without trying to get rid of them, avoid them, or replace them; one of the six principles of ACT

Acceptance and commitment therapy (ACT): Learning to let difficult thoughts and feelings just *be* by staying in the present moment, noticing what's happening without trying to change those thoughts or feelings, and moving in the direction of what matters to the client

Adolescence: Period of development, roughly from 10 to 24 years of age, where brain-body-behavior changes are rapidly underway, which primes young people for learning, renders them highly sensitive to social experiences, and promotes desire for independence

Affirmations: Positive statements about the client's characteristics or behaviors that help reinforce change behaviors

Bibliotherapy: Using published literature about stuttering to help clients better understand their own experiences

Change: Overt and covert behaviors that are personally important to the client; for many adolescents who stutter, it involves (1) learning ways to talk and stutter more easily, (2) developing more positive thoughts and feelings about stuttering, and (3) reducing avoidances

Change journey: The process that a client goes through as they learn new ways to think about and act upon stuttering

Cinematherapy: Using films about stuttering to help clients better understand their own experiences

Comfort zone: Situations in which one feels equipped to readily act and succeed; can be expanded by taking small steps just outside one's comfort zone

Defusion: Separating oneself from one's thoughts by looking *at* thoughts rather than engaging or embodying them; one of the six principles of ACT

Disclosure: Sharing with others the fact that one stutters

Easing out: When in a moment of stuttering, releasing tension and gently and mindfully transitioning to the next sound

Hierarchy: Stepwise progression through linguistic and situational contexts of increasing difficulty used to help clients generalize new behaviors

Holding and tolerating: Volitionally continuing to hold tension in a moment of stuttering for longer than usual to desensitize the person to difficult feelings that arise in that moment and to develop behavioral self-awareness in the moment

Motivational interviewing: Strengthening the client's motivation for and commitment to their goals by eliciting and exploring their own reasons for change

Mindfulness: Staying in the present moment and being nonjudgmentally aware of present moment experiences

Safe stuttering space: A situation or context in which the client feels that the environment is open to and accepting of stuttering

Solution-focused brief therapy (SFBT): A style of counseling that focuses on the client's strengths and resources for change that is important to them, rather than focusing on their problems

Stages of change: Five discrete phases of readiness to change that people move through dynamically as they shift how they think about a target behavior

Strengths: Personal attributes that help the client make value-driven decisions in their everyday life

Struggle: Avoidance and escape behaviors that interfere with the speaker's ability to move directly into, and stay easily within, stutters

Therapeutic alliance: Unwavering rapport between the client and clinician that is based on a mutual trust and respect; it develops from the clinician's curiosity about the client's experience with stuttering and showing that "it's ok to stutter" through their mindful use of accepting verbal and nonverbal language

Thinking traps: Processing information in a negative way where the person can feel "trapped" in a cycle of negative thinking

Voluntary stuttering: When a stutterer or nonstutterer imitates a moment of stuttering; also known as *pseudostuttering* or *stuttering on purpose*

INTRODUCTION

This chapter will introduce you to the unique aspects of stuttering therapy with adolescents. You have already learned some ways to establish a strong therapeutic relationship with your client, and this is arguably the most important aspect of adolescent stuttering therapy. Adolescents thrive on feeling heard and validated, so your primary responsibility is to situate your adolescent client in the metaphorical driver's seat as you listen deeply and validate their experiences from the passenger's side. This foundation of unwavering rapport will help your adolescent client feel safe, valued, empowered, and socially connected. And from here, **change** is possible.

In this chapter, once we establish common ground on the unique challenges and opportunities for young people, we will explore some therapy approaches and activities that are well-suited for helping adolescents codevelop their therapy goals, learn ways to stutter more easily, develop healthier thoughts and feelings about themselves and stuttering, and reduce avoidance of sounds, words, and situations. This is all in service of helping adolescents cultivate responsibility and autonomy over their ***change journey***—the process that an adolescent goes through as they learn new ways to think about and act upon stuttering.

BACKGROUND ON ADOLESCENCE

Adolescence has historically been thought to "begin in biology and end in culture"—that it is bookended by the onset of puberty on one side, and the achievement of culturally expected milestones of adulthood on the other (things like marriage and gainful employment) (Conger & Peterson, 1984). Contemporary models of adolescence harness recent neurobiological evidence that reveals that puberty is starting earlier and earlier, and neurological development continues well into one's 20s. This has inspired recent calls to expand the age range of adolescence to be 10 to 24 years (Sawyer et al., 2018).

What makes adolescence such a unique period of one's life that it warrants its own literature base, its own research questions and methods, its own approach to stuttering therapy? Because adolescents are not simply older children nor younger adults, so regarding them is a disservice to the exceptional challenges and possibilities that are unique to this period of great risk and opportunity.

The challenges of adolescence stem from the drastic changes in social-emotional networks in the brain that render adolescents exceptionally sensitive to their social world. While highly active limbic regions are amplifying emotional experiences, the less mature prefrontal regions are still developing self-regulation abilities (Shulman et al., 2016). During this time, adolescents are shifting their dependence on their parents to their peers instead, and this shift toward peers happens at a time when social fears and worries naturally escalate. In fact, social anxiety typically begins around 13 years of age (Kessler et al., 2007), and there is evidence that reveals higher rates of social anxiety among people who stutter than those in the general population (Bernard et al., 2022). Therefore, it is reasonable to expect the adolescent years to be a particularly vulnerable and tumultuous time for those who stutter. The common, intense desire to fit in is challenged by stuttering—a part of them that sets them apart from their peers. On top of the great lengths that many young people who stutter go to hide this part of themselves, they may not be particularly receptive to well-intentioned clinicians recruited to help them. Some young people view clinicians as extensions of their parents—*here is another adult telling me what to do*—and this attitude of not needing or wanting help can strain a budding therapeutic relationship.

Adolescence is simultaneously a time of tremendous possibilities. Those same neurobiological changes that make adolescence a difficult time also prime them for learning, particularly self-directed learning. In fact, the surge in neuroplasticity we see during the adolescent years is second only to that observed in the first 3 years of life (Cohen Kadosh et al., 2013). It is a time when identities and lifelong habits take root as young people make sense of who they are and find their place in the world. This is a crucially pivotal time for young people to have supportive experiences that allow them to flourish and develop healthy ways of coping, because toxic environments and experiences can have long-lasting damaging effects on their livelihood (Steinberg, 2014). Clinicians can help facilitate these positive experiences by working *with* adolescents' natural tendencies for independence, novelty seeking, exploration, and peer connection.

SETTING THE TONE FOR THERAPY

From the outset of therapy, the clinician's primary mission is to establish a strong therapeutic relationship that is based on mutual trust and respect. To earn an adolescent's trust, take genuine interest in understanding what they like and care about—what they like and dislike about school, what they do in their time outside of school, what their family is like, who their friends are, what they're looking forward to or nervous about. Take notes and use these details in conversations that follow, as that signals to the adolescent that you are invested in them, and you truly care about them as people.

Creating a Safe Stuttering Space

Clinicians must not only set an honest tone that stuttering is ok but also demonstrate that this is true. There is underestimated power in four simple words: "it's okay to stutter." Say this often and *mean it* by the intentional use of verbal and nonverbal actions. Keep neutral eye contact, facial expressions, and body language, especially during moments of stuttering. Nod along naturally. It's helpful not to remind them to use their "speech tools" when they are just sharing about their life and not intentionally practicing a new skill; offering such reminders sends the message that you are more concerned about how they talk rather than themselves as people. If they are practicing some sort of speech change during a structured activity later in the session, then that confined activity would be an acceptable time to offer guidance and reminders in a supportive, nonpunitive way. If, in conversation, you notice that the client is spontaneously fluent—that they are speaking easily and fluently without control or conscious effort—it is often *not* helpful to comment on this because the ease was not the result of anything they were doing intentionally. Regardless of how the client delivers their message and how much they stutter, it is always useful to praise them for sharing their ideas. Many young people come to avoid sharing what's on their mind—the little things that aren't necessary like anecdotes, jokes, etc.—to minimize the cost: *if I don't talk, then I won't stutter.* If after a conversational turn with some tough stutters, you may offer some validation like, "I appreciate that you stuck with it. You have lots of great ideas and I want to hear them." Together, these listening practices send the message to the adolescent that you care about *what* they have to say and that you are not hyperfocused on *how* they say it. Ultimately, we want our adolescent clients to share whatever is on their mind and feel safe letting us in.

As a clinician who stutters myself, I have found that stuttering openly and confidently can be one of the quickest and most powerful ways to establish a bond with teens who stutters, many of whom have never met someone else who stutters before. They may feel an instantaneous connection with you since there is an unspoken understanding that know what stuttering is like, and they may feel relieved to know an adult who stutters who survived adolescence.

For all clinicians (those who do and those who don't stutter), you can show your client that it's ok to stutter by confidently putting stuttering in your own mouth. This is often called "**voluntary stuttering**" or "pseudostuttering." First, ask the adolescent if it's ok for you to try to voluntary stutter like them, explaining that doing so will help you better understand how they stutter. Once the client has consented, have them teach you how they stutter and try to voluntary stutter in that way, learning their pattern by attending to where and how tension builds and how it can release. Eventually, you will model ways of stuttering more easily—easier bounces, easier blocks. As you try to help clients generalize a new communication skill outside the therapy room (whether it's stuttering openly, maintaining eye contact while stuttering, **easing out** of a stutter, or something else the client finds important), always offer to do it first and then offer to take turns while the skill is still new. This sends a clear message to the client that you're not afraid of stuttering and that you are also willing to take the same risks that you are asking them to take. This inspires mutual trust and respect.

Focusing on "What's Right" With the Client

Psychologist Kelly Wilson (2009) argued that clients are best served when they are valued as "a sunset to be appreciated rather than a problem to be solved" (p. 15). Clinicians can do a lot of good by focusing on the client's **strengths** and values—those qualities that already reside within the client that motivate how they live their day-to-day and make choices. In line with positive psychology (Seligman, 2012), **motivational interviewing** (Miller & Rollnick, 2012), and **solution-focused brief therapy (SFBT)** (De Shazer et al., 2021), we can focus on "what's right" with the client, rather than on their deficits or problems.

Early in the therapeutic relationship, clinicians can ask their clients: "What do you think you're good at?" and "What would your family and friends say you're good at?" Another way to tap into the client's innate abilities is to prompt them: "I'd like you to think of another time in your life when you learned a new skill or made some sort of change. Perhaps you learned how to speak Spanish, or how to play basketball, or how to drive a car. What kind of skill have you learned? What happened? How did you manage to learn that new skill? What does that show you about yourself?" Clinicians may help clients recognize the incredible dedication and problem solving that already exists within them. This type of dialogue aligns with principles of motivational interviewing, where clients bring to conscious awareness their natural abilities that allow them to do hard things.

To extend this conversation, you can also have the client complete a "signature strengths" assessment to identify their top five character strengths (freely available at www.viacharacter.org). This facilitates the client's self-knowledge and helps them focus on their positive attributes. Then, in conversations that unfold over your therapy sessions, you can help them identify times that they activated those character strengths. Week to week, as they share constructive shifts in their life, you can point out positive things about them that you've noticed (eg, "It seems like you care a lot about your friends," "I can tell that you're a hard worker," "You figured out a way to take care of yourself."). Sharing these observations often helps adolescents build their own ability to recognize and appreciate these strengths within themselves.

Codeveloping Goals Guided by the Client's Readiness to Change

Goals and outcomes should be developed collaboratively between the clinician and adolescent. Involving young clients in the process sends the message that the clinician's role is more facilitative than authoritarian, which bolsters the client's autonomy, investment, and independence that are blossoming at this time in their life. To do this, you pose open-ended questions to elicit what the adolescent wants to change. These open-ended questions can blend principles from SFBT and motivational interviewing to elicit the adolescent's "best hopes" or "preferred future" (SFBT terms).

In Table 16.1, when adolescents are asked what they want to be different, many of them will reply with something along the lines of "I want to be more fluent" or "I don't want to stutter as much." This is an invitation to explore what meaning the client has attributed to *fluency* on a deeper level. First, it's important to validate their desire for talking to be easier through reflecting what they said and the underlying feeling. You can gently reframe the client's language to help them start focusing on *ease* and *communication* over fluency. For example, you may reply: "Stuttering can be really hard sometimes. It's normal to want talking to be easier. I'm here to support you in exploring what easier talking sounds and feels like." This sets the tone for the collaborative journey that lies ahead. Using the client's language within SFBT-style questions can be useful to dive a bit deeper: "If you were more fluent (or if you weren't stuttering as much), what would that look like?

TABLE 16.1 Discussion Prompts for Identifying What and How Adolescents Can Make Changes That Are Personally Meaningful

Topic	Example Question to Ask
What they want to change	■ What would you like to see different about stuttering or how you live with it? I'm interested in what you want, not what you think your parents or teachers might want for you.
Why this change is important to them	■ What are the pros or benefits of making this change? ■ What are the cons or drawbacks of making this change?
How ready are they to make this change	■ What makes you think that this might be a good time to make this change?
What steps they can take to make this change	■ The steps I plan to take in changing are... ■ The ways other people can help me are... ■ I will know that my plan is working if... ■ Some things that could interfere with my plan are... ■ What I will do if the plan isn't working...

What would you be doing instead?" Perhaps they share that they would participate more in school, be more outgoing, or have better friendships. From these responses, you may say something like "It seems like participating in school is important to you. Do you think it's possible to participate more in school even if you still stutter?" This helps them focus on what's important to them rather than on how fluent they are. It also plants seeds of **acceptance** where they start to consider that they can achieve what they want, with stuttering still a part of who they are. Additional SFBT-style prompts you can offer are: "What would more fluency/less stuttering mean to you? What difference would that make? How would you be different? How would your life be different?" These questions also open up possibilities that they can achieve their goals even if they still stutter (Rodgers et al., 2020).

When confronted with the question about what they want to change, some adolescents may not know what they want or have difficulty expressing it. In this case, you can offer some evidence-based domains of change that Dr. Tricia Zebrowski and I have identified in our research (Rodgers et al., 2021; Zebrowski et al., 2021). Based on our interviews with adolescents who stutter and stuttering specialists, we found three overarching behavior changes that are relevant to many teens who stutter:

1. Making speech changes to talk or stutter more easily
2. Developing more positive thoughts and feelings about stuttering
3. Reducing avoidance of sounds, words, situations

The clinician can offer these three behavior changes and then ask them: "On a scale of 1-5, how important is each of these behaviors to you? Which one do you think you're most ready to start with?"

A prominent theory of behavior change known as the *transtheoretical model* (commonly known as the ***stages of change***) suggests that a person's readiness to change hugely impacts their engagement in the change process and, ultimately, how durable their change is over time. In this theory, as seen in Figure 16.1, there are five stages of change, ranging from precontemplation (where the person is not at all ready to change) to maintenance (where they have stuck to a new behavior for at least 6 months). People tend to move through the stages dynamically or nonlinearly, meaning they can make progress, regress, and then progress again—multiple times over. As people re-cycle through the stages, they tend to move through the stages more quickly with each cycle and the change that results tends to be more durable. More information about the stages of change and its application to adolescent stuttering therapy can be found in papers by Zebrowski et al. (2021) and Rodgers et al. (2021). Research has shown that it's best to start a change journey with the target behavior that the client is most ready to change or finds most important to their well-being (Prochaska et al., 1994). Once they have started to make changes in that primary domain and start noticing signs of progress, they will likely feel more confident that they can address other domains that at first seemed too far out of reach.

STUTTERING WITH GREATER EASE

Most young people who stutter want talking to be easier. They may think that stuttering itself is what makes talking hard. But in reality, stuttering does not have to be hard nor does it have to make talking hard. Vivian Sisskin, a well-known stuttering specialist and pioneer of *Avoidance Reduction Therapy for Stuttering* (ARTS), distinguishes stuttering from **struggle** (Sisskin, 2023). Stuttering is not inherently struggled. Often, it is all the things that stutterers do to *avoid* stuttering that makes stuttering and talking struggled. For example, one

Stages of Change
I don't see a problem here.
I don't feel good about stuttering, but I don't know what to do about it. There are important reasons why I want to change, but also important reasons holding me back.
I want to do something about this. Let me look online to see what options are out there. Maybe my parents can help me find a speech therapist, too.
I'm making changes to how I communicate and cope with stuttering. It's taking a lot of time and energy.
I've been making changes for a while and I'm feeling more confident that I can stick to them.
Precontemplation
Contemplation
Preparation
Action
Maintenance

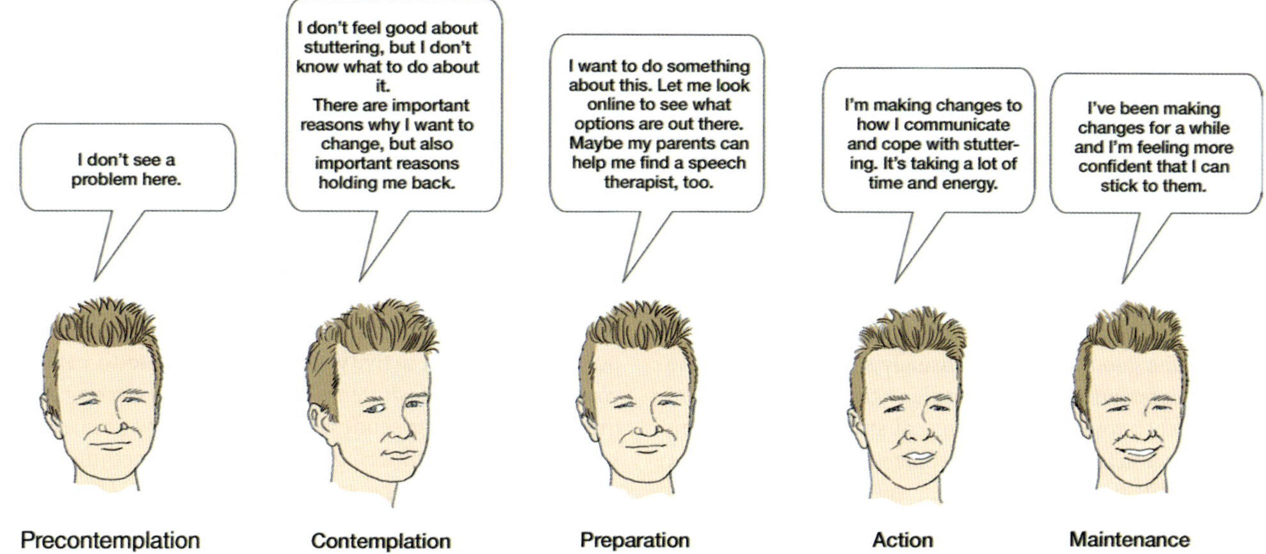

Figure 16.1 Five stages of change, which adolescents who stutter can move through dynamically.

teen that I worked with realized that he physically braced for upcoming stutters by pressing his lips together right before a target sound he knew he would stutter on, even if the target sound wasn't produced bilabially. This often altered the target sound that came out and would impact his intelligibility. That's an example of struggle. With this struggle versus stutter distinction in mind, one of our aims when working with young people who stutter is to guide them in figuring out ways to reduce struggle so they can stutter with greater ease. They can do this by learning about the physiology of talking and stuttering, identifying when and how they stutter, and then figuring out ways to work *with* their speech mechanism rather than fight against it.

Learning About the Speech Mechanism

One of the most important precursors to making any sort of behavioral speech changes is to learn how the speech mechanism works to produce talking and stuttering. A helpful way to start this discussion is to find or make an age-appropriate drawing of the speech mechanism that includes everything from the diaphragm up—lungs, vocal folds, articulators (tongue, teeth, lips, jaw), nose, and don't forget the brain that decides what to say and directs parts of the speech mechanism to move in certain ways. Creative clients may be interested in making a 3D model of the speech mechanism using modeling clay, Legos, origami paper, household objects, or other resourceful materials.

Once a common vocabulary about speech anatomy has been established, it's time to understand how the different parts work together. It's useful to start by explaining how the parts work together seamlessly most of the time to produce easy, fluent speech: The brain sends a signal to the body to inhale, which sends the diaphragm down to make room for the lungs to fill up with air. Once we've inhaled, we start talking as we exhale. The air moves up from the lungs into the windpipe and then through the vocal folds, which starts their vibration so that the voice can turn on. The air then moves into the mouth where the articulators shape the air to make different sounds.

Once the teen understands the path of airflow, it's helpful to explore with them where and how different sounds are made. Have them produce different sounds: labials /p, b, m, w, f, v/, alveolars /t, d, n, l, s/, velars /k, g/, and those that occur at the vocal folds including vowels and /h/. The clinician should model each one first, producing each of these sounds easily and then increase the tension by, say, 25% → 50% → 75%. When playing around with different tension levels, this is a natural time to talk about and experiment with the three core behaviors of stuttering—repetitions, prolongations, and blocks. From single sounds, you can start producing single words and simple phrases with the same approach (first easily, then gradually adding tension). In the spirit of Dr Dean Williams (one of the renowned giants of stuttering therapy at the University of Iowa from the 1950s to 1980s), prompt the client to really "feel what you're doing"—recruiting their cognitive and physical attention so they are moving mindfully and intentionally. This is educational, kinesthetic, and desensitizing as it builds their behavioral awareness of where and how they may get stuck when they stutter. Try to tap into your own curiosity and creativity to make this activity engaging and interesting for your adolescents; model the type of intrigue and excitement that the complexity of speech production deserves! A video of Dean Williams working with a teen is available on Lippincott Connect. It is titled, "Dean Williams helps a student stutter more easily."

Identifying Moments of Stuttering

Once the adolescent has developed a clear understanding of speech anatomy and physiology, and has experimented with modifying tension on different target sounds and words, it's time to help them identify when and how they actually stutter. Many young clients (and adults who are new to therapy, too) will initially have difficulty with identifying stutters on the fly, so we need to scaffold initial skill acquisition to help them become good observers. I usually start *away* from the client (understanding other people's stuttering) and then gradually work toward their own real stutters. Perhaps you could watch YouTube videos of people who stutter and work together to identify stutters in their speech by raising your finger when you see one. Then, pause the video and you and the client both try to imitate the stutter, followed by brief description of where in the speech mechanism it was produced and what type of stutter it was (repetition, prolongation, block). Once the client has showed that they are able to identify moments of stuttering in these recordings of others and can describe where and how they are produced, the next step could be you producing pseudostutters in conversation with the client, prompting them to raise a finger when they notice you pseudostutter, and then describing where and how you pseudostuttered. You do not need to make your pseudostutters really hard and struggled. I once had a 13-year-old client tell me that she was uncomfortable when her previous clinician pseudostuttered because the clinician did it with a lot of physical struggle; the client thought, "is that what *I* look like when I stutter?" So, before you pseudostutter with a client, it is helpful to gauge their comfort with you pseudostuttering and if they give you the go-ahead, know that you can make your point by pseudostuttering confidently and without a lot of struggle.

After the client has demonstrated success with identifying your pseudostutters, it's time to move to the client's own stutters. Some clients are willing to be videorecorded in the session and then watching it back right away with the clinician and identifying their own stutters offline. However, watching recordings of oneself can be confrontational and uncomfortable, even for people who *don't* stutter. So, if the client does not want to do this step, then by all means skip it and move to the last step where the client tries to identify their own stutters as close to in real-time as possible. Have them try to raise their finger when they notice themselves stuttering. The type of stimuli you use to elicit a conversational turn from the client in this activity depends on how frequently they stutter. For clients who stutter very often, you may get real stutters by eliciting shorter phrases. For clients who stutter less frequently, you may need to elicit longer responses or increase the communicative stress by having them explain something complex or take a stance about a controversial topic. Ensure that the topics and stimuli are relevant to their life—their interests, hobbies, school topics.

Two notes about semantics here. First, in the spirit Dean Williams, it is useful to talk about stuttering as something the speaker *does*, not something that *happens to them*. If stuttering is something they do, they can do something different about it; if stuttering is something that happens *to* them, then they likely feel at the mercy of stuttering, which robs them of making any choices about it. This type of active language is not intended to blame the client for the stuttering, but rather to instill a sense of autonomy. Second, if you are not a person who stutters and you are stuttering on purpose during an activity, it is more accurate to call what you're doing *pseudostuttering* or *voluntary stuttering* rather than stuttering. This sends a subtle signal to your client that you respect their stuttering experience as something that is unique to them and the stuttering community. Often, well-intentioned listeners and clinicians will attempt to console people who stutter or normalize stuttering by saying things like, "everyone stutters sometimes." Everyone is *disfluent* sometimes, but not everyone *stutters* sometimes.

Holding, Tolerating, Then Easing Out

Once the adolescent has demonstrated knowledge of when, where, and how they stutter, they can start to figure out ways to reduce tension in moments of stuttering to ease out gently. At this stage, it's helpful to stay in stutters for longer than usual so that they have time to turn their attention inwards and focus on how it feels in the moment. Most people who stutter will do whatever they can to get out of stutters as quickly as they can; stuttering can feel uncomfortable, stressful, embarrassing, and so of course they want to get out of it as soon as they can. But a big part of desensitizing oneself to those negative thoughts and emotions amid a stutter is to stay in it for longer than they have to. This act of progressive desensitization increases their comfort with stuttering, which in turn will help them stutter more easily.

To stay in a stutter, the person is guided to volitionally keep the tension in that spot to keep the stutter going. Many teens find it helpful to close their fist as a visual and physical way of "catching the stutter" and then keeping their fist closed as they keep the stutter going. This is what I mean by "**holding and tolerating**." Then, as they slowly unfurl their fingers and open their fist, they slowly reduce the tension in their articulators and ease into the next sound. As they ease into the next sound, the teen is guided to really elongate this moment and focus their attention on how the smooth transition to the next sound *feels*. It's as if they are putting this moment under a microscope so they can study it and understand it.

I have found that learning how to hold, tolerate, and ease out works best when teens begin with voluntary stutters. Once they have gotten a hang of how to do it with fake stutters, they can move to doing it with real stutters. If they miss a moment of real stuttering, they can go back into the target word using a voluntary stutter and practice it that way.

At first, many adolescents will feel very uncomfortable with this activity. After all, they thought they were coming to you so they could learn how to stutter *less* and here you are telling them to stutter *more*. It's important to offer a very strong rationale for why you are asking them to hold and tolerate. I may say something like this: "Our therapy room is a safe place to explore moments of stuttering—not by fighting them, but by learning how to work *with* them so that eventually they become less scary and easier to move through. So we're going to try to hold onto stutters—both fake ones and real ones—for longer than we need to or longer than feels natural. Something like this [model an example, synchronizing your verbal model with your fist closing and opening as described in the previous paragraph]. By taking our time in these moments, we are giving our body and brain enough time to tune in and learn. It may feel odd or uncomfortable to stay in stutters longer than you're used to, especially if you're wanting them to be *shorter* not longer. But this is an important step in teaching your body and brain that you can be brave and courageous when stuttering. The more you do this, the less scary stuttering will be and in time, you'll be able to make the stutters shorter." The use of analogies can be particularly useful here. For example, it can be helpful to do something you're afraid of (eg, flying without your parents, learning how to drive) by taking small steps toward it in a safe way. If there's an example from the client's own life that you can draw on, this would make the point more effectively.

Using Hierarchies to Level Up

For those who want to stutter more easily, the ultimate goal is to be able to do so across interactions and situations in the "real world." But how does a new behavior become reliable and engrained? By systematically practicing it in situations of increasing difficulty. This applies to all populations that clinicians serve, not just those who stutter. In the world of stuttering therapy, we often talk about "hierarchies" to help clients gradually work their way up to using new communication behaviors in more challenging situations.

There are two types of hierarchies that are relevant for stuttering therapy: *linguistic hierarchies* and *situational hierarchies*. A linguistic **hierarchy** is similar to that which is used in traditional articulation therapy where new sounds are acquired in isolation, then words, then phrases, then structured conversation, and finally unstructured conversation. A linguistic hierarchy is most useful within stuttering therapy sessions when clients are first learning to hold, tolerate, and ease out of stutters; it offers a structured roadmap for how to practice the new skill in increasingly complex utterances.

While a common linguistic hierarchy is applicable to lots of people, a situational hierarchy is highly unique to each client and therefore should be created together with the client to ensure that it is personally relevant to them. A situational hierarchy is a list of social interactions that are ordered from easiest or least stressful, to hardest or most stressful. These can include certain people (eg, talking to specific family members, peers) or certain contexts (eg, talking in specific classes, giving class presentations, ordering at a restaurant, talking on the phone). A situational hierarchy is useful within and outside therapy sessions because the people and contexts on the hierarchy likely exist outside the therapy room (eg, talking to a teacher or coach, giving a class presentation).

A savvy clinician uses both linguistic and situations hierarchies to support gradual skill development in an intentional way that feels safe to the teen. Both types of hierarchies are effectively visualized using a staircase or a ladder that can make the process concrete for teens. The process can also be gamified to make it more engaging for teens; once they have "beaten" a level, they move to the next level in their hierarchy. Over time, it's likely that their **comfort zone** will expand and they will approach harder situations with a bit more confidence. It's important to tune into the client's comfort level. While it's appropriate to gently nudge when it is clear that the teen is capable and ready for a new challenge, do not ask teens to do something that is too stressful for them at that moment as that damages the trust you have worked so hard to establish. This is described in greater detail in the section "Expanding Comfort Zone" toward the end of the chapter. Across all challenges, always offer to model first either in a role play or real scenario as you shouldn't ask your client to do something that you yourself are not willing to model. Also, always offer to be there as a support person as appropriate or feasible; your presence as a trusted partner can minimize the scariness of doing something new.

DEVELOPING HEALTHIER THOUGHTS AND FEELINGS ABOUT STUTTERING

Behaviors can be both overt and covert. There are behaviors that are visible to others, and there are behaviors that are invisible to others like thoughts, feelings, and memories (Ciarrochi et al., 2005). Thus, addressing how a young person thinks and feels about communication is a behavioral goal within our scope of practice (American Speech-Language-Hearing Association, n.d.).

My perspective is that negative thoughts and feelings about stuttering are typical reactions to an atypical stressor—that they arise because young stutterers are learning how to navigate a fast-paced society that is often unwelcoming to people who need more time to do anything, including talking. And this is unfolding at a period in their life when social approval is paramount to their well-being. Repeated experiences with being interrupted, teased, bullied, told to talk differently, or reminded to "slow down, think about what you want to say" when stuttering has nothing to do with fast speech rate or incoherent language, can easily break the spirit of adolescents who are striving to fit in. It's easy to place blame on the stuttering or the stutterer for these negative experiences—*if they didn't stutter, none of these negative things would happen*—but we can flip the narrative and conceive that negative thoughts and feelings are evoked by the immediate and historical environment, not something pathological about the stutterer (Gerlach-Houck et al., 2023). As such, I have found that a counseling approach that is *trauma-informed* (Goldstein, 2022) and grounded in ***acceptance and commitment therapy* (ACT)** (Beilby & Byrnes, 2012) helps young people understand and navigate their inner experiences.

There is an old Buddhist saying that "pain is inevitable, suffering is optional." In Figure 16.2, the adolescent on the left is experiencing pain when difficult experiences arise; they are noticing difficult or painful thoughts and feelings. The adolescent on the right is suffering; they are making judgments and generating narratives about how bad things seem. This escalation can get in the way of their ability to notice things objectively and identify a productive way forward. Our task is to help adolescents learn to notice and make room for their inner experiences rather than trying to suppress them and to discover new ways of coping that honor, rather than belittle, what they are going through. Carl Rogers, a renowned humanistic psychologist who advocated for the power of client-centered therapy, argued that for a person to flourish, they need an environment that offers genuineness (openness and self-disclosure), acceptance (being treated with unconditional positive regard), and empathy (being listened to and understood) (Rogers, 1951). With these tenets in mind, let's explore ways to work with adolescents' inner stuttering experiences.

De-Mystifying Stuttering Through Education

Often times, our emotions about things that are hard and painful fog our ability to think rationally about it. For example, if you are afraid of flying and you go on an airplane, you may be so consumed by your own anxiety and worry that you don't realize that flying is actually one of the safest modes of transportation and may be the only feasible way for you to get to that faraway place you're going. An adaptive way of coping with something scary is to learn about it

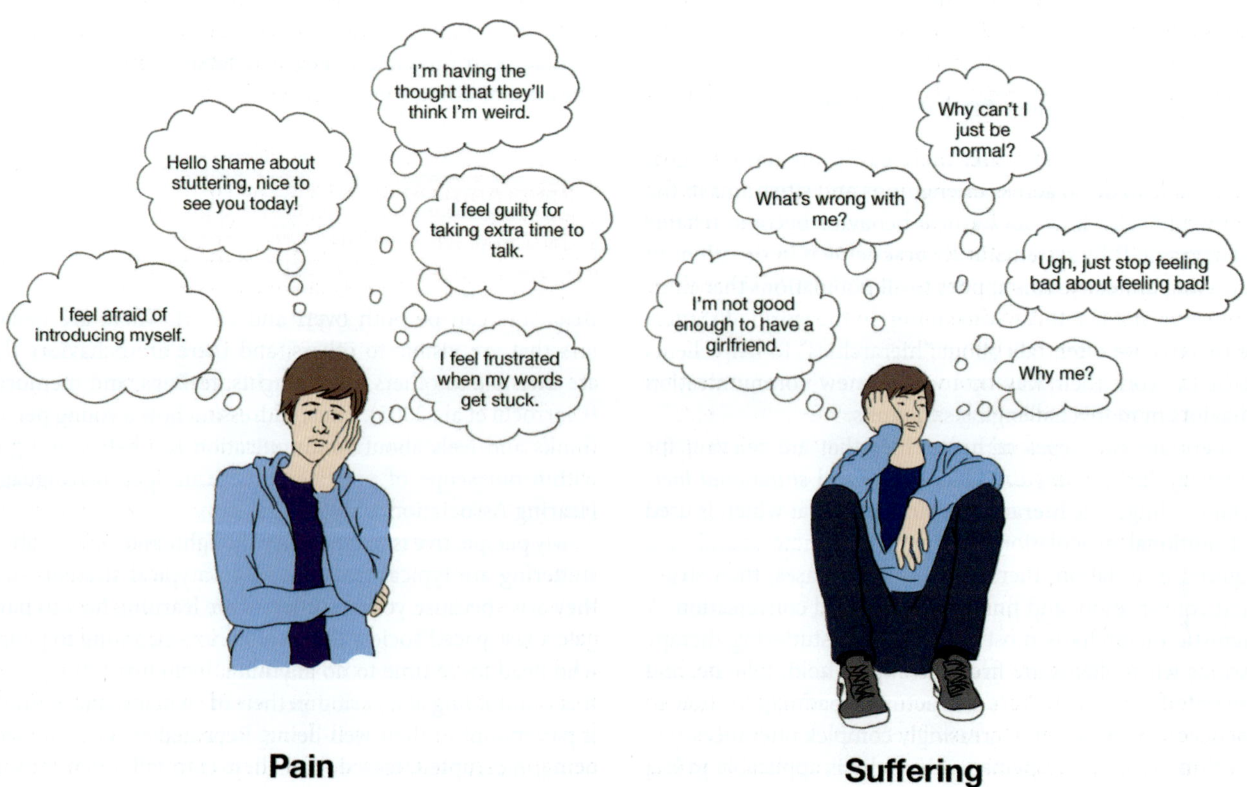

Figure 16.2 Adolescents can experience pain about stuttering (*left*), which can escalate to suffering (*right*).

and hopefully come to a point where you befriend it. You may choose to educate yourself about how safe air travel really is and how to handle stressful situations in flight. The same applies to stuttering; adolescents may experience a lot of anxiety and worry about stuttering and may not know a lot about it or believe commonly held misconceptions about it.

It is helpful to spend time learning about stuttering: how many people in the world stutter, the fact that stuttering exists in every culture around the globe, what causes it, what contributes to its variability, etc. There are plenty of websites that offer such information, just make sure that you vet the resources you find as there is plenty of misinformation floating around. Of course, learning about how the speech mechanism produces speech and stuttering (as described earlier in this chapter) also counts as learning about stuttering.

It is also helpful to learn about other people's experiences with stuttering, which can help normalize what the young person is going through. For adolescents who enjoy reading, you can do **bibliotherapy** where you both read a section of a book on your own and then at your next session discuss what resonated with the client (Gerlach & Subramanian, 2016). There are fictional books and memoirs about people who stutter. *Paperboy* is appropriate for middle-schoolers, while *Out With It* and *Life on Delay* are appropriate for older adolescents (*Life on Delay* contains mature content so it would only be appropriate for those who are at least 18 years old). There are also several great documentaries and YouTube videos about stuttering that you can use for **cinematherapy** (Azios et al., 2020). Feature-length documentaries like *My Beautiful Stutter, The Way We Talk,* and *When I Stutter* include adolescents who stutter. There are lots of shorter YouTube videos available as well, and I encourage you to find some that share healthy messages about stuttering rather than perpetuating misconceptions. Similar to bibliotherapy, you can have them watch a film on their own (or with their parents or a friend, if the teen is open to that) and then come to the next session ready to share what resonated with them. Adolescents who are savvy with social media can find numerous influencers who stutter on TikTok, Instagram, or other platforms who share their experiences with stuttering. Together, these avenues invite adolescents to learn about stuttering from others who stutter, which helps normalize their inner experiences.

Reframing "Success" and Celebrating Small Steps

Because many young people who stutter and their parents seek speech therapy to become more fluent, they often gauge how successful therapy is by how fluent they become. Despite how rampant this perspective is, it can be harmful to young people's well-being because they are being asked to control something that is quite uncontrollable and highly variable. When the success of therapy hinges on how much the young person stutters, they are more likely to conceal their stuttering because hiding it is the only way to not do it as often (Gerlach-Houck et al., 2023). And research has shown that the more one conceals their stuttering, the higher psychological distress they experience (Gerlach et al., 2021).

While young people cannot control *when* they stutter, they can make some choices about *how* they stutter and communicate. Through the process of codeveloping therapy goals and outcomes, which was described earlier, you can help adolescents and their parents consider "success" more holistically. For example, perhaps success means being more open about stuttering, communicating effectively by stuttering more easily and keeping eye contact, or being true to who they are. From there, you can help the teen identify and clarify their values around that vision of success. If "being true to who they are" resonates with them, help them explore their values surrounding communication, relationships, and self-growth and then help them see that they can make decisions that align with those values. This is inspired by ACT, where a client's values represent a "compass that guides people through the storms and confusing times of life and toward the things they care about" (Hayes & Ciarrochi, 2015). Values are most helpful when they are stated as actions. For example, some commonly valued activities that contribute to well-being include "connecting with others," "giving to others and having a positive influence," "embracing the moment," "challenging myself and learning," and "caring for myself." Not all of these are equally relevant to all adolescents, so this list is not intended to be prescriptive. However, this list can provide a launching point for how values are usefully worded. The website https://www.therapistaid.com/therapy-worksheets/values/adolescents has several useful activities for facilitating discussions about values with adolescents. Over time, adolescents make value-driven decisions and experience cohesion between *who I am* and *what I do*. This allows them to feel successful in being true to who they are, rather than hinging their success on how much they stuttered in a given situation.

In addition to reframing "success" to be more holistic, we can also help young people notice small signs of progress. We all have had experience with wanting to change something quickly (eg, get fit, lose weight, feel better), and perhaps feeling discouraged that change, in fact, takes a long time and a lot of dedication. *It is a marathon, not a sprint*, after all. One helpful thing that we can do to keep morale up and stay the course is noticing and celebrate small steps in the desired direction. For example, if one of your client's goals is to be more open about stuttering, you wouldn't withhold praise until they are open about stuttering all the time with everyone they meet. You would applaud small things they do that show they're being more open. For example, perhaps they talked to one of their teachers about reasonable classroom accommodations for oral participation, disclosed their stuttering to a new friend via text or SnapChat, or shared a post about stuttering on their social media. There are also creative ways to open up about stuttering. I once had a 17-year-old client who painted an amazing self-portrait about what stuttering felt like, and a 14-year-old who created and performed a dance solo about what stuttering meant to her. All of these examples are invitations to praise proactive movement toward their goal of being more open about stuttering. Understand that these are no small feats and likely take a lot of courage, as young people discover ways of being open about stuttering that they may have hidden for a very long time. By celebrating these small successes, we can help create a sort of ripple effect where adolescents believe they are capable of doing hard things and are inspired to keep the momentum going.

Identifying "Thinking Traps"

A common approach to changing how one thinks and feels is *cognitive-behavioral therapy* (CBT). In CBT, people learn how their thoughts, feelings, and bodily sensations motivate their behavior. While there is a lot of high-level research evidence supporting the efficacy of CBT, even applied specifically to people who stutter (Menzies et al., 2008) some practitioners believe that CBT can gaslight clients into thinking that their thoughts are dysfunctional or irrational. However, there are certain aspects of CBT that remain productive in helping adolescents become more aware of how they think and feel so they can develop healthier ways of coping, if done in a respectful way that uses empowering, rather than disempowering or pathologizing, language. One of these aspects is ***thinking traps*** (my preferred terminology rather than "cognitive distortions" or "irrational thoughts" which is commonly used in the CBT literature). Thinking traps are styles of processing information in a negative way, and they can sometimes make someone feel "trapped" in a vicious cycle of negative thinking. Table 16.2 summarizes some common thinking traps that I have discussed with teens who stutter.

These cognitive behaviors usually occur because of the teen's past experiences that have shaped how they view the world. It's not because something is wrong with them; it is their brain's way of trying to protect them from incoming threat. This is an important thing to help young people understand, especially when they feel guilty for thinking negatively or get into a vicious cycle where they start to feel bad about feeling bad. If you are interested in learning more about this topic, Google "thinking traps" or "cognitive distortions" and you'll find plenty of relevant websites.

To introduce this topic to your teen, you can select a few thinking traps that seem relevant to them based on what they've shared with you. Discuss the names, descriptions, and examples for each one. Perhaps you come up with some additional examples and have the teen identify what type of thinking trap they are. The teen can also come up with other examples themselves. Artistic clients may enjoy drawing pictures or cartoons of the thinking traps they experience. To help teens navigate through thinking traps, we can help them develop skills to play "devil's advocate." Often, this involves examining the facts about a situation and exploring alternative

TABLE 16.2 Thinking Traps

Name	Description	Example
All or Nothing Thinking	Seeing things as black or white	You ordered lunch and think that it went terribly because of how much you stuttered
Overgeneralization	Taking one outcome and thinking it accurately predicts a future similar experience	You introduce yourself and stutter on your name, so the next time you introduce yourself you believe you'll get stuck
Mental Filter	Paying attention to one piece of information from a situation and ignoring additional information	While giving a class presentation, you see one person in class giggling and you really focus on them, instead of noticing all the other people in the room who look engaged
Fortune Telling	Predicting an outcome about something without real evidence that it's true	You want to ask someone to Homecoming, but you believe they won't want to go with you because you stutter
Mind Reading	Assuming what someone else is thinking	You're talking to someone and when you start to stutter the listener gives you "the look," so you assume they're uncomfortable or judging you

conclusions they can draw. By exploring alternatives, the teen may realize that there are more helpful ways of thinking about something that allow them to be resilient and to keep moving forward. An alternative would be cognitive **defusion**, which is an ACT approach that is summarized in the next section.

Accepting and Letting Go of Difficult Thoughts and Emotions

While the basis of CBT is to help people control difficult thoughts and emotions, ACT offers a somewhat more humanistic approach that recognizes that pain is an inevitable part of building a meaningful life. With ACT, people learn to let difficult thoughts and emotions just *be*, without avoidance or control, by staying in the present moment, noticing what's happening without trying to change their thoughts or feelings, and moving in the direction of what matters to them (Black, 2022). True ACT is an embodied experience, where experiential activities and metaphors help clients gain a visceral understanding of the skills. There are six principles of ACT that help teens develop this sort of cognitive flexibility: present moment (stay here), self as context (notice yourself), acceptance (let it be), defusion (let it go), values (choose what matters), and committed action (do what matters). It is outside the scope of this chapter to dive into each one of these principles in detail, but let's cover a few that are specifically dedicated to accepting and letting go of difficult thoughts and feelings about stuttering. If you are interested in developing your ACT knowledge, I highly recommend the book *ACT for Adolescents: Treating Teens and Adolescents in Individual and Group Therapy* by Turrell and Bell (2016).

First, they can learn to stay in the present moment and become aware of those present moment experiences. This is commonly known as ***mindfulness***. This may be particularly important for teens who stutter because it's often difficult for them to pay attention objectively to the momentary physical experience of stuttering, and/or they find themselves not fully present when talking to others because they are thinking about stuttering. For example, have you ever had the experience where someone is talking to you, and you realize that even though you've been standing right in front of them, looking into their eyes while they are talking, you were actually thinking about something else, so afterward you don't remember what they said? This often happens to teens who stutter, especially if they are ruminating about some stuttering that just happened or anxiously planning what they're going to say next or how they'll say it. Mindfulness activities to increase their present moment awareness can be helpful to build this skill. You can guide them in eating a sour gummy worm mindfully (a teen-friendly alternative to the common "raisin exercise" for which you can find scripts online), 5-5-5 exercise where they are prompted to notice five things they see, hear, and feel at any moment, or short guided mindfulness meditations to help them build their capacity for nonjudgmental present moment awareness. The book *5-Minute Mindfulness Meditations for Teens* by Nicole Libin might be a good addition to your clinical bookshelf if you'd like to guide your adolescent clients in short guided meditations. There are also prerecorded ones available online; I particularly like the ones by Tara Brach, although they tend to be closer to 15 to 20 minutes each.

Another relevant domain is acceptance—letting private experiences just be there without trying to do anything like get rid of them, avoid them, or replace them. The attempt to suppress or control difficult thoughts and feelings can actually amplify them and make them harder to cope with. For younger teens, you can do a glitter bottle activity where you get a bottle, fill it with a combination of clear glue and water, have the client add some scoops of glitter or metallic confetti, and then seal the lid. Have the client shake the bottle so the glitter is swirling all around in the water. You tell the client that the goal is to get the glitter to go back to the bottom of the bottle. They realize that they can't do anything to *make* the glitter go down, they have to just wait for the glitter to settle. If they try to turn the bottle, the glitter will go the opposite direction and will take longer to settle. Our thoughts and feelings are like the glitter in the bottle; often, the most helpful thing we can do is wait for the thought or feeling to settle on its own without trying to control it in any way.

An additional experiential activity that works for fostering acceptance is using a Chinese finger trap. Have the client put their index fingers into each end of the finger trap. If they try to pull their fingers out using brute strength, they will get even more stuck. This is often what happens in the physical moment of stuttering, and it happens with our thoughts and feelings too. The way to get out of the trap is to relax into it and actually bring their fingers together, which at first seems counterintuitive. This activity is so relevant to stuttering—both in demonstrating the benefit of easing out of physical tension rather than pushing harder, and the value of accepting thoughts and feelings—that it may be worthwhile to purchase a bag of these inexpensive finger traps so you have them handy whenever the right teachable moment arises with your clients.

The last idea I'll share for fostering acceptance is to help the teen learn to say hello to their thought and feelings. This works best if they are able to infuse some humor into it. For example, "Hello fear about stuttering, you're looking fabulous today!" or "Hey worries about what others think of me, it's so nice to see you again!" This type of dialogue can help teens welcome and soften thoughts and feelings that they may have historically wanted to avoid or may have felt consumed by. It is also a process of "name it to tame it," a phrase dubbed by psychologist Dr. Dan Siegel who suggests that labeling a feeling can help ground us when we're feeling emotionally overwhelmed or disconnected (Siegel, 2010).

The final domain I'll describe here is *defusion*—stepping back and getting some separation from one's thoughts.

It involves looking *at* thoughts rather than engaging or embodying them, because thoughts are simply something the brain does, they are not who we are. ACT practitioners help clients become unstuck from difficult inner experiences through various exercises and metaphors. A common one is using the carrier phrase *"I'm having the thought that..."* For example, if a teen who stutters tells you that they can't introduce themselves, you could offer a reframe like "You're having the thought that you can't introduce yourself." Or if a teen shares that when they're stuttering, they worry that others will think they are weird, they could learn to defuse by saying "I'm having the thought that they'll think I'm weird." Then, they can practice saying *thank you* to their mind for being so helpful and working so hard to solve the problem (again, having a sense of humor can be helpful here). This creates some distance between the teen and their thoughts, and with enough practice, they start to realize that their thoughts are not facts and that they themselves are not their thoughts. Other defusion activities involve mindfulness visualizations where the teen can either imagine standing on the shore of a beach and placing their difficult thought/feeling on a wave and watching it roll back out to sea, or perhaps they imagine that they are a clear blue sky looking down at their thoughts that are clouds passing by below them.

There are many, many more creative ways of guiding teens to develop their ability to accept and let go of difficult internal experiences. These ACT-inspired ones that I introduced here are all in service of strengthening their emotional intelligence so they feel equipped to handle difficult experiences as they arise. By helping adolescents identify and understand their range of cognitive and emotional reactions to stuttering, they learn to make space for challenges rather than get into a power struggle with them. These efforts will help them make peace with the inevitable ups and downs of their stuttering experiences.

Creating Affirmations

In helping adolescents approach everyday experiences with a more positive orientation, some may be open to focusing on an affirmation at the start of each day and/or in challenging situations. **Affirmations** are positive statements about the adolescent's characteristics or behaviors and are useful to reinforce change behaviors (Epton et al., 2015). Adolescents may disengage if they sense the affirmation is overly cheerleader-like or disingenuous (eg, "I feel on top of the world" when they are actually feeling stressed or upset). It's important that affirmations are honest and specific about target changes—for example, "I make space for stuttering," "My stuttering does not define me," "My stuttering makes me unique," "I am an effective communicator," "I have important ideas to share," "I am becoming my best self," "I am always learning more about who I am," and "Let me be seen" to name a few. Affirmations can be developed with the adolescent in a therapy session and then written down for them to take with them into their week. Make sure you have discussed a clear plan for how the affirmations will be used—for instance, written in their planner and revisited at the start of each school day, said internally at the start of each class period or before certain interactions, etc.

Finding Community

One of the most powerful ways to combat the loneliness and isolation that often accompanies stuttering is to get involved in the stuttering community (Gerlach et al., 2019). In doing so, the teen feels, perhaps for the first time, that they are not alone—that they are *not* the only one in the world who stutters, although it often feels like that. All adolescents who stutter, regardless of their age, their background, or how they stutter, would benefit from meeting other people who stutter, although the right timing will be unique to each of them. Some adolescents need time to understand their own stuttering and their own experience before they are willing to meet other stutterers. As their clinician, know that this process takes time and you are encouraged not to pressure the teen to meet other stutterers if they indicate they don't want to yet; doing so may backfire in unintended ways.

There are several established stuttering communities that you can introduce the teen to. The two most common ones are FRIENDS (The National Association for Young People Who Stutter; www.friendswhostutter.org) and NSA (The National Stuttering Association; www.westutter.org). At the time of this writing, FRIENDS offers free monthly virtual support groups for teens. The NSA has some local chapters for families and some that are specifically for teens; both are supported by the Teen Advisory Council, which is an advisory board comprised of teens who stutter. Both FRIENDS and NSA offer an in-person annual convention that both usually take place in July (thankfully on different weekends). If there is no local NSA chapter in your area and you are interested in starting one, reach out to the NSA office and they will help get you started. It's relatively easy to get a new chapter off the ground logistically and as long as there are families of teens who stutter in your area who are interested in participating, you are encouraged to launch a chapter in your area. Metaphorically, you'll receive big returns on your investment.

There are also numerous summer camps that have popped up all over the country for kids and teens who stutter. Camp SAY (NY), Camp Shout Out (MI), Camp Words Unspoken (MA), and Camp More (OR), to name a few. There are also some summer programs affiliated with university clinics, like UISPEAKS (University of Iowa), Colorado Speaks (University of Colorado at Boulder), Camp Dream.Speak.Live (University of Texas at Austin), and CSTEP (Texas State University). If a university in your area has a speech clinic, you could reach out to them to inquire about summer programming for young people who stutter. If the clinic doesn't have a summer program yet (or even a local support group that meets throughout the year), you could broach the idea of collaborating to start one.

REDUCING AVOIDANCE OF SOUNDS, WORDS, AND SITUATIONS

Most adolescents who stutter will admit that the stuttering experience is filled with daily mental gymnastics. Aside from the looming sense of worry about impending stuttering and rumination about how past interactions went, many teens find themselves in interactions where they are actively scanning ahead to figure out ways to not stutter—constantly updating current plans depending on how the moment and context unfold. This avoidance happens at the level of certain sounds the teen thinks is challenging to say, words they have historically had difficulty saying, or situations they don't want to stutter in. These mental gymnastics of avoiding triggering sounds, words, and situations is what often contributes to mental load and fatigue, rather than the stuttering itself, and it is cognitively and emotionally exhausting. Thus, one of our responsibilities is helping adolescents become more aware of how their own mental gymnastics works and figuring out ways they can reduce that mental load so they can communicate more freely.

Talking Openly About Stuttering and Increasing Disclosure

Stuttering is often an isolating experience. Not only do adolescents sometimes feel like the only person in their world who stutters, but because of their increasing desire for independence, they may feel like stuttering is something they have to, or want to, deal with on their own. While in some ways this may feel safe and comfortable because they are not sharing their vulnerability with others, it can come to feel like a very heavy burden to carry solo. For many adolescents, choosing at least one safe person to open up to about stuttering (other than you, the clinician) can be life changing. This can be a family member, a close friend, or other trusted confidante. The intention behind this task is multifold. First, connecting with a trusted listener about our hurt and vulnerabilities can be cathartic if we are met with empathy. Healing and authenticity happen in empathetic space. Second, it can help the adolescent build their skills and confidence in self-advocacy. Perhaps they choose to tell their parents what is helpful or unhelpful about how their parents attempt to support them, or they want to vent to a friend about recent interpersonal challenges that they want to address. Talking this out with someone the teen trusts can open opportunities to live more authentically and proactively.

While it's helpful (albeit scary) to talk to someone new about stuttering, disclosing one's stuttering to new listeners offers great rewards. Self-disclosure is the act of overtly telling or showing that one is a person who stutters. Many people assume that self-disclosure is verbal, but there are other creative ways to share one's stuttering identity such as through putting a stuttering sticker on their water bottle or laptop, wearing a stuttering T-shirt or hat, posting about it on social media, sharing a creative artifact they created like a slam poem or painting about stuttering. There is a growing body of literature on stuttering self-disclosure, some of which has revealed that nonapologetic **disclosures** are perceived most favorably by listeners (Byrd et al., 2017). I imagine that nonapologetic disclosures also benefit speakers because not apologizing for something out of one's control can increase their sense of self-worth.

For adolescents for whom talking about stuttering and/or self-disclosing is challenging, it could be helpful to discuss, script out, and/or role play a variety of disclosures. In my experience, for young people who stutter, the trick is to figure out a way to disclose naturally at a time that doesn't draw attention to themselves. If the teen has a good sense of humor, help them tap into that; using humor can ease an otherwise tense or nervous moment for them.

Expanding Comfort Zone

Everyone has situations that are within and outside their comfort zone, and those zones look different for each person. Situations within our comfort zone invite us to act right away, as we feel safe and equipped to meet the demands of the situation with the skills we have now. Not all situations outside our comfort zone are equally difficult. Some situations may perhaps feel doable now, although it requires courage, while other situations feel wholly out the realm of possibility because they are too stressful. A little bit of stress can be helpful and facilitate growth, while a lot of stress is a signal that the body (including the mind) is not equipped to handle the demands of the situation and needs safety. This can be visualized as a three-tiered ring with comfort zone at the core, surrounded by the stretch zone, and enclosed by the stress zone. As seen in Figure 16.3, as one's capacity for self-regulation and agency increase in the face of challenge, their stress zone shrinks, which allows increased comfort and adaptability with a wider range of behaviors and situations. I have found it incredibly helpful to discuss this graphic with teens and guide them to share situations that are in their comfort, stretch, and stress zones for them right now. This introduces the importance of understanding one's body. Another useful metaphor is borrowed from Vivian Sisskin's work with ARTS, wherein adolescents identify self-imposed "stop signs" in their everyday life—things like words they don't want to say, situations they don't want to experience, events they don't want to attend, emotions they don't want to feel (Sisskin & Goldstein, 2022). With compassionate guidance, teens identify stop signs they can safely roll on through and what that might look like.

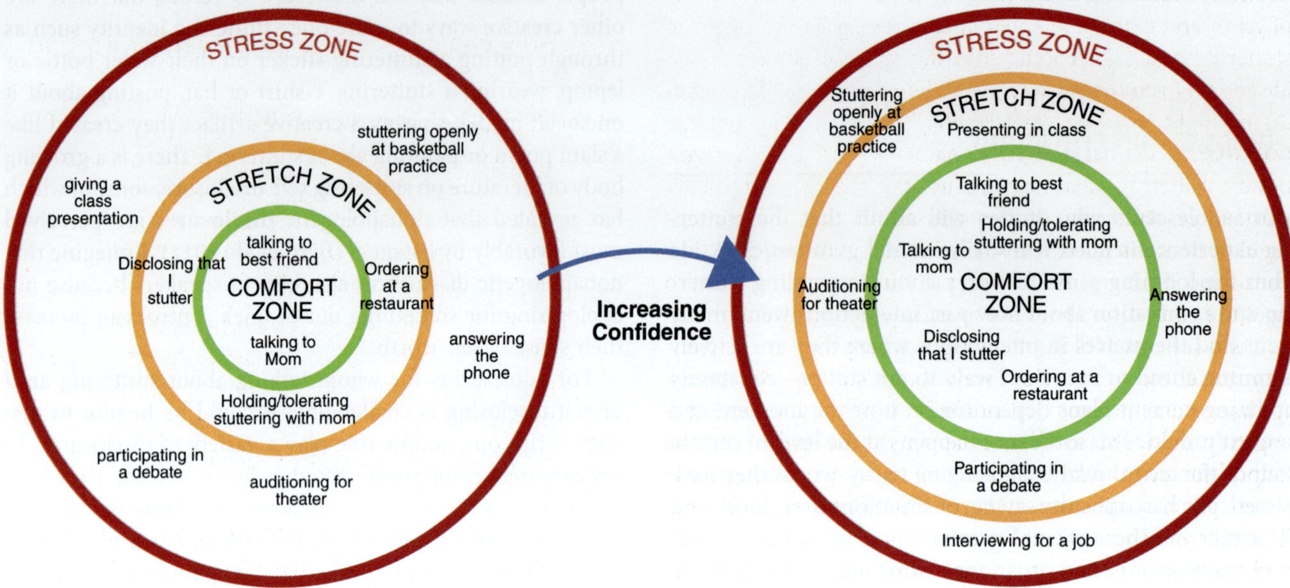

Figure 16.3 Comfort, stretch, and stress zones fluctuate depending on one's confidence.

As they tell you about situations they encounter and avoid in subsequent sessions, you can ground the discussion in this visual of the three-tiered comfort zone. You are encouraged to validate how hard some things feel now and be intentional about your language to facilitate growth mindset. *You're not quite ready to do that yet, and that's ok. I know it feels out of reach right now, but it won't always be. What's a small thing you could do to step into your stretch zone, or safely roll this stop sign?* It's important to recognize that pushing adolescents (all clients, really) into their stress zone, even if you think they're capable of doing it or that it would be good for them, is counter-productive. Our goal is to help adolescents tune into their body and make decisions that facilitate self-growth, in their desired direction, when they decide the time is right for them. This is a life skill that will help them learn how to direct their own behaviors and changes, with a focus on stepping into their stretch zone if it moves them toward a value-driven direction.

The situational hierarchy discussed previously in the section on "Using Hierarchies to Level Up" can also be situated in this comfort-stretch-stress zone context. Identify which steps on the hierarchy constitute each of the three zones. Then, you and the client can cocreate weekly opportunities that are guided by the hierarchy or the zones. Make sure that you are in consensus about what constitutes a "success," focusing on doing the hard thing regardless of how much they stuttered. Perhaps success means that they ordered exactly what they wanted instead of ordering what was easy to say, or that they asked a follow-up question when they normally woudn't have, or that they answered the phone instead of letting it go to voicemail. Clients can record their observations about those opportunities in a journal or on a note on their phone and bring them back to the therapy session to discuss with you. If they are hung up on how much they stuttered, try to redirect their focus on the fact that they felt afraid and did it anyways, and that's what matters most. (Notice the use of "and" not "but"—"you felt afraid *and* still did it"; this contrasts with "you felt afraid *but* still did it," which discounts the feeling of fear.) If they are hung up on how other people reacted or behaved, try to help them separate their own self-worth from other people's evaluations of them (whether perceived or actual). Offer lots of verbal praise for trying to take advantage of opportunities even if it didn't go exactly according to their plan, and perhaps help the teen identify something they can do for themself as a reward. Over time, these efforts compound to expand one's comfort and stretch zones.

Voluntary Stuttering

The methods for using voluntary stuttering in the therapy setting were discussed previously in the section on "Identifying Moments of Stuttering." Voluntary stuttering is also sometimes called *pseudostuttering, fake stuttering,* or *stuttering on purpose* (although I like to say stuttering *with* purpose). In a nutshell, you and the client both practice voluntary stuttering in situations of increasing difficulty, starting in simple, structured therapy activities and working up to opportunities outside the therapy room (eg, ordering at a coffee shop, asking a store clerk a question in person and on the phone, with a family member). Use the client's individualized linguistic and situational hierarchy to guide this process.

Voluntary stuttering is a form of exposure therapy, which is a common psychotherapeutic method for addressing fears and avoidances. In the context of stuttering therapy, voluntary stuttering helps adolescents do the thing they are so often afraid of doing: stuttering. Voluntary stuttering is done supportively with the intention of (1) exposing the teen to the physical and emotional experience of being in a moment of stuttering and (2) stepping into the space of stuttering-as-identity. *If I voluntary stutter when I don't have to, I am claiming my right to stutter and accepting the identity of someone who stutters. I'm not hiding that part of myself.* Together, voluntary stuttering often helps reduce the client's reactivity to, and fear of, stuttering, thereby allowing them to better self-regulate in moments of real stuttering and feel equipped to go ahead and "let it rip". As their fear of stuttering goes down, so does the compulsion to avoid sounds, words, and situations.

I will say that adolescents will greet the prospect of voluntary stuttering with varying levels of openness or willingness. It's important that your rationale for voluntary stuttering is cogently delivered so they understand why this would be helpful for them. And even with the most articulate, clearly stated pitch, some teens still won't be on board. That's ok. That tells you about where they are in their stuttering journey and there is no need to push them too hard. Remember, the more you push, the more they'll resist.

SUMMARY

- Adolescence is a period of great risk and opportunity rooted in neurobiological changes of puberty; clinicians are encouraged to work with adolescents' increasing desire for independence and social connection.
- A crucial ingredient in an effective therapeutic experience is to create a **safe stuttering space**.
- Therapy goals should be developed collaboratively with the client through solution-focused discussions about what changes are important and achievable to them. Behavior changes can be both overt (observable to others) and covert (changes to thoughts and feelings).
- Learning to stutter in an easier way involves learning about the speech mechanism to understand how stuttering works, then practicing holding, tolerating, and easing out of moments of stuttering. Clinicians who model desired behaviors (including voluntary stutters) show their clients that they are willing to do new, scary things too which facilitates mutual respect and can be motivating for the client.
- Cognitive-behavioral therapy and ACT are useful ways to help adolescents develop healthier thoughts and feelings about stuttering.
- To help clients reduce situational avoidance, you can help clients identify their values so they can make value-driven decisions bolstered by their strengths, affirmations, and rolling self-imposed stop signs when they are ready.

STUDY QUESTIONS

1. How can clinicians create a safe stuttering space?
2. What is unique about adolescents, which makes it different than working with children and adults?
3. What are some common behavior changes that adolescents who stutter and clinicians believe are important?
4. How can you guide an adolescent client through the process of desensitization and learning to ease out of moments of stuttering?
5. How are CBT and ACT similar? How are they different?
6. What are some ways to help adolescents who stutter reduce avoidance?

SUGGESTED PROJECTS

1. Visit www.viacharacter.org, create a free account, and complete the *Signature Strengths for Adults* assessment, which should take around 10 to 15 minutes. Click "Skip and get your free results." List your top five strengths, describe each of them.
2. Write a script for how you would teach an adolescent about speech anatomy and physiology, and how you would guide them through experiencing easiness and tension in different areas of the speech mechanism.
3. Think of a time in your life when you wanted to change something about yourself (eg, lose weight, stop drinking soda, floss your teeth daily, manage your anxiety). Reflect on how ready you think you were to make that change at that time, and generate a list of pros and cons of the target behavior. This exercise is intended to help you reflect on how hard it is to change parts of yourself, and it may help you empathize with how difficult the change journey is for adolescents who stutter.
4. Think of a challenge that you'd like to achieve. Make a situational hierarchy for yourself to help you work systematically toward meeting that challenge.
5. Listen to a guided meditation, perhaps one by Tara Brach that's freely available on her website and as a podcast. Then, find a guided meditation that would be appropriate for adolescents—one that either (1) helps them tune into their body or (2) integrates visualization to help them experience letting go of difficult experiences.
6. Fill in a comfort-stretch-stress zone diagram for yourself.
7. Research stuttering support groups or camps that would be available to adolescents in your area—either local or national opportunities.

SUGGESTED READINGS

Damour, L. (2023). *The emotional life of teenagers: Raising connected, capable, and compassionate adolescents*. Ballantine Books.

For those who are broadly interested in adolescence, Dr Damour summarizes the science of adolescents' emotional experiences and how adults involved in adolescents' lives can effectively support them.

Hallett, K., & Donelan, J. (2019). *Trauma treatment toolbox for teens: 144 trauma-informed worksheets and exercises to promote resilience, growth, and healing*. PESI Publishing & Media.

This workbook provides practical worksheets that clinicians can use to help teens (not restricted to those who stutter) understand how their brain and body work and help them develop adaptive coping strategies.

Hayes, L., & Ciarrochi, J. (2015). *The thriving adolescent: Using acceptance and commitment therapy and positive psychology to help teens manage emotions, achieve goals, and build connection*. New Harbinger.

Intended for therapists, counselors, and teachers, this book uses a strength-based approach to supporting adolescence as they navigate challenges.

Hendrickson, J. (2023). *Life on delay: Making peace with a stutter*. Alfred A. Knopf.

A raw memoir by journalist John Hendrickson who expertly weaves together his own experiences and voices from others in the field as he seeks closure on painful stuttering experiences dating back to his early childhood. Contains mature content, so recommended for those who are at least 18 years old.

Preston, K. (2013). *Out with it: How stuttering helped me find my voice*. Atria Books.

Another outstanding memoir, Katherine Preston takes readers on a journey from her search for a stuttering cure to ultimately embracing her stuttered voice and identity.

17

Treatment of Adults: Advanced Stuttering

Chapter Outline

Chapter Objectives

After studying this chapter, readers should be able to:

- Describe some of the behavioral, cognitive, and emotional characteristics of stuttering in adults
- Explain what components of advanced stuttering may be learned, thus making them candidates for unlearning
- Describe three fluency goals that are appropriate for adults who stutter
- Explain how classical conditioning principles can be used to help individuals unlearn old responses that account for many stuttering behaviors and attitudes
- Explain why fears and other emotions must be dealt with in treatment, along with changing how the individual speaks
- Explain what is accomplished in the first stage of treatment, "exploring stuttering"
- Describe how the clinician can help the client deal with feelings associated with stuttering
- Delineate some of the important principles that must be followed to transfer a

new behavior from the therapy room to outside situations

- Explain how voluntary stuttering may help a person who stutters
- Give several examples of how a person who stutters can be open about their stuttering
- Indicate some of the things the client must do to maintain fluency gains after treatment
- Describe the situations in which you would consider recommending controlled fluency as an option for a client to consider

Key Terms

Approach behavior: Consciously going toward something that was previously feared (or still is feared). Part of the reason that stuttering persists is that the individual avoids stuttering and avoids saying feared words and entering feared situations, causing the fear to continue. By deliberately approaching feared words and situations again and again, fear diminishes and so does stuttering

Becoming your own clinician: By including the client in decision-making regarding therapy as much as possible right from the beginning, clients may begin to recognize themselves as their own clinicians. However, near the termination of therapy, the client becomes more and more able to give themselves assignments to maintain the desired outcomes they achieved working with the clinician. But more discussion of the client becoming their own clinician may be needed as they move toward taking on sole responsibility for this role

Catch and release: A term some clients and clinicians use to label staying in the stutter and letting the fear and tension go so that the word can be finished easily and smoothly

Controlled fluency: A style of speaking that improves fluency by modifying certain elements of speech, including speaking more slowly, pausing, using easy onsets at the beginnings of words, using light contacts of articulators, and employing proprioception (becoming aware of the movements of articulators)

Counterconditioning: A way of decreasing a response such as fear of stuttering by pairing the previously feared stimulus (eg, stuttering) with a positive stimulus (eg, praise). The Wikipedia description of counterconditioning has a link to one of the pioneers of counterconditioning, Mary Cover Jones. The description of Jones' use of counterconditioning to help a boy named Peter reduce his fear of rabbits is a gem and will help readers understand counterconditioning via a straightforward example

Deconditioning: Similar to counterconditioning except that instead of a positive stimulus, the previously feared stimulus (stuttering) is paired with a neutral stimulus (no negative consequence)

Easier stuttering: A mild form of stuttering that neither interferes with communication nor bothers the speaker or listener

Exploring stuttering: Activities that help the client get in contact with the experience of stuttering without the negative emotions usually associated with stuttering. It is a type of approach behavior that can achieve **deconditioning**, thereby decreasing fear

Spontaneous fluency: Speech without stuttering that doesn't require thinking about it

Staying in the stutter: Going right into the stutter, without any avoidance, and then prolonging the articulatory posture and sound associated with the moment of "stuckness." The purpose is to extinguish or reduce the threat and fear associated with the experience of being stuck. The clinician's praise and acceptance of the client's staying in the stutter are very important in extinguishing these emotions

Voluntary stuttering: Stuttering on purpose or at least producing speech in a way that mimics stuttering, with the aim of reducing fear of stuttering and potentially advertising one's stutter to one's audience with the idea of doing it when and where it suits the speaker

AN INTEGRATED APPROACH

Individuals with advanced stuttering are usually adults who have been stuttering for many years. Their patterns, which are well entrenched, consist of blocks, repetitions, and prolongations that are usually accompanied by tension and struggle, as well as escape and avoidance behaviors. Typically, these individuals have developed negative anticipations about speaking situations and listener reactions. Sometimes, their stuttering has been such an important factor in their lives that they have chosen occupations beneath their abilities (Van Riper, for example, worked as a farmhand, digging potatoes, after he earned his Master's degree in English literature from the University of Michigan). Adults with advanced stuttering sometimes turn down promotions if more speaking is required than in their present positions and will often not participate fully in group discussions, team meetings, and conversations. In rare instances, some adults who stutter hide their stuttering by avoiding words or situations so completely that they don't show the usual signs of stuttering. Their stuttering is sometimes referred to as "interiorized" or "covert."

Because the complex patterns of advanced stuttering involve behaviors, emotions, and cognitions, treatment is most effective if it targets all of these areas. These patterns are so deeply etched into the brain that treatment is best if it is intense, is long-lasting, and provides training for long-term maintenance. My approach to treatment is a brew blended from many sources. I have tried to integrate these procedures so that clients reduce their negative emotions and avoidances and learn to respond differently, with more fluent stuttering to old cues that have always triggered tense and struggled stuttering (see Fig. 17.1).

Our integrated approach to stuttering in adults is illustrated above, using an example of a highly motivated young

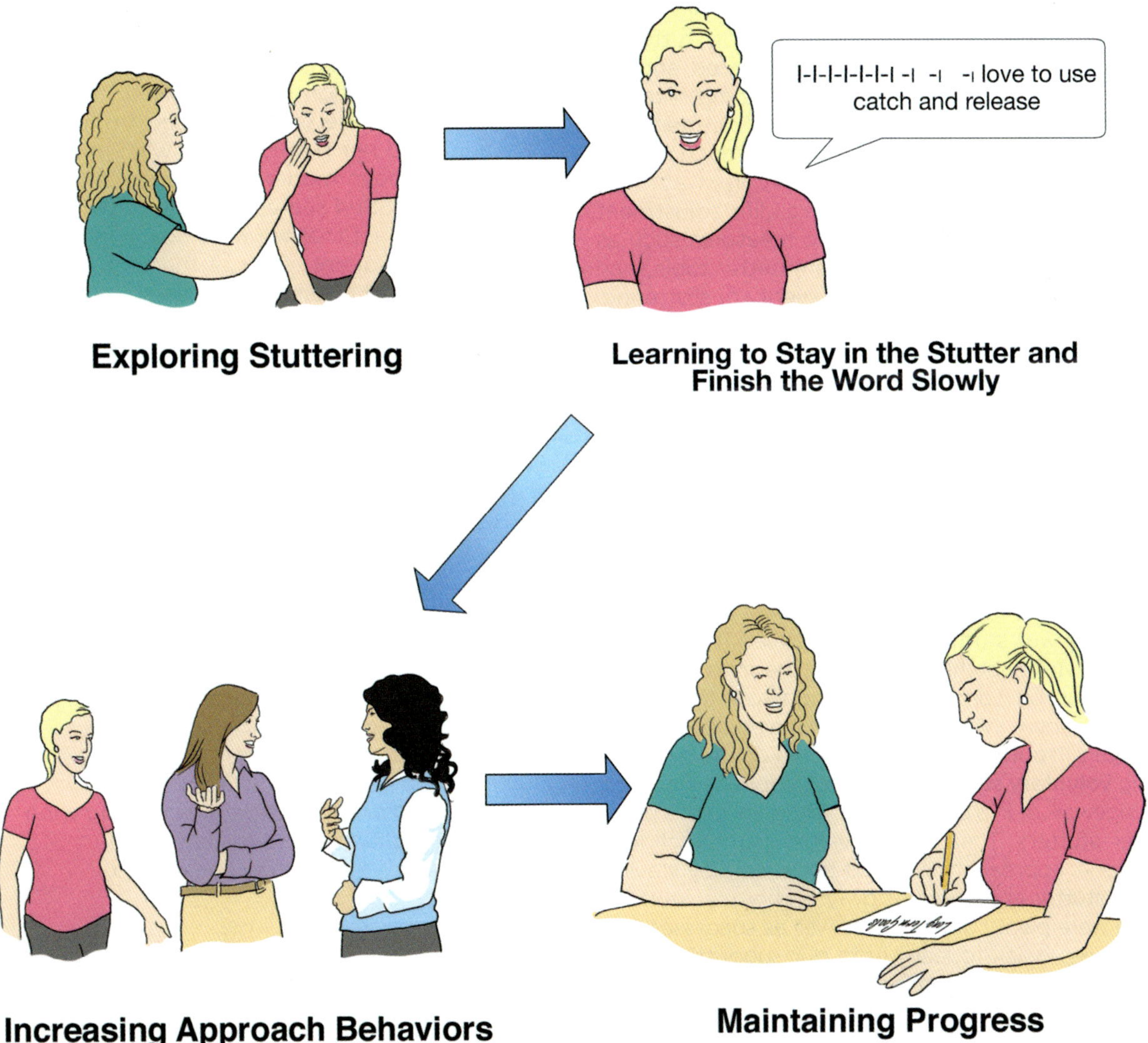

Figure 17.1 Elements of an integrated approach to treatment.

Case Example

Malisa

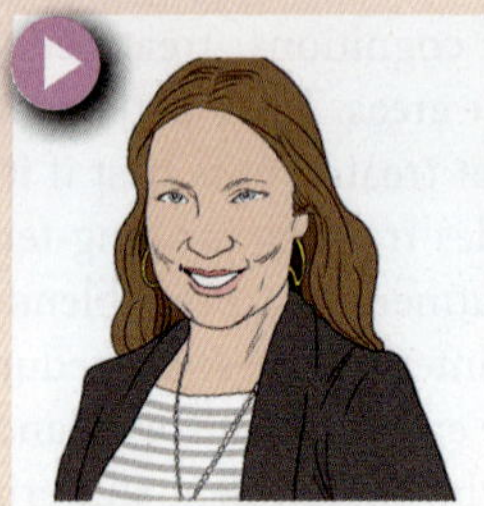

In the fall semester several years ago, a young woman named Malisa, an elementary school teacher in Vermont, came to us for help with her stuttering. She reported having difficulty talking to the parents of her students, introducing herself to new people, and making telephone calls. In addition to teaching, Malisa is a poet and she felt that her stuttering was keeping her from reading her poetry aloud at public gatherings. Malisa had a family history of stuttering and, in fact, had no memory of speaking without stuttering, even as a child. Our initial evaluation measures showed that her frequency of stuttering in conversation was 7.4% syllables stuttered, and her rating on the SSI-4 was severe. More importantly, the Overall Assessment of Speakers' Experience of Stuttering (OASES, a measure of how much impact stuttering has on the individual's daily life) was moderate. In assessing a client's overall life adjustment before, during, and after therapy, measures such as OASES and the Erickson S-24 are better tools than assessments of frequency and severity of stuttering.

Two of my graduate students and I worked with Malisa during the fall and spring semesters. We began by helping her explore her stuttering and her feelings about it, through having her feel what she was doing when she stuttered, watching herself in the mirror when she stuttered, and discussing stuttering experiences and accompanying feelings, both in the past and present. After several weeks, we progressed to having Malisa stay in the moment of stuttering—learning to tolerate the frustration of being stuck—then gradually reduce the tension and slowly finish the word on which she was stuttering. She practiced these easier stutters while watching herself in the mirror with us in the clinic, on video playback, and also in the nearby student center. When our work involved speaking to strangers in public, the clinician would do the task first, using **voluntary stuttering**, as they stopped people on the sidewalk or in a building and asked questions using easier stutters. Then, Malisa would gamely choose someone, approach them, and try to employ staying in the stutter and ending slowly on her real stutters. There were plenty of failures as well as successes, but Malisa was quick to learn from our suggestions and worked diligently, in both her sessions with us and her assignments to practice at home.

The first five or six sessions focused not just on stuttering behaviors but most importantly on feelings associated with stuttering. Malisa's fear of stuttering diminished as she learned more about her stuttering, explored past experiences and feelings, and repeatedly sought out opportunities to practice. Once Malisa was making changes in her overlearned stuttering patterns as well as in her feelings and attitudes, we introduced some elements of "**controlled fluency**"—easy onsets, proprioception, flexible rate, and pausing. After practice on using these in her fluent speech, we helped Malisa employ them to deal with anticipated stutters. Again, Malisa was a quick learner and was successful in turning some of her stutters into easier, briefer stutters so that she felt comfortably in control. Malisa also worked on voluntary stuttering and letting listeners know that she stuttered.

By the middle of the spring semester, she was doing well, but still had some challenges when the stress was high or when she was caught by surprise. By the end of the spring semester, in May, after a total of 21 sessions, Malisa's percent syllables stuttered in conversation had decreased (from 7.4) to 1.4. Her SSI-4 score had decreased from severe to very mild, and her OASES score was "mild/moderate" (having been moderate). The percent syllables stuttered and SSI-4 scores may well have been influenced by the fact that we were now a familiar audience. In an eloquent letter of thanks to the clinic, Malisa wrote, "The last two semesters of work with you and (the two graduate students) have been pivotal in changing my outlook and stuttering behavior.... To be confident in 'voice' is a life skill with far-reaching effects." She added that she had just published a poem in a literary journal and was able to read it in public, not with complete fluency, but in a way that made her proud. Here is one of her poems about stuttering:

A stutterer introduces herself
or not, if the syllables come without sound
and the mouth pantomimes
the onset M in white gloves.

She begins with her lips open
so the penned up can slip out
to grass before morning's milking.
Let it always be a county fair in May.
Let moored breath beckon a wheedling wind
before the thunder of big-top speech.
Everyone will look up, necks exposed,
and wait
as the clouds roll in.

So the fluency's flexible,
may a maundering farm hand amble
the meandering mile, and consonants
become malleable when struck
or stuck by the jaw.

But if blocked again again again,
the repetitions of Ma- Ma- Ma-
might call to mind the bleat
of judged goats in the grandstand and
you will feel ashamed
of your adolescent associations.
A trick trap door's underfoot
for moments like this.

Or, if you're kinder sort, maybe instead
you'll hear the infant summoning
Mother (the first sensible uttering)
and notice she's pretty
though her message is mazy.

And if the confusion continues
in this casual meeting of strangers,
I suggest you generously
let her build momentum or cancel
the conversation completely.
Some carousels are silent.
She's looking away.

Letting beginning be easy as ice cream—
licking maple creamees
melty at noon under the oak,
make light contact with your eyes
and her tongue will make light contact
in her mouth. And her larynx will release
the mechanical latch holding back
the tin tine that plays
the music of mute clowns.
The melody holds most of the meaning anyway
and red lipstick smears all the M's.

Reprinted from her book *Handing Out Apples in Eden* (2014, Wind Ridge Books) with permission of the author.

adult. If any of the terminology used in this description is not clear at first, it will become clear after reading about the treatment process later in the chapter.

Author's Beliefs

The assertions that follow are not facts but rather my inferences about advanced stuttering and its treatment. The reader should keep in mind that it is filtered through my own experiences as a person who has stuttered since age 3, who received therapy at age 21 from Charles Van Riper, and who has had both successes and failures over the 50 years he has worked as a stuttering therapist.

Nature of Stuttering

As I described in Chapter 6, I believe that the origins of advanced stuttering arise from a physiological predisposition for inefficient neural activation patterns for speech and a vulnerable temperament interacting with environmental influences to produce and exacerbate core behaviors of, typically (but not always), repetitions. In the early stages, a child may react to these repetitions with a response of increased tension, pushing, and hurry. This, in essence, trying hard *not* to stutter. As a reactive child continues to experience and respond to the core behaviors, a negative spiral worsens the stuttering. Increased tension and struggle become more and more alarming to the child, and the child then pushes harder to get words out. Soon, they try to cope by adding a variety of escape behaviors, which are reinforced through operant conditioning, via the reward of finishing the word after deploying an escape behavior such as an eyeblink or a head nod. During this same period, negative feelings—such as frustration, fear, and shame—become associated with stuttering. These feelings generalize through classical conditioning to more and more words and situations. Finally, the child begins to avoid feared words and situations, with fear perpetuated through intermittent reinforcement. If these underlying processes continue until an individual reaches young adulthood, the client will enter the stage of advanced stuttering.

Because increased tension, speeding up of speech rate, secondary behaviors, and feelings and attitudes are learned, they can be modified. The tension, speeding up, escape, and avoidance behaviors are all things the stutterer does to keep from stuttering or to hide the stuttering; once the person can learn to let the stutter out in the open, stuttering becomes easier and easier. Because the handicapping behaviors of stuttering result from operant and classical conditioning principles, these same principles can be used to make changes. However, because predisposing physiological factors contribute to these behaviors and also because many years of learning have reorganized the brain in people with advanced stuttering, *complete* unlearning may not be possible. Thus, it is crucial to help individuals with advanced stuttering learn how to stutter more easily and cope with residual disruptions in speech if they are going to maintain improvements in their comfort with speaking.

Speech Behaviors Targeted for Therapy

In this section, I include both *new* behaviors, which need to be learned, and *old* behaviors, which need to be reduced or eliminated. In most individuals with advanced stuttering, well-learned tension and speeding-up responses are cued by anticipated and actual stuttering. They are typically accompanied by a considerable overlay of other learned secondary behaviors. To cope with these learned behaviors and to stutter more easily, individuals with advanced stuttering need to decrease their fear of stuttering and eliminate their escape and avoidance behaviors. Then, they can learn to respond to actual or anticipated stuttering by going right into the stutter without using starters or other delaying techniques. Once in the stuckness of the stutter, they need to learn to stay in the stuck posture while producing appropriate airflow and/or sound. When they are able to "be present" in the stutter and—with much help from the clinician—tolerate the moment of "stuckness," the tension will reduce. The muscles will relax and they will be able to move slowly through the rest of the word. The slow, loose finish of the word will be reinforced by the relief of finishing the word. Whew!

The above description is a *new* behavior that can be learned with guidance and support from the clinician. When learned and practiced, it gives the client a new feeling of being in control of their stuttering. Then, the client can relinquish more and more of their maladaptive *old* behaviors. These old behaviors include escape and avoidance maneuvers that keep the stuttering "hot" and bar the way to making changes that can help them flourish as a communicator. But also, as the client feels they have a tool that works (staying in the moment of stuttering and remaining calm)—a tool that gives them some control—their emotions will change as well. Note that I advocate only this single tool to respond to stuttering, making it easier for the client to decide what to do under stress. They don't have to choose among four or five different strategies. I will talk more about this in the sections to come on treatment procedures.

Fluency Goals

The ultimate goal that many people with advanced stuttering have in mind when they start therapy is spontaneous "fluency" in all situations or, in other words, normal speech. In my experience, most individuals with advanced stuttering do not reach this level of fluency, and that's fine, especially if the person embraces the idea that making speaking easier rather than simply making it more fluent for the sake of the listeners is key. After treatment, clients may have periods of **spontaneous fluency**, lasting from a few hours to a month or more, but usually some stuttering returns, especially in stressful situations. At these times, I want clients to have an option.

For those individuals who stutter who want to speak confidently, communicate easily, and feel comfortable in their speech, I want them to have the freedom to go directly into stutters, keep the sound or airflow going for a few seconds, remain calm, and then end the word slowly. How they achieve these kinds of stutters will be explained when I describe the nuts and bolts of therapy.

Sometimes individuals who have been in therapy with me will have days and times when they can't get a handle on their stuttering. At those times, I would like them to just talk, without hiding or avoiding their stuttering. Ideally, at these times, they would just focus on communicating with their conversational partner, listening well, and saying what they want to say when they want to say it—stuttering be damned!

Feelings and Attitudes

I believe that most adults with advanced stuttering typically have strong negative feelings and attitudes toward their stuttering and toward themselves when they begin therapy. I give these emotions and cognitions substantial attention throughout therapy. From the beginning, the client and I work together as a team to explore their fears of getting stuck on certain sounds and words, as well as fears of situations that have been humiliating to them in the past. We also work to uncover feelings of shame and inadequacy that years of stuttering have spawned. Even after many therapy sessions, these negative emotions and attitudes will rise up again as we transfer the client's newly learned tool of stuttering management to the outside world. Our direct work on feelings and attitudes, combined with the client's successes in feeling some control over their stuttering, reduces these negative emotions. This change is critical if our clients are to break free of morbid self-consciousness and be able to focus on the back-and-forth of good communication.

I believe that one of the clinician's major weapons for attacking negative emotions is *extinction*. As I described in Chapters 5 and 6, classical conditioning has linked many stuttering stimuli to negative emotions, and extinction will weaken those links. For example, when an individual sees an upcoming "bugaboo" word (like their name, when they anticipate introducing themselves), they dread it. But when they are accompanied in this situation by a supportive clinician whom they trust, and the clinician has taught them to use a tool that helps them stutter more fluently, they may feel substantially less dread. They know that the clinician is right there by their side and will accept them no matter what happens. The client knows that the clinician will praise them for even going into the situation and will applaud them for just *trying* to stutter more easily. Thus, because they face their fear, the link weakens. This is extinction. When this happens again and again—when the client experiences a situation that has previously been humiliating but is now followed by a feeling of pride—they are more and more likely to not anticipate disaster when introducing themselves.

You can see from this example that the client-clinician relationship is key. I think that when the client learns that the clinician is strong and knowledgeable, and that the clinician has the client's best interest at heart, the client can move mountains, or at least they can learn to stutter more easily, both in the therapy room and outside, both for now and for the long term.

Maintenance Procedures

Despite the important role of extinction in therapy, it is clear from research that extinction of fear responses is vulnerable to "spontaneous recovery" (Bouton, 2016). The mind and body don't truly and totally eliminate the over-learned responses to the deeply etched memories of how awful stuttering had been to them. Thus, maintenance routines used by the client are vital to keep old tension, struggle, escape, and avoidance responses from returning under stress and with the passage of time. Effective maintenance depends, in part, on clients becoming their own clinicians, which should begin early in therapy. Clients learn to evaluate their own performance in mastering the skill of stuttering more easily and to monitor their fears and avoidances. I gradually shift more and more of the responsibility for therapy planning to clients as they improve, and it is important for them to have a realistic understanding of what they should expect in terms of their long-term fluency. Thus, clients need to understand the purpose of going right into the stutter and **staying in the stutter**, calming themselves, until negative emotion and tension are reduced and then finishing the word slowly and easily. In this way, an easy stutter is reinforced by the relief of completing the utterance and the pride in controlling what had felt uncontrollable before. It is also important that clients appreciate the relationship between regular practice of what they have learned in therapy and the attainment of their goals.

Clinical Methods

Like the approach described for intermediate stuttering with school-age children, my management for advanced stuttering in adults begins with exploring behaviors, cognitions, and emotions to decrease negative emotion associated with stuttering. My clinical relationship with the client is paramount in helping the client get in touch with their feelings and accept those feelings. We work together on the client's emotional responses—particularly those that started in childhood and that are still strong. Much sharing about feelings and attitudes, much work on becoming open and accepting of one's stuttering is needed. When the time is right, I help the client learn to go right into the stuckness of the stutter and learn to tolerate the moment of stuttering to reduce the fear, and to finish easily. Then, I help the individual transfer and stabilize those skills with hierarchies of more and more challenging situations, voluntary stuttering, and seeking out feared words and feared situations. The measures I use to assess progress will be described shortly.

Clinical Procedures: Reducing Fear and Learning to Stutter More Easily

Procedures described here for working with advanced stuttering in adults borrow liberally from many clinicians, especially my own therapist, Van Riper (1973a). I am also indebted to numerous colleagues in the field, as well as to my students and clients who have generously shared their ideas.

Key Concepts

1. *Treatment of adults usually takes a long time, demands considerable motivation, and must maintain a focus on many fronts.* As you may remember from Chapters 13 and 14, treatment of preschool children can be as brief as a few months. But the older individual has been stuttering for many years, and much fear-based and unhelpful learning has taken place. Therefore, as you will see, my approach has many stages, each subsequent stage building on the former and requiring continuing hard work on changing behaviors and emotions. There are exceptions; some rare clients are so ready to change and so emotionally robust that treatment feels like sailing with the wind at your back. Their treatment is discussed in the section titled "Learning and Generalizing Controlled Fluency."
2. *Treatment should be tailored to each client's needs.* Although it would be easier if one sequence of treatment fit all clients, stuttering therapy is not so simple. Each person's biological makeup and life experiences differ; therefore, individuals require different therapy ingredients in their overall recipe for their success. Of the procedures presented in this section, *going directly into the stutter without avoidance, staying in the stutter, calming oneself, and releasing it slowly and loosely* are the heart of learning to stutter more easily. But in order for it to work, the client must not be hampered by overwhelming fears of stuttering or of listener reactions. To deal with these fears, most clients will need to confront, explore, and accept their stuttering with the clinician's support.

   A clinician just learning how to carry out stuttering therapy may want to go through each step of treatment just as I have described them. An experienced clinician may want to work with the client to reorder the steps to suit the client or may omit steps that the client and clinician believe the client doesn't need, or add new steps, as needed.
3. *Successful outcome of treatment depends, in part, on increasing* ***approach behaviors*** *and reducing avoidance.* Evidence from treatment outcome research suggests that a successful long-term outcome related to speech behaviors is associated with positive communication attitudes and low levels of avoidance (eg, Guitar, 1976; Guitar & Bass, 1978; Langevin et al., 2006). Thus, work in these areas may not only improve the speaker's quality of life but also the observed fluency of speech. Work on attitudes, negative emotions, and avoidances takes two forms in an integrated approach to therapy. First, direct work on decreasing fear and avoidance can be effective in reducing overt stuttering (Van Riper, 1958). Neurophysiologically, the emphasis on approach activities may "kindle" emotional regulation by the left hemisphere, which, in turn, may "dampen" the avoidance and fear responses regulated by the right hemisphere (Davidson, 1984; Kinsbourne, 1989; Kinsbourne & Bemporad, 1984). Second, confronting stuttering by going right into the stutter, staying there with an attitude that reduces fear, and finishing the word slowly and loosely will positively affect attitudes and emotions through repeated experiences of feeling in control in situations where feelings of helplessness previously prevailed.

4. *Adults who stutter may continue to have speech-processing deficits after treatment and may need to continue to deal with them.* Brain imaging research suggests that even after successful treatment, adults who stutter are likely to continue to show abnormally low activity in left-brain regions that are highly active for speech processing in nonstutterers (Ingham et al., 2018; Neumann et al., 2003). Thus, the treatment procedures described in the following pages include work on new responses to residual stuttering in a way that is comfortable for both the speaker and listener and that doesn't interfere with communication.
5. *Measurements of progress and outcome are important.* To assess a client's progress and outcome in terms of their feelings and attitudes about communication, I use the Modified Erickson Scale of Communication Attitudes (S-24), which was also described in Chapter 11. This measure has been adapted for repeated use and has been shown to be predictive of treatment outcomes (Andrews & Craig, 1988; Andrews & Cutler, 1974; Guitar & Bass, 1978). If a client shows more negative attitudes than the average normal speaker, it is a cue to continue working on attitudes and feelings, as well as approach behaviors and ensure that the client has mastered the use of easy stuttering in most situations. Evidence for the validity and reliability of these measures can be found in Chapter 11. I also suggest the OASES-A (Yaruss & Quesal, 2016) to evaluate a client's perceptions of and their reactions to the stuttering, as well as how stuttering affects their quality of life. In addition, the SSI-4 (Riley, 2009) is a valuable tool to assess the severity of stuttering at the beginning of treatment as well as during treatment and after.

Beginning Therapy

There are several issues I deal with in the first therapy sessions. The first is to understand what treatment goals the client has. The form "Personal Aims for Stuttering Treatment" (Fig. 9.1) gives me a glimpse of the client's initial hopes for what they can achieve in treatment. Frequently, we have discussed this in a preliminary way during the evaluation, but once treatment actually gets under way, it is important to revisit this topic and to clarify for both the client as well as the clinician what they are working toward. During this discussion, I bring up the options of spontaneous fluency, controlled easy stuttering, or open stuttering that the client seeks to accept and be comfortable with. This latter goal aligns with the neurodiversity movement that espouses the philosophy that stutterers are just a different version of typical speakers, with a different, but acceptable, way of talking. I also discuss how important it may be for the client to communicate easily in various situations. In this discussion, we talk about various situations in their life that are likely to be affected by stuttering, and we explore what level of fluency is important in each of them. We look for situations in which the client is satisfied with their fluency and discuss what the speech is like at such times. We try to find levels of stuttering or fluency that would be good targets to shoot for. It is also important to find out if the client feels that they just want to feel more accepting and open about their current stuttering, so that they don't hide or avoid it. This choice suggests working on feelings and attitudes—a critical part of an integrated approach to stuttering therapy, as you will discover in the next sections on clinical procedures.

A second issue the client and I deal with early on is to make a map of a possible course of treatment. Mindful of what the client's aims are, I provide brief descriptions of the stages of treatment we can go through, matching treatment to the client's present situation and their desires for improvement. The general plan I would describe is first for the client to get to know what they do when they stutter, including their behaviors, their thoughts, and their feelings about their stuttering and about listener reactions. If the client wants to learn to *stutter more easily* as well as work on communicating effectively, I let them know that the next steps involve the confrontation of their stuttering with the aim of changing it to an easier form that would feel in control. Gradually, with my support, the client would seek out formerly feared words and situations and replace old avoidance behaviors with a more assertive attitude and a more confident, more relaxed approach to those stutters that remain. Finally, in the later stages of this treatment orientation, I would help the client work out a plan to use their new **easier stuttering** in more and more situations and to gradually become their own clinician so that they can diagnose and repair their speech if more severe stuttering creeps back in.

Exploring and Changing Stuttering

The aim of this first phase of treatment is to help the client become more objective about their stuttering and to lift the clouds of dread and mystery that surround it. Objectivity is fostered through procedures that help the client learn about their pattern of stuttering behaviors—what they do and why—and learn that their current stuttering behaviors are OK for now. They are an acceptable, understandable response to the feelings of frustration, shame, and being out of control. But they and the clinician can work together to change that. One of the clinician's first goals can be to help the client change how they feel about their stuttering as they see it more objectively and feel more accepting of it via the clinician's acceptance, support, and encouragement. The clinician should keep in mind that as important as these steps are, the relationship with the client is even more important. As I've said before, the client must experience the clinician as accepting, but at the same time confident in the client's ability to change. Thus, the clinician shouldn't be afraid to challenge the client to try new ways of thinking and behaving. As this process goes on, the client will likely become more optimistic. They realize that stuttering consists of behaviors that they can control, and they feel supported by the clinician's belief in

TABLE 17.1 Steps in Exploring and Changing Stuttering

Step	Activities	Goals
Understanding stuttering	Provide handout and discuss the elements of the client's stuttering with them. Clinician shows deep acceptance of client as they are now and shares the perspective that there is a logic behind what the client currently does in their core, escape, and avoidance behaviors.	To gain an understanding what has been mysterious and scary; beginning of desensitization
Approaching, exploring, and changing stuttering in the treatment room	Clinician and client examine client's stuttering behaviors. They then catch and hold stutters. Clinician showers client with positive feedback as they stay in a stutter and learn to feel what they're doing physically when they stutter. Clinician coaches client to feel tension reduce until the word can be completed. Via the clinician's modeling and coaching, client learns to end stutter slowly and loosely.	Continuing desensitization. Beginning of learning to modify stutters
Approaching and exploring stuttering outside of the treatment room	Client and clinician observe stuttering and client's reactions to it outside the clinic. As the stuttering is studied, client tries to catch, hold, and slowly release stutters outside of the treatment room. Continuing discussion of how client feels about their stuttering. Audio recording by client of their stuttering in various situations followed by discussions with clinician.	Continuing desensitization. Client learns that they can tolerate their stuttering with more and more listeners. Client learns to stay in stutter until they can reduce tension and finish the word with a feeling of control

their ability to change. All through this procedure, the clinician remains accepting of the goals the client has set. These goals may be aiming for their stuttering to stay, but with comfort and openness about it. They may be OK with some stuttering remaining, but they want an experience of mostly feeling in control of it and it not being a burden to them. Or they may want total fluency. If this last goal has been verbalized by the client, the clinician should accept it. It often happens that clients who at first want total fluency, become accepting of some remaining stuttering

Steps in the exploration process are outlined in Table 17.1.

Understanding Stuttering

I begin by explaining why we want to explore their stuttering with them. I often use a handout called "Understanding Your Stuttering." This handout and six others that explain aspects of the treatment program are available on *Lippincott Connect*.

As we discuss the client's stuttering, I also find out from them about other activities that they have worked on previously and improved, like skiing, painting, golf, photography, or anything else that required a positive attitude and practice. We discuss how emotions and attitudes can get in the way of new learning and may perpetuate old behaviors. I draw an analogy between the skills that the client has worked on and the task before us, which is to learn to modify stuttering and thereby increase fluency, if that's their goal. We discuss the idea that if the client can learn what they're doing when they stutter, then they may feel more objective and optimistic about their stuttering and realize they can change what they're doing toward easier and potentially more fluent speech. I try to convey the idea, which will be repeated in many forms, that they have learned to speak in an inefficient way that is at least in part influenced by their desire not to stutter. However, despite years of harder stuttering, they can now learn to replace it with an easier stuttering that incidentally may be seen by listeners as more fluent. This process begins by getting to know what they do when they stutter. As we're doing this, I blanket them with feelings of "what you are doing is OK, but we can work together to get rid of the extra junk in your stuttering and make it simpler and more comfortable."

Approaching, Exploring, and Changing Stuttering in the Treatment Room

The goal is for the client to make the first steps toward *approaching* their stuttering, rather than backing away from it. I also encourage the client, when I think they're ready, to take the big step of changing how they stutter, to make it easier. As we begin studying the client's stuttering, I often use an illustration or model of the speech mechanism to show the client the structures associated with speaking and how they function in spontaneous fluency and in stuttering. The client needs to learn about the core, escape, and avoidance components of their stuttering and, to some degree, why they occur. The client should also feel that the clinician is genuinely interested in them and in their speech and accepting of where they are now. Because approach behaviors are thought to be regulated by the left hemisphere, activation of approach behaviors may dampen negative emotions that are right-hemisphere based (Davidson, 1984; Kinsbourne, 1989;

Kinsbourne & Bemporad, 1984). Hence, these approach activities are meant, in part, to decrease the client's fear of stuttering.

The activities associated with this step involve examining moments of stuttering as they occur in the treatment room. Thus, I encourage them to stutter. I explain to a client that one of the aims of our work is to reduce the client's fear of stuttering. For years, they have been feeling "trapped" in the stuckness of stutters, helpless and struggling, with little or no reliable way to escape. I explain that they are like most people who stutter; the very act of struggling to escape from stutters increases their muscle tension and consequently the feeling of being stuck. But being able to stop struggling and be "present" in the experience of being trapped reduces their tension and perhaps provides more positive sensory feedback to the brain, allowing them to move forward in speech. I usually try to have the client feel tension at first and then notice that the tension gradually decreases while they're holding the posture and I am coaching them to stay in the sound and then finishing the word.[1] For some clients, this step in therapy is difficult and requires much practice and encouragement. The tension response is probably not a conscious deliberate action, and reducing the tension is not so much an act of will and effort as it is an emotional "letting go." It may take much experimentation, as well as acceptance and support, when this letting go is hard to come by. If you can get some change in the client's tension as you encourage the client to temporarily accept the discomfort of the stutter, then you can spend some time exploring with the client what they did or what they felt or what they thought, as the tension was reduced. This is similar to what Dean Williams achieves with the young client illustrated in the video titled "Dean Williams Helps a Student Stutter More Easily." This is available on *Lippincott Connect* with the Chapter 17 videos.

Progress on this step can be assessed by the client's movement up the hierarchy for this activity. The hierarchy goes from them controlling my pseudostuttering with a hand signal (to give them a model of how to hold a stutter and feel in control while doing it), all the way to them holding onto a stutter for several seconds in a conversation while maintaining good eye contact and staying relaxed.

I use Handout 2—"Holding onto the Stutter"—to provide the client the rationale for the activities associated with this step. It is available in *Lippincott Connect.* I also explain the procedure to the client in person and then carry out the activity. You can also watch a video of a 9-year-old child learning to hold onto his stutter on *Lippincott Connect, "CM Trial Therapy"* after minute 2:26.

When I think the client understands the task, I talk about something of interest, such as our self-help group or the overall course of stuttering therapy. I put in some really obvious voluntary stutters that would be easy for me to hold onto, such as voiced continuant consonants like /l/ or /r/. The purpose of this is to model for the client a good example of holding onto a stutter the way I want them to do. If they don't immediately signal me to hold onto my stutter, I explain again how they should do that. Then, I get back into voluntarily stuttering so the client can catch one, and when the client signals that they notice that I am in a stutter, I prolong the sound and continue to maintain the tension I have, gradually letting the tension go so that the pitch of my voice goes down as my vocal folds relax while I am staying calm and unhurried. I emphatically praise the client's catching my stutters because even someone else's voluntary stutters may be hard for a sensitive client to bear. As we go along and discuss my stutters and what I'm doing physically when I stutter, I use a large array of different sounds and I try to stutter in the manner that they do. Then, we reverse roles and I show them how to hold onto their stutters.

After I get the client's OK to interrupt them, I ask them to talk about hobbies, work, or their school—anything easy for them to talk about. As the client talks, I watch for one of their more severe stutters and then signal them to hold onto it. I focus on severe stutters at first because mild stutters may go by so quickly that the client cannot hold the stutters as they are occurring. This process may take some coaching and practice because people who are not trained in our field (most clients) may not understand how to hold onto the exact sound that is being stuttered. Particularly hard are plosives, and the client may need extra coaching to stay right in a /b/ or /p/ that is stuttered (by producing it as the fricative counterpart to those stops), *without going on to the next vowel sound.* It is important, as you have the client hold onto a stutter, for them to have airflow and/or voicing appropriate for the sound they're stuck on. The clinician's model—when the clinician shows the client how to hold onto a stutter—should demonstrate airflow and/or voicing. This is easier when the sound is a voiced continuant, as I indicated earlier. Plosives, such as /p/, can be held by keeping the lips only slightly in contact and allowing airflow to continue until tension is reduced and the transition into the next sound can be made slowly and loosely. A held-onto /p/ has the sound of air swishing through the lips. The sound /b/ can be held by also keeping the lips only slightly in contact and allowing voicing to happen while the lips vibrate. That sound will be sort of like the buzzing of a bee.

Some clients appear to have tight laryngeal closures as their major form of "stuckness" in a block. They may require a little extra work as you explore with them what they are doing to hold back sound and/or airflow. As they and you explore, they may find that your demonstrated acceptance

[1]Staying in a stutter but gradually reducing the tension (or letting tension reduce itself) before finishing the word is essentially what Van Riper called a "pullout." At first, emphasis is on staying in the stutter; then, once that is mastered, the client can learn to reduce tension and finish the word. Whereas Van Riper's pullout is a deliberate act of reducing tension, for me, having the client stay in a stutter and tolerate it and feeling what they are doing results in a nonconscious letting go of tension, as negative emotion subsides. It may also occasionally result in a point where conscious control seems to be regained.

and support of them during the stutter allows the block to release so that sound or airflow can begin. Remember, the tension in the block is happening because the client is resisting it (probably nonconsciously), as a response to the threat of stuckness. Your acceptance of the client's being stuck will allow them to stop reacting to it, accept the momentary stuckness, and then the tension will subside. If necessary, you can help the client discover whether vocal fry (voicing that sounds like something frying in a pan on the stove and actually results from very slow vibrations of the vocal folds) can help get voicing going.

I show genuine interest and curiosity in the client's stuttering and make observations about it such as "I noticed on that one it looked like you squeezed your vocal folds" (or you may want to use the word "throat" instead) "trying to get the word out." I also ask questions like, "Is that how you usually stutter on words that start with 'b?" As we explore stuttering together, I use my interest and acceptance to begin the process of *desensitization* or reducing the fear associated with stuttering. During this activity, I continue to teach the client about different components of stuttering, including core, escape, and avoidance behaviors, particularly as they apply to the client's stuttering. We have touched on components of the client's stuttering before, but our continued discussion of the client's stuttering behaviors, suffused with my acceptance and even humor about them, helps to drain some of the client's shame about their stuttering. This activity continues at a pace suited to a client's comfort talking about their stuttering. When the client is relatively comfortable examining their stuttering, I may use a mirror to help them explore and confront their stuttering, as depicted with a female client in Figure 17.2.

Another aspect of staying in the stutter is to maintain natural eye contact with the listener when holding onto the stutter. This may be very hard for some clients who frequently look away from the listener because they feel ashamed. When eye contact can be learned and practiced, it creates a confident feeling in the speaker themselves and enhances the social connection between speaker and listener. It enables the speaker and listener to assess the emotional state of each other. Thus, if the person who stutters maintains a calm demeanor and has natural eye contact with the listener, the listener is usually put at ease and is likely to telegraph that "everything is OK" back to the person stuttering. In that way, eye contact can become a means of enlisting an ally in a difficult moment.

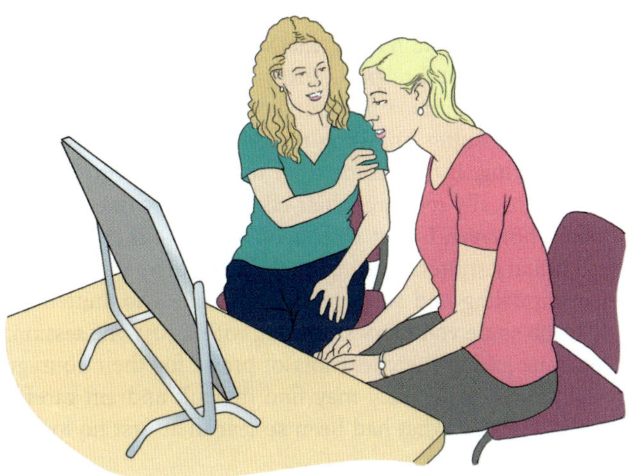

Figure 17.2 Exploring stuttering with the help of a mirror.

Note that while we work on approaching stuttering and exploring it, I am especially pleased when they can follow my instructions to "stay in the stutter."[2] When the client stays in their stutters, they learn that when they can tolerate the "stuckness," and stay in it, their physical tension drains away. This is a key experience. It is the discovery that they themselves have the power to control what happens when they stutter—even if that control involves trying to "do" as little as possible but tolerate what is happening.

As indicated earlier, an important sequel of learning to catch and hold onto stutters is to allow physical tension to be released to the point (and beyond) where the stutter becomes unstuck and the word finished. As I mentioned, some clients call this "**catch and release**," the phrase used to describe catching a fish and letting it go. It is not only releasing the block but it is letting go of the fear. Note that the release of the word must be done only after the tension is reduced to near-normal speech levels, so it doesn't feel stuck any more. This process involves powerful learning (operant conditioning). The relief felt by the client when they can release and finish the word using an easy stutter *reinforces* the reduction of tension to normal levels.

If the client is able to reliably produce easy stutters on feared words for a period of days or weeks, these become more automatic. Then, for many clients, because of the operant conditioning—the reinforcement of finishing the word with little tension—the reduction of tension occurs *just as they start* saying the word. Van Riper's term for this, when it is done deliberately, is "preparatory set."

Approaching and Changing Stuttering Outside the Treatment Room

After the client has many experiences in the therapy room "catching" their stutters, holding onto them, feeling what they're doing physically, and describing what they feel they're doing, we make plans to transfer this learning of easier stuttering to real-world situations. The client and I build a hierarchy of situations that begin with those that are least threatening.

[2]When I ask a client to "stay in the stutter," I am borrowing a technique from the late Dean Williams, who was a master stuttering clinician at the University of Iowa. Dean was able to work temporary miracles by having a client stay in a moment of stuttering, feel what they were doing, and reduce the tension (or the tension just reduced itself). When a client did this, he often became suddenly very fluent. See the video titled "Dean Williams Helps a Student Stutter More Easily" on Lippincott Connect

In the beginning, the clinician provides as much support as possible. It helps to emphasize to the client, as they transfer their catch and release strategy to the world outside the treatment room, that they only have this single tool to focus on. Some other approaches load the client with so many possible strategies that they are confused about which to use.

In my experience with my own stuttering and with many clients, I have found that the transfer of easier stuttering to the outside world is facilitated with the use of voluntary stutters. These are stutters done deliberately, using the familiar prolongation (holding) of the target sound and posture, followed by a slow release of the word. Voluntary stutters will be discussed at length in the next section. Not every client is willing to engage in voluntary stuttering before working on catching and releasing real stutters outside the therapy room. Thus, the clinician and client together decide when and if to use voluntary stuttering as a tool for transferring easier stuttering to a client's everyday life.

Using Voluntary Stuttering

One of the techniques I teach—at first in the treatment room—to prepare the client to transfer of easier stuttering to situations outside the therapy room is *voluntary stuttering*, touched upon in the previous section. This can be a very potent strategy for reducing tension and avoidance and thereby facilitating the transfer of catch and release. By using voluntary stuttering, the client is performing an approach behavior, which is intended to decrease fear and tension. This makes it more likely that the client will be able to use easier stutters successfully. Every clinician should be familiar with voluntary stuttering. The handout that I give to clients in this stage of therapy explains the whys and wherefores of voluntary stuttering. It is Handout 3: Voluntary Stutters, available on *Lippincott Connect*.

Here's one client's comments on how it felt to him when he started using voluntary stuttering (he calls it "pretend stuttering"):

Just sharing a brief description and a few thoughts regarding my feeling and experience while doing a strong pretend stutter.

As mentioned, when I produce a strong or a very intense pretend stutter, with significant stuckness in the first syllable, I feel the following:

- *Both physical and emotional relief at the end and softer part of the word/sound. Almost as if something very tense in my body and my mind, which was stuck, has been released.*
- *The physical relief is felt mostly in the chest, the neck, and around the mouth.*
- *The more intense the stuckness in the beginning, the greater the relief.*
- *If it's very intense, it almost feels as if my brain confuses it for a real stutter. Regardless of my (or my brain's) interpretation, the tension in the chest and neck are real.*
- *Lastly, although in the beginning there's no relief, mostly tension—there's some satisfaction because you are creating the stuckness and you control it.*

When I first introduce voluntary stuttering to clients, many think I am crazy. After all, they came to therapy to rid themselves of stuttering, not to do more of it. At this point, I explain the rationale behind voluntary stuttering: stuttering is perpetuated by fear of stuttering, and reducing this fear will reduce the stuttering. An analogy often helps. For instance, suppose a person wanted to overcome a fear of dogs that causes the person to freeze and be unable to move when in the presence of a dog or to run away. Overcoming the fear could not be done by running away from dogs. Instead, the person would have to begin seeking out contact with dogs with knowledge of how to approach them. The best way to do this would be to have the guidance of someone who was an expert on dogs and was not afraid of them and who would guide the person's contact with dogs in a series of small steps.

For example, the first step might involve only looking at puppies in a pet store; the next step might be talking to a clerk about the puppies. Then, the person might briefly pet a puppy and then perhaps pick up the puppy and hold it for a short period. This process would need to be repeated over and over again with gradually larger and larger dogs. Eventually, the person would learn how to approach a dog in a friendly way—after verifying with the owner that the dog is unafraid and friendly toward strangers. As the person learned how to approach and make friends with dogs, their fear would gradually decrease.

This same process can be used with stuttering. With the clinician's guidance, the client first learns to stutter on purpose in the safety of the therapy room and realize that they have nothing to fear. They'll learn that voluntary stuttering frees them from the need to be perfectly fluent and enables them to use easier stutters because they are less afraid and no longer feel a need to avoid stuttering. The success of this process depends a great deal on the clinician being comfortable with stuttering. Thus, clinicians need to desensitize themselves to stuttering by practicing voluntary stuttering themselves until the experience of voluntary stuttering and the experience of negative listener reactions do not bother them.

After explaining the rationale behind voluntary stuttering, I teach clients how to stutter voluntarily. First, I model the sort of "catch and release" that we have been working on, remaining calm and relaxed. Then, I encourage the client to attempt some voluntary stuttering on words that they would typically not stutter on, using the catch and release style of easy stuttering. If they come close to doing it appropriately, I enthusiastically reinforce their efforts. If they find this too difficult, however, I do it with them and have them shadow my voluntary stuttering using catch and release. With appropriate modeling and support, most people who stutter are able to do some voluntary stuttering within just one session. I continue giving the client lots of praise for their courage in doing something they may find difficult and am careful to point out that what had been so fearful at first no longer seems so scary.

After the client becomes comfortable using voluntary stuttering with catch and release in the clinic, it is time for them to move out into the world. First, the client and I establish a hierarchy of situations in which they can use voluntary stuttering. The clinician should always go into situations with the client and be the first to use voluntary stuttering during the beginning steps of the hierarchy. I ask the client to rate my listeners on a scale that reflects a range of qualities. For example, a "10" might be someone who laughs or looks away, and a "1" might be someone who is attentive and listens patiently, or you could reverse the scale if that makes more sense to you. The client may want to continue using this rating system when it is their turn to practice voluntarily stuttering as well, because it can countercondition old emotions of feeling victimized and helpless. Clearly, when you are in the position of evaluating someone else (in this case, the listener), the power dynamic has changed in favor of the evaluator.

I voluntarily stutter in situations such as asking directions from strangers or getting information from store clerks, and I remain calm as I do it. If all of my listeners are patient and understanding, I ask the client to choose listeners for me whom they feel might be more difficult. Once, when I was working with a 12-year-old girl who stuttered, she chose a large group wearing motorcycle paraphernalia (a biker gang perhaps) walking in a shopping mall for me to stutter to. As it turned out, they were as polite as any listeners I've ever stuttered to. I think the girl was impressed and more willing than ever to stutter to strangers.

After I've completed several of these encounters where the client chooses the person to whom I stutter with voluntaries, it is the client's turn to stutter voluntarily with strangers. We then continue to alternate turns, which provides additional **counterconditioning** as the client and I compare our ratings of listeners and take turns choosing listeners for each other. In time, a client's feelings of assertiveness and exploration usually increase, which diminishes feelings of fear and avoidance.

I am careful not to allow a client to get in "over their head" with listeners who may be too difficult. I also lavish praise on each of the client's attempts, acknowledging how difficult it can be, and try to be sensitive to how much they want to discuss each event. After a good workout with store clerks, for example, I may suggest that we take a break for a snack at a restaurant, where we can practice voluntary stuttering with the server and enjoy the counterconditioning effects of having a snack while doing something that was previously unpleasant. If we've had a bad listener, together we try to come up with a reason that person might have responded in an unfriendly way, such as that they'd found a parking ticket on their car or worse, their car had been towed.

The client and I continue working together on voluntary stuttering until they feel comfortable. Then, they work their way through the rest of the situations in their hierarchy (such as voluntary stuttering with friends and relatives) on their own. The client has to continue putting voluntary stuttering into their speech in each situation until their fear subsides before going on to the next situation. I check clients' progress during therapy sessions, commending them when they are successful while supporting, encouraging, and counseling them when they run into problems. Voluntary stuttering is a procedure that clients will continue to use throughout active treatment and maintenance.

Continuing to Transfer Voluntary Stutters to the Outside World

Once I'm satisfied that the client understands and can use voluntary stuttering, I begin transfer by making a phone call myself to a store to ask what their hours are, with plenty of voluntary stutters. If the client is more afraid of making phone calls than face-to-face transfer activities, I might begin with something easier by bringing into the room someone whom the client doesn't know to use voluntary stuttering with. Or, if the client is OK with phone calls, I can begin with calls to randomly chosen stores. I put in a handful of voluntary stutters, similar to the client's real stutters, but with the catch and release strategy, making them end as easy stutters. We discuss my voluntary stutters as well as the listeners' reactions. This works really well if I can do it with the cell phone speaker turned on so the client can hear how the listener responds. When they're ready, the client makes a phone call and tries to catch their real stutters and release them slowly. Immediately afterward, we discuss the client's stutters and the listeners' reactions. Many listeners, of course, are patient and even encouraging. A few, who may be confused or anxious, may answer abruptly or even hang up. We celebrate these negative reactions, acting as though they were trophies given for having a hard time but surviving it, even triumphing over it. This positive way of responding to what could be a negative experience puts a completely different spin on negative listener reactions. These experiences desensitize the client to their own stuttering and to listener reactions.

If a client is having a particularly hard time dealing with a less than positive listener reaction, you may want to share with them an interesting video clip of a TED Talk about dealing with rejection.[3] The speaker, who was not someone who stuttered, describes how he desensitized himself to the pain of someone responding negatively to him. This video could lead to a fruitful discussion of listener reactions in which your client could express his feelings about them honestly.

The expressing of feelings is a vital part of therapy. As I work with an adult, I try to attend to the client's emotions so that therapy can keep moving forward. Perhaps I should better say "lurching forward in fits and starts." *Therapy is rarely simple and predictable, and experienced clinicians know they must tolerate a messy process.* I discussed dealing with emotions in Chapter 12, and some points are worth repeating. Wherever behavior change is going on, emotions bubble up. Stuttering therapy is no exception. The clinician should

---

[3]You can access the video online at https://ed.ted.com/featured/VdQTGGdx/

expect emotions and even try to elicit them so that the clinician can listen and accept them, just as they accept the person who stutters and their stuttering. Feelings of frustration, anger toward the self and toward the clinician, and hostility toward listeners are all common. When the client talks about their feelings, sometimes stuttering worsens, but the clinician should just accept whatever stuttering accompanies the expression of feelings, rather than "doing therapy" on the stuttering that comes out when feelings are vented. Not every clinician is a natural in dealing with feelings, but they, like their clients, can learn to increase their ability to do so. It may take consistent reviewing of recordings of therapy sessions for most clinicians to recognize when a client is expressing feelings and to become alert enough to encourage the client to discuss them further. Sometimes emotions come in the disguise of resistance—refusing to work on stuttering outside the therapy room, doing assignments half-heartedly, and other signs of holding back. Such resistance is often a sign that, as Van Riper has pointed out, "the basic disorder is being affected" (Van Riper, 1958). He meant that the resistance is a sign that the client is feeling emotionally vulnerable and you are reaching the heart of their emotional sensitivity. You can often move clients forward, out of this emotional kind of "stuckness," by expressing acceptance of whatever is going on for them and their holding back and letting them know that it's not uncommon for someone who stutters to have times when progress bogs down. Deeply learned habits are notoriously hard to change so the client must make a determined effort to change them. As we'll see, as assignments move outside of the therapy room, change becomes harder, and the clinician's support becomes even more important than before.

For any assignments I might give, I usually carry them out first, modeling the sort of conversational interaction I have in mind, modeling voluntary stutters. If we are walking outside on a sidewalk, I'll ask someone passing by what time it is or where a certain building or store is. I put in a few voluntary stutters and maintain a calm demeanor with good eye contact. Then, the client and I discuss my stutters and the listener's reactions. At this point if the client is game, we plan a speaking opportunity for them. Figure 17.3 illustrates the client using stutters with a stranger. If the client is not game, then I ask them to pick a situation for me to do more stuttering in, and I carry out more voluntary stuttering while they listen and watch. Even if the client is only observing, they usually gain a lot by seeing my calm manner even while having severe (voluntary) stutters and by noticing that most listeners are very patient. If the client continues to resist approaching strangers and difficult situations, their feelings about this should be explored back in the therapy room. When the client is ready—either in this session or a later one—he goes into a planned situation and uses their typical speech, fluent or not. Most often, there will be some natural stutters that we can discuss immediately on the sidewalk or in a store.

Sometimes when we go into situations outside the clinic together, I use my cell phone to record our work for further

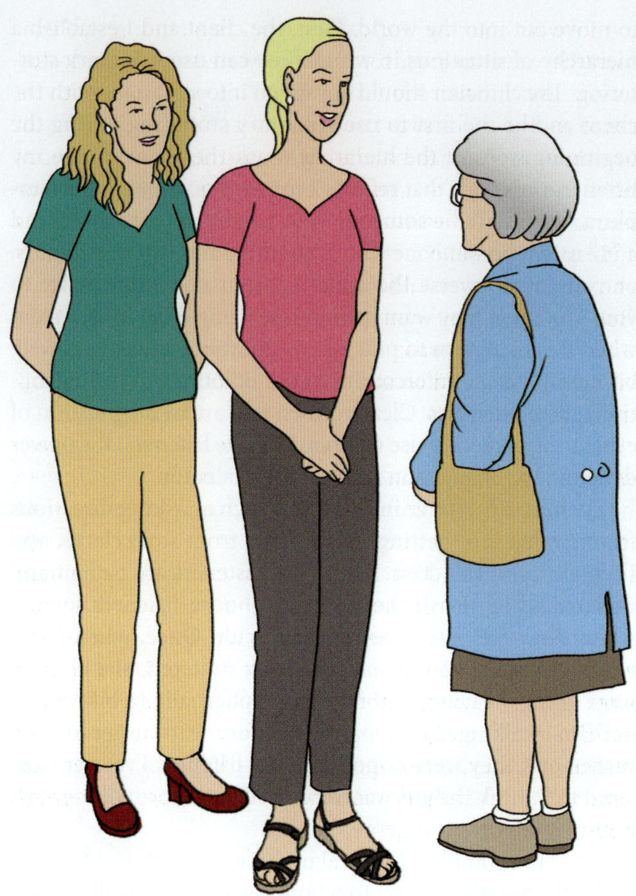

Figure 17.3 Transferring easier stutters in conversation with a stranger.

discussion. Any small portable recorder will do. When the client is doing well, we record their stutters and listen to them again, back in the clinic. I always ask listeners if they mind if we record them, explaining what we are working on. This not only makes the recording process very ethical but also promotes openness about stuttering. After we have recorded some of the client's easier (real) stuttering, we return to the clinic and listen to the recordings, discussing not only what the client was doing but also how they were feeling. If this goes well, I then ask the client to record some samples of their stuttering at home or at work and write down their observations about their stuttering when they later listen to it and finally share it with me.

In the next session, when the client brings a recording back, I respond enthusiastically. Remember that one goal of treatment is to activate "approach" behaviors and lessen avoidance behaviors. Recording stutters at home or at the office is, indeed, an approach behavior. If a client has been unable to carry out this task, they and I do the task together and record their stuttering in a situation outside the room or on the telephone.

During the sessions in which the client and I analyze their typical stuttering, I also look for stutters that are mild, brief, and forward-moving and call the client's attention to them. I ask the client to look for them in their samples collected outside and in their stuttering in the therapy room. As we attend to these, I let the client know that these are models of how they can learn to handle their stutters. In fact, they can make them more like natural speech, so that neither they nor their listeners will particularly notice them or hear them as stutters. They will, in fact, become similar to the way persons who don't stutter would handle disruptions in their speech (Boehmler, personal communication, 2004). Another thing to watch for and praise is the client finishing their stutters with greatly reduced tension. In some clients, it happens naturally; in others, it must be practiced and reinforced.

The client and I develop transfer activities, or sometimes we call them simply "challenges," that continue to strengthen the client's approach attitudes and behaviors but that are not beyond their present capacity. The best challenges will be those that help the client feel that they are confronting hard speaking situations and succeeding. As they gather these victories, their confidence swells. These accomplishments will feel particularly powerful if they can record them or take notes and share them with the clinician. It helps if the client and clinician keep in touch by telephone or e-mail between treatment sessions. Not every client will stay in touch, but some will do it regularly and others will be in touch intermittently.

Teaching the Client to Evaluate and Reinforce Their Behavior

An important component of treatment is helping the client learn to observe, evaluate, and reward their own efforts to change. This is vital for generalizing the changes the client is making to their everyday behavior, and it should start early in treatment. A chapter by Finn (2007) provided an introduction to this process. Finn described the process as comprised of several steps:

1. Training the client to observe their behavior. In this stage of treatment, it is recording the stuttering and making notes on listeners' reactions. The clinician can work with the client in outside situations (with debriefing in the treatment room) to teach them how to carry out this assignment. They can decide together how many times the client should do this between sessions.
2. Training the client to self-evaluate their work. The client and clinician can together evaluate the frequency and quality of the client's recordings and observations of listener reactions.
3. Training the client to reinforce themselves when they achieve a targeted goal. For example, the client may want to reward themselves each time they record their stuttering and take notes on listeners' responses. The client knows best what would truly be reinforcing, so deciding what to use for reinforcement should be a discussion led by the client. Finn suggested, as many have, that effective rewards are often things that the client is likely to do. Examples are drinking a favorite beverage, eating a favorite food, or taking the time to read a magazine or book. The client might want to give themselves an instant reward such as a point or token that is counted toward a total that must be achieved before a tangible reward is collected. I keep myself motivated to run several miles every other day by eating a small pastry smeared with homemade red marmalade, after my run.

Positive reinforces can be coupled with mild punishments to be most effective. The chapter by Finn (2007) and the references he provided are a rich source of ideas about how to incorporate self-management into treatment. Self-management can be used in each stage of treatment, and this will prepare the client to become their own clinician when treatment is finished.

Increasing Approach Behaviors

Reducing Fear of Listeners' Reactions

The goal of this step is for the client to continue to reduce avoidance, self-consciousness, and shame about their stuttering through further "approach" activities, such as being open about their stuttering. Until a few years ago, I had clients work on being open about their stuttering much earlier in therapy, but I have found that this is often a difficult step for most people who stutter. It has been easier for clients to tackle approaching previously difficult situations after they have learned how to stutter more easily. Success can be seen if clients are going into situations they previously avoided and if they are reporting greater comfort despite some remaining stuttering. This step and the next can be the most difficult part of treatment for many clients, who often require encouragement and support from the clinician. It may help to remind them of where they are in the progression of treatment and to review the rationale for confronting fears associated with their stuttering. It may help even more if the client rewards themselves generously after each time they are open about their stuttering. The major activity of this step involves the client talking to others about their stuttering, which I initiate by giving them a handout on discussing stuttering with others—Handout 4: Discussing Stuttering Openly—available on *Lippincott Connect*.

A few people with advanced stuttering will find these assignments easy, but most will not. I make sure that a client feels they and I are working as a team and that I am supportive and empathetic. I usually help them make lists of the situations in which they will begin to be open about their stuttering and then model an example for them. For example, if commenting on stuttering during a telephone call is on their list, I would call a store, produce a voluntary stutter, and immediately make a comment, such as "Wow, looks like I'm really stuttering more than usual today." Recently, when working with a young man who was quite sensitive and reluctant to talk openly about his stuttering, I had him video record me as I interviewed three different people on a busy shopping street. After getting permission to video record, I asked them a variety of questions about stuttering and found that each gave positive, supportive answers. The young man seemed impressed that the public was, after all, not uptight about stuttering. He then asked to do the next interview and carried it off with great success. Exercises such as this can help clients test reality and find out that much of their anxiety and disapproval about stuttering is in their minds rather than in those of the listeners. However, I prepare clients for the possibility that there will be a negative listener reaction (although this is rare) by expressing the hope that at least one listener will be impatient or rejecting so that we can see if we can retain our calm under stress. I also mention that many of their interviews about stuttering will help some of their listeners to think positively about stuttering. In doing so, they are also helping the world to become a better place for people who stutter.

Often, by using a hierarchy of situations, stress can be increased slowly and dealt with. A client and I plan a hierarchy of tasks in which the client is open about their stuttering. We might go, for example, from a casual comment they might make to a store clerk about having a stuttery day all the way up to telling a group of people that they (the client) stutter and sometimes it's better and sometimes it's worse, but that's just the way it is. In psychological terms, reductions in negative emotions that are associated with less stressful tasks will generalize to more stressful tasks. Consequently, when a client gets to the more stressful tasks, they will no longer be as difficult.

After the client completes the assignments on their hierarchy, they discuss the outcomes with me. I diligently give them a great deal of praise for confronting their fears and discussing their stuttering openly. At times, I may need to encourage or even push the client to move on to the next step; however, I need to be sensitive to the intensity of their feelings so that I don't expect too much too soon. Ultimately, the client needs to be in control of the amount of stress under which they put themselves.

The client will probably never completely finish with this activity because discussing their stuttering openly will always be an important, but perhaps intermittently difficult, strategy for them, not only during therapy but possibly throughout their lifetime. It can help them maintain their improved fluency long after therapy has ended. Thus, I get the client started on their hierarchy and then move on to the next step. Even as they work on other strategies, they will find it valuable to continue to be open about their stuttering. I encourage the client to keep a written record of their progress up this hierarchy so that they may refer to it if, after termination of therapy, they begin to hide their stuttering and old fears creep back in. Using their old records and seeing their old victories may motivate them to try anew to stutter openly, comment on their stutters, and reestablish their freedom to work on their stuttering in difficult situations.

Using Feared Words and Entering Feared Situations

Using feared words (words with sounds they fear they will stutter on) and entering feared situations are important approach behaviors that help clients continue their progress in managing their stuttering. Some clients will have accomplished a great deal in this area during the transfer of getting directly into the stutter and staying in it until tension is reduced. However, most will benefit from practice in seeking out remaining fears. I use a handout—Handout 5: Using Feared Words and Entering Feared Situations—available on *Lippincott Connect*, to begin teaching this step and supplement it with examples and discussion.

After the client has read the handout, I answer any questions they may have. I then encourage them to not use any postponements or word avoidances when in therapy from then on. When I think they deliberately use a word or sound that they appeared to want to avoid, I strongly reinforce this approach behavior. I also set up activities in which the client purposefully has to say feared words that we had previously identified and the client uses easier stutters when producing these words. These activities may involve them reading word lists and text that are loaded with their feared words or involve their composing sentences with these words. I warmly praise them each time they do not postpone or avoid a feared word, especially when they successfully use easy stutters. Sometimes, they may be unable to stutter easily—their old habits may have shanghaied them. However, I am accepting of these occasions and let them know that I understand how hard it can be. This will help the client become more comfortable saying these words and will reduce their tendency to want to avoid them.

To help the client eliminate their use of avoidances outside the clinic, I assist them in setting up a hierarchy of word and situation avoidances they commonly use in daily life. Like most hierarchies, it should be sequenced from least to most difficult for the client. By using this strategy, the client's fears will be kept at just the right level—not too hard, not too easy. A typical step in the hierarchy is the client's deliberate use of certain feared words throughout the day. How often should they use these feared words? They have to be used over and over until the client no longer wants or needs to avoid them.

Another step in the hierarchy has the individual entering situations that they usually avoid in daily life (Fig. 17.4).

As before, they need to enter these situations until they lose their motivation to avoid them. Many of the assignments can be completed as the client goes through their daily routine and will not take any extra time out of their day. For instance, they just need to answer the telephone whenever it rings with the feared "hello," said using an easy stutter, or introduce himself to a different person each day and try to use easy stutters. Saying "hello" with an easy

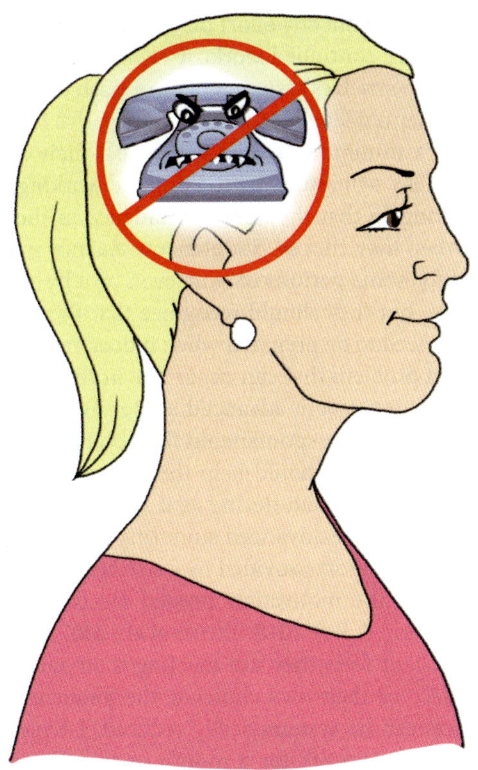

Figure 17.4 The client reduces fear and avoidance by approaching previously feared situations.

stutter can be challenging. You need to let out some air for the "h" sound and then get the vowel "e" to start slowly, perhaps with some "vocal fry" at the beginning. It will sound like "hhhhhhhhhh(air going out mouth like a whisper)... eeeeeee(started with a gravelly sound, if needed)llloow." Other assignments to practice feared words and sounds may have to be created, and they may need to go out of their way to perform them. For example, the client may have to shop for an item whose name contains one of their feared sounds or fabricate reasons for making telephone calls to local businesses. When I was trying to get over my fear of words beginning with the /l/ sound, I went into many stores asking about *l*uggage, *l*ocks, and *l*ampshades.

To help the client get started on an outside hierarchy, it is helpful for me to join them for some of the assignments. Once they have the idea how they might do this, they will complete the assignments by themselves and discuss their progress and any problems with me during regular therapy sessions. I make sure that they keep on track in completing their hierarchy and provide them with the necessary support and sometimes gentle nudging to help them do so. After the client has worked through as many situations as they and I think are sufficient, it is appropriate for them to complete the Modified Erickson Scale of Communication Attitudes (see Chapter 11). This will give us an indication of whether or not there are still situations that might benefit from being approached and mastered.

Like discussing stuttering openly, eliminating the use of avoidances is a strategy that individuals will need to use throughout therapy and beyond. So, once a client has begun outside assignments successfully, it is time to move on to steps that will create the foundation for long-term change. Self-evaluation and self-reinforcement are crucial elements in a client's learning to decrease avoidance. As described in an earlier section, these behaviors need to be explicitly trained.

Maintaining Improvement

The goal of this last phase of therapy is to help clients generalize their improvement—that is, transferring their *reduced* negative feelings, attitudes, avoidances, and, possibly, increased fluency to all remaining speaking situations and maintaining this improvement following termination of therapy. I introduce the following procedures during this phase: (1) **becoming your own clinician** and (2) establishing long-term fluency goals. A handout on this work—Handout 6: Becoming Your Own Clinician—is available on *Lippincott Connect.*

Becoming Your Own Clinician

If clients with advanced stuttering are going to generalize the changes they are making to all speaking situations and maintain this improvement, I believe that they must assume responsibility for their own therapy. The literature on self-management provides helpful guidance for fostering this transition. The article "Self-Regulation and the Management of Stuttering" (Finn, 2003) referred to earlier, is a good example. Finn pointed out that having clients set their own goals is a key element of success. I would also highlight the importance of teaching clients to formulate their own plans that target specific behaviors for specific changes. An article in *Time* (Ripley, 2005, 2008) on surviving disasters suggests that survivors of September 11 and other catastrophes often had developed a plan of action beforehand so that they were not affected by the common human response to unexpected stress—"freezing" or being unable to move. Plans made by clients before stressful situations arise will help them take action when they have opportunities to use catch and release and other strategies that will help them stutter more easily and feel in control of their speech.

By this time, clients are probably getting close to completing their everyday speaking situation hierarchy. I point out to them, however, that completing this hierarchy is not enough and that they need to pursue any other situations that are still giving them trouble. I ask them the following kinds of questions: Are you avoiding talking in any situations? Are you still afraid while talking in some situations? Are you unable to successfully use easy stuttering when anticipating stuttering in some situations? Are you hesitant to use voluntary stuttering in some situations?

If clients are still avoiding some situations, I remind them of the importance of using feared words and entering feared situations. It will also help them to prepare to be open about their stuttering in feared situations. I may have them reread the handout and then prepare assignments to overcome their current avoidances. I try not to assume any more responsibility than is necessary. I try to ask helpful questions but want them to figure out on their own what they need to do. As time goes on, I will gradually have the client assuming more and more responsibility for planning their own assignments.

If they are having difficulties using easy stutters to replace their old tense stutters that they still push through too quickly in some situations, I explore the nature of their difficulties with them and help them determine what types of assignments they need to work on to be successful. Maybe they need more practice in some less difficult situations before they can reasonably expect to be successful in the more difficult situations. Perhaps they need to further reduce their speech rate and muscle tension in these difficult situations so that their motor control does not break down as readily. I have found that some clients strive to be as fluent as possible in all situations; however, others are happy with some residual stuttering if it doesn't interfere with their communication. From my perspective, all of this is great; clients' goals are ultimately their own. During all of our discussions, I try to keep in mind that my goal is to help the client become independent in meeting their own goals. So, I gradually become less directive and less of a therapist than a consultant. Throughout this phase of therapy, the client should be working daily on outside assignments and discussing their progress with me during therapy sessions.

Establishing Long-term Fluency Goals

Before therapy ends, it is very important for a client to be aware of what they can expect in terms of fluency after termination from therapy. By having realistic goals, they can substantially decrease the possibility of becoming disappointed and frustrated with their speech and not developing feelings that may lead to relapse. To begin this topic, I share with them Handout 7: Establishing Long-Term Goals that can be found on *Lippincott Connect*.

I make sure that the client understands the concepts of spontaneous fluency, easy stuttering, and not-so-easy stuttering that is comfortable for them. When I am convinced that they understand what is meant by these terms, I explore with them the types of fluency they currently have in various everyday speaking situations. If they are unsure of whether they have achieved the levels of fluency they want in various situations, they give themselves assignments to help them find out whether or not they are satisfied with the types of fluency they have in these situations. If they are satisfied, then they have met their goals, and the end of therapy is near. They can continue working along the lines discussed in the previous section on "Becoming Your Own Clinician."

I have observed a couple of problems that can occur with clients' fluency expectations or goals. First, many clients experience a great deal of spontaneous fluency at this point in therapy. They expect and want this spontaneous fluency to last forever without any effort on their part. It can last, but that will require continued work. A client will need to continue giving themselves assignments—or push themselves, as they encounter old fears—to keep their negative feelings and attitudes at a minimum and to extinguish their avoidance behaviors. They will also need to continue working on their easy stuttering so that they have confidence in their ability to use it when they choose. Spontaneous fluency may sometimes and for some periods of time even be a by-product of these efforts, but they should recognize that they will probably always need to be prepared when it doesn't occur.

A second problem that can occur late in therapy involves clients with more severe advanced stuttering. These clients may fail to achieve any spontaneous fluency. For these clients in particular, therapy should help them accept and become comfortable with their stuttering as it is and be open about it. Clients with severe advanced stuttering may benefit especially from the support provided by a self-help group to help them maintain the motivation needed for continued self-therapy (Trichon & Raj, 2018; Yaruss et al., 2007).

Once a client feels they are meeting their fluency goals and have become their own clinician, the frequency of therapy contacts can be systematically reduced. I typically fade contacts to once a week for a month or two, then to once a month for several months, and finally to once a semester for 2 years. This gradual transition provides the client with some continued support. For example, if they are doing well, I reinforce their feelings, and if they are having a few problems, I can help them find solutions. Of course, if they have relapsed completely, they can re-enroll in therapy. Ultimately, as I say "goodbye," when we formally discontinue therapy, I commend them for all their hard work and let them know that if they ever need me again, I am available to them.

Throughout the fading process, I assess their speech using the OASES, the Erickson S-24, the Stutterer's Self-Rating of Reactions to Speech Situations, and the SSI-4, that are all presented in Chapter 11. The process of us mutually analyzing the client's stuttering, emotions, and attitudes, as well as working on areas that need further practice helps to keep them focused on using easier stuttering. It also increases the chances that their easy stuttering will become more and more automatic.

A series of eight video clips of therapy with an adult is available in the Chapter 17 videos section of Lippincott Connect. The videos show the initial evaluation, initial therapy sessions, and ending in sessions that focus on maintaining the fluency attained in treatment.

Clinical Procedures: Learning and Generalizing Controlled Fluency

This section is *not* meant for most clients, but for those *rare* clients who come to us with little fear of stuttering, are comfortable with themselves, and have good social-conversational skills. The description on *Lippincott Connect* details the procedures to teach an adult how to use Controlled Fluency, a different speech pattern to generate fluency, which is then shaped to sound like normal speech and transferred to everyday life. If you are convinced that negative emotions and attitudes are not a problem for a client, you may want to try using controlled fluency with them. In my experience, an intensive period of therapy (eg, 4-6 hours/day for several days in a row) can be a good way to teach controlled fluency skills before beginning generalization. However, a less intense approach—an hour or two per week with daily home assignments—can be used if needed.

An example of the effectiveness of teaching controlled fluency to selected clients comes to mind. I recently had a "reunion lunch" with a client I had not seen for more than 30 years and was impressed with how fluent she was and how comfortable she was with her remaining very mild stuttering. I'll refer to her as "Jean." Jean had come to our university clinic for treatment for her moderate-to-severe stuttering. She told us that she had participated in hypnotherapy to recall an event in her childhood that precipitated her stuttering. Despite recalling that event, her stuttering hadn't changed. Now she wanted to manage her stuttering because it was interfering with her work and her social life. She seemed, to us, to be well adjusted and happy with herself. My student clinicians and I began teaching Jean controlled fluency using a device with a microphone and earphones that delayed the auditory feedback she heard while speaking (this is commonly called "delayed auditory feedback"). This kind of feedback forced Jean to speak very slowly, prolonging each sound. She was entirely fluent while talking this way. As we worked together, with Jean doing most of the talking in conversation with the clinicians, we reduced the amount of delay in her feedback, little by little. This allowed Jean to gradually increase her speech rate. On the first day (a Thursday), we worked together for about 6 hours and Jean finished the workout with fluent but very robotic-sounding speech. She then went home and returned the next day, Friday, speaking fluently but slowly. We then worked with her for another 6 hours to shape her fluency so that she sounded like a typical speaker, although her speech sounded somewhat precise and careful. That was at the end of the day on Friday. We asked her to return to our clinic after the weekend, and we cautioned her that some of her stuttering would probably have come back by then, and we would work on that.

On Monday, Jean came back to the clinic, saying that she was essentially fluent and many of her friends had commented on it. Over the next 6 months, we stayed in touch, primarily by phone, and she reported continued fluency. She told us that she planned to move from Vermont to Colorado. She did move and got married and reported continuing fluency. After that, we lost touch for 30 years. Then, I became curious about how she was doing and used the internet to find her and arrange a meeting when she was back in Vermont for a visit. We met at a restaurant near her home and she told me that those 2 days of therapy 30 years before had changed her life. Although she occasionally had a stutter or two, it was not an issue for her and she was also able to speak well and easily in all situations. I think her success was at least in part due to her robust temperament and her lack of significant negative emotions associated with her stuttering, even when she stuttered severely throughout her school years and on her job afterward, until she came to our clinic for therapy. She is an example of a client benefitting from learning controlled fluency and generalizing it mostly by herself. Now read the material on controlled fluency available on *Lippincott Connect*.

OTHER APPROACHES

Avoidance Reduction Therapy

Sisskin (2018) has written an excellent chapter on her avoidance reduction approach, which is based on the work of Joseph and Vivian Sheehan (1984), with whom she worked and practiced avoidance reduction therapy. The heart of the therapy is to help clients reduce both noticeable features of stuttering and negative thoughts and feelings that make up the struggle related to stuttering. These are learned behaviors, and they can be changed. One of the "mantras" of this approach is that clients are taught to do less, rather than more. That is, they are supported to shed the behaviors they have been using to hide and avoid stuttering and let go of "mental gymnastics" related to potential listener reactions. Clients eventually are free to go ahead and stutter openly without trying to hold their stuttering back, conceal it, or feel ashamed of it. But to get there, clients are guided to face their fear of stuttering, embrace their identity as a stutterer/person who stutters, and resist the stigma they have internalized since childhood. Many of the elements of Sisskin's therapy are similar to the integrated approach described in this textbook—which is pleasing for us both—but her approach discourages efforts to *control* stuttering. In other words, she believes clients can show their stuttering openly, without struggle, fear, or shame by letting go of control and gradually, according to their fear hierarchy, experiencing the feeling of *loss of control*. Sisskin believes that anticipated loss of control is what may motivate avoidance and concealment among many who stutter. In my stuttering modification approach, the feeling of control, achieved by holding onto a moment of stuttering openly, being present and calm and then ending the stutter slowly and loosely, is celebrated. I can't help but think that both approaches work because they both reduce the threat (nonconscious) and fear (conscious) of stuttering. In addition to her fine chapter, Sisskin describes how her approach is applied to school-age children (Sisskin & Goldstein, 2022) and demonstrates her approach in a video titled "Avoidance Reduction Therapy in a Group Setting" (2017) available from the Stuttering Foundation.

Pharmacological Approaches

The use of medications for stuttering has a long history, preceding even the Greeks' and Romans' use of wine to soothe the muscular tension and emotional turmoil of those who stuttered. In the current climate, medications may not be widely administered for stuttering, but some stutterers with severe symptoms—especially those who have not been able to get adequate relief from traditional therapy—may benefit from the latest medications *combined with* the best behavioral approaches. Personally, I experience so much satisfaction from managing my stuttering, that I wouldn't want to take a magic potion that made my stuttering disappear.

At one time (the 1960s), there was some hope that an antipsychotic drug called haloperidol, which blocked receptors for the neurotransmitter dopamine, might prove to be effective. In a later review of pharmacological approaches to stuttering, Brady (1991) discussed a number of studies on haloperidol. Several authors (Prins et al., 1980; Rosenberger, 1980; Swift et al., 1975) who studied haloperidol suggested that its effectiveness might result from diminishing the uptake of dopamine, because dopamine could interfere with fluency if it were produced in excess. Although haloperidol seemed to work directly on stuttering symptoms, rather than through overall sedative or tranquilizing mechanisms, major side effects have contraindicated its use. These side effects included drowsiness, sexual dysfunction, excess movement of limbs, and the risk of a permanent, neurologically based movement disorder: tardive dyskinesia. When I worked in Australia, I participated in a haloperidol trial and found that it reduced the tension in my stuttering, allowing blocks to seemingly melt in my mouth, but the side effects were hard to bear. I was always on the verge of falling asleep, and my legs were beset with uncontrollable wiggling.

The effectiveness of haloperidol in treating some stutterers, prompted a number of researchers (eg, Alm, 2004) to suggest that the basal ganglia may be implicated as a causal factor in stuttering. The section in Chapter 6 (Theories About Stuttering) titled "Stuttering as a Problem in the Cortico-basal Ganglia-Thalamocortical Loop" (the BG loop) details possible dysfunctions in the BG loop that interfere with the proper timing of syllable production. The neurotransmitter dopamine (in exactly the right amount) regulates the critical activation and inhibition of movement for speech—the "go" signal for a new syllable and the "stop" signal to inhibit that syllable after it has been produced. Excess dopamine will disrupt the timing of this activation and inhibition cycle so that the inappropriate stoppages and activation of motor movements of stuttering occur. The effectiveness of haloperidol in reducing stuttering comes from the fact that it reduces excess dopamine. But because haloperidol has bad side effects, researchers have looked for other dopamine-reducing drugs.

As a substitute for haloperidol, Maguire et al. (2004) tested *olanzapine*, another dopamine antagonist, which doesn't have the side effects that haloperidol does. In a double-blind study, olanzapine was reported to significantly ($P < .05$) reduce stuttering compared with the placebo on each of the following three measures: the SSI-3, the clinician's global impression, and the participant's self-rating of stuttering. The only side effect noted was a tendency for weight gain but that was minimized via counseling about diet and exercise. But the search for other drugs continued. Maguire et al. (2010) described their model of the action of the neurotransmitter dopamine in the etiology of stuttering and presented an update study on the effect of a new drug called *pagoclone*. In a separate publication, Maguire et al. (2010) showed that pagoclone reduced stuttering in 88 patients by 19.4%, whereas a placebo group of 44 patients reduced stuttering by only 5.1% in an 8-week trial. When this trial was over and all patients were offered continued use of pagoclone, the entire group showed a reduction of 40% after a year of treatment. The only significant side effect of pagoclone was headache, experienced by about 12% of the pagoclone patients. However, the search for other even more effective drugs for stuttering goes on. Maguire et al. (2020) reported on recent studies of the drugs *ecopipam* and *deutetrabenazine*, both of which reduce the excess dopamine intake in the basal ganglia and thus reduce stuttering. Both drugs have fewer side effects than previously studied dopamine antagonists.

In summary, although case studies appearing in the literature (eg, Brady & Ali, 2000) frequently report the success of a variety of medications, large-scale double-blind studies most frequently support drugs that interfere with the uptake of dopamine, especially olanzapine and pagoclone. New experiments with even newer drugs should appear in the literature by the time this textbook is published. Readers can use Google Scholar to look them up, using a search phrase such as "medications that reduce stuttering." At this time and for most individuals who stutter, medication for stuttering has not proven any more effective than traditional treatment. LaSalle, Ames, & Maguire (2022) suggested that future studies should compare groups of stutterers who receive (1) traditional speech therapy, (2) medication for stuttering, and (3) the combination of speech therapy and medication.

For more detailed information about current (and historical) medications for stuttering, I recommend the chapter in Zebrowski et al. (2022) titled "Pharmacological Considerations for the Treatment of Stuttering" by LaSalle et al. (2022). This chapter describes the hypothetical role of excess dopamine in stuttering and the "two-loop hypothesis" regarding dysfunction in the basal ganglia that results in mistiming of syllable activation and syllable inhibition networks going among the basal ganglia, the cerebral cortex, and speech musculature.

Treatment and Support Groups

My description of treatment groups will, to some extent, draw on my own experience as a client in one of Van Riper's stuttering modification treatment groups (see Van Riper (1958) for a description of his group therapy) and my experience as a clinician in fluency-shaping therapy groups (Guitar, 1976). Manning and DiLollo (2018) provided a good description of group stuttering therapy in their chapter on treatment of adolescents and adults.

Among the benefits of group therapy is the mutual support that its members experience as they face the challenges of confronting and changing their stuttering. An effective group leader will facilitate extensive interaction among group members so that they encourage each other, share hopes and fears, and provide a safe haven for trying out new behaviors. Many of us in Van Riper's group paired up to do some of our beyond-clinic assignments together. We were able to give each other helpful feedback, both in our group sessions and when we went out together to work on our speech in shopping areas and restaurants. Seeing each other's stuttering made ours more bearable, and vying with each other to bring back "trophies" of successful changes in our speech was healthy competition. The techniques we were taught and the changes we made in our behaviors, feelings, and attitudes were, I suspect, much the same as would have occurred in individual therapy, but the group made the road we had to travel less lonely and more fun. Van Riper measured the outcome of his treatment 5 years after the end of therapy, using the following five criteria: (1) the client's speech must be at or below 0.5 on the Iowa Scale of Severity of Stuttering (Sherman, 1952; this scale is a 1 to 7 scale requiring perceptual judgments of severity); (2) the client must not be avoiding words or situations; (3) stuttering must not be interfering with the client's social or vocational adjustment; (4) the client's word and situation fears must be close to zero; and (5) the client's stuttering must present no concern to themselves or others (Van Riper, 1958). The seven members of our group had our ups and downs, and several of us have had some additional therapy, but most of us did fairly well, but not perfectly, in terms of Van Riper's criteria.

The fluency-shaping groups I worked with in Australia as a clinician (Guitar, 1976; Howie & Andrews, 1984) focused first on learning a prolonged speech pattern to replace stuttering and shaping conversational speech to sound essentially normal. Group members then generalized their fluency to their natural environments. In this approach, the group functioned primarily as a setting in which conversational speech could be practiced. Treatment in a group promoted an efficient use of the clinician's time as well as opportunities for members to practice using fluent speech in the give-and-take of a conversation among six people. Results of treatment varied widely for individuals (Guitar, 1976), but the overall group mean of percent syllables stuttered went from 14% before treatment to 3.9% a year after treatment, with essentially normal mean speech rates (Howie & Andrews, 1984). Subsequent modifications of the program brought follow-up stuttering percentages to even lower levels (1-2 %SS) (Andrews & Craig, 1982).

Support or self-help groups differ from treatment groups because their main function is to provide an atmosphere in which members can freely share their feelings and develop a sense of connectedness to others who stutter, and they can provide an excellent opportunity for maintenance of improvement made in formal therapy. In my experience, getting together with others who stutter and sharing experiences, especially triumphs and frustrations, gives us a great opportunity to continue working on strategies that we have found helpful, as well as feel the support and encouragement of others. Probably the most important part of the group experience is sharing and mutual support, rather than specific work on techniques. Our group at the University of Vermont, which has been running for more than 50 years, is a mix of support and therapy. Participants share their experiences, comment supportively on each other's techniques, and give themselves speech assignments, both for that meeting and for the 2 weeks in between meetings. Group members often bring funny stories to tell the group. There is much therapeutic humor, directed both at stuttering and at difficult listeners.

Ramig (1993) surveyed 62 self-help participants and found that 49 of them believed that their fluency had improved "at least somewhat" as a result of attending meetings regularly. The majority of respondents felt that the group experience improved their feelings about themselves, as well as their comfort in their personal and work environments. Information about the return rate of the survey was not available. Ramig did note that there is a paucity of research on the impact of self-help groups on the lives of people who stutter, and he gave 17 suggestions for designing studies on self-help groups.

An excellent review of self-help groups as a supplement to traditional therapy was presented in a chapter by Yaruss et al. (2007). This chapter lists several national self-help groups for stuttering organizations and provides evidence of benefit to participants gathered by self-report studies. A chapter by Trichon and Raj (2018) gives a history of the stuttering self-help movement and an update on national self-help meetings, international self-help organizations, and internet-based peer support for stuttering. The National Stuttering Association provides excellent mentoring for people who want to start their own self-help groups, including assistance in setting up a website. For an example, see the University of Vermont stuttering group's website.[4]

A study by Tichenor and Yaruss (2019) about self-help groups for adults provides data that show that adult stutterers who attend these groups, compared to those who don't, feel more open and comfortable about their stuttering and are less likely to try to hide their stuttering or avoid situations in which they may stutter. In a study by Gerlach et al. (2019) of young stutterers who attended an annual meeting of the self-help group "Friends" showed more positive scores on the OASIS after versus before the event. The authors of both studies recommend self-help groups as an effective addition to traditional stuttering therapy.

---

[4]www.burlingtonstutters.org

SUMMARY

- Advanced stuttering is characterized by repetitions, prolongations, and blocks, accompanied by overlearned patterns of tension, struggle, and escape and avoidance behaviors. Clients will also typically have negative attitudes, feelings, and beliefs about stuttering and about speaking.
- I believe that because these behaviors are so well-learned, treatment must focus on helping people who stutter learn new stuttering management skills as responses to old cues that would otherwise still tend to elicit struggle and avoidance behaviors.
- Treatment begins by helping the client confront and understand their stuttering and, in the process, decreasing fear and shame. Then, the clinician teaches stuttering management skills (going directly into stutters, holding onto them with voicing and/or airflow, and, as fear and tension decrease, finishing the word slowly and loosely). When these skills are done well, they are termed "easy stutters."
- The client first learns stuttering management skills in the clinic and then generalizes them into their daily life. They practice them in many situations with the clinician's support and then on their own. They also learn to voluntarily stutter and be open about their stuttering to other people.
- For many clients, continued work is needed on increasing approach behaviors and decreasing avoidance behaviors. For all clients, the responsibility for managing their own speech is gradually transferred to them over the course of treatment.
- A variety of other treatments are available for advanced stuttering, including controlled fluency, individual and group approaches, intensive and non-intensive treatment, and medication. Knowing about these options can give you a wider range of options to offer your clients, especially those who need something more or something different from the integrated approach offered in this chapter.

STUDY QUESTIONS

1. Summarize the main differences between *intermediate stuttering in school-age children, stuttering in adolescents,* and *advanced stuttering in adults* and the treatment approaches used for them.
2. How does "**exploring stuttering**" help a client decrease their fear and shame associated with stuttering? What is the clinician's role in this process?
3. Do you think it is a treatment failure if a client has mild stuttering after treatment? Explain the reasoning behind your answer.
4. How does "catch and release" help extinguish fear of stuttering.
5. If a client has kept their stuttering a hidden secret all their life, how do you motivate them to be more open about it?
6. Many clients are reluctant to use voluntary stuttering. What are some reasons you could give them as to why it may be helpful? Are there any clients with whom you would not use it?
7. Imagine yourself being an individual who stutters who is in search of a place to share your experiences and get support. How do you look for one in your town or city? Does National Stuttering Association or Stuttering Home Page or the Stuttering Foundation have suggestions to find a group near you?
8. Which clients would be most suited for treatment with a pharmacological approach?
9. What do you think are the most valid measures of the benefits of a treatment approach?

SUGGESTED PROJECTS

1. Choose a behavior of yours that you would like to change, and develop a self-therapy plan to explore your present behavior, identify the change you would like to make, and develop a hierarchy to practice the new behavior. Report on your success.
2. Write out a conversation that you could have with a new adult client to describe the possible course of treatment (see the section on "Beginning Therapy"). Make your discussion both challenging and inspirational.
3. If you are someone who *doesn't* stutter, your biggest fear in doing voluntary stuttering is probably that you will be unable to stutter convincingly, and a listener will unmask you. Confront that fear by stuttering to several listeners, and see if that decreases your fear.
4. Watch a session of the Van Riper videos (available from stutteringhelp.org) (eg, the session on desensitization), and see if you can determine what made him so effective as a stuttering therapist.

SUGGESTED READINGS

Fraser, M. (2010). *Self-therapy for the stutterer* (11th ed.). Stuttering Foundation.

This self-help book contains a sequenced program for an adult who stutters to use, either on his own or with the help of a clinician or supportive friend. It describes many of the techniques you have been reading about in this book. In addition, it contains many personal and inspirational messages for the reader. I recommend it not only to individuals who stutter but also to clinicians so that they may get another perspective on adult stuttering therapy.

Guitar, B., & Guitar, C. (2005). *If you stutter: Advice for adults (DVD).* Stuttering Foundation.

This video presents a broad spectrum of treatment approaches, and many of them are demonstrated by adults who have benefited from stuttering therapy.

Guitar, B., & McCauley, R. (Eds.) (2010). *Treatment of stuttering: Established and emerging interventions.* Lippincott Williams & Wilkins.

This book has four approaches for adults and adolescents who stutter: two behavioral treatments, one involving the SpeechEasy device, and one on pharmacological therapy. Each chapter is illustrated with a video that depicts the treatment process as well as before- and after-therapy interviews with clients.

Hendrickson, J. (2023). *Life on delay: Making peace with a stutter.* Alfred A. Knopf.

This is an enthralling memoir by the author of a 2019 Atlantic magazine article, based on his interview with President Biden, "What Joe Biden Can't Bring Himself to Say." In Life on Delay, Hendrickson paints a painful and vivid picture of what it is like to have a severe stutter that shackles spoken communication in a devastating way. Hendrickson is particularly articulate when he interviews famous musicians and other artists about how they've coped (and not) with their stuttering.

Manning, W., & DiLollo, A. (2018). *Clinical decision making in fluency disorders* (4th ed.). Plural Publishing.

An excellent and sensible book about stuttering therapy by knowledgeable clinicians. It has the added benefit of being written by individuals who stutter and who have largely recovered. Their clinical experiences are shared throughout the book, putting readers in the shoes of the authors' many clients.

National Stuttering Association. Website: www.westutter.org

This site contains a wealth of information for adolescents and adults who stutter, including basic information about the nature of stuttering and treatment opportunities. A DVD, Transcending Stuttering, about the struggle and triumph of many individuals who stutter, is among NSA's recent offerings.

Shapiro, D. (2011). *Stuttering intervention: A collaborative journey to fluency freedom.* Pro-Ed.

This book is a thoughtful account of working with people who stutter, written by an experienced clinician who stutters himself. Shapiro is particularly eloquent on the feelings that affect people who stutter.

Stuttering Foundation. Website: www.stutteringhelp.org

Background information on stuttering and its treatment are provided. Books, videos, and lists of clinicians who specialize in stuttering are offered on this site.

Stuttering Home Page: www.mnsu.edu/comdis/kuster/stutter.html

Developed by Judy Kuster at Mankato State University, the Stuttering Home Page offers a wide variety of helpful pages and links. On this site, the user can connect to chat rooms and access an annual online conference and its archives, the latest research, and commentary by people who stutter. Links to stuttering sites in other countries are also provided.

Van Riper, C. (1975). *Therapy in action (DVD).* Stuttering Foundation.

This nine-session DVD shows a master clinician conducting stuttering modification treatment with an adult who stutters. Van Riper takes this young man from the assessment to the final treatment meeting in seven sessions. There are then 1-year and 20-year follow-up interviews. Van Riper introduces each session describing what he has planned for the session and then follows the session with a commentary on what was accomplished.

18

Treatment of Atypical Fluency Disorders

Chapter Outline

Chapter Objectives

After studying this chapter, readers should be able to:

- Describe the evaluation and treatment of acquired neurogenic stuttering
- Describe trial therapy for psychogenic stuttering and how that may be continued beyond the initial trial
- Describe the evaluation of cluttering and concomitant problems
- Describe why motivation is a major issue in the treatment of cluttering
- Describe the treatment of cluttering

Key Terms

Delayed auditory feedback (DAF): Hearing one's own voice a half-second or so after speaking. This is usually done via a computer program, with the client speaking into a microphone and hearing themselves through headphones. It typically forces a client to speak more slowly and temporarily but dramatically reduces stuttering

Fluency-inducing or fluency-enhancing conditions: Speaking conditions that usually cause a person who stutters to speak much more fluently. Examples are speaking in a rhythmic or staccato manner, speaking under loud masking noise so the client can't hear their own voice, and speaking while very relaxed

Functional stuttering: This is a subcategory of functional neurological disorders in that there are no structural issues with the brain nor any neurological disease associated with the stuttering. The origins are thought to be "biopsychosocial," meaning that psychological issues have affected biological function. This category of stuttering was formerly called "psychogenic stuttering." Psychological stress or trauma may be the origin of this stuttering

Lowest common denominator (LCD): This is an attempt to define cluttering, in terms of its most salient characteristics. The current definition was proposed by St. Louis and Schulte (2011). The benefit would be that clinicians and researcher would share a common view of cluttering

Malingering: Pretending to stutter in order to fool someone. For example, a person who doesn't stutter who committed a crime may pretend to stutter to claim innocence

Pacing: A treatment technique in which each individual syllable is spoken separately, sometimes accompanied by physical movement such as tapping a finger as each syllable is spoken

Prolonged speech: A treatment for stuttering that induces the client to stretch out sounds, start words with a gentle onset of phonation, and touch the articulators lightly when producing consonants

Trial therapy: A brief treatment for stuttering carried out during the evaluation to identify treatment techniques that seem particularly effective. Some trial therapies may take longer to have an effect than others

INTRODUCTION

This chapter describes assessment and treatment for three fluency disorders that were discussed in Chapter 8 on Atypical Disfluency. These disorders are neurogenic stuttering, functional (formerly psychogenic) stuttering, and cluttering. The first two are similar to developmental stuttering in some ways but require somewhat different approaches for treatment. The third, cluttering, may co-occur with developmental stuttering but is treated quite differently.

ACQUIRED NEUROGENIC STUTTERING

Nature

As you will remember from Chapter 8, where it is discussed in detail, the onset of acquired neurogenic stuttering is associated with a neurological injury or condition. Stroke, traumatic brain injury, and neurodegenerative diseases are often causal factors. A comparison of developmental stuttering with neurogenic stuttering is shown in Table 18.1.

Diagnosis and Evaluation

Cruz et al. (2018), Helm-Estabrooks (1999), Junuzovic-Zunic et al. (2021), and Ringo and Dietrich (1995) provide a framework for assessing acquired neurogenic stuttering and distinguishing it from other disorders. These authors suggest that the following procedures are important not only for evaluating individual cases but also for gathering data that may make a contribution to the literature.

1. A complete case history reflecting:
   - Onset of stuttering and its association with other neurological or psychological signs
   - The client's level of concern, anxiety, or fear about their stuttering
   - Extent to which stuttering interferes with communication
   - Changes in stuttering since onset
   - The client's own history and family's history of speech, language, or learning problems
   - Neurological and psychological health history

   This information can be gathered initially through a case history and then supplemented during the interview.
2. Direct assessment of speech:
   - The Stuttering Severity Instrument (Riley, 2009) should be administered, and speech should be video recorded during conversation and reading samples.
   - Stuttering in speech samples should be analyzed for
     - Proportion of stuttering on function (grammatical) words versus content (substantive) words. More stuttering on function words suggests neurogenic stuttering.

TABLE 18.1 Comparative Characteristics of Neurogenic Stuttering Compared With Developmental Stuttering

Characteristic	Developmental Stuttering	Neurogenic Stuttering
Etiology	Deficits in the speech production areas of the brain	Specific injuries or disease processes in neural pathways for speech
Onset	Usually in early childhood between ages 2 and 5 years	Often in adulthood, after brain injury or disease process
Development or change over time	If it does not disappear in early childhood, stuttering usually gets gradually more severe during childhood and adolescence	Stuttering usually remains similar to what it was like on onset
Types of stuttering behavior	Repetitions, prolongations, and blocks	Most often repetitions, but sometimes also prolongations or blocks
Frequency of stuttering	Almost always below 45% syllables stuttered	Similar to frequency of developmental stuttering
Secondary behaviors	Beyond early childhood, tension and struggle often observed, along with escape and avoidance behaviors	Typically, very few secondary behaviors or none
Emotional response to stuttering	Beyond early childhood, frequently notable emotional reactions such as struggle, embarrassment, and shame	Usually little emotional response to stuttering, except occasional frustration
Locus of stutters	Stutters tend to occur on syllables at beginnings of words and at beginnings of phrases More stuttering on content words than function words	Stutters occur at many locations in words and phrases Stutters may occur just as often on function as on content words
Response to fluency-inducing conditions such as swinging arm or choral reading	Stuttering markedly reduced in fluency-inducing conditions	Sometimes no improvement with fluency-inducing conditions
Adaptation effect: repeated reading of a passage	Adaptation frequently seen—stuttering frequency and severity decrease with repeated reading of passage	Adaptation often does not change the frequency or severity of stuttering
Treatment	Stuttering modification or fluency-shaping treatments can make substantial improvements	Pacing (speaking one syllable at a time) can be helpful, as can slowing speech rate

- ☐ Presence of stuttering on noninitial syllables, such as in these words "exciteme-me-ment," "cowb-b-b-oy," and "canister-er-er." More stuttering on noninitial syllables suggests neurogenic stuttering.
- ☐ Documentation of secondary (ie, escape and avoidance) behaviors such as eye blinks, head nods, and use of "um" to get a word started. *Absence* of secondary behaviors suggests neurogenic stuttering.
- ☐ The same short passage should be read aloud six times to determine if stuttering is reduced progressively through the repeated readings. See Chapter 1 for more information and references for this *adaptation* procedure. Lack of adaptation suggests neurogenic stuttering.
- ☐ Speaking in a variety of **fluency-inducing** conditions should be explored, especially speaking in a rhythm while swinging an arm, speaking while listening to loud masking noise, and speaking slowly under **delayed auditory feedback (DAF)** set at a maximum delay. If fluency-inducing conditions do not increase fluency, this suggests neurogenic stuttering.

3. Other assessment components:
   - Helm-Estabrooks (1999) recommended using the Aphasia Diagnostic Profiles (Helm-Estabrooks, 1992) to exclude the possibility that the stuttering actually reflects language formulation problems.
   - Helm-Estabrooks (1999) also recommended that if other neurological problems are present and might interfere with treatment, neuropsychological testing would be important for assessing the client's capabilities.
   - De Nil et al. (2007) also strongly suggested testing for other disorders that may affect communication or treatment. These include dysarthria, aphasia, motor disorders, cognitive disorders, and chronic pain. These authors also provide an assessment battery that includes measures of attitudes about stuttering, including the S-24 (Andrews & Cutler, 1974) and the Locus of Control for Behavior (Craig et al., 1984).
   - Administering the Overall Assessment of Speaker's Experience of Stuttering (OASES) would provide information about the extent to which the stuttering affects the client's life.
   - I would add to this list of assessment targets the distinction between stuttering-like disfluencies (repetitions of sounds, syllables and monosyllabic words, prolongations, or blocks) versus typical disfluencies (multisyllable word repetitions, phrase repetitions, interjections, revision-incomplete phrases) (Theys et al., 2013).

The information gathered from the above procedures can be used to improve our understanding of neurogenic stuttering, to differentially diagnose neurogenic stuttering (ie, distinguish it from other fluency disorders), and to help in planning treatment. The data on the client's and relatives' handedness and history of speech, language, or learning problems are primarily used to determine if a client might have a predisposition for stuttering. Left-handedness or ambidexterity as well as a history of speech or language problems in a family may predispose an individual for stuttering (Geschwind & Galaburda, 1985). If a client began to stutter or if previous stuttering recurred or worsened in association with the occurrence of neurological problems, neurogenic stuttering should be suspected. On the other hand, stuttering that appeared in conjunction with psychological stress or trauma may be of psychogenic origin (**functional stuttering**). Sometimes these etiologies are difficult to sort out and are discussed further in the section on functional stuttering.

It is difficult to be *certain* that an individual has neurogenic stuttering rather than disfluencies caused by other impairments. A diagnosis of neurogenic stuttering can be more certain if other signs of neuropathology are shown. As indicated earlier, every effort needs to be made to rule out cognitive and memory problems, language formulation problems (such as in aphasia), and emotional distress as the *source* of a client's disfluencies. Sometimes a combination of neurogenic and psychogenic issues may contribute to disfluencies, as I describe in a section on stuttering related to military experience in Chapter 8.

Considerations for Treatment

Helm-Estabrooks (1999) suggested several criteria for determining which clients have the potential to benefit from treatment. She noted that some neurogenic stuttering is quite mild and may not result in a handicap that warrants treatment. Other individuals, whose stuttering may be a serious handicap, may have other health problems that are far more serious, such as a progressive neurological disorder. A third consideration is the extent to which other neurological problems, such as dementia, may interfere with treatment. If a client does have severe and persistent stuttering, is motivated to undergo treatment, and has adequate cognitive and linguistic abilities to benefit from treatment, then several treatment options are available.

Treatment Approaches

Because individuals with neurogenic stuttering do not usually have the cognitive and emotional involvement (eg, fear, shame, and negative feeling about self) that characterize developmental stuttering in adults, treatment is often entirely behavioral. An exception is when the neurological etiology of the stuttering is known and can be treated by surgery or drugs. De Nil et al. (2007) noted that not all patients with neurogenic stuttering need treatment because, as Helm et al. (1980) have indicated, neurogenic stuttering may appear and then gradually improve without treatment.

1. **Behavioral treatments.** Many of the treatments (or components thereof) that have been used for developmental stuttering have also been used for neurogenic stuttering with some success.
   - ***Pacing.*** This is essentially a technique of speaking one syllable at a time, so that each syllable is spoken separately, without the usual coarticulation across syllables. As a result, speech is produced more slowly and with a strong, staccato rhythm. This treatment was developed by Helm (1979) for patients with palilalia (ie, rapid repetition of whole words and phrases) but has been used for neurogenic stuttering as well (Helm-Estabrooks, 1999). To facilitate pacing, especially in those patients who have difficulty slowing their speech, pacing devices can be used. One example is a pacing board (Helm-Estabrooks & Kaplan, 1989) (see Fig. 18.1); another is a molded form that fits over the patient's index finger and makes tapping more distinct (Rentschler et al., 1984). With either of these devices, the patient moves a finger from place to place, timing each syllable with a finger movement. Helm-Estabrooks (1999) suggested that pacing could begin with a device and progress to simply tapping rhythmically on the thigh to produce fluent speech.

     Theys and De Nil (2022) note that pacing and similar treatment approaches may be better-suited to neurogenic stutterers than traditional therapies that try to

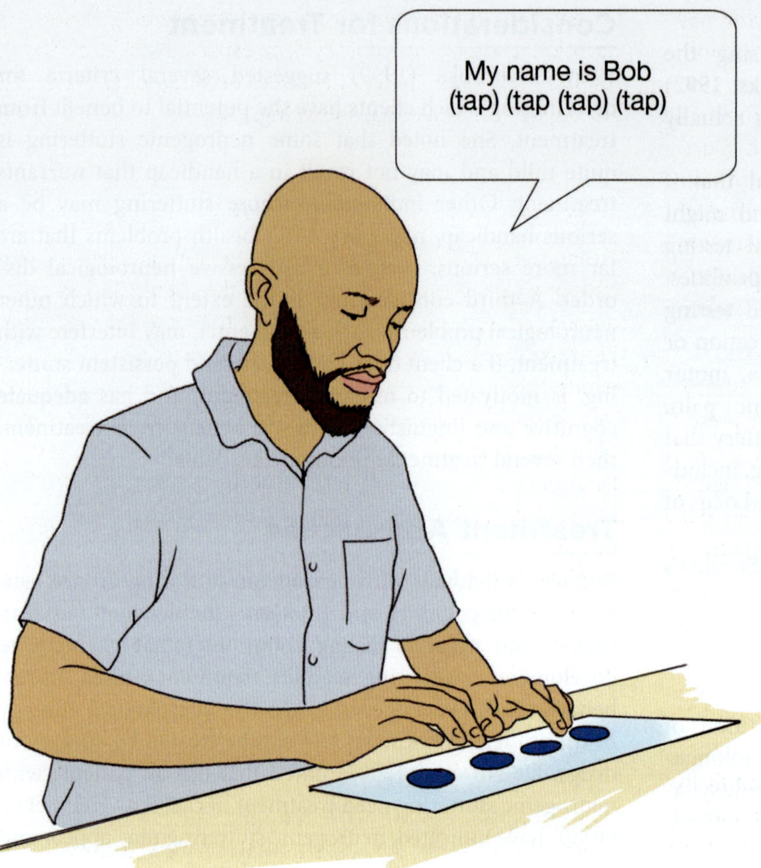

Figure 18.1 Patient with acquired neurogenic stuttering using a pacing board to talk fluently by speaking one word at a time and tapping with finger on circles on board.

teach clients to slow their speech rates. Such slowing would require constant monitoring of speech and tax these clients' cognitive abilities.

- *Auditory masking and DAF.* Rentschler et al. (1984), Marshall and Starch (1984), and Helm-Estabrooks (1999) reported that masking and DAF can be used as therapeutic tools to induce fluency in neurogenic stuttering, and in some cases, fluency can then be generalized.
- *Slow rate and easy onset.* Market et al. (1990) conducted a survey of clinicians who had worked with acquired neurogenic stuttering and found that many of them reported success with fluency-shaping tools, such as slow rate and easy onset.
- *Stuttering modification.* Only a modest percentage of the clinicians surveyed by Market et al. (1990) reported that they had used such stuttering modification tools as light contacts, preparatory sets, cancellations, and pullouts.
- *Electromyographic biofeedback for tension reduction.* Reports by Helm-Estabrooks (1986) and Rubow et al. (1986) suggested that training patients to relax muscles with the help of biofeedback can be effective in reducing neurogenic stuttering.

2. **Neurosurgery.** Sometimes when a neurological problem requires surgical intervention, the surgery resolves or improves stuttering. Cases reported by Donnan (1979) and Jones (1966) suggested that for whatever reason, surgery that resolved a neurological problem may also resolve stuttering. Andy and Bhatnager (1992) reported on four patients who were improved by surgical implantations of electrodes to stimulate the thalamus for other neurological conditions. The implication is that some disturbance in neurological functioning can result in stuttering, and when the neurosurgery changes this neurological functioning, stuttering can be resolved. This finding is consistent with recent evidence suggesting that brain structure and function may be aberrant in developmental stuttering (eg, Chang, 2014; Chang & Guenther, 2020; Chang, Angstadt, et al., 2017; Chang, Zhu, et al., 2015; Cykowski et al., 2010).
3. **Medications.** As I described in Chapter 14, a number of drugs such as haloperidol, olanzapine, and pagoclone have been tried with varying degrees of success with developmental stuttering. These medications have not been tried, as far as I know, with neurogenic stuttering. Rather, case studies have reported that drugs for seizure disorders, schizophrenia, depression, anxiety, Parkinson disease, and

asthma can *precipitate* stuttering in individuals who have not stuttered previously (Baratz & Mesulam, 1981; Duffy, 2013; Elliott & Thomas, 1985; McClean & McClean, 1985; Nurnberg & Greenwald, 1981; Quader, 1977). In most of these cases, stuttering is reduced or eliminated when drug dosage is adjusted or an alternative drug is used. In other studies, drugs have been given for other symptoms and have relieved stuttering (Perino et al., 2000; Turgut et al., 2002). There is no evidence that there are drugs for clients with neurogenic stuttering that are effective, without serious side effects.

Overall, there is no clear consensus about effective treatments for neurogenic stuttering, and few studies present evidence of the long-term effectiveness of treatment. In part, this may be because the many different etiologies of neurogenic stuttering and the relative rarity of this disorder pose significant barriers to long-term group studies of treatment of neurogenic stuttering.

FUNCTIONAL (PSYCHOGENIC) ACQUIRED STUTTERING

Functional acquired stuttering is a specific condition fitting in the category of functional speech disorders (FSDs), which are, in turn, a subtype of functional neurological disorders (FNDs), a group of conditions that may be difficult to diagnose, but that present with positive clinical features rather than as disorders defined by exclusion (Utianski and Duffy, 2021). FNDs can involve a variety of symptoms (eg, paralysis, gait disturbances, pseudo seizures), with speech symptoms occurring in about 25% to 50% of cases. Affecting women more frequently than men, FNDs tend to occur in individuals between 7 and 50 years and to be associated with disruptions in brain network activity and activity supporting the idea that symptoms are not the result of volitional **malingering**. In their 2021 article on FSDs, Utianski and Duffy review current thinking on the disorder and review four cases seen at the Mayo Clinic, including one in which stuttering was a symptom.

Nature

Our understanding of functional stuttering may be enhanced by a notable book titled *The Body Keeps the Score: Brain, Mind, and Body in the Healing of Trauma* (van der Kolk, 2014). The author describes his clinical and research work as a psychiatrist that began by helping Vietnam war veterans with posttraumatic stress disorder (PTSD) and, later, individuals who experienced trauma as children or adults. He details what research tells us about changes in the brain after trauma and how brain scans after successful treatment show a return to more typical brain functions. For example, trauma appears to upset the balance between the rational brain (prefrontal cortex, particularly the medial prefrontal cortex) and the emotional brain (the limbic system, especially the amygdala). Table 18.2 delineates the differences between developmental stuttering and functional stuttering.

Diagnosis and Evaluation

Functional stuttering is believed to be associated with psychological stress or trauma. Often the client will report an emotional event close to the time of the onset of stuttering. However, there may also be signs of neurological issues, in which case there is a possibility that the stuttering is the first indication of a neurological disorder. Therefore, a multidisciplinary approach, involving neurology, psychiatry, and speech-language pathology (SLP), may be needed, especially if a client has specific neurological signs, such as headache, dizziness, or numbness of extremities in addition to the stuttering.

Note: If the clinician can maintain an interested, curious, accepting attitude during the evaluation, the client is more likely to reveal vital information about the emotions associated with the stuttering. Baumgartner (1999) noted that clients' expression of feelings may be accompanied by increased fluency, which is a possible sign of psychogenic basis for the stuttering.

The evaluation should include the following:

1. A complete case history obtained either exclusively in an interview or via a questionnaire followed up with an interview. The case history should obtain information concerning:
   - Onset of stuttering, including circumstances surrounding onset, such as whether it occurred during prolonged or acute stress/trauma. The nature and pattern of the stuttering when it first started should be determined
   - Changes in *stuttering* since onset and whether there have been times of complete fluency
   - Current *pattern* of stuttering, its situational variability, and its impact on the client's life
   - Whether the *individual* stuttered prior to the onset of the current stuttering at any time and if so, the nature and pattern and the extent of recovery of this earlier stuttering
   - Family history of stuttering and other speech, language, or learning problems
2. A motor speech disorder, such as apraxia or Parkinson disease, should be ruled out. The text Motor Speech Disorders (Duffy, 2020), for example, provides guidance for a motor speech exam. If clients show signs of language or cognitive problems, these should be further tested.
3. Analysis of stuttering. Samples should be obtained of the client's conversational speech and reading aloud so that baseline measures of stuttering severity can be made with the SSI-4, and the patterns of stuttering can be examined. As mentioned above, unusual struggle behaviors, especially if they are independent of moments of stuttering, are signs of possible psychogenicity of stuttering.

TABLE 18.2 Comparative Characteristics of Functional Stuttering Compared With Developmental Stuttering

Characteristic	Developmental Stuttering	Functional Stuttering
Etiology	Deficits in the speech production areas of the brain	Response to emotional stress
Onset	Usually in early childhood between ages 2 and 5 years	Late childhood or adulthood, soon after emotional stress
Development or change over time	If it does not disappear in early childhood, stuttering usually gets gradually more severe during childhood and adolescence	Stuttering usually remains similar to what it was like at onset
Types of stuttering behavior	Repetitions, prolongations, and blocks	May be similar to developmental stuttering. Alternatively, may consist of very rapid repetitions. Unusually steady eye contact is sometimes evident
Frequency of stuttering	From mild to severe. Almost always below 45% syllables stuttered	Usually high frequency
Secondary behaviors	Beyond early childhood, tension and struggle often observed, along with escape and avoidance behaviors	May consist of unusual or severe blocks
Emotional response to stuttering	Beyond early childhood, frequently notable emotional reactions such as struggle, embarrassment, and shame	Usually little emotional response to stuttering. In some cases, client may smile during stuttering
Locus of stutters	Stutters tend to occur on syllables at beginnings of words and at beginnings of phrases More stuttering on content words than function words	Stutters occur at many locations in words and phrases Stutters may occur just as often on function as on content words
Response to fluency-inducing conditions such as swinging arm or choral reading	Stuttering markedly reduced in fluency-inducing conditions	Sometimes, no improvement with fluency-inducing conditions. In some cases, stuttering becomes more severe
Adaptation effect: repeated reading of a passage	Adaptation frequently seen—stuttering frequency and severity decrease with repeated reading of passage	Adaptation often does not change the frequency or severity of stuttering
Treatment	Stuttering modification or fluency-shaping treatments can make substantial improvements	Treatment should be accompanied by strong suggestion that it will help. Intensive fluency-shaping (such as prolonged speech) may be immediately beneficial

4. **Trial therapy** should be carried out. If the client immediately becomes fluent with trial therapy, functional stuttering may be suspected. An example of trial therapy is described in the section on functional stuttering in Motor Speech Disorders (Duffy, 2020) and in Duffy's chapter in Roth et al. (2011). This approach has the clinician put their hands on the thyrohyoid area (the throat near the larynx), feel for tension, and have the speaker talk while the clinician pulls the thyroid cartilage down to a more relaxed position. The client can be told that they are maintaining excessive tension in this area; the clinician can then guide them through a hierarchy of producing vowels, single words, sentences, and conversation in a very relaxed and slow style. A functional basis of the stuttering is supported

if the client becomes very fluent in this trial treatment. While individuals with developmental stuttering can be noticeably helped by trial therapy, it will usually not generalize to fluency during the remainder of the session. The clinician should be careful to explain the client's fluency to them, relating it to the relaxation that counteracts the excess tension developed as a response to stress.

Another approach to trial therapy, called controlled fluency[1], involves beginning very mindful slow talking that gradually speeds up but keeps the client highly aware of their articulator movements. The steps are as follows: (1) the clinician models a very slow, stretched out style of talking with plenty of pausing and easy onsets of each word. As an example of how slow to go, the sentence "My name is (pause) Nelson" should take 10 seconds to produce. (2) The clinician should model this style of speaking and have the client shadow the clinician's model, saying the same words along with the clinician. If the client does not produce the phrase fluently, the clinician should coach the client to make their speech more like the clinician's. (3) See if the client can produce their own short phrases without the clinician's model. If the client can talk fluently this way for several minutes while talking about a simple topic like what their favorite foods are, this suggests possible functional stuttering.

Considerations for Treatment

Individuals who are able to decrease their stuttering dramatically in trial therapy and whose psychological adjustment is adequate are often good candidates for stuttering therapy. Even though they may need psychotherapy eventually, speech therapy may well start immediately. On the other hand, clients who are unable to improve fluency during trial therapy and/or who are dysfunctional because of psychological issues may benefit from receiving psychotherapy concurrently with (or prior to) stuttering therapy. Individuals who resist the idea that their stuttering may have a stress-related basis and who do not improve with trial therapy may not be good candidates for treatment or may need extended treatment.

Treatment Approaches

In Chapter 17, we described the treatment for a young woman (Jean) whose stuttering started after a traumatic childhood event, a possible sign of functional stuttering. Jean had come to our clinic with moderately severe stuttering that had burdened her since she experienced an emotionally upsetting incident when she was 5 years old. As an adult, she had forgotten what had happened to her but prior to her visit to our clinic, she was able, with the help of a hypnotherapist, to recall the incident and talk about it. However, this did not change her stuttering. Upon reading van der Kolk's book, I considered that perhaps recalling the incident and talking about it with the hypnotherapist was not enough to relieve Jean's stuttering, much as many of van der Kolk's trauma patients were not helped by "talk therapy." Rather, most effective therapies for his trauma patients involved them getting in touch with their bodies, their movements, and their breathing. Jean's therapy with us, as you will recall, involved talking for 6 hours a day over 2 days while she was listening to herself via DAF. As she learned to match the rate of her speech to the feedback delay and speak fluently, she needed to speak very slowly and be aware of her articulator movements. This may have increased her bodily awareness of speaking fluently. With us, Jean didn't talk about the incident in her childhood, but about her job, her social life, and other nonemotional topics. Perhaps the intense experience of talking mindfully for 12 hours had allowed her mind and body to undo the "freezing" (a term used by van der Kolk) of her speech that resulted in stuttering. As you may remember from my description in Chapter 17, Jean became fluent after these 2 days of **prolonged speech** therapy and we have followed her for more than 30 years and found that she remained fluent.

One approach for trial therapy (controlled fluency) involves talking very slowly but fluently, at about 40 syllables per minute. Once the client is fluent at this very slow rate of speech, their speaking rate can be very gradually increased, but ensuring that fluency is maintained as speech rate is increased. If this is effective in producing temporary fluency, it can be used as a treatment for functional stuttering, as in the case of Jean, described previously.

Alternatively, treatments used for developmental stuttering may be appropriate for functional stuttering (Baumgartner, 1999; Duffy, 2020; Mahr & Leith, 1992; Roth et al., 1989). For example, Roth et al. (1989) suggested that approaches such as easy onset, light contact, and easy repetitions can work with functional stuttering. Weiner (1981) employed desensitization combined with vocal control therapy, an approach that emphasizes adequate respiratory support, gentle onsets, and optimal vocal resonance. Transfer was carried out using a hierarchy of easy-to-difficult situations. Unfortunately, no group studies of long-term treatment outcomes for therapy with psychogenic stuttering have been reported.

Treatment for neurogenic and/or functional stuttering in active military personnel or veterans can follow the guidelines given in the preceding section on treatment of functional stuttering. However, different treatment approaches may be needed if these don't work. In his book, *The Body Keeps the Score,* the psychiatrist Bessel van der Kolk (2014) describes his work at the Massachusetts Mental Health Center with former soldiers who suffered from PTSD. It is clear that many are not helped by "talk therapy" but require more innovative treatments for these individuals who have been traumatized.

---

[1]See section on controlled fluency on the Lippincott Connect in the material on Chapter 17.

van der Kolk believes that "For real change to take place, the body needs to learn that the danger has passed..." (p. 21). It may be that for those with functional stuttering who are not helped by our current therapies, unorthodox approaches described in van der Kolk's book, such as eye movement desensitization and reprocessing, yoga, Pilates, and neurofeedback would be effective.

Summary and Conclusions

In the past 10 years, there has been an increasing acceptance of the idea that disfluencies associated with psychological trauma and stress may be a unique type of stuttering. The main diagnostic markers are (1) stuttering onset that occurs in late adolescence or adulthood, although it can begin earlier, as I described in my client Jean; (2) stuttering onset that is associated with prolonged or acute stress; (3) unusual struggle behaviors that may not always be associated with moments of stuttering; (4) stuttering that increases in fluency-inducing conditions; and (5) dramatically improved fluency during trial treatment. Compared with neurogenic stuttering, there is relatively little known about the speech characteristics observed in psychogenic stuttering (such as the linguistic loci of stutters), nor is there consensus on the common types of core behaviors associated with this disorder.

MALINGERING

Although malingering (faking a disorder to receive some benefit) is not psychogenic/functional, I think it would be helpful for me to describe this manifestation of stuttering in close proximity to my discussion of neurogenic and functional stuttering since all three of these most often occur with adult onset, which makes it important to differentially diagnose them. Also, who knows? You may someday be asked to testify in court if malingering stuttering is suspected. Table 18.3 indicates the differences between developmental stuttering and malingering.

Case reports by Shirkey (1987) and Seery (2005) described protocols that they used to attempt to distinguish between developmental, neurogenic, or psychogenic stuttering, versus malingering. In each case, the person in question had been accused of a crime during which he spoke fluently but claimed he was innocent because he stuttered so severely that he could not have been that individual. Their approaches were similar and the suggestions given here combine their reports. An additional report by the neuropsychologists Binder et al. (2012) detailed three cases of possible malingered, neurogenic, or psychogenic stuttering that were evaluated after mild brain injury resulted in lawsuits or workers' compensation claims. Seery's protocol was used, along with other neuropsychological assessment procedures, to evaluate the claims of these clients.

The following diagnostic procedures may be helpful for differentiating malingering from developmental stuttering, although evidence gained in this way may not be foolproof. I use the term "client" here for the individual who may or may not be malingering.

Develop a good working relationship with the client and elicit a speech sample to later analyze while, at the same time, gathering information about the client's history and experience as someone who stutters. Questions about the onset and development of the stuttering may help determine if—as in typical developmental stuttering—the client's stuttering onset was in childhood, the client experienced negative listener reactions, and the client was self-conscious about his stuttering.

The speech sample should be analyzed to determine the frequency of stuttering, secondary behaviors, the types of stutters, the variability of stuttering, and the loci of stutters. In malingering, the frequency of stuttering may be more than 45%, above the range expected for developmental stuttering (Seery, 2005). Other aspects of the stuttering that may indicate malingering are stereotyped and very severe types of stuttering, lack of secondary behaviors, and presence of good eye contact throughout the sample.

In the client's description of their stuttering onset and development, the time of onset may be unusual in cases of malingering, with onset typically in adulthood and a high level of consistency over time, but neurogenic and psychogenic stuttering may also show such features as onset in adulthood and little change in stuttering over a long period of time.

The clinician should have the client speak under fluency-inducing conditions, such as speaking in time to an arm swing or finger tapping, reading in unison with the clinician, and speaking in a slow, prolonged manner, either in response to DAF or in following the clinician's model of slow, prolonged speech. An individual who is malingering is likely to improve little or less than expected in these conditions that will usually create fluency in those with typical developmental stuttering. However, clients with neurogenic or psychogenic stuttering may also show less improvement than expected.

Obtain information from the client's friends and relatives about whether the client stutters with them and what the client's stuttering is like. Try to determine if the client is significantly more fluent with them than they have been in this interview. If someone is malingering by showing very severe and consistent stuttering in the interview, it is likely that friends and relatives will report less severe and less consistent stuttering in their interactions with the client—or no stuttering at all.

Readers who are tasked with evaluating a client suspected of malingered stuttering should consult the articles referred to in this section, especially Seery's report (2005) and her Table 1 that summarizes the characteristics of developmental, neurogenic, psychogenic, and malingered stuttering.

TABLE 18.3 Comparative Characteristics of Malingering Compared With Developmental Stuttering

Characteristic	Developmental Stuttering	Malingering
Etiology	Deficits in the speech production areas of the brain	Attempt to gain benefit by appearing to stutter. May fake more severe stuttering than is actually the case
Onset	Usually in early childhood between ages 2 and 5 years	Adulthood, sometimes after an accident to claim compensation or after a crime to claim innocence
Development or change over time	If it does not disappear in early childhood, stuttering usually gets gradually more severe during childhood and adolescence	Stuttering usually remains similar to what it was like on onset
Types of stuttering behavior	Repetitions, prolongations, and blocks	May be similar to developmental stuttering, but also may have unusual symptoms
Frequency of stuttering	From mild to severe. Almost always below 45% syllables stuttered	Sometimes, high frequency of stuttering
Secondary behaviors	Beyond early childhood, tension and struggle often observed, along with escape and avoidance behaviors	May appear like developmental, but also may be very rote, with the same type of stutter in each instance
Emotional response to stuttering	Beyond early childhood, frequently notable emotional reactions such as struggle, embarrassment, and shame	Typically little emotional response to stuttering. No shame or embarrassment
Locus of stutters	Stutters tend to occur on syllables at beginnings of words and at beginnings of phrases More stuttering on content words than function words	Stutters occur at many locations in words and phrases Stutters may occur just as often on function as on content words
Response to fluency-inducing conditions such as swinging arm or choral reading	Stuttering markedly reduced in fluency-inducing conditions	Usually, no improvement with fluency-inducing conditions
Adaptation effect: repeated reading of a passage	Adaptation frequently seen—stuttering frequency and severity decrease with repeated reading of passage	Adaptation often does not change the frequency or severity of stuttering
Treatment	Stuttering modification or fluency-shaping treatments can make substantial improvements	Treatment inappropriate

CLUTTERING

Nature

As you've read in Chapter 8, cluttering is characterized by a rapid rate of speech in many (but not all) utterances, accompanied by reduced intelligibility—because words are often jammed together so that some sounds may be omitted and others slurred together. In addition, the speaker may produce many nonstuttering disfluencies (such as whole word and phrase repetitions) and may put in many inappropriate pauses.

St. Louis and Schulte (2011) suggested a **"lowest common denominator" (LCD)** definition of cluttering meant to include aspects of speech that individuals who clutter

TABLE 18.4 Comparison of Developmental Stuttering With Cluttering

Etiology	Developmental Stuttering	Cluttering
Etiology	Probably neurophysiological (anomalies in left hemisphere) exacerbated by temperament and environment	Neurological anomalies appear to consist of overactivity in premotor cortex pre-SMA (supplementary motor area) and basal ganglia. These suggest a problem in planning and execution of speech-motor control
Typical onset	Usually ages 2-5, with some onsets in school years	May be present in preschool years, but often not diagnosed until problem interferes with school performance
Speech characteristics	Single-syllable whole-word repetitions, part-word repetitions, prolongations, and blocks. Frequency is usually more than 3% syllables stuttered. Secondary behaviors (escape and avoidance) common. Pattern varies somewhat	Excess of normal disfluencies, lack of intelligibility, especially during rapid bursts of speech. May slur syllables and leave out others entirely
Client's level of concern	Client typically shows frustration and embarrassment about stuttering, as well as fear of speaking	Frequently unaware of problem, except when listeners tell him they can't understand what he's said
Other diagnostic information	Frequency and severity are often variable from day to day and situation to situation	Often accompanied by stuttering, as well as language, attention, auditory processing, writing, and reading problems, and other learning disabilities
Treatment	School-age children and adults benefit from integration of behavioral, affective, and cognitive focus of stuttering therapy	Increase awareness of cluttering, particularly fast speech rate. Help client self-regulate speech rate and fluency. Improve awareness of listener cues and language skills such as narrative organization and pragmatics

will manifest at some time when they talk: "Cluttering is a fluency disorder wherein segments of conversation in the speaker's native language typically are perceived as too fast overall, too irregular, or both. The segments of rapid and/or irregular speech rate must further be accompanied by one or more of the following: (1) excessive 'normal' disfluencies; (2) excessive collapsing or deletion of syllables; and/or (3) abnormal pauses, syllable stress, or speech rhythm." (pp. 241-242) Table 18.4 lists the difference between developmental stuttering and cluttering.

Diagnosis and Evaluation

The process of evaluating a client for possible cluttering differs for different ages (school age vs. adult) and will vary depending on the setting in which the evaluation takes place (eg, school vs. university or hospital clinic). In many cases, especially with school-age children, a multidisciplinary approach to evaluation is important and may involve the SLP, classroom teacher, special educator, psychologist, and audiologist. In the following section, I give some general guidelines that reflect information gleaned from several sources, including Myers and St. Louis (1986, 2007), St. Louis (1996), Scaler Scott (2020, 2022), St. Louis et al. (2003), and van Zaalen et al. (2011).

Case History and Interview

The case history can be filled out by a client (or parent) beforehand and used as a guideline for the interview. Among the important areas to be covered in the case history and interview are the following:

- *The client's, parents', and/or teachers' perceptions of the problem.* What aspects of the cluttering "syndrome" are the presenting problem (from the viewpoint of the person completing the form and participating in the interview)? Because the individual who clutters is themselves often unaware of their own speech, an adult or adolescent may report that their problem is that people say they are sometimes hard to understand. It should be ascertained, however, how cluttering affects the client. For example, do they have a hard time in school, social situations, or their job because people don't always understand them?

- *How long the problem has existed.* In some cases, cluttering might have begun in preschool years, but it is usually not until the school years that listeners tell them that they're mumbling or talking too fast, or that they simply can't understand them. Nonetheless, it is useful to gather information about the individual's speech and language development—whether it was delayed, advanced, or atypical.
- *When and where the problem appears.* Cluttering can be variable, so it's important to understand which situations are particularly troublesome. This may depend on the listeners and the demands of the situation. Some children may do well when they are reading or giving one-word answers but may lose intelligibility during narratives. Adults who clutter may be fluent and intelligible when speaking to close friends, but their intelligibility may suffer when speaking in more demanding situations.
- *Background on the individual and their family.* It is helpful in understanding a client's cluttering to view it in a larger perspective, including whether other members of the client's extended family clutter or have other communication or learning problems; whether the client has other problems, such as stuttering, that interfere with communication; and whether the client has received treatment for their communication problem(s) and how successful treatment has been.
- *Reasons for seeking treatment at this time.* A major determinant of success in cluttering therapy is the client's motivation. It is important to find out from the case history or interview whether the client is aware of their cluttering and whether it bothers them enough to undertake the hard work that successful therapy will require.
- *Other problems.* The case history and interview should determine if the client has any of the other problems that often accompany cluttering, such as receptive or expressive language difficulties, articulation problems, central auditory processing deficits, attention deficit/hyperactivity, reading problems, or learning disabilities.

Direct Assessment of Speech

The client's speech should be examined on a variety of tasks in a variety of situations. Cluttering, like stuttering, varies a great deal so it is easy to gain a false impression from a small sample of speech gathered in the clinic. Extensive information about assessment of cluttering can be obtained from the website for the International Cluttering Association (you can find this with Google or another search engine). On their website, go to the Information menu and choose "Cluttering Assessment"; this link provides information for clinicians to use to evaluate individuals who clutter as well as guidelines for self-assessment by individuals who consider themselves as having cluttering as a disorder.

Recording of Speech

The client should be digitally audio or video recorded for 15 or 20 minutes while performing a number of speaking tasks, including

- A narrative about a topic not related to his speech, such as describing what they did on their last vacation or foods that they love. A topic that really engages the client, like a favorite movie or video game, will more likely result in cluttering.
- Reading a passage appropriate for the client's reading level.
- A conversation in which the client talks about something that really interests them.
- Many clients will speak in a more guarded, controlled way in a clinic interview, so it will be more valid to obtain a recording of the client talking with friends or family.
- van Zaalen et al. (2011) also recommend that older clients should be asked to produce words that may be difficult, such as "statistical" or "chrysanthemum," as well as words with differing stress patterns such as the sequence "apply," "application," and "applicable" to assess their ability to handle complex phonological sequences and changing linguistic stress patterns. These authors also recommend retelling a story.

Analysis of Speech

After the recording has been made, the speech samples should be analyzed to assess speech rate in syllables per minute using the procedures described in Chapter 9. Many individuals who clutter can reduce their overly fast rate when they try; therefore, the narrative and reading samples may show slower rates than do conversation samples. If it is the clinician's impression during the evaluation that the client's speech rate was not slower during narrative or reading compared to conversation (as would be expected for most speakers), they should ask the client to engage in a narrative task and try to speak at a slow, normal rate. The client's ability to slow their speaking rate may be a good prognostic sign, because much of cluttering therapy is focused on slowing a client's speaking rate. The various samples can be compared to the speech rate norms for different ages that were given in Chapter 9.

Many individuals who clutter don't speak at a consistently fast rate, but at a relatively normal rate with sudden bursts of rapid speech. Assessment, therefore, should include measures of speech rate during these bursts and how frequently they occur. A comparison may be made between the client's articulatory rate (ie, syllables per second with pauses less than 250 ms included) during fast bursts of speech and during regular speech. The articulatory rates of typical adults in conversation are six to seven syllables per second (St. Louis et al., 2003).

Analysis of Cluttering

When evaluating a client with suspected cluttering (or suspected stuttering, for that matter), analysis of speech samples should also include separate counts of typical disfluencies and stuttering-like disfluencies (see Chapter 7 for this distinction). The number of syllables that are normally disfluent and the number that are stuttered can be expressed as a proportion of the total number of syllables spoken in the sample. These measures will reflect the proportions of stuttering and cluttering in the client's speech. Some clients have both stuttering and cluttering in their speech, but one usually predominates. It has been suggested that when stuttering is mixed with cluttering, a client's cluttering may not be noticed until his stuttering is substantially reduced by therapy (Bakker, 2002; St. Louis et al., 2003).

Analysis of Meaningful Versus Extraneous Syllables

When I evaluate a client with cluttering, I find it useful to calculate the ratio of the number of syllables spoken that are part of the intended message, if that can be reliably discerned, to the number of syllables spoken that are extraneous to the message. For example, in the utterance, "Well, you see, I think, I think the, the, the sky is well is blue" (15 syllables), we can assume that the speaker meant to convey "I think the sky is blue" (six syllables). Thus, nine syllables, or 60% of the utterance, are extraneous, which undoubtedly detracts from the speaker's communicative effectiveness. This measure may be helpful also in assessing a client's progress in therapy.

Analysis of Intelligibility

The intelligibility of a sample should be assessed by having one or more listeners unfamiliar with the client gloss (ie, interpret) each word and each utterance. The percentage of words and of utterances that are understood can be calculated, providing pretherapy measures of a client's intelligibility.

Language Assessment

The language skills of clients who clutter may be affected by the disorder or as a result of concomitant language disorder. However, many clinical researchers believe that cluttering is separate from language disorders so that language may not be affected in some individuals who clutter. Wiig (2002) suggested that many aspects of the language of people with cluttering can be effectively tested using the Clinical Evaluation of Language Fundamentals (CELF-3) (Semel et al., 1995). Almost certainly this applies to the CELF-5 (Wiig et al., 2013), which is appropriate for individuals from 5 to 21 years old. This test assesses "the relationships among semantics, syntax/morphology, and pragmatics, and the interrelated domains of receptive and expressive language." Wiig suggested that it be administered in such a way that a client's responses could be timed, because under time pressure, which simulates everyday conversational situations, the scores of a client who clutters might well be lower.

It may also be helpful to assess a client's pragmatic behaviors in the videotaped conversational sample described above. Pragmatic skills that may be lacking include appropriate turn taking, supplying complete information to the listener, and repairing communication when it breaks down.

Other aspects of language assessment are described in van Zaalen et al. (2011) and Myers and St. Louis (2007).

Assessment of Cluttering Characteristics

Clients may exhibit a variety of traits that are part of the cluttering syndrome. The clinician may find it helpful to use Daly's Predictive Cluttering Inventory (2006). This checklist evaluates a client in four areas: pragmatics, speech-motor control, language cognition, and motor coordination for writing. It can be used for assessing areas of deficit as well as for treatment planning. These ratings help the clinician determine which cluttering characteristics are most salient and are, therefore, most in need of treatment.

Assessment of Coexisting Disorders in Domains Other Than Communication

In the process of gathering information about a client, the clinician may become aware of challenges that affect communication but are not the province of only the SLP. These may include auditory processing disorders, attention deficit disorder, hyperactivity, reading difficulties, social adjustment problems, illegible handwriting, and learning disabilities (Ward & Scott, 2011). These challenges may best be assessed with the help of other specialists, such as an audiologist, psychologist, learning specialist, reading specialist, and the classroom teacher.

Considerations for Treatment

Because clients who clutter are often not aware of their problem and are often surprised when listeners don't understand them, they rarely seek treatment. Indeed, those who do seek treatment are often referred by someone else. Some individuals who clutter, however, can be motivated to work hard in therapy and can make good progress. Two positive prognostic signs are the ability to speak without cluttering if asked to do so and a specific reason for improving, such as getting or keeping a job or receiving a promotion at work. Children who clutter can often be engaged in games and activities that will create motivation for their work in treatment.

With cluttering, keeping the client in treatment and focusing on a problem that may not, at first, feel like a problem to the client, can be a challenge. Thus, an important motivation for this work with individuals who clutter may come from an effective client-clinician relationship. Sønsterud (2019) has written about this relationship in cluttering therapy, referring to it as the working alliance. She and her colleagues have shown that an effective working alliance between client and clinician can contribute to successful outcomes in stuttering therapy (Sønsterud et al., 2019) and she suggests that such an alliance may help cluttering therapy achieve better results. If you are interested in studying your alliance with a client who stutters, you may wish to download (via a browser) a form titled Working Alliance Inventory–Short Revised (Items copyright © Adam Horvath). It probably makes most sense to ask the client to complete the form only after you have worked together for several sessions. Of particular importance is that the client feels that you and they agree on the goals you and they are working toward.

Treatment Approaches

The evaluation procedures described above should indicate if there are areas that are particular challenges for the client. Treatment can then focus on these areas. Lanouette (2011), Myers (2002, 2011), Myers and St. Louis (2007), and Scaler Scott (2022) outlined several cluttering therapy strategies that they have explored in their work with cluttering over several years. I describe them in the following section with some minor changes:

1. Increase the client's awareness of their speech rate and their ability to decrease rate.
   - Simulate various speaking rates by having the client move their arm or walk at slow, medium, and fast tempos. Then, teach the client to attend to their sensory feedback while they are doing this so that they learn the feeling of these rates.
   - Alternate between speaking and moving various body parts or walking at various rates while attending to sensory feedback.
   - Use movements and walking paced by fast and slow music (Fig. 18.2).
   - With children, engage in activities in which they can get speeding tickets or, perhaps to start with, give speeding tickets to the clinician for speaking too fast.
   - Teach clients to attend to various verbal and nonverbal cues from a listener that indicate they are speaking too quickly or cannot be understood. For example, listeners may frown or show puzzlement on their faces or repeatedly ask the speaker to repeat themselves.
   - For readers, put symbols at periods and commas, such as red or yellow lights, to help them slow their speech rate at relevant places in a text.
   - Teach phrasing and pausing in conversational speech.
   - Use the concept of a speedometer for children and ask them to speak at 75 miles per hour and then at 35 miles per hour.
   - Teach clients to speak with strong stress patterns by reciting or reading poetry, for example.
2. Improve linguistic skills.
   - Teach clients to chunk and sequence their thoughts by having them write a story or narrative on cards, sequence them, and then tell the story aloud using the cards.
   - Involve clients in skits and plays so that they learn to follow a script and use turn taking.

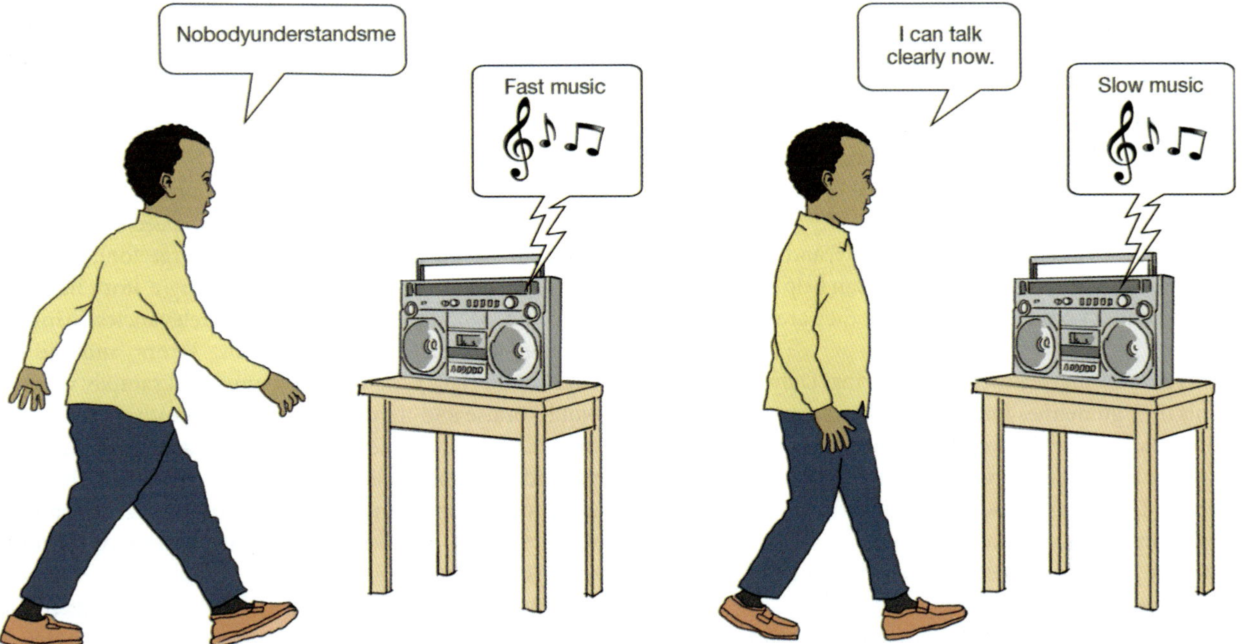

Figure 18.2 Child walking and talking rapidly and then walking slowly and timing speech to slow walking movements as an activity for children in treatment for cluttering. Fast and slow music are used to help timing of walking and talking.

- Teach them such pragmatic skills as turn taking in conversation and staying on topic in conversation.
- Teach them how to use complex sentences with subordinate clauses.

3. Facilitate fluency.
   - Use DAF to help clients learn to speak in a slower, more fluent manner.
   - Use DAF to teach proprioception, by having clients speak at a normal rate under maximal delay (ie, 250 ms) by ignoring auditory feedback and focusing on the feeling of the articulators moving.
4. Increase the client's knowledge and awareness of cluttering.
   - Teach clients about the disorder of cluttering using Daly and Burnett-Stolnack's (1995) checklist to help the client learn which cluttering behaviors they have.
   - Have the client transcribe and analyze a recording of their cluttered speech.
   - Help the client become aware of their thought processes when they are talking in fast bursts of disorganized speech.

Further suggestions for treatment were presented by St. Louis et al. (2003), which included:

1. Rather than admonish the client to "slow down," have them match the clinician's speech rate using a computer-based program to display the clinician's and client's utterances. I have used Visi Pitch for this, but there may be computer apps available for playing the clinician's model and the client's speech simultaneously.
2. To help clients achieve their potential to use normal speech, have them imagine themselves (ie, in their mind's eye and ear) speaking effectively and have them use positive self-talk to strengthen their visual and auditory images. It may help also for the client and clinician to video record the client's best and worst speech and play these samples back to them to remind them of the range of their options. Perhaps playing only the client's *best* speech would be more motivating and put a positive spin on therapy.
3. When working on intelligibility and organization, begin with short utterances that are spoken clearly and then gradually increase length and complexity while ensuring high quality of fluency, articulation, rate, and organization. Video recording and replaying them can help clients establish an auditory-visual image of what they are aiming for.

In his chapter on treatment of cluttering, Daly (1986) provides his own guidelines for many of the treatment strategies described earlier. He believes that video feedback and analysis of audio samples are crucial for increasing a client's self-awareness. Daly also advocates helping clients learn to use relaxation exercises, mental imagery, and positive self-talk. His chapter has many references, which can help clinicians learn more about these activities.

There are very few studies of the treatment outcomes of cluttering therapy, and the ones that do exist consist of only one or two cases. A special edition of the *Journal of Fluency Disorders* (vol. 21, nos. 3–4, September–December 1996) on cluttering has a number of case studies. For example, data on a person who both cluttered and stuttered treated in a 3-week intensive smooth speech program indicated that the client's stuttering and speech rate were reduced to near-normal limits and that the gains appeared to be retained 10 months after treatment.

A report on a case study of the treatment of a teen who cluttered suggested two possible strategies to reduce overcoarticulation—the condensing of syllables so much that they become unintelligible (Healy et al., 2015). The two strategies were (1) having the client overarticulate their speech so that syllables were produced much more precisely and clearly and (2) having the client pause at natural places as they talked to slow their overall speech rate. Both strategies worked initially to reduce overcoarticulation, but only the pausing was used by the teen outside of the clinic.

One of the clients who was seen in our university clinic was treated for cluttering. Here are some details of his treatment. This young man, whom I shall call Alex, was an undergraduate who was referred to us by the Office of Student Services and Support. Alex had been diagnosed with—in addition to cluttering—attention deficit hyperactivity disorder, as well as problems in visual acuity, organizational skills, and handwriting. His scores on the Predictive Cluttering Inventory (Daly, 2006) were 85/198 where any score between 80 and 120 indicates a mix of stuttering and cluttering. His score on the Overall Assessment of the Speaker's Experience of Stuttering (OASES) was 3.11, which indicated moderate/severe impairment.

Many aspects of treatment focused on helping Alex increase his awareness of his speech and his cluttering. He did not recognize how his rate of speech, omission of sounds and syllables, and narrative disorganization made him substantially unintelligible to listeners. He also did not pick up cues from listeners that they did not understand something he said, nor did he notice when listeners were signaling him that they were very busy or were frustrated that he wasn't giving them a turn to talk.

Early in the semester, his clinician used playback of audio/video recordings to teach Alex to self-evaluate his intelligibility. As he improved, the clinician brought in unfamiliar listeners to increase stress and generalize Alex's increasing ability to evaluate and self-correct his speech. At times, his clinician would make transcripts (in large font, because of his visual acuity problem) of his retelling a story he read, to have him "see" the extra sounds and irrelevancies he inserted. He then retold the story, correcting errors, and the clinician would replay the recorded improved sample, which she would praise and they would discuss. Another step in Alex's hierarchy was to go to a room with strangers who had been primed to occasionally nonverbally convey that they didn't understand something he said or that, after a period, they were too busy to talk or they wished to talk. With the clinician's guidance, Alex began to recognize listener cues and respond appropriately. Going further up the generalization hierarchy, Alex visited classes in which he talked, learned self-advocacy strategies (saying "give me a second to think about that"), talked with strangers around campus, and practiced job interviews. When he decided to stop therapy, Alex was gainfully employed and had become much more able to communicate effectively. At the end of his first semester in therapy, his scores on the OASES had improved from 3.11 to 2.72, which showed only moderate impairment.

Summary and Conclusions

Cluttering is a disorder with a probable neurological etiology. It is characterized by an excess of disfluencies, rapid rates of speech that often occur in momentary bursts, and lack of intelligibility (that comes from overcoarticulation—jamming sounds and syllables together), especially during bursts with increased rate. Although there is relatively little research on the nature and treatment of cluttering, there is some consensus that it isn't viewed as a problem until a child has reached school age. Evaluation procedures include (1) obtaining background information to determine, among other things, whether or not the client is aware of the problem and is motivated to undergo therapy; (2) direct assessment of speech on several different tasks to measure (i) frequency and type of disfluencies and (ii) speech rate and intelligibility overall as well as during fast bursts of speech; (3) language testing, particularly pragmatics and other aspects of expressive language; and (4) assessment of other possible concomitant disorders. Treatment should address the interdependent qualities of speech rate, fluency, intelligibility, and expressive language. Although many clinicians report success with motivated clients, there is little outcome data on a particular treatment approach for cluttering.

Because cluttering often co-occurs with stuttering, the disorders appear to be related in some as yet undetermined way. Given the strong effect of slow speaking on stuttering and cluttering alike, it is possible that subgroups of individuals who stutter and those who clutter have difficulty maintaining a slow enough speech rate to reach their capacity to synchronize the elements of language and speech output. Perhaps each disorder has a particular level of processing at which such dyssynchrony occurs.

The most important goal for treatment of cluttering is improved communication. Using a working alliance to bring agreement on this goal, the client, with the clinician's support, may be able to discover what they need to change to make their spoken utterances understood and appreciated by the listener.

STUDY QUESTIONS

1. If you had only one activity you could do with a client to differentiate neurogenic from psychogenic stuttering, which activity would you choose and why?
2. After reading about neurogenic stuttering, do you think that Canter's three categories of neurogenic stuttering are adequate? Why or why not?
3. Name four characteristics of stuttering behavior that appear to distinguish neurogenic stuttering from developmental stuttering.
4. What are contraindications (if any) for treatment of neurogenic stuttering?
5. If an adult-onset client had evidence of a neurological disorder, would you rule out psychogenic stuttering? Why or why not?
6. Compare the reported treatment success of psychogenic stuttering and neurogenic stuttering.
7. What are the contraindications (if any) for treatment of psychogenic stuttering?
8. What are the two most salient problems in cluttering?
9. Why might language and learning problems be related to the speech problems of cluttering?
10. What are the contraindications (if any) for treatment of cluttering?

SUGGESTED READINGS

Neurogenic Stuttering

De Nil, L., Jokel, R., & Rochon, E. (2007). Etiology, symptomatology, and treatment of neurogenic stuttering. In E. Conture, & R. F. Curlee (Eds.), *Stuttering and related disorders of fluency* (3rd ed., pp. 326–343). Thieme Medical Publishers.

This chapter covers prevalence and incidence of neurogenic stuttering in detail not seen elsewhere. The authors also present a critical review of the reported speech characteristics of neurogenic stuttering and indicate how different etiologies (eg, stroke vs head wound) may produce different speech characteristics.

Duffy, J. (2020). *Motor speech disorders* (4th ed.). Elsevier, Mosby.

This book provides excellent coverage of the nature of neurogenic and functional stuttering as well as their management. Duffy is particularly good at describing etiologies of these disorders and the other conditions with which they may be associated. His sections on management reflect his extensive clinical experience.

Ringo, C. C., & Dietrich, S. (1995). Neurogenic stuttering: An analysis and critique. *Journal of Medical Speech-Language Pathology*, 3, 111–122.

This article is particularly useful in that it critically examines characteristics of neurogenic stuttering that have been proposed by various authors since Canter's (1971) seminal publication about differential diagnosis of neurogenic stuttering. Each of seven characteristics is examined in light of evidence that it is present in neurogenic stuttering in a way that is different from its manifestation in developmental stuttering. Suggestions are made to standardize the data to be collected and reported on individual cases.

Psychogenic Stuttering

Baumgartner, J. (1999). Acquired psychogenic stuttering. In R. F. Curlee (Ed.), *Stuttering and related disorders of fluency* (2nd ed., pp. 269–288). Thieme Medical Publishers.

This chapter is an excellent starting place for anyone interested in learning about psychogenic (functional) stuttering. Baumgartner has been writing about this topic for several years and has first-hand clinical experience with individuals who have functional stuttering, thus making the chapter a solid source for information.

Roth, C. R., Aronson, A. E., & Davis, L. J. (1989). Clinical studies in psychogenic stuttering of adult onset. *Journal of Speech and Hearing Disorders*, 54, 634–646.

This journal article examines the records of 12 patients who were evaluated and treated for psychogenic (functional) stuttering. Because the subjects were patients at the Mayo Clinic, they were examined thoroughly for psychological/psychiatric and neurological functioning in a standardized way, providing substantial evidence of the psychogenic/functional nature of the stuttering. A case study is given to illustrate how stuttering can appear as a conversion reaction to emotional conflict. Clinical recommendations are given.

Utianskia, R. L., & Duffy, J. R. (2022). Understanding, recognizing, and managing functional speech disorders: Current thinking illustrated with a case series. *American Journal of Speech-Language Pathology, 31*, 1205–1220.

This is a significant publication, describing a new categorization of FSDs that includes functional stuttering. Note that FSD is a subcategory of FNDs. The publication also highlights the recent creation of the FNDs Society, a multidisciplinary group that is focused on helping clients with FNDs (and FSDs) and that sponsors a website to share information. This article explains FSDs in detail, including hypotheses about the biopsychosocial etiology for them. Four cases of FSDs are presented with particulars of diagnostic and treatment procedures.

Malingering

Seery, C. (2005). Differential diagnosis of stuttering for forensic purposes. *American Journal of Speech-Language Pathology, 14*, 284–297.

Although this article appears to be a case study, the background and protocols for evaluation are thorough and insightful. It is a must read for anyone who will be evaluating a case of suspected malingering of stuttering.

Cluttering

Kuster, J. *Online resources on cluttering: The other fluency disorder.* http://www.mnsu.edu/comdis/kuster/cluttering.html

This web page is a treasure trove of useful resources on cluttering. Among them are videos, assessment techniques, computer-assisted cluttering instruments, treatment suggestions, links to support groups, and an extensive section on research.

Myers, F. L., & St. Louis, K. O. (2007). *Cluttering [DVD]*. The Stuttering Foundation.

This video provides excellent examples of cluttering in several young adults, as well as clear guidelines for evaluation and treatment.

Myers, F. L., & St. Louis, K. O. (Eds.) (1986). *Cluttering: A clinical perspective*. Singular Publishing Group, Inc.

This book, with an interesting forward by Charles Van Riper, is the first text on cluttering since the classic text on cluttering by Deso Weiss (1964). Chapters by the authors and other clinicians working with cluttering provide an overview of the disorder as well as practical suggestions for evaluation and treatment.

Scaler Scott, K., Sønsterud, H., & Reichel, I. (2022). Cluttering: Etiology, symptomatology, identification, and treatment. In P. Zebrowski, J. Anderson, & E. Conture (Eds.), *Stuttering and related disorders of fluency* (4th ed.). Thieme.

This chapter provides good information on the nature of cluttering and also details about evaluation and treatment of cluttering. An added bonus is their discussion of treatment of concomitant disorders, the working alliance, and future directions for treatment of stuttering. Another bonus is a detailed description of diagnosis and treatment of a real client who was a junior in high school.

St. Louis, K., & Schulte, K. Defining cluttering: The lowest common denominator. In: D. Ward, K. Scaler Scott (Eds.). *Cluttering: Research, intervention, and education.* Psychology Press; 2011.

This chapter examines the many different aspects of cluttered-speech and suggests a "LCD" that designate three signs of cluttering as typical of all or most clutterers: (1) rapid sounding speech, (2) overarticulation, and (3) excessive typical disfluencies.

St. Louis, K. O. (Ed.) (1996). Research and opinion on cluttering: State of the art and science (special issue). *Journal of Fluency Disorders, 21*(3–4), 171–374.

This special issue of Journal of Fluency Disorders is rich with case studies of evaluations and treatments of individuals who clutter. It is, therefore, one of the few sources with data on treatment outcome, although the heterogeneity of the cases and the manner in which they are studied highlight the fact that research on cluttering is in its infancy. The cases studies are bracketed by overviews of the disorder at the beginning and critical reviews at the end that summarize the case studies and call attention to the poverty of credible data. A chapter by Myers is particularly valuable for its annotated list of publications on cluttering between 1964 and 1996.

St. Louis, K. O., Raphael, L. J., Myers, F. L., & Bakker, K. (2003, Nov 18). Cluttering updated. *The ASHA Leader*, 4–5, 20–22.

This article, which is available online at www.asha.org, provides a clear synopsis of how to identify and evaluate cluttering, as well as specific suggestions for treating the core behaviors. For those who know little about cluttering, this publication is an excellent place to begin.

Ward, D. (2017). *Stuttering and cluttering: Frameworks for understanding and treatment* (2nd ed.). Taylor and Francis.

This is the second edition of a scholarly and clinical book on the nature and treatment of both cluttering and stuttering.

Ward, D., & Scott, K. S. (Eds.) (2011). *Cluttering: A handbook of research, intervention and education.* Psychology Press.

This is a rich compendium of international authors discussing the nature of cluttering, as well as assessment and treatment. The two chapters on treatment have excellent overall organization as well as many ideas for specific activities. There are several chapters that describe clients with cluttering who also have other disorders such as Down syndrome, learning disabilities, and autism spectrum disorders.

Bibliography

Abbs, J. H. (1996). Mechanisms of speech motor execution and control. In N. Lass (Ed.), *Principles of experimental phonetics* (pp. 93–111). Mosby.

Abi-Habib, M. (2022, January 16). Horror in board games: Recalling a wartime childhood. *New York Times*, 10.

Accordi, M., Bianchi, R., Consolaro, C., Tronchin, F., DiFilippi, R., Pasqualon, L., & Croatto, L. (1983). L'Eziopatogenesi della balbuzie: Studio stadstico su 2801 casi. *Acta Phoniatrica Latina, 5*, 171–180.

Achenbach, T. M. (1988). *Child behavior checklist for ages 2-3*. University of Vermont.

Adams, M. (1977). A clinical strategy for differentiating the normally non-fluent child and the incipient stutterer. *Journal of Fluency Disorders, 2*(2), 141–148.

Adams, M. (1990). The demands and capacities model I: Theoretical elaborations. *Journal of Fluency Disorders, 15*, 135–141.

Adams, M., & Hayden, P. (1976). The ability of stutterers and nonstutterers to initiate and terminate phonation during production of an isolated vowel. *Journal of Speech and Hearing Research, 19*, 290–296.

Adams, M., & Runyan, C. M. (1981). Stuttering and fluency: Exclusive events or points on a continuum? *Journal of Fluency Disorders, 6*, 197–218.

Adani, S., & Cepanec, M. (2019). Sex differences in early communication development: Behavioral and neurobiological indicators of more vulnerable communication system development in boys. *Croatian Medical Journal, 60*(2), 141–149.

Ahern, G. L., & Schwartz, G. E. (1985). Differential lateralization for positive and negative emotion in the human brain: EEG spectral analysis. *Neuropsychologia, 23*(6), 745–755.

Ajdacic-Gross, V., Bechtiger, L., Rodgers, S., Muller, M., Kawohl, W., von Kanel, R., & Howell, P. (2018). Subtypes of stuttering determined by latent class analysis in two Swiss epidemiological surveys. *PLoS One, 13*(8), e0198450.

Alfonso, P. J., Story, R. S., & Watson, B. C. (1987). The organization of supralaryngeal articulation in stutterers' fluent speech production: A second report. *Annual Bulletin Research Institute of Logopedics and Phoniatrics, 21*, 117–129.

Allen, G. D., & Hawkins, S. (1980). Phonological rhythm: Definition and development. In G. H. Yeni-Komshian, J. F. Kavanagh & C. A. Ferguson (Eds.), *Child phonology* (Vol. 1, pp. 227–256). Academic Press.

Allen, S. (1988). *Durations of segments in repetitive disfluencies in stuttering and nonstuttering children (Unpublished manuscript)*. University of Vermont.

Allman, J. M., Hakeem, A., Erwin, J. M., Nimchinsky, E., & Hof, P. (2001). The anterior cingulate cortex: The evolution of an interface between emotion and cognition. *Annals of the New York Academy of Sciences, 935*, 107–117.

Alm, P. A. (2004). Stuttering and the basal ganglia circuits: A critical review of possible relations. *Journal of Communication Disorders, 37*, 325–396.

Alm, P. A. (2005). On the causal mechanism of stuttering. *PhD thesis*. University of Lund.

Alm, P. A., & Risberg, J. (2007). Stuttering in adults: The acoustic startle response, temperamental traits, and biological factors. *Journal of Communication Disorders, 40*, 1–41.

Amato Maguire, M., Onslow, M., Lowe, R., O'Brian, S., & Menzies, R. (2022). Searching for Lidcombe Program mechanisms of action: Inter-turn latency. *Clinical Linguistics & Phonetics*, 1–13.

Ambrose, N., Cox, N., & Yairi, E. (1997). The genetic basis of persistence and recovery in stuttering. *Journal of Speech, Language, and Hearing Research, 40*, 556–566.

Ambrose, N., Yairi, E., & Cox, N. (1993). Genetic aspects of early childhood stuttering. *Journal of Speech and Hearing Research, 36*(4), 701–706.

Ambrose, N. G., & Yairi, E. (1999). Normative data for early childhood stuttering. *Journal of Speech, Language and Hearing Research, 42*, 895–909.

Ambrose, N. G., Yairi, E., Loucks, T., Seery, C., & Throneberg, R. (2015). Relation of motor, linguistic and temperament factors in epidemiologic subtypes of persistent and recovered stuttering: Initial findings. *Journal of Fluency Disorders, 45*, 12–26.

American Speech-Language-Hearing Association (n.d.) Counseling for professional service delivery. (Practice portal). Retrieved December 23, 2022 from www.asha.org/Practice-Portal/Professional-Issues/Counseling-For-Professional-Service-Delivery/

Amster, B., & Klein, E. (2018). *More than fluency: The social, emotional, and cognitive dimensions of stuttering*. Plural Publishing.

Anderson, J., & Conture, E. G. (2000). Language abilities of children who stutter: A preliminary study. *Journal of Fluency Disorders, 25*(4), 283–304.

Anderson, J., & Ofoe, L. C. (2019). The role of executive function in developmental stuttering. *Seminars in Speech and Language, 40*(4), 305–319.

Anderson, J., Pellowski, M., & Conture, E. G. (2001, November). *Temperament characteristics of children who stutter. Paper presented at the Annual meeting of the American Speech-Language Hearing Association*. New Orleans, LA.

Anderson, J., Pellowski, M., Conture, E. G., & Kelly, E. (2003). Temperamental characteristics of young children who stutter. *Journal of Speech, Language and Hearing Research, 46*, 1221–1233.

Anderson, J. D., Pellowski, M. W., & Conture, E. G. (2005). Childhood stuttering and disassociations across linguistic domains. *Journal of Fluency Disorders, 30*, 219–253.

Andrews, G., & Craig, A. (1982). Stuttering: Overt and Covert measurement of the speech of treated subjects. *Journal of Speech and Hearing Disorders, 47*, 96–99.

Andrews, G., & Craig, A. (1988). Prediction of outcome after treatment for stuttering. *British Journal of Disorders of Psychiatry, 153*, 236–240.

Andrews, G., & Cutler, J. (1974). Stuttering therapy: The relation between changes in symptom level and attitudes. *Journal of Speech and Hearing Disorders, 39*, 312–319.

Andrews, G., & Harris, M. (1964). *The syndrome of stuttering*. W. Heinemann Medical Books.

Andrews, G., Hoddinott, S., Craig, A., Howie, P., Feyer, A.-M., & Neilson, M. (1983). Stuttering: A review of research findings and theories circa 1982. *Journal of Speech and Hearing Disorders, 48*, 226–246.

Andrews, G., Howie, P., Dozsa, M., & Guitar, B. (1982). Stuttering: Speech pattern characteristics under fluency-inducing conditions. *Journal of Speech and Hearing Research, 25*, 208–216.

Andrews, G., & Ingham, R. (1971). Stuttering: Considerations in the evaluation of treatment. *British Journal of Communication Disorders, 6*, 129–138.

Andrews, G., Morris-Yates, A., Howie, P., & Martin, N. (1991). Genetic factors in stuttering confirmed. *Archives of General Psychiatry, 48*(11), 1034–1035.

Andrews, G., & Tanner, S. (1982). Stuttering treatment: An attempt to replicate the regulated-breathing method. *Journal of Speech and Hearing Disorders, 47*, 138–140.

Andy, O. J., & Bhatnager, S. C. (1992). Stuttering acquired from subcortical pathologies and its alleviation from thalamic perturbation. *Brain and Language, 42*(4), 385–401.

Arenas, R., & Zebrowski, P. (2013). The effects of autonomic arousal on speech production in adults who stutter: A preliminary study. *Speech, Language and Hearing, 16*(3), 176–185.

Arnott, S., Onslow, M., O'Brian, S., Packman, A., Jones, M., & Block, S. (2014). Group Lidcombe Program treatment of early stuttering: A randomized controlled trial. *Journal of Speech Language and Hearing Research, 57*, 1606–1618.

Arthur, G. (1952). *Arthur adaptation of the Leiter International Performance Test*. Western Psychological Services.

Ayres, J. J. B. (1998). Fear conditioning and avoidance. In W. O'Donohue (Ed.), *Learning and behavior therapy*. Allyn and Bacon.

Azios, M., Irani, F., Bellon-Harn, M., Swartz, E., & Benson, C. (2020). The utility of cinematherapy for stuttering intervention: An exploratory study. *Seminars in Speech and Language, 41*(5), 400–413.

Azrin, N., & Nunn, R. (1974). A rapid method of eliminating stuttering by a regulated breathing approach. *Behavior Research and Therapy, 124*, 279–286.

Baer, D. (1990). The critical issue in treatment efficacy is knowing why treatment was applied. In L. B. Olswand, C. K. Thompson, S. F. Warren & N. J. Minghetti (Eds.), *Treatment efficacy research in communication disorders* (pp. 35–48). ASHA.

Baker, D. J. (1967). The amount of information in the Oral Identification of Forms by normal speakers and selected speech-defective groups. In J. F. Bosma (Ed.), *Symposium of oral sensation and perception* (pp. 287–293). Thomas.

Bakhtiar, M., Zhang, C., & Ki, S. S. (2019). Impaired processing speed in categorical perceptions: Speech perception of children who stutter. *PLoS One, 14*(4), e0216124. 10.1371/journal.pone.0216124

Bakker, K. (2002, November). *Putting cluttering on the map: Looking back/Looking ahead. Paper presented at the Annual meeting of the American Speech Language Hearing Association*. Atlanta.

Bangert, K. J., & Finestack, L. H. (2020). Linguistic maze production by children and adolescents with attention deficit/hyperactivity disorder. *Journal of Speech, Language and Hearing Research, 63*(1), 274–285.

Bankson, N., & Bernthal, J. (1990). *BBTOP: Bankson—Bernthal test of phonology* (2nd ed.). Pro-Ed.

Barasch, C. T., Guitar, B., McCauley, R. J., & Absher, R. G. (2000). Disfluency and time perception. *Journal of Speech, Language, and Hearing Research, 43*, 1429–1439.

Baratz, R., & Mesulam, M. (1981). Adult-onset stuttering treated with anticonvulsants. *Archives of Neurology, 38*, 132–133.

Barrett, L., & Howell, P. (2021). Altered sensory feedback in speech. In M. J. Ball (Ed.), *Manual of clinical phonetics* (p. 19). Routledge.

Bates, E., Appelbaum, M., Salcedo, J., Saygin, A. P., & Pizzamiglio, L. (2003). Quantifying dissociations in neuropsychological research. *Journal of Clinical and Experimental Neuropsychology, 25*, 1128–1153.

Battle, D. E. (2012). *Communication disorders in multicultural and international populations* (4th ed.). Elsevier/Mosby.

Bauerly, K. R., & De Nil, L. F. (2015). Nonspeech sequence learning under single and dual task conditions in adults who stutter. *Canadian Journal of Speech-Language Pathology and Audiology, 39*, 116–132.

Baumgartner, J. M. (1999). Acquired psychogenic stuttering. In R. Curlee (Ed.), *Stuttering and related disorders of fluency* (2nd ed., pp. 269–288). Thieme.

Beal, D. S., Gracco, V., Brettschneider, J., Kroll, R. M., & De Nil, L. F. (2013). A voxel-based morphology (VBM) analysis of regional grey and white matter volume abnormalities within the speech production network of children who stutter. *Cortex, 49*(8), 2151–2161.

Beal, D. S., Gracco, V. L., Lafaille, S. J., & De Nil, L. F. (2007). Voxel-based morphometry of auditory and speech-related cortex in stutterers. *Neuroreport, 18*(2), 1257–1260.

Beck, J. S. (1995). *Cognitive therapy: Basics and beyond*. Guilford Press.

Beilby, J., Brynes, M. L., & Yaruss, J. S. (2012). Acceptance and Commitment Therapy for adults who stutter: Psychosocial adjustment and speech fluency. *Journal of Fluency Disorders, 37*(4), 289–299.

Beilby, J., & Byrnes, M. L. (2012). Acceptance and commitment therapy for people who stutter. *Perspectives on Fluency and Fluency Disorders, 22*(1), 34–46.

Beilby, J., & Yaruss, J. S. (2018). Acceptance and Commitment Therapy for stuttering disorder. In B. Amster & E. Klein (Eds.), *More than fluency: The social, emotional, and cognitive dimensions of stuttering.* Plural Publishing.

Beitchman, J., Nair, R., Clegg, M., & Patel, P. (1986). Prevalence of speech and language in 5-year-old kindergarten children in Ottawa-Carleton region. *Journal of Speech and Hearing Disorders, 51*, 98–110.

Benito-Aragon, C., Gonzalez-Sarmiento, R., Liddell, T., Diez, I., Uquillas, F. D. O., Ortiz-Teran, L., & Sepulcre, J. (2020). Neurofilament-lysosomal genetic intersections in the cortical network of stuttering. *Progress in Neurobiology, 184*, 1017–1018.

Bernard, R., Hofslundsengen, H., & Norbury, F. C. (2022). Anxiety and depression symptoms in children and adolescents who stutter: A systematic review and meta-analysis. *Journal of Speech, Language, and Hearing Research, 65*(2), 624–644.

Berk, L. E. (1991). *Child development* (2nd ed.). Allyn & Bacon.

Bernstein Ratner, N. (1981). Are there constraints on childhood disfluency? *Journal of Fluency Disorders, 6*, 341–350.

Bernstein Ratner, N. (1997). Stuttering: A psycholinguistic perspective. In R. F. Curlee & G. M. Siegel (Eds.), *Nature and treatment of stuttering: New directions* (2nd ed., pp. 99–127). Allyn & Bacon.

Bernstein Ratner, N. (2005). Evidence-based practice in stuttering: Some questions to consider. *Journal of Fluency Disorders, 30*(3), 163–168.

Bernstein-Ratner, N. (1995). Treating the child who stutters with concomitant language and phonological impairment. *Language, Speech and Hearing in Schools, 26*(2), 180–186.

Bernstein Ratner, N., & MacWhinney, B. (2018). Fluency Bank: A new resource for fluency research and practice. *Journal of Fluency Disorders, 56*, 69–80.

Bernstein Ratner, N., & Sih, C. C. (1987). Effects of gradual increases in sentence length and complexity on children's dysfluency. *Journal of Speech and Hearing Disorders, 52*, 278–287.

Bernstein Ratner, N., & Silverman, S. (2000). Prenatal perceptions of children's communicative development at stuttering onset. *Journal of Speech, Language and Hearing Research, 43*, 1252–1263.

Bernthal, J., & Bankson, N. (1998). *Articulation and phonological disorders* (4th ed.). Allyn & Bacon.

Bernthal, J., Bankson, N., & Flipsen, P. (2022). *Articulation and phonological disorders: Speech sound disorders in children* (9th ed.). Pearson.

Berry, M. (1938). A study of the medical history of stuttering children. *Speech Monographs, 5*, 97–114.

Berry, R. C., & Silverman, F. H. (1972). Equality of intervals on the Lewis-Sherman-scale of stuttering severity. *Journal of Speech and Hearing Research, 15*, 185–188.

Beurskens, R., Helmich, I., Rein, R., & Boch, O. (2014). Age-related changes in prefrontal activity during walking and dual-task situations: A fNIRS study. *International Journal of Psychophysiology, 92*(3), 122–128.

Biancarosa, G., Kennedy, P. C., Park, S., Otterstedt, J., Gearin, B., Ives, C., & Yoon, H. (2020). *DIEBELS: Dynamic indicators of basic early literary skils* (8th ed.). Amplify Education.

Bijleveld, H., Lebrun, Y., & van Dongen, H. (1994). A case of acquired stuttering. *Folia Phoniatrica et Logopedica, 46*, 250–253.

Binder, L., Spector, J., & Youngjohn, J. (2012). Psychogenic stuttering and other acquired nonorganic speech and language abnormalities. *Archives of Clinical Neuropsychology, 27*(5), 557–568.

Black, J. W. (1951). The effects of delayed sidetone on vocal rate and intensity. *Journal of Speech and Hearing Disorders, 16*, 56–60.

Black, T. D. (2022). *ACT for treating children: The essential guide to Acceptance and Commitment Therapy for kids.* New Harbinger Publications.

Blood, G. W. (1985). Laterality differences in child stutterers: Heterogeneity, severity levels, and statistical treatment. *Journal of Speech and Hearing Disorders, 50*, 66–72.

Blood, G. W., Blood, I., Tellis, G., & Gabel, R. (2001). Communication apprehension and self-perceived communication competence in adolescents who stutter. *Journal of Fluency Disorders, 263*, 161–178.

Blood, G. W., & Blood, I. M. (1989). Multiple data analysis of dichotic listening advantages of stutterers. *Journal of Fluency Disorders, 14*, 97–107.

Blood, G. W., Ridenour, V. J., Qualls, C. D., & Hammer, C. S. (2003). Co-occurring disorders in children who stutter. *Journal of Communication Disorders, 36*(6), 427–448.

Bloodstein, O. (1948). *Conditions under which stuttering is reduced or absent.* (Unpublished doctoral dissertation). University of Iowa.

Bloodstein, O. (1950). Hypothetical conditions under which stuttering is reduced or absent. *Journal of Speech and Hearing Disorders, 15*, 142–153.

Bloodstein, O. (1960a). The development of stuttering: I. Changes in nine basic features. *Journal of Speech and Hearing Disorders, 25*, 219–237.

Bloodstein, O. (1960b). The development of stuttering: II. Developmental phases. *Journal of Speech and Hearing Disorders, 25*, 366–376.

Bloodstein, O. (1961). Stuttering in families of adopted stutterers. *Journal of Speech and Hearing Disorders, 26*, 395–396.

Bloodstein, O. (1974). The rules of early stuttering. *Journal of Speech and Hearing Disorders, 39*, 379–394.

Bloodstein, O. (1975). Stuttering as tension and fragmentation. In J. Eisenson (Ed.), *Stuttering: A second symposium* (pp. 1–95). Harper & Row.

Bloodstein, O. (1987). *A handbook on stuttering* (4th ed.). National Easter Seal Society.

Bloodstein, O. (1993). *Stuttering: The search for a cause and a cure.* Allyn & Bacon.

Bloodstein, O. (1995). *A handbook on stuttering* (5th ed.). Singular.

Bloodstein, O. (1997). Stuttering as an anticipatory struggle reaction. In R. F. Curlee & G. M. Siegel (Eds.), *The nature and treatment of stuttering: New directions* (2nd ed., pp. 169–181). Allyn & Bacon.

Bloodstein, O. (2001). Incipient and developed stuttering as two distinct disorders: Resolving a dilemma. *Journal of Fluency Disorders, 26*, 67–73.

Bloodstein, O. (2002). Early stuttering as a type of language difficulty. *Journal of Fluency Disorders, 27*, 163–167.

Bloodstein, O., & Gantwerk, B. (1967). Grammatical function in relation to stuttering in young children. *Journal of Speech and Hearing Research, 10*, 786–789.

Bloodstein, O., & Ratner, N. B. (2008). *A handbook on stuttering* (6th ed.). Thomson Delmar Learning.

Bloodstein, O., Ratner, N. B., & Brundage, S. (2021). *A handbook on stuttering* (7th ed.). Plural.

Bloom, L. (1970). *Language development: Form and function MIT.* Research Monograph series #59. MIT Press.

Bluemel, C. S. (1932). Primary and secondary stuttering. *Quarterly Journal of Speech, 18*, 187–200.

Bluemel, C. S. (1957). *The riddle of stuttering.* Interstate Publishing Co.

Boberg, E., Yeudall, L., Schopflocher, D., & Bo-Lassen, P. (1983). The effect of an intensive behavioral program on the distribution of EEG alpha power in stutterers during the processing of verbal and visuospatial information. *Journal of Fluency Disorders, 8*, 245–263.

Boehme, G. (1968). Stammering and cerebral lesions in early childhood: Examinations of 802 children and adults with cerebral lesions. *Folia Phoniatrica, 20*, 239–249.

Boey, R., Van de Heyning, P., Wuyts, F., Heylen, L., Stroap, R., & De Bodt, M. (2009). Awareness and reactions of young stuttering children aged 2 - 7 years old towards their speech disfluency. *Journal of Communication Disorders, 42*(5), 334–346.

Boey, R., Wuyts, F., Van de Heyning, P., De Bodt, M., & Heylen, L. (2007). Characteristics of stuttering-type disfluencies in Dutch-speaking children. *Journal of Fluency Disorders, 32*(4), 310–329.

Bolat, N., & Yalcin, O. (2017). Factitious disorder presenting with stuttering in two adolescents: The importance of psychoeducation. *Noro Psikiyatri Arsivi, 54*(1), 87–89.

Bolles, R. C. (1970). Speech-specific defense reactions and avoidance learning. *Psychological Review, 77*, 32–48.

Boone, D., McFarlane, S., Von Berg, S., & Zraick, R. (2014). *The voice and voice therapy.* Pearson Education.

Borden, G. J. (1983). Initiation versus execution time during manual and oral counting by stutterers. *Journal of Speech and Hearing Research, 26*, 389–396.

Bosshardt, H.-G. (1999). Effects of concurrent mental calculation on stuttering, inhalation and speech timing. *Journal of Fluency Disorders, 24*, 43–72.

Bosshardt, H.-G. (2002). Effects of concurrent cognitive processing on the fluency of word repetition: Comparison between persons who do and do not stutter. *Journal of Fluency Disorders, 27*, 93–113.

Bosshardt, H.-G. (2006). Cognitive processing load as a determinant of stuttering: Summary of a research programme. *Clinical Linguistics and Phonetics, 20*, 371–385.

Bothe, A. (2004). *Evidence-based treatment of stuttering: Empirical bases and clinical applications.* Erlbaum.

Botterill, W., & Kelman, E. (2010). Palin parent-child interaction. In B. Guitar & R. J. McCauley (Eds.), *Treatment of stuttering: Established and emerging interventions* (pp. 63–90). Wolters Kluwer.

Bouton, M. (2016). *Learning and behavior: A contemporary synthesis* (2nd ed.). Sinauer Associates, Inc.

Boyce, W. T., Chesney, M., Alkon-Leonard, A., Tschann, J., Adams, S., Chesterman, B., Cohen, F., Kaiser, P., Folkman, S., & Wara, D. (1995). Psychobiologic reactivity to stress and childhood respiratory illness: Results of two prospective studies. *Psychosomatic Medicine, 57*, 411–422.

Boyle, M. P. (2017). Personal perceptions and perceived public opinion about stuttering in the United States: Implications for anti-stigma campaigns. *American Journal of Speech Language Pathology, 26*(3), 921–938.

Brady, J., & Ali, Z. (2000). Alprazolam, citalopram, and clomipramine for stuttering. *Journal of Clinical Psychopharmacology, 202*, 287.

Brady, J. P., & Berson, J. (1975). Stuttering, dichotic listening, and cerebral dominance. *Archives of General Psychiatry, 32*, 1449–1452.

Brady, J. P. (1991). The pharmacology of stuttering: A critical review. *American Journal of Psychiatry, 148*, 1309–1316.

Branigan, G. (1979). Some reasons why successive single word utterances are not. *Journal of Child Language, 6*, 411–421.

Braun, A., Varga, M., Stager, S., Schulz, G., Selbie, S., Maisog, J., Carson, R. E., & Ludlow, C. L. (1997a). Altered patterns of cerebral activity during speech and language production in developmental stuttering: An H215O positron emission tomography study. *Brain, 120*, 761–784.

Braun, A. R., Varga, M., Stager, S., Schulz, G., Selbie, S., Maisog, J. M., Carson, R. E., & Ludlow, C. L. (1997b). A typical lateralization of hemispherical activity in developmental stuttering: An H2 15 0 positron emission tomography study. In W. Hulstijn, H. F. M. Peters & P. H. H. M. van Lieshout (Eds.), *Speech production: Motor control, brain research and fluency disorders* (pp. 279–292). Elsevier.

Brayton, E. R., & Conture, E. G. (1978). Effects of noise and rhythmic stimulation on the speech of stutterers. *Journal of Speech and Hearing Research, 21*, 285–294.

Briley, P. M., Merlo, S., & Ellis, C. (2021). Sex differences in childhood stuttering and coexisting developmental disorders. *Journal of Developmental and Physical Disabilities, 34*, 505–527. 10.1007/s10882-021-09811-y

Brosch, S., Haege, A., & Johannsen, H. (2002). Prognostic indicators for stuttering: The value of computer-based speech analysis. *Brain and Language, 82*, 75–87.

Brosch, S., Haege, A., Kalehne, P., & Johannsen, S. (1999). Stuttering children and the probability of remission: The role of cerebral dominance and speech production. *International Journal of Pediatric Otorhinolaryngology, 47*, 71–76.

Brown, S. F. (1937). The influence of grammatical function on the incidence of stuttering. *Journal of Speech Disorders, 2*, 207–215.

Brown, S. F. (1938a). A further study of stuttering in relation to various speech sounds. *Quarterly Journal of Speech, 24*, 390–397.

Brown, S. F. (1938b). Stuttering with relation to word accent and word position. *Journal of Abnormal Social Psychology, 33*, 112–120.

Brown, S. F. (1938c). The theoretical importance of certain factors influencing the incidence of stuttering. *Journal of Speech Disorders, 3*, 223–230.

Brown, S. F. (1943). An analysis of certain data concerning loci of "stutterings" from the viewpoint of general semantics. *Papers from the Second American Congress of General Semantics, 2*, 194–199.

Brown, S. F. (1945). The loci of stutterings in the speech sequence. *Journal of Speech Disorders, 10*, 181–192.

Brown, S. F., Ingham, R. J., Ingham, J., Laird, A. R., & Fox, P. T. (2005). Stuttered and fluent speech production: An ALE meta-analysis of functional neuroimaging studies. *Human Brain Mapping, 25*(1), 105–117.

Brown, S. F., & Moren, A. (1942). The frequency of stuttering in relation to word length during oral reading. *Journal of Speech Disorders, 7*, 153–159.

Brundage, S., & Bernstein Ratner, N. (1989). The measurement of stuttering frequency in children's speech. *Journal of Fluency Disorders, 14*, 351–358.

Brundage, S., Ratner, N. B., Boyle, M. P., Eggers, K., Everard, R., Franken, M. C. J., & Yaruss, J. S. (2021). Clinical focus: Consensus guidelines for the assessments of individuals who stutter across the lifespan. *American Journal of Speech-Language Pathology, 30*, 2379–2393.

Brutten, G. J., & Shoemaker, D. J. (1967). *The modification of stuttering*. Prentice-Hall.

Brutten, G. J., & Vanryckeghem, M. (2007). *Behavior Assessment Battery for school-age children who stutter*. Plural Publishing.

Bryngelson, B. (1935). Sideness as an etiological factor in stuttering. *Journal of Genetic Psychology, 47*, 204–217.

Buck, S., Lees, R., & Cook, F. (2002). The influence of family history of stuttering on the onset of stuttering in young children. *Folia Phoniatrica et Logopedica, 54*, 117–124.

Budde, K. S., Barron, D. S., & Fox, P. T. (2014). Stuttering, induced fluency, and natural fluency: A hierarchical series of activation likelihood estimation meta-analysis. *Brain and Language, 139*, 99–107.

Burman, D. D., Bitan, T., & Booth, J. R. (2008). Sex differences in neural processing of language among children. *Neuropsychologia, 46*(5), 1349–1362.

Byrd, C. T., Bedore, L. M., & Ramos, D. (2015). The disfluent speech of bilingual Spanish-English children: Considerations for differential diagnosis of stuttering. *Language, Speech & Hearing Services in Schools, 46*(1), 30–43.

Byrd, C. T., Croft, R., Gkalitsiou, Z., & Hampton, E. (2017). Clinical utility of self-disclosure for adults who stutter: Apologetic versus informative statements. *Journal of Fluency Disorders, 54*, 1–13.

Byrd, C. T., Werle, D., Coalson, G. A., & Eggers, K. (2020). Use of monolingual English guidelines to assess stuttering in bilingual speakers. *Journal of Monolingual and Bilingual Speech, 2(1)*, 1–23.

Byrd, C. T., Wolk, I., & Davis, B. L. (2007). Role of phonology in childhood stuttering and its treatment. In E. Conture & R. Curlee (Eds.), *Stuttering and related disorders of fluency* (3rd ed., pp. 168–182). Thieme.

Calkins, S. D., & Fox, N. A. (1994). Individual differences in the biological aspects of temperament. In J. E. Bates & T. D. Wachs (Eds.), *Temperament: Individual differences at the interface of biology and behavior* (pp. 199–217). American Psychological Association.

Callan, D. E., Kent, R. D., Guenther, F. H., & Vorperian, H. K. (2000). An auditory-feedback based neural network model of speech production that is robust to developmental changes in the size and shape of the articulatory system. *Journal of Speech, Language, and Hearing Research, 43*, 721–736.

Campbell, P., Constantino, C., & Simpson, S. (Eds.) (2019). *Stammering pride and prejudice: Difference not defect*. J & R Press.

Canter, G. (1971). Observations on neurogenic stuttering: A contribution to differential diagnosis. *British Journal of Communication Disorders, 6*, 139–143.

Caplan, D. (1987). *Neurolinguistics and linguistic aphasiology*. Cambridge University Press.

Caruso, A. J., Abbs, J. H., & Gracco, V. L. (1988). Kinematic analysis of multiple movement coordination during speech in stutterers. *Brain, 111*, 439–455.

Caruso, A. J., Chodzko-Zajko, W., Bidinger, D., & Sommers, R. (1994). Adults who stutter: Responses to cognitive stress. *Journal of Speech and Hearing Research, 37*, 746–754.

Caruso, A. J., Chodzko-Zajko, W., & McClowry, M. (1995). Emotional arousal and stuttering: The impact of cognitive stress. In C. W. Starkweather & H. F. M. Peters (Eds.), *Stuttering: Proceedings of the first world congress on fluency disorders*. International Fluency Association.

Chang, S.-E. (2010). Similarities in speech and white matter characteristics in idiopathic developmental stuttering and adult-onset stuttering. *Journal of Neurolinguistics, 23*(5), 455–469.

Chang, S.-E. (2014). Research update in neuroimaging studies of children who stutter. *Seminars in Speech and Language, 35*, 67–79.

Chang, S. E., Angstadt, M., Chow, H., Etchell, A., Garnett, E., Choo, A. L., & Sripada, C. (2018). Anamalous network architecture of the resting brain in children who stutter. *Journal of Fluency Disorders, 55*, 46–67.

Chang, S.-E., Erickson, K., Ambrose, N. G., Hasegawa-Johnson, M., & Ludlow, C. L. (2008). Brain anatomy differences in childhood stuttering. *NeuroImage, 39*(3), 1333–1344.

Chang, S.-E., & Guenther, F. H. (2020). Involvement of the cortico-basal ganglia-thalamocortical loop in developmental stuttering. *Frontiers in Psychology, 10*, 3088. 10.3389/fpsyg.2019.03088

Chang, S.-E., Horowitz, B., Ostuni, J., Reynolds, R., & Ludlow, C. L. (2011). Evidence of left inferior frontal-premotor structural and functional connectivity deficits in adults who stutter. *Cerebral Cortex, 21*(11), 2507–2518.

Chang, S.-E., Kenny, M., Loucks, T., & Ludlow, C. L. (2009). Brain activation abnormalities during speech and non-speech in stuttering speakers. *NeuroImage, 46*(1), 201–212.

Chang, S.-E., & Zhu, D. (2013). Neural network connectivity difference in children who stutter. *Brain, 136*(12), 3709–3726.

Chang, S.-E., Zhu, D. C., Choo, A. L., & Angstadt, M. (2015). White matter neuroanatomical differences in young children who stutter. *Brain, 138*(3), 694–711.

Chase, C. H. (1996). Neurobiology of learning disabilities. *Seminars in Speech, Language and Hearing, 17*(3), 173–181.

Cheadle, O., Sorger, C., & Howell, P. (2018). Identification of neural structures involved in stuttering using vibrotactile feedback. *Brain and Language, 180-182*, 50–61.

Chen, H., Xu, J., Zhou, Y., Gao, Y., Wang, G., Xia, J., & Sun, Y. (2015). Association study of stuttering candidate genes GNPTAB, GNPTG and NAGPA with dyslexia in Chinese population. *BMC Genetics, 6*(7), 1–7.

Chmela, K. (2004). *Working with preschoolers who stutter [DVD]*. Stuttering Foundation of America.

Chmela, K. A., & Reardon, N. A. (2001). *The school-aged child who stutters: Working effectively with attitudes and emotions: A workbook*. Stuttering Foundation of America.

Choi, D., Conture, E. G., Walden, T. A., Jones, R. M., & Kim, H. (2016). Emotional diathesis, emotional stress and childhood stuttering. *Journal of Speech, Language and Hearing Research, 59*(4), 616–630.

Choo, A. L., Burnham, E., Hicks, K., & Chang, S.-E. (2016). Dissociations among linguistic, cognitive, and auditory-motor neuroanatomical domains in children who stutter. *Journal of Communication Disorders, 61*, 29–47.

Chow, H., & Chang, S.-E. (2017). White matter developmental trajectories associated with persistence and recovery of childhood stuttering. *Human Brain Mapping, 38*(7), 3345–3359.

Chuang, C. K., Fromm, D. S., Ewanowski, S. J., & Abbs, J. H. (1980, November). *Nonspeech articulatory sensori-motor control differences between stutterers and nonstutterers. Paper presented at the Annual Meeting of the American Speech and Hearing Association.* Detroit, MI.

Ciarrochi, J., Robb, H., & Godsell, C. (2005). Letting a little non-verbal air into the room: Insights from acceptance and commitment therapy. Part 1: Philosophical and theoretical underpinnings. *Journal of Rational-Emotive and Cognitive-Behavior Therapy, 23*(2), 79–106.

Clarke-Stewart, A., & Friedman, S. (1987). *Child development: Infancy through adolescence.* John Wiley & Sons.

Cohen Kadosh, K., Linden, D. E. J., & Lau, J. Y. F. (2013). Plasticity during childhood and adolescence: Innovative approaches to investigating neurocognitive development. *Developmental Science, 16*(4), 574–583.

Cohen, M. S., & Hanson, M. L. (1975). Intersensory processing efficiency of fluent speakers and stutterers. *British Journal of Disorders of Communication, 102,* 111–122.

Colburn, N., & Mysak, E. D. (1982a). Developmental disfluency and emerging grammar. I. Disfluency characteristics in early syntactic utterances. *Journal of Speech and Hearing Research, 25,* 414–420.

Colburn, N., & Mysak, E. D. (1982b). Developmental disfluency and emerging grammar. II. Co-occurrence of disfluency with specified semantic-syntactic structures. *Journal of Speech and Hearing Research, 25,* 421–427.

Colcord, R. D., & Adams, M. R. (1979). Voicing duration and vocal SLP changes associated with stuttering reduction during singing. *Journal of Speech and Hearing Research, 22,* 468–479.

Coleman, T. J. (2000). *Clinical management of communication disorders in culturally diverse children.* Allyn & Bacon.

Conger, J. J., & Peterson, A. C. (1984). *Adolescence and youth: Psychological development in a changing world.* Harper & Row.

Conrad, C. (1996). Fluency in multicultural populations. In L. Cole & V. R. Deal (Eds.), *Communication disorders in multicultural populations.* American Speech-Language-Hearing Association.

Constantino, C., Manning, W. H., & Nordstrom, S. N. (2017). Rethinking covert stuttering. *Journal of Fluency Disorders, 53,* 26–40.

Conture, E. G. (1982). *Stuttering.* Prentice-Hall.

Conture, E. G. (1990). *Stuttering* (2nd ed.). Prentice-Hall.

Conture, E. G. (2001). Assessment and evaluation. In E. G. Conture (Ed.), *Stuttering: Its nature, diagnosis and treatment.* Allyn & Bacon.

Conture, E. G. (2001a). *Stuttering: Its nature, diagnosis, and treatment.* Allyn & Bacon.

Conture, E. G. (2010). *Stuttering and your child: Questions and answers* (4th ed.). Stuttering Foundation.

Conture, E. G., Louko, L., & Edwards, M. L. (1993). Simultaneously treating stuttering and disordered phonology in children. *American Journal of Speech-Language Pathology, 2,* 72–81.

Conture, E. G., McCall, G. N., & Brewer, D. W. (1977). Laryngeal behavior during stuttering. *Journal of Speech and Hearing Research, 20,* 661–668.

Conture, E. G., & Walden, T. A. (2012). Dual diathesis-stressor model of stuttering. In L. Bellakova & Y. Filatova (Eds.), *Theoretical issues of fluency disorders* (pp. 94–127). National Book Center.

Cooper, E. B., & Cooper, C. S. (1993). Fluency disorders. In D. E. Battle (Ed.), *Communication disorders in multicultural organizations* (pp. 189–211). Andover Medical Publishers.

Cordes, A. K. (1994). The reliability of observational data: I. Theories and methods for speech-language pathology. *Journal of Speech and Hearing Research, 37,* 264–278.

Cordes, A. K., & Ingham, R. J. (1999). Effects of time-interval judgment training on real-time measurement of stuttering. *Journal of Speech, Language and Hearing Research, 42,* 862–879.

Coster, W. (1986). *Aspects of voice and conversation in behaviorally inhibited and uninhibited children.* (Unpublished doctoral dissertation). Harvard University.

Coulter, C., Anderson, J., & Conture, E. G. (2009). Childhood stuttering and dissociations across linguistic domains: A replication and extension. *Journal of Fluency Disorders, 34*(4), 257–278.

Cox, N., & Yairi, E. (2000, November). *Genetics of stuttering: Insights and recent advances. Paper presented at the Annual meeting of the American Speech-Language-Hearing Association.* Washington, DC.

Craig, A. (2014). Anxiety and stuttering [Special Issue]. *Journal of Fluency Disorders, 40,* 1–140.

Craig, A., Franklin, J., & Andrews, G. (1984). A scale to measure locus of control of behavior. *British Journal of Medical Psychology, 57,* 173–180.

Craig, A., Hancock, K., Tran, Y., Craig, M., & Peters, M. (2002). Epidemiology of stuttering in the community across the entire life span. *Journal of Speech Language and Hearing Research, 45,* 1097–1105.

Craig, A., & Tran, Y. (2014). Trait and socil anxiety in adults with chronic stuttering: Conclusions following meta-analysis. *Journal of Fluency Disorders, 40,* 35–43.

Cross, D. E., & Cooke, P. (1979). Vocal and manual reaction times of adult stutterers and nonstutterers. (Abstract). *American Speech-Language and Hearing Association, 21,* 693.

Cross, D. E., & Luper, H. L. (1979). Voice reaction time of stuttering and nonstuttering children and adults. *Journal of Fluency Disorders, 4,* 58–77.

Cross, D. E., & Luper, H. L. (1983). Relation between finger reaction time and voice reaction time in stuttering and nonstuttering children and adults. *Journal of Speech and Hearing Research, 26,* 356–361.

Cross, D. E., Sweet, J., & Bates, D. (1985, November). *Mental imagery and stuttering: Electroencephalographic and physiological characteristics. Paper presented at the Annual Meeting of the American Speech and Hearing Association.* Washington, DC.

Cruz, C., Amorim, H., Beca, G., & Nunes, R. (2018). Neurogenic stuttering: A review of the literature. *Revista de Neurología, 66*(2), 59–64.

Crystal, D. (1987). Towards a bucket theory of language disability: Taking account of interaction between linguistic levels. *Clinical Linguistics and Phonetics, 1,* 7–22.

Culatta, R., & Goldberg, S. (1995). *Stuttering therapy: An integrated approach to theory and practice.* Allyn & Bacon.

Cullinan, W. L., & Springer, M. T. (1980). Voice initiation times in stuttering and nonstuttering children. *Journal of Speech and Hearing Research, 23,* 344–360.

Curlee, R. (1984). Stuttering disorders: An overview. In J. M. Costello (Ed.), *Speech disorders in children* (pp. 227–260). College-Hill Press.

Curlee, R. (1993). Identification and management of beginning stuttering. In R. Curlee (Ed.), *Stuttering and related disorders of fluency* (pp. 1–22). Thieme Medical Publishers.

Curry, F., & Gregory, H. H. (1969). The performance of stutterers on dichotic listening tasks thought to reflect cerebral dominance. *Journal of Speech and Hearing Research, 12*, 73–82.

Cykowski, M. D., Fox, P. T., Ingham, R. J., Ingham, J. C., & Robin, D. A. (2010). A study of the reproducibility and etiology of diffusion anisotropy differences in developmental stuttering: A potential role for impaired myelination. *NeuroImage, 52*(4), 1495–1504.

Daliri, A., & Max, L. (2018). Stuttering adults' lack of pre-speech auditory modulation normalizes when speaking with delayed auditory feedback. *Cortex, 99*, 55–68.

Dalton, P., & Hardcastle, W. J. (1977). *Disorders of fluency*. Elsevier.

Daly, D. A. (1986). The clutterer. In K. St. Louis (Ed.), *The atypical stutterer*. Academic Press.

Daly, D. A. (2006). Predictive cluttering inventory.

Daly, D. A., & Burnett-Stolnack, M. L. (1995). Identification of and treatment planning for stuttering clients: Two practical tools. *The Clinical Connection, 8*, 15.

Damian, S. (2014). *Voice: A stutterer's odyssey*. Behler Publications.

Daniels, D. E. (2008). Working with people who stutter of diverse cultural backgrounds: Some ideas to consider. *Perspectives on Fluency and Fluency Disorders, 18*, 95–100.

Daniels, D. E., Gabel, R., & Hughes, S. (2012). Recounting the K-12 school experiences of adults who stutter: A qualitative analysis. *Journal of Fluency Disorders, 37*(2), 71–82.

Darley, F. L., & Spriestersbach, D. (1978). *Diagnostic methods in speech pathology* (2nd ed.). Harper & Row.

Davenport, R. W. (1977). *Dichotic ear preferences of stuttering adults*. (Unpublished doctoral dissertation). Iowa State University.

Davidson, R. J. (1984). Affect, cognition, and hemispheric specialization. In C. E. Izard, J. Kagan & R. Zajonc (Eds.), *Emotion, cognition and behavior*. Cambridge University Press.

Davidson, R. J. (1995). Cerebral asymmetry, emotion, and affective style. In R. J. Davidson & K. Hugdahl (Eds.), *Brain asymmetry* (pp. 361–387). MIT press.

Davis, D. M. (1940). The relation of repetitions in the speech of young children to certain measures of language maturity and situational factors: Parts II & III. *Journal of Speech Disorders, 5*, 235–246.

Davis, M., & Guitar, B. (1976). *Speech rate of elementary school children in Vermont*. (Graduate student research paper). University of Vermont.

De Nil, L. F. (1995, November). *Linguistic and motor approaches to stuttering: Exploring unification. Paper presented at the Annual Meeting of the American Speech-Language-Hearing Association*. Orlando, FL.

De Nil, L. F., & Abbs, J. H. (1991). Kinaesthetic acuity of stutterers and nonstutterers for oral and non-oral movements. *Brain, 114*, 2145–2158.

De Nil, L. F., & Brutten, G. J. (1991). Speech-associated attitudes of stuttering and normally fluent children. *Journal of Speech and Hearing Research, 34*, 60–66.

De Nil, L. F., Jokel, R., & Rochon, E. (2007). Etiology, symptomatology, and treatment of neurogenic stuttering. In E. Conture & R. Curlee (Eds.), *Stuttering and related disorders of fluency* (3rd ed., pp. 326–343). Thieme.

De Nil, L. F., Kroll, R. M., & Houle, S. (1998, November). *A PET study of neural activation changes following stuttering treatment. Paper presented at the Annual Meeting of the American Speech-Language-Hearing Association*. San Antonio.

De Nil, L. F., Kroll, R. M., Houle, S., Ludlow, C. L., Braun, A. R., Ingham, R. J., & Wu, J. (1995, November). *Advances in stuttering research using positron emission tomography brain imaging. Paper presented at the Annual meeting of the American Speech-Language-Hearing Association*. Orlando, FL.

De Nil, L. F., Kroll, R. M., Kapur, S., & Houle, S. (2000). A positron emission tomography study of silent and oral single word reading in stuttering and nonstuttering adults. *Journal of Speech, Language, and Hearing Research, 43*, 1038–1053.

De Nil, L. F., Kroll, R. M., Lafaille, S. J., & Houle, S. (2003). A positron emission tomography study of short- and long-term treatment effects on functional brain activation in adults who stutter. *Journal of Fluency Disorders, 28*, 357–380.

De Nil, L. F., Theys, C., & Jokel, R. (2017). Stroke-related acquired neurogenic stuttering. In P. Coppens & J. L. Patterson (Eds.), *Aphasia rehabilitation: Clinical challenges* (pp. 173–201). Jones & Bartlett Learning.

De Shazer, S., Dolan, Y., Korman, H., Tepper, T., McCollum, E., & Berg, I. K. (2021). *More than miracles: The state of the art of solution-focused brief therapy*. Routledge.

de Sonnerville-Koedoot, C., Bouwmans, C., Franken, M. C. J., & Stolk, E. (2015a). Economic evaluation of stuttering therapy in preschool children: The RESTART-study. *Journal of Communication Disorders, 58*, 106–118.

de Sonnerville-Koedoot, C., Stolk, E., Rietveld, T., & Franken, M. C. J. (2015b). Direct versus indirect therapy for preschool children who stutter: The RESTART randomized trial. *PLoS One, 10*(7), e0133758.

Decker, B., Guitar, B., & Solomon, A. (2018). Corpus callosum demylenination associated with acquired stuttering. *BMJ Case Reports, 21*, 2018. 10.1136/bcr-2017-223486

Dehqan, A., Bakhtiar, M., Panahi, S., & Ashayeri, H. (2008). Relationship between stuttering severity in children and their mothers speaking rate. *Sao Paulo Medical Journal, 126*(1), 29–33.

DeJoy, D. A., & Gregory, H. H. (1985). The relationship between age and frequency of disfluency in preschool children. *Journal of Fluency Disorders, 10*, 107–122.

Denworth, L. (2021). The stuttering mind. *Scientific American, 325*, 56–63.

Dietrich, S., Barry, S. J., & Parker, D. E. (1995). Middle latency auditory responses in males who stutter. *Journal of Speech and Hearing Research, 38*, 5–17.

Dinoto, A., Busan, P., Formaggio, E., Bertolotti, C., Menichelli, A., Stokelj, D., & Manganotti, P. (2018). Stuttering-like hesitation in speech during acute/post-acute phase of immune encephalitis. *Journal of Fluency Disorders, 58*, 70–76.

DiSimoni, F. G. (1974). Preliminary study of certain timing relationships in the speech of stutterers. *Journal of the Acoustical Society of America, 56*, 695–696.

Doidge, N. (2007). *The brain that changes itself*. Penguin Books.

Doidge, N. (2016). *The brain's way of healing*. Penguin Books.

Dolcos, F., & McCarthy, G. (2006). Brain systems mediating cognitive interference by emotional distraction. *Journal of Neuroscience, 26*(7), 2072–2079.

Dollaghan, C., & Campbell, T. F. (1998). Nonword repetition and child language impairment. *Journal of Speech, Language and Hearing Research, 41*(5), 1136–1146.

Donaher, J. (2011). *ADHD and children who stutter*. Presentation at Oxford Dysfluency Conference. Video by Stuttering Foundation.

Donaher, J., Healey, C., & Soffer, S. (n.d.). ADHD and stuttering. Available as free downloadable brochure from Stuttering Foundation.

Doneva, S. P. (2019). Adult stuttering and attentional ability: A meta-analytic review. *International Journal of Speech-Language Pathology* 10.1080/17549507.2019.1665710

Donnan, G. A. (1979). Stuttering as a manifestation of stroke. *Medical Journal of Australia, 1*, 44–45.

Douglas, E., & Quarrington, B. (1952). The differentiation of interiorized and exteriorized secondary stuttering. *Journal of Speech and Hearing Disorders, 17*(4), 377–385.

Douglass, J. E., Schwab, M., & Alvardo, J. (2018). Covert stuttering: Investigation of the paradigm shift from covertly stuttering to overtly stuttering. *American Journal of Speech-Language Pathology, 27*, 1235–1243.

Douglass, L. C. (1943). A study of bilaterally recorded electroencephalograms of adult stutterers. *Journal of Experimental Psychology, 32*, 247–265.

Dowling, M. (2014). *Young children's personal, social and emotional development* (4th ed.). Sage Publications.

Drayna, D. (1997). Genetic linkage studies of stuttering: Ready for prime time? *Journal of Fluency Disorders, 22*, 237–241.

Duffy, J. (2013). *Motor speech disorders: Substrates, differential diagnosis and management* (3rd ed.). Elsevier.

Duffy, J. (2015). Diagnosis and management of acquired functional speech disorders. *Online video course*. MedBridge, Inc.

Duffy, J. (2016). Functional speech disorders: Clinical manifestations, diagnosis and management. In M. Hallet, J. Stone & A. Carson (Eds.), *Functional neurologic disorders. Handbook of Clinical Neurology* (Vol. 139). Academic Press.

Duffy, J. (2020). *Motor speech disorders: Substrates, differntial diagnosis, and management* (4th ed.). Evolve Learning Resources for Students and Lecturers, a division of Elsevier.

Dunn, D. (2018). *Peabody picture vocabulary test* (5th ed.). Pearson.

Dworzynski, K., Remington, A., Rijsdijk, F., Howell, P., & Plomin, R. (2007). Genetic etiology in cases of recovered and persistent stuttering in an unselected, longitudinal sample of young twins. *American Journal of Speech-Language Pathology, 6*(2), 169–178.

Edelman, G. (1992). *Bright air, brilliant fire: On the matter of mind.* Basic Books.

Edwards, M. L., Stone, J., & Lang, A. E. (2014). From psychogenic movement disorder to functional movement disorder: It's time to change the name. *Movement Disorders, 29*(7), 849–852.

Eggers, K. (2012). *Temperamental characteristics of children with developmental stuttering.* Tilburg University.

Eggers, K., Millard, S. R., & Kelman, E. (2021). Treatment and the impact of stuttering in children aged 8 - 14 years. *Journal of Speech, Language and Hearing Research, 64*(2), 417–432.

Eggers, K., van Eerdenbrugh, S., & Byrd, C. T. (2020). Speech disfluencies in bilingual Yiddish-Dutch speaking children. *Clinical Linguistics & Phonetics, 35*(6), 576-592.

Egolf, D. B., Shames, G. H., Johnson, P. R., & Kasprisin-Burrelli, A. (1972). The use of parent-child interaction patterns in the treatment of young stutterers. *Journal of Speech and Hearing Disorders, 37*(2), 222–232.

Eisenberg, N., & Sulik, M. J. (2012). Emotion-related self-regulation in children. *Teaching of Psychology, 39*(1), 77–83.

Elliott, R. L., & Thomas, B. J. (1985). A case report of alprazolam-induced stuttering. *Journal of Clinical Psychopharmacology, 5*, 159–160.

Ellis, B. J., & Boyce, W. T. (2008). Biological sensitivity to context. *Current Directions in Psychological Science, 5*, 183–187.

Ellis, J. B., Finan, D., & Ramig, P. R. (2008). The influence of stuttering severity on acoustic startle response. *Journal of Speech, Language and Hearing Research, 51*(4), 836–850.

Embrechts, M., & Ebben, H. (1999). A comparison between the interactions of stuttering and nonstuttering children and their parents. In K. L. Baker, L. Rustin & F. Cook (Eds.), *Proceedings of the Fifth Oxford Dysfluency Conference, 7th-10th July, 1999* (pp. 125–133). Kevin Baker.

Epton, T., Harris, P. R., Kane, R., van Koningsbruggen, G. M., & Sheeran, P. (2015). The impact of self-affirmation on health-behavior change: A meta-analysis. *Health Psychology, 34*(3), 187.

Erickson, R. (1969). Assessing communication attitudes among stutterers. *Journal of Speech and Hearing Research, 12*, 711–724.

Etchell, A., Civier, O., Ballard, K., & Sowman, P. (2017). A systematic literature review of neuroimaging research on developmental stuttering between 1995 and 2016. *Journal of Fluency Disorders, 55*, 6–45.

Etchell, A., Johnson, B. W., & Sowman, P. (2014a). Behavioral and multimodal neuroimaging evidence for a deficit in brain timing networks in stuttering: A hypothesis and theory. *Frontiers in Human Neuroscience, 8*, 487.

Etchell, A. C., Johnson, B. W., & Sowman, P. F. (2014b). Beta oscillations, timing, and stuttering. *Frontiers in Human Neuroscience, 8*, 1036.

Ezrati-Vinacour, R., Platzky, R., & Yairi, E. (2001). The young child's awareness of stuttering-like disfluency. *Journal of Speech Language and Hearing Research, 44*, 368.

Fagan, M. K. (2002). *Stuttering, social-cognitive, and emotional development.* Unpublished manuscript. Columbia, MO.

Fagnani, C., Fibiger, S., Skytthe, A., & Hjelmborg, J. (2011). Heritability and environmental effects for self-reported periods with stuttering: A twin study from Denmark. *Logopedics Phoniatrics Vocology, 36*(3), 114–120.

Fanselow, M. (1994). Neural organization of the defensive behavior system responsible for fear. *Psychonomic Bulletin & Review, 1*(4), 429–438.

Felsenfeld, S. (1997). Epidemiology and genetics of stuttering. In R. F. Curlee & G. Siegel (Eds.), *The nature and treatment of stuttering: New directions* (2nd ed., pp. 3–23). Allyn & Bacon.

Felsenfeld, S., Kirk, K., Zhu, G., Statham, D., Neale, M., & Martin, N. (2000). A study of the genetic and environmental etiology of stuttering in a selected twin sample. *Behavior Genetics, 305*, 359–366.

Femrell, L., Avfall, M., & Lindstrom, E. (2012). Two-year follow-up of the Lidcombe Program in ten Swedish-speaking children. *Folia Phoniatrica et Logopedica, 64*, 248–253.

Fibiger, S. (1971). *Stuttering explained as a physiological tremor* (pp. 2–3). Quarterly Progress and Status Report: Speech Transmission Laboratory.

Fibiger, S. (1972). Further discussion on stuttering explained as a physiological tremor. *Quarterly Progress and Status Report: Speech Transmission Laboratory.*

Findlay, K., & Shenker, R. (2014, November). *Establishing benchmarks for linguistically diverse populations: Treatment time for the Lidcombe Program. Paper presented at the Annual meeting of the American Speech-Language and Hearing Association.* Orlando, FL.

Fineberg, N. A., Reghunandanan, S., Kolli, S., & Atmaca, M. (2014). Obsessive-compulsive (anankastic) personality: Toward the ICD-11. *Revista Brasileira de Psiquiatria, 36*, S40–S50.

Finn, P. (2003). Self-regulation and the management of stuttering. *Seminars in Speech and Language, 24*, 27–32.

Finn, P. (2007). Self-control and the treatment of stuttering. In E. Conture & R. Curlee (Eds.), *Stuttering and related disorders of fluency* (3rd ed., pp. 344–359). Thieme.

Fish, C. H., & Bowling, E. (1962). Effect of amphetamines on speech defects in the mentally retarded. *California Medicine, 96*(2), 109–101.

Fish, C. H., & Bowling, E. (1965). Stuttering: The effect of therapy with D-amphetamines and a tranquilizing agent, Trifluoperazine: A preliminary report on an uncontrolled study. *California Medicine, 103*(5), 337–339.

Flechsig, P. (1927). *Meine myelogenetische Hirnlehre*. Julius Springer.

Flinker, A., Korzeniewska, A., Shestyuk, A. Y., Franaszczuk, P. J., Dronke, N. F., Knight, R. T., & Crone, N. E. (2015). Redefining the role of Broca's area in speech. *PNAS, 112*(9), 2871–2875.

Forster, D. C., & Webster, W. G. (2001). Speech-motor control and interhemispheric relations in recovered and persistent stuttering. *Developmental Neuropsychology, 19*(2), 125–145.

Foundas, A. L., Bollich, A. M., Corey, D. M., Hurley, M., & Heilman, K. M. (2001). Anomalous anatomy of speech-language areas in adults with persistent developmental stuttering. *Neurology, 57*, 207–215.

Foundas, A. L., Bollich, A. M., Feldman, S., Corey, D. M., Hurley, M., Lemen, L. C., & Heilman, K. M. (2004). Aberrant auditory processing and atypical planum temporale in developmental stuttering. *Neurology, 63*(9), 1640–1646.

Fowlie, G. M., & Cooper, E. B. (1978). Traits attributed to stuttering and nonstuttering children by their mothers. *Journal of Fluency Disorders, 34*, 233–246.

Fox, N., & Davidson, R. (1984). Hemispheric substrates of affect: Developmental model. In N. Fox & R. Davidson (Eds.), *The psychobiology of affective development*. Lawrence Erlbaum Associates.

Fox, P. T. (2003). Brain imaging in stuttering: Where next? *Journal of Fluency Disorders, 284*, 265–272.

Fox, P. T., Ingham, R. J., Ingham, J. C., Hirsch, T. B., Downs, J. H., Martin, C., Jerabek, P., Glass, T., & Lancaster, J. L. (1996). A PET study of the neural systems of stuttering. *Nature, 382*, 158–162.

Fox, P. T., Ingham, R. J., Ingham, J. C., Zamarripa, F., Xiong, J.-H., & Lancaster, J. L. (2000). Brain correlates of stuttering and syllable production: A PET performance-correlation analysis. *Brain, 123*, 1985–2004.

Franken, M. C. J., Kielstra-van der Schalk, C. J., & Boelens, H. H. (2005). Experimental treatment of early stuttering. *Journal of Fluency Disorders, 30*(3), 189–199.

Frankenburg, W., & Dodds, J. (1967). The Denver Developmental Screening Test. *Journal of Pediatrics, 71*(2), 181–191.

Fraser, M. (2010). *Self-therapy for the stutterer* (11th ed.). Stuttering Foundation.

Frattali, C. (1998). *Measuring outcomes in speech-language pathology*. Thieme.

Freeman, F. J., & Ushijima, T. (1975). Laryngeal activity accompanying the moment of stuttering: A preliminary report of EMG investigations. *Journal of Fluency Disorders, 1*, 36–45.

Freeman, F. J., & Ushijima, T. (1978). Laryngeal muscle activity during stuttering. *Journal of Speech and Hearing Research, 21*, 538–562.

Frigerio-Domingues, C., & Drayna, D. (2017). Genetic contributions to stuttering: The current evidence. *Molecular Genetics and Genomic Medicine, 5*(2), 95–102.

Gabbard, C. (2016). *Lifelong motor development*. Wolters Kluwer.

Gaines, N. D., Runyan, C. M., & Meyers, S. C. (1991). A comparison of young stutterers' fluent versus stuttered utterances on measures of length and complexity. *Journal of Speech and Hearing Research, 34*, 37–42.

Gainotti, G. (2019). The role of the right hemisphere in emotional and behavioral disorders of patients with frontotemporal lobar degeneration: An updated review. *Frontiers in Aging Neuroscience, 11*, 55.

Games, D., Paul, D., & Reeves, N. (2014). Oral reading fluency measures and accommodations for school-age students who stutter. *Perspectives on Fluency and Fluency Disorders, 24*(2), 38–45.

Garfinkel, H. A. (1995). Why did Moses stammer? and, was Moses left-handed? *Journal of the Royal Society of Medicine, 88*, 256–257.

Garnett, E., Chow, H., & Chang, S. E. (2019). Neuroanatomical correlates of childhood stuttering: MRI indices of white and grey matter development that differentiate persistence versus recovery. *Journal of Speech, Language and Hearing Research, 62*(8S), 2986–2998.

Gattuso, R., & Leocata, A. (1962). L'haloperidol nella terapia della balbutzie. *La Clinica Otorinolaringoiatrica, 14*, 227–234.

Gendlin, E. (1981). *Focusing*. Bantam Books.

Gerlach, H., Chaudoir, S. R., & Zebrowski, P. (2021). Relationships between stigma-identity constructs and psychological health outcomes among adults who stutter. *Journal of Fluency Disorders, 70*, 105842.

Gerlach, H., Hollister, J., Caggiano, L., & Zebrowski, P. (2019). The utility of stuttering support organization conventions for young people who stutter. *Journal of Fluency Disorders, 47*, 1–12.

Gerlach, H., & Subramian, A. (2016). Qualitative analysis of bibliotherapy as a tool for adults who stutter and graduate students. *Journal of Fluency Disorders, 47*(1), 1–12.

Gerlach-Houck, H., Kubart, K., & Cage, E. (2023). Concealing stuttering at school: "When you can't fix it···the only alternative is to hide it". *Language, Speech & Hearing Services in Schools, 54*(1), 96–113.

Geschwind, N., & Galaburda, A. M. (1985). Cerebral lateralization: Biological mechanisms, associations, and pathology: I. A hypothesis and a program for research. *Archives of Neurology, 42*, 429–459.

Gibson, E. (1972). Reading for some purpose. In J. F. Kavanaugh & I. Mattingly (Eds.), *Language by ear and by eye*. MIT Press.

Gibson, G. (2008). The environmental contribution to gene expression profiles. *Nature Reviews Genetics, 9*, 575–581.

Gildston, P. (1967). Stutterers' self-acceptance and perceived parental acceptance. *Journal of Abnormal Psychology, 721*, 59–64.

Gillam, R. B., Logan, K. J., & Pearson, N. A. (2009). *TOCS: Test of childhood stuttering*. Pro-Ed.

Goldman, R., & Fristoe, M. (2015). *GFTA-3: Goldman-Fristoe test of articulation*. Pearson Assessment.

Goldman-Eisler, F. (1968). *Psycholinguistics: Experiments in spontaneous speech.* Academic Press.

Goldstein, C. (2022). *Understanding stuttering therapy through a trauma-informed lens* https://www.redefiningstammering.couk/understanding-stuttering-therapy-through-a-trauma-informed-lens

Goodhue, R., Onslow, M., Quine, S., O'Brian, S., & Hearne, A. (2010). The Lidcombe Program of early stuttering intervention: Mothers' experiences. *Journal of Fluency Disorders, 35*(1), 70–84.

Goodman, R. (1997). The strengths and difficulties questionnaire: A research note. *Journal of Child Psychology and Psychiatry and Allied Disciplines, 38,* 581–586.

Gordon, P. A., Luper, H. L., & Peterson, H. A. (1986). The effects of syntactic complexity on the occurrence of disfluencies in 5 year old stutterers. *Journal of Fluency Disorders, 11,* 151–164.

Gottwald, S. (2010). Stuttering prevention and early intervention: A multidimensional approach. In B. Guitar & R. J. McCauley (Eds.), *Treatment of stuttering: Established and emerging interventions* (pp. 91–117). Lippincott Williams & Wilkins.

Gottwald, S., & Starkweather, C. W. (1984, November). *Stuttering prevention: Rationale and method. Paper presented at the Annual meeting of the American Speech and Hearing Association.* San Francisco, CA.

Gottwald, S., & Starkweather, C. W. (1999). Stuttering prevention and early intervention: A multiprocess approach. In M. Onslow & A. Packman (Eds.), *Handbook of early stuttering intervention* (pp. 53–82). Singular.

Gray, C. (1994). *Comic strip conversations: Colorful, illustrated interactions with students with autism and related disorders.* Jensen Public Schools.

Gray, C. (2010). *The new social story book.* Future Horizons.

Gray, J. A. (1987). *The psychology of fear and stress* (2nd ed.). Cambridge University Press.

Greenspan, S. I. (1993). Making time for your child. *Parents* (August), 111–114.

Guenther, F. H. (1994). A neural network model of speech acquisition and motor equivalent speech production. *Biological Cybernetics, 72*(1), 43–53.

Guenther, F. H. (2007). Neuroimaging of normal speech production. In R. J. Ingham (Ed.), *Neuroimaging in communication sciences and disorders* (pp. 1–51). Plural Publications.

Guenther, F. H. (2016). *Neural control of speech.* MIT Press.

Guenther, F. H., Ghosh, S. S., & Tourville, J. A. (2006). Neural modeling and imaging of the cortical interactions underlying syllable production. *Brain and Language, 96*(3), 280–301.

Guenther, F. H., & Hickok, G. (2015). The human auditory system. In G. G. Celesia & G. Hickok (Eds.), *Handbook of clinical neurology: Fundamental organization and clinical disorders.* Elsevier.

Guitar, B. (1976). Pretreatment factors associated with the outcome of stuttering therapy. *Journal of Speech and Hearing Research, 19,* 590–600.

Guitar, B. (1978). Between parent and stuttering child. *WMU Journal of Speech, Language and Hearing, 14*(1), 3–5.

Guitar, B. (1997). Therapy for children's stuttering and emotions. In R. F. Curlee & G. M. Siegel (Eds.), *Nature and treatment of stuttering: New directions* (2nd ed., pp. 280–291). Allyn & Bacon.

Guitar, B. (1998). *Stuttering: An integrated approach to its nature and treatment* (2nd ed.). Lippincott Williams & Wilkins.

Guitar, B. (2000). Emotion, temperament and stuttering: Some possible relationships. In K. L. Baker, L. Rustin & F. Cook (Eds.), *Proceedings of the Fifth Oxford Dysfluency Conference, 7th-10th July, 1999* (pp. 1–6). K. L. Baker.

Guitar, B. (2003). Acoustic startle responses and temperament in individuals who stutter. *Journal of Speech, Language, and Hearing Research, 46*(1), 233–240.

Guitar, B. (2004). Burn your textbooks! Evidence-based practice in stuttering treatment. In A. Packman, A. Meltzer & H. F. M. Peters (Eds.), *Theory, research and therapy in fluency disorders: Proceedings of the Fourth World Congress in Fluency Disorders* (pp. *21–27*). Nijmegan University Press.

Guitar, B., & Bass, C. (1978). Stuttering therapy: The relation between attitude change and long-term outcome. *Journal of Speech and Hearing Disorders, 43,* 392–400.

Guitar, B., & Conture, E. (2015). *The child who stutters: To the pediatrician* (5th ed.). Stuttering Foundation.

Guitar, B., & Fraser, J. (2007). Stuttering: Basic clinical skills [DVD]. Stuttering Foundation.

Guitar, B., & Grims, S. (1977, November). *Developing a scale to assess communication attitudes in children who stutter. Paper presented at the Annual meeting of the American Speech-Language-Hearing Association.* Atlanta.

Guitar, B., & Guitar, C. (2003). Stuttering and your child: Help for parents. Stuttering Foundation.

Guitar, B., & Guitar, C. (2005). If you stutter: Advice for adults [DVD]. Stuttering Foundation.

Guitar, B., Guitar, C., & Fraser, J. (2010). Stuttering and your child: Help for families [DVD]. Stuttering Foundation.

Guitar, B., Guitar, C., Neilson, P. D., O'Dwyer, N. J., & Andrews, G. (1988). Onset sequencing of selected lip muscles in stutterers and nonstutterers. *Journal of Speech and Hearing Research, 31,* 28–35.

Guitar, B., Kazenski, D., Howard, A., Cousins, F., Fader, E., & Haskell, P. (2015). Predicting treatment time and long-term outcome of the Lidcombe Program: A replication and reanalysis. *American Journal of Speech-Language Pathology, 24,* 533–544.

Guitar, B., Kopff-Schaefer, H., Donahue-Kilburg, G., & Bond, L. (1992). Parent verbal interaction and speech rate. *Journal of Speech and Hearing Research, 35,* 742–754.

Guitar, B., & Marchinkowski, L. (2001). Influence of mothers' slower speech rate on their children's speech rate. *Journal of Speech Language and Hearing Research, 44*(4), 853–861.

Guitar, B., & McCauley, R. J. (2010). *Treatment of stuttering: Established and emerging interventions.* Lippincott Williams & Wilkins.

Guitar, B., & Reville, J. (1997). *Easy talker: A fluency workbook for school-age children.* Pro-Ed Publishers.

Guttormsen, L., Kefalianos, E., & Naess, K.-A. (2015). Communication attitudes in children who stutter: A meta-analytic review. *Journal of Fluency Disorders, 46,* 1–14.

Habib, M., Daquin, G., Milandre, L., Royere, M. L., Rey, M., Lanteri, A., Salamon, G., & Khalil, R. (1995). Mutism and auditory agnosia due to bilateral insular damage: Role of the insula in human communication. *Neuropsychologia, 333,* 327–339.

Hadders-Algra, M., & Forssberg, H. (2002). Development of motor function in health and disease. In H. Lagercrantz, M. L. Hanson, P. Evrard & C. H. Rodeck (Eds.), *The newborn brain: Neuroscience and clinical applications.* Cambridge University Press.

Hagenaars, M. A., Oitzl, M., & Roelofs, K. I. (2014). Updating freeze: Aligning animal and human research. *Neuroscience and Biobehavioral Revews, 47*, 165–176.

Hakim, H. B., & Bernstein Ratner, N. (2004). Nonword repetitions abilities of children who stutter: An exploratory study. *Journal of Fluency Disorders, 29*, 179–199.

Hall, J. W., & Jerger, J. (1978). Central auditory function in stutterers. *Journal of Speech and Hearing Research, 21*, 324–337.

Hall, N., Garbarino, J., & Bernstein Ratner, N. (2022). Language and phonological consideration. In P. Zebrowski, J. Anderson & E. Conture (Eds.), *Stuttering and related disorders of fluency* (4th ed., pp. 215–226). Thieme.

Hall, N., Wagovich, S., & Bernstein Ratner, N. (2007). Language consideration in childhood stuttering. In R. Curlee & E. G. Conture (Eds.), *Stuttering and related disorders of fluency* (3rd ed., pp. 153–167). Thieme.

Hampton, A., & Weber-Fox, C. (2008). Non-linguistic auditory processing in stuttering: Evidence from behavior and event-related brain potentials. *Journal of Fluency Disorders, 33*(4), 253–273.

Han, T.-U., Park, J., Domingues, C., Moretti-Ferreira, D., Paris, E., Sainz, E., & Drayna, D. (2014). A study of the role of the FOXP2 and CNTNAP2 genes in persistent developmental stuttering. *Neurobiology of Disease, 69*, 23–31.

Hannley, M., & Dorman, M. F. (1982). Some observations on auditory function and stuttering. *Journal of Fluency Disorders, 7*, 93–108.

Harrison, E., Bruce, M., Shenker, R., & Koushik, S. (2010). The Lidcombe Program for school-age children who stutter. In B. Guitar & R. J. McCauley (Eds.), *Treatment of stuttering: Established and emerging interventions* (pp. 150–166). Lippincott Williams & Wilkins.

Harrison, E., & Onslow, M. (2010). The Lidcombe Program for preschool children who stutter. In B. Guitar & R. J. McCauley (Eds.), *Treatment of stuttering: Established and emerging interventions* (pp. 118–149). Lippincott, Williams & Wilkins.

Hayes, L. L., & Ciarrochi, J. (2015). *The thriving adolescent: Using acceptance and commitment therapy and positive psychology to help teens manage emotions, achieve goals and build connection.* New Harbinger Publications.

Hayhow, R. (2009). Parents' experience of the Lidcombe Program of early stuttering intervention. *International Journal of Speech-Language Pathology, 11*(1), 20–25.

Haynes, W. O., & Hood, S. B. (1978). Disfluency changes in children as a function of the systematic modification of linguistic complexity. *Journal of Communication Disorders, 11*, 79–33.

Healy, K. T., Nelson, S., & Scaler Scott, K. (2015). A case study of cluttering treatment outcomes in a teen. *Procedia - Social and Behavioral Sciences, 193*, 141–146.

Helliesen, G. G. (2002). *Forty years after therapy: One man's story.* Apollo Press.

Helm, N. A. (1979). Management of palilalia with a pacing board. *Journal of Speech and Hearing Disorders, 44*, 350–353.

Helm, N. A., Butler, R. B., & Canter, G. (1980). Neurogenic acquired stuttering. *Journal of Fluency Disorders, 5*, 269–279.

Helm-Estabrooks, N. (1986). Diagnosis and management of neurogenic stuttering in adults. In St. Louis (Ed.), *The atypical stutterer.* Academic Press.

Helm-Estabrooks, N. (1992). *Aphasia diagnostic profiles.* Applied Symbolix.

Helm-Estabrooks, N. (1999). Stuttering associated with acquired neurological disorders. In R. Curlee (Ed.), *Stuttering and related disorders of fluency* (2nd ed., pp. 255–268). Thieme.

Helm-Estabrooks, N., & Kaplan, E. (1989). *Boston stimulus boards.* Applied Symbolix.

Hendrickson, J. (2020). What Joe Biden can't bring himself to say. *Atlantic.*

Hendrickson, J. (2022). I stutter, but I need you to listen https://www.youtube.com/watch?v=m0EwMIwfSl

Hendrickson, J. (2023). *Life on delay: Making peace with a stutter.* Alfred A. Knopf.

Hennessey, N., Dourado, E., & Beilby, J. (2014). Anxiety and speaking in people who stutter: An investigation using the emotional Stroop Task. *Journal of Fluency Disorders, 40*, 44–57.

Herndon, G. (1967). A study of the time discrimination abilities of stutterers and nonstutterers. *Speech Monographs, 34*, 303–304.

Hickok, G., Houde, J., & Rong, F. (2011). Sensorimotor integration in speech processing: Computational basis and neural organization. *Neuron, 69*(3), 407–422.

Hickok, G., & Poeppel, D. (2007). The cortical organization of speech processing. *Nature Reviews Neuroscience, 8*, 393–402.

Hilger, A., Zelaznik, H. N., & Smith, A. (2016). Evidence that bimanual motor timing performance is not a significant factor in developmental stuttering. *Journal of Speech Language and Hearing Research, 59*, 674–685.

Hill, D. (2003). Differential treatment of stuttering in the early stages of development. In H. H. Gregory, J. Campbell, C. Gregory & D. Hill (Eds.), *Stuttering therapy: Rationale and procedures* (pp. 142–185). Allyn & Bacon.

Hill, H. (1954). An experimental study of disorganization of speech and manual responses in normal subjects. *Journal of Speech and Hearing Disorders, 19*, 295–305.

Hillman, R. E., & Gilbert, H. R. (1977). Voice onset time for voiceless stop consonants in the fluent reading of stutterers and nonstutterers. *Journal of the Acoustical Society of America, 61*, 610–611.

Hiscock, M., & Kinsbourne, M. (1977). Selective listening asymmetry in preschool children. *Developmental Psychology, 133*, 217–224.

Hiscock, M., & Kinsbourne, M. (1980). Asymmetry of verbal-manual time sharing in children: A follow-up study. *Neuropsychologia, 18*, 151–162.

Hodson, B. W. (2004). *Hodson assessment of phonological patterns (HAPP-3)* (3rd ed.). LinguiSystems.

Hodson, B. W., & Paden, E. P. (1991). *A phonological approach to remediation: Targeting intelligible speech.* Pro-Ed.

Holland, A. L., & Nelson, R. L. (2020). *Counseling in communication disorders: A wellness perspective* (3rd ed.). Plural Publishing.

Hollister, J., Van Horne, A., & Zebrowski, P. (2017). The relationship between grammatical development and disfluencies in preschool children who stutter and those who recover. *American Journal of Speech-Language Pathology, 26*(1), 1–13.

Holloway, J. L., Allen, M. T., Myers, C. E., & Servatius, R. J. (2014). Behaviorally inhibited individuals demonstrate significantly enhanced conditioned response acquisition under non-optimal learning conditions. *Behavioural Brain Research, 261*, 49–55.

Hood, L. (1987, November). *Middle latency responses in stutterers. Paper presented at the Annual meeting of the American Speech-Language-Hearing Association.* New Orleans, LA.

Horovitz, L. J., Johnson, S. B., Pearlman, R. C., Schaffer, E. J., & Hedin, A. K. (1978). Stapedial reflex and anxiety in fluent and disfluent speakers. *Journal of Speech and Hearing Research, 214*, 762–767.

Horowitz, A. (2009). *Inside of a dog: What dogs see, smell, and know*. Scribner.

Howell, P., El-Yaniv, N., & Powell, D. J. (1987). Factors affecting fluency in stutterers when speaking under altered auditory feedback. In H. F. M. Peters & W. Hulstijn (Eds.), *Speech motor dynamics in stuttering* (pp. 361–369). Springer.

Howell, P., & Van Borsel, J. (2011). *Multilingual aspects of fluency disorders*. Multicultural Matters.

Howie, P. M. (1981). Concordance for stuttering in monozygotic and dizygotic twin pairs. *Journal of Speech and Hearing Research, 24*, 317–321.

Howie, P. M., & Andrews, G. (1984). Treatment of adult stutterers: Managing fluency. In R. Curlee & W. Perkins (Eds.), *Nature and treatment of stuttering: New directions* (pp. 425–445). College-Hill Press.

Hubbard, C. P., & Yairi, E. (1988). Clustering of disfluencies in the speech of stuttering and nonstuttering preschool children. *Journal of Speech and Hearing Research, 312*, 228–233.

Hughes, S. (2014). Bullying: What speech-language pathologists should know. *Language, Speech & Hearing Services in Schools, 45*, 3–13.

Humphrey, D. R., & Reed, D. J. (1983). Separate cortical systems for control of joint movement and joint stiffness: Reciprocal activation and coactivation of antagonist muscles. *Advances in Neurology, 39*, 347–372.

Ingham, R. J. (1979). Comment on stuttering therapy: The relation between attitude change and long-term outcome. *Journal of Speech and Hearing Disorders, 44*, 397–400.

Ingham, R. J. (1999). Performance-contingent management of stuttering in adolescents and adults. In R. Curlee (Ed.), *Stuttering and related disorders of fluency* (2nd ed., pp. 200–211). Thieme Medical Publishers.

Ingham, R. J. (2001). Brain imaging studies of developmental stuttering. *Journal of Communication Disorders, 34*, 493–516.

Ingham, R. J. (2003). Brain imaging and stuttering: Some reflection on current and future developments. *Journal of Fluency Disorders, 28*(4), 411–420.

Ingham, R. J., Cordes, A. K., & Finn, P. (1993a). Time-interval measurement of stuttering: Systematic replication of Ingham, Cordes & Gow (1993). *Journal of Speech and Hearing Research, 36*, 503–515.

Ingham, R. J., Cordes, A. K., & Gow, M. (1993b). Time-interval measurement of stuttering: Modifying interjudge agreement. *Journal of Speech and Hearing Research, 36*, 503–515.

Ingham, R. J., Fox, P. T., & Ingham, J. C. (1995, November). *A report on a functional-activation and functional-lesion PET study of stuttering in adults. Paper presented at the Annual Meeting of the American Speech-Language-Hearing Association.* Orlando, FL.

Ingham, R. J., Gow, M., & Costello, J. M. (1985). Stuttering and speech naturalness: Some additional data. *Journal of Speech and Hearing Disorders, 502*, 217–219.

Ingham, R. J., Ingham, J. C., Bothe, A., Wang, Y., & Kilgo, M. (2015). Efficacy of the Modifying Phonation Intervals (MPI) stuttering treatment program with adults who stutter. *American Journal of Speech-Language Pathology, 24*, 256–271.

Ingham, R. J., Ingham, J. C., Euler, H. A., & Neumann, K. (2018). Stuttering treatment and brain research in adults: A still unfolding relationship. *Journal of Fluency Disorders, 55*, 106–119.

Ingham, R. J., Ingham, J. C., Finn, P., & Fox, P. T. (2003). Towards a functional neural systems model of developmental stuttering. *Journal of Fluency Disorders, 284*, 297–318.

Ingham, R. J., Wang, Y., Ingham, J., Bothe, A., & Grafton, S. (2013). Regional brain activity change predicts responsiveness to treatment for stuttering in adults. *Brain and Language, 127*(3), 510–519.

International Classification of Functioning, *Disability, and health*. (2001)

Ito, T. (1986). Speech dysfluency and the acquisition of syntax in children 2-6 years old. *Folia Phoniatrica, 38*, 310. (Abstract).

Iverach, L., O'Brian, S., Jones, M., Block, S., Lincoln, M., Harrison, E., & Onslow, M. (2009). Prevalence of anxiety disorders among adults seeking speech therapy for stuttering. *Journal of Anxiety Disorders, 23*(7), 928–934.

Jafari, H., Mohamadi, M., Haghjoo, A., & Heidari, M. (2019). Newly recognized stuttering in three young children following the Hojedk earthquake in Iran. *Prehospital and Disaster Medicine, 34*(4), 456–457.

Jaffe, J., & Anderson, S. W. (1979). Prescript to Chapter 1: Communication rhythms and the evolution of language. In A. W. Siegman & S. Feldman (Eds.), *Of speech and time: Temporal speech patterns, interpersonal contexts*. Lawrence Erlbaum Associates.

James, W. (1890). *The principles of psychology*. Holt & Co.

Jancke, L., Hanggi, J., & Steinmetz, H. (2004). Morphological brain differences between adult stutterers and non-stutterers. *BMC Neurology, 4*, 23.

Janssen, P., Kraaimaat, F., & Brutten, G. (1990). Relationship between stutterers' genetic history and speech associated variables. *Journal of Fluency Disorders, 8*, 39–48.

Jensen, P. J., Sheehan, J. G., Williams, W. M., & LaPointe, L. L. (1975). Oral-sensory-perceptual integrity of stutterers. *Folia Phoniatrica, 272*, 106–115.

Johnson, K. N., Walden, T. A., Conture, E. G., & Karrass, J. (2010). Spontaneous regulation of emotions in pre-school children who stutter: Preliminary findings. *Journal of Speech, Language and Hearing Research, 53*(6), 1478–1495.

Johnson, W. (1944). The Indians have no word for it: II. Stuttering in adults. *Quarterly Journal of Speech, 30*, 456–465.

Johnson, W. (1955). A study of the onset and development of stuttering. In W. Johnson & R. R. Leutenegger (Eds.), *Stuttering children and adults*. University of Minnesota Press.

Johnson, W. (1942). A study of the onset and development of stuttering. *Journal of Speech Disorders, 7*, 251–257.

Johnson, W.; and Associates (1959). *The onset of stuttering*. University of Minnesota Press.

Johnson, W., & Brown, S. (1935). Stuttering in relation to various speech sounds. *Quarterly Journal of Speech, 21*, 481–496.

Johnson, W., Darley, F., & Spriestersbach, D. (1952). *Diagnostic manual in speech correction: A professional training workbook*. Harper & Brothers.

Johnson, W., & Inness, M. (1939). Studies in the psychology of stuttering: XIII. A statistical analysis of the adaptation and consistency effects in relation to stuttering. *Journal of Speech Disorders, 4*, 79–86.

Johnson, W., & Knott, J. R. (1937). Studies in the psychology of stuttering: I. The distribution of moments of stuttering in successive readings of the same material. *Journal of Speech Disorders, 2*, 17–19.

Johnson, W., & Moeller, D. (1967). *Speech handicapped school children*. Harper & Row.

Johnson, W., & Rosen, L. (1937). Studies in the psychology of stuttering: VII. Effects of certain changes in speech pattern upon frequency of stuttering. *Journal of Speech Disorders, 2*, 105–109.

Johnson, W., & Solomon, A. (1937). Studies in the psychology of stuttering: IV. A quantitative study of expectation of stuttering as a process involving a low degree of consciousness. *Journal of Speech Disorders, 2*, 95–97.

Jokel, R., De Nil, L. F., & Sharpe, K. (2007). Speech disfluencies in adults with neurogenic stuttering associated with stroke and traumatic brain injury. *Journal of Medical Speech-Language Pathology, 15*(3), 243–261.

Jones, J. E., & Niven, P. (1993). *Voices and silences*. Charles Scribner's Sons.

Jones, M., Onslow, M., Harrison, E., & Packman, A. (2000). Treating stuttering in young children: Predicting treatment time in the Lidcombe Program. *Journal of Speech Language and Hearing Research, 43*, 1440–1450.

Jones, M., Onslow, M., Packman, A., Williams, S., & Ormond, T. (2005). Randomized control trial of the Lidcombe programme of early stuttering intervention. *BMJ, 331*, 659.

Jones, R., Choi, D., Conture, E. G., & Walden, T. A. (2014). Temperament, emotion, and childhood stuttering. *Seminars in Speech and Language, 35*(2), 114–131.

Jones, R. K. (1966). Observations on stammering after localized cerebral injury. *Journal of Neurology, Neurosurgery and Psychiatry, 29*, 192–195.

Jossinger, S., Sares, A., Zislis, A., Sury, D., Gracco, V., & Ben-Shachar, M. (2022). White matter correlates of sensorimotor synchronization in persistent developmental stuttering. *Journal of Communication Disorders, 95*(1), 106169.

Junuzovic-Zunic, L., Sinanovic, O., & Majic, B. (2021). Neurogenic stuttering: Etiology, symptomatology and treatment. *Medicinski Arhiv, 75*(6), 456–461.

Jurgens, U. (1979). Vocalization as an emotional indicator. *Behavior, 69*(1), 88–117.

Jurgens, U. (1994). The role of the periaqueductal grey in vocal behaviour. *Behavioural Brain Research, 62*(2), 107–117.

Juste, F. S., & Furquim de Andrade, C. R. (2011). Speech disfluency types of fluent and stuttering individuals: Age effects. *Folia Phoniatrica et Logopedica, 63*(2), 57–64.

Kagan, J. (1981). *The second year: The emergence of self-awareness*. Harvard University Press.

Kagan, J. (1989). Temperamental contributions to social behavior. *American Psychologist, 44*, 668–674.

Kagan, J. (1994a). The realistic view of biology and behavior. *The Chronicle of Higher Education, 5*, A64.

Kagan, J. (1994b). *Galen's prophecy: Temperament in human nature*. Basic Books.

Kagan, J., Reznick, J. S., & Snidman, N. (1987). The physiology and psychology of behavioral inhibition in children. *Child Development, 58*, 1459–1473.

Kagan, J., & Snidman, N. (1991). Temperamental factors in human development. *American Psychologist, 468*, 856–862.

Kang, C., Riazuddin, S., Mundorf, J., Krasnewich, D., Friedman, P., Mulliken, J., & Drayna, D. (2010). Mutations in the lysosomal enzyme-targeting pathway and persistent stuttering. *New England Journal of Medicine, 362*(8), 677–685.

Karlin, I. W. (1947). A psychosomatic theory of stuttering. *Journal of Speech Disorders, 12*(3), 319–322.

Karniol, R. (1992). Stuttering out of bilingualism. *First Language, 12*(38), 255–283.

Karrass, J., Walden, T. A., Conture, E. G., Graham, C. G., Arnold, H. S., & Hartfield, K. N. (2006). Relation of emotional reactivity and regulation to childhood stuttering. *Journal of Communication Disorders, 32*, 402–423.

Kay, D. (1964). The genetics of stuttering. In G. Andrew & M. Harris (Eds.), *The syndrome of stuttering* (pp. 132–143). The Spastics Society Medical Education and Information Unit.

Kefalianos, E., Onslow, M., Ukoumunne, O. C., Block, S., & Reilly, S. (2017). Temperament and early stuttering development: Cross-sectional findings from a community cohort. *Journal of Speech, Language and Hearing Research, 60*(4), 772–784.

Kell, C., Neumann, K., von Kriegstein, K., Posenenske, C., von Gudenberg, A., Euler, H. A., & Giraud, A.-L. (2009). How the brain repairs stuttering. *Brain, 132*(10), 2747-2760.

Kelly, E. (1994). Speech rates and turn-taking behaviors of children who stutter and their fathers. *Journal of Speech and Hearing Research, 37*, 1284–1267.

Kelly, E., & Conture, E. G. (1992). Speaking rates, response time latencies, and interrupting behaviors of young stutterers, nonstutterers, and their mothers. *Journal of Speech and Hearing Research, 35*, 1256–1267.

Kelly, E., Smith, A., & Goffman, L. (1995). Orofacial muscle activity of children who stutter. *Journal of Speech and Hearing Research, 38*, 1025–1036.

Kelman, E., & Nicholas, A. (2008). *Practical intervention for early childhood stammering: Palin PCI*. Speechmark.

Kelman, E., & Nicholas, A. (2020). *Palin parent-child interaction therapy for early childhood stammering*. Routledge.

Kelman, E., & Whyte, A. (2012). *Understanding stammering or stuttering: A guide for parents, teachers and other professionals*. Jessica Kingsley Publishers.

Kent, R. D. (1981). Sensorimotor aspects of speech development. In R. D. Alberts & M. R. Peterson (Eds.), *The development of perception: Psycho-biological perspectives*. Academic Press.

Kent, R. D. (1984). Stuttering as a temporal programming disorder. In R. F. Curlee & W. H. Perkins (Eds.), *Nature and treatment of stuttering: New directions* (pp. 283–301). College-Hill Press.

Kent, R. D. (1985). Developing and disordered speech: Strategies for organization. *ASHA Reports, 15*, 29–37.

Kent, R. D. (1993). Speech intelligibility and communicative competence in children. In A. P. Kiser & D. B. Gray (Eds.), *Enhancing children's communication: Research foundations for intervention* (Vol. 2, pp. 223–229). Brooks Publishing.

Kent, R. D. (2000). Research on speech motor control and its disorders: A review and prospective. *Journal of Communication Disorders, 33*, 391–428.

Kent, R. D., & Perkins, W. (1984). *Oral-verbal fluency: Aspects of verbal formulation, speech motor control and underlying neural systems*. (Unpublished manuscript).

Kent, R. D., & Vorperian, H. K. (1995). Anatomic development of the craniofacial-oral-laryngeal systems: A review. *Journal of Medical Speech-Language Pathology, 3*, 145–190.

Kent, R. D., & Vorperian, H. K. (2007). In the mouths of babes: Anatomic motor and sensory foundations of speech development. In R. Paul (Ed.), *Language disorders from a developmental perspective: Essays in honor of Robin Chapman*` (pp. 56–80). Lawrence Erlbaum.

Kent, R. D., & Vorperian, H. K. (2013). Speech impairment in Down syndrome: A review. *Journal of Speech, Language and Hearing Research, 56*, 178–210.

Kenyon, E. L. (1942). The etiology of stammering: Fundamentally a wrong psychophysiologic habit in control of the vocal cords for the production of an individual speech sound. *Journal of Speech Disorders, 7*, 97–104.

Kessler, R. C., Amminger, G. P., Aguilar-Gaxiola, S., Alonso, J., Lee, S., & Ustun, T. B. (2007). Age of onset of mental disorders: A review of recent literature. *Current Opinion in Psychiatry, 20*(4), 359–364.

Kidd, K. K. (1977). A genetic perspective on stuttering. *Journal of Fluency Disorders, 2*, 259–269.

Kidd, K. K. (1984). Stuttering as a genetic disorder. In R. Curlee & W. Perkins (Eds.), *Nature and treatment of stuttering: New directions* (pp. 149–169). College-Hill Press.

Kidd, K. K., Heimbuch, R. C., Records, M. A., Oehlert, G., & Webster, R. L. (1980). Familial stuttering patterns are not related to one measure of severity. *Journal of Speech and Hearing Research, 23*, 539–545.

Kidd, K. K., Kidd, J. R., & Records, M. A. (1978). The possible causes of the sex ratio in stuttering and its implications. *Journal of Fluency Disorders, 3*, 13–23.

Kidd, K. K., Reich, T., & Kessler, S. (1973). A genetic analysis of stuttering suggesting a single major locus. *Genetics, 74*(2 (Pt. 2)), 137.

Kikuchi, Y., Okamoto, T., Ogata, K., Hagiwara, K., Umezaki, T., & Kenjo, M. (2017). Abnormal auditory synchronization in stuttering: A magnetoencephalographic study. *Hearing Research, 344*, 82–89.

Kim, K. S., Daliri, A., Flanagan, J. R., & Max, L. (2020). Dissociated development of speech and limb sensorimotor learning in stuttering: Speech auditory-motor learning is impaired in both children and adults who stutter. *Neuroscience and Behavioral Physiology, 451*, 1–211.

Kinsbourne, M. (1989). A model of adaptive behavior related to cerebral participation in emotional control. In G. Gianotti & C. Caltagirone (Eds.), *Emotions and the dual brain*. Springer-Verlag.

Kinsbourne, M., & Hicks, R. (1978). Functional cerebral space: A model for overflow, transfer and interference effects in human performance: A tutorial review. In M. Kinsbourne (Ed.), *Asymmetrical function of the brain* (pp. 345–362). Cambridge University Press.

Kinsbourne, M. B., & Bemporad, E. (1984). Lateralization of emotion: A model and the evidence. In N. A. Fox & R. J. Davidson (Eds.), *The psychology of affective development*. Lawrence Erlbaum Associates.

Kirschbaum, C., Pirke, K. M., & Hellhammer, D. H. (1993). The 'Trier Social Stress Test': A tool for investigating psychobiological stress responses in a laboratory setting. *Neuropsychobiology, 28*, 76–81.

Kleinow, J., & Smith, A. (2000). Influences of length and syntactic complexity on the speech motor stability of the fluent speech of adults who stutter. *Journal of Speech, Language, and Hearing Research, 432*, 548–559.

Kloth, S., Janssen, P., Kraaimaat, F., & Brutten, G. (1995). Speech-motor and linguistic skills of young stutterers prior to onset. *Journal of Fluency Disorders, 20*, 157–170.

Kloth, S., Janssen, P., Kraaimaat, F., & Brutten, G. (1998). Child and mother variables in the development of stuttering among high-risk children: A longitudinal study. *Journal of Fluency Disorders, 23*, 217–230.

Kloth, S. A. M., Kraaimaat, F. W., Janssen, P., & Brutten, G. J. (1999). Persistence and remission of incipient stuttering among high-risk children. *Journal of Fluency Disorders, 244*, 253–265.

Knott, J. R., Johnson, W., & Webster, M. J. (1937). Studies in the psychology of stuttering: II. A quantitative evaluation of expectation of stuttering in relation to the occurrence of stuttering. *Journal of Speech Disorders, 2*, 20–22.

Kolk, H., & Postma, A. (1997). Stuttering as a covert repair phenomenon. In R. F. Curlee & G. M. Siegel (Eds.), *Nature and treatment of stuttering: New directions* (2nd ed., pp. 182–203). Allyn & Bacon.

Kraft, S. J. (2010). *Genome-wide association study of persistent developmental stuttering*. (PhD dissertation). University of Illinois.

Kraft, S. J., Ambrose, N. G., & Chon, H. (2014). Temperament and environmental contributions to stuttering severity in children: The role of effortful control. *Seminars in Speech and Language, 35*, 80–94.

Kraft, S. J., Lowther, E., & Beilby, J. (2019). The role of effortful control in stuttering severity in children: Replication study. *American Journal of Speech-Language Pathology, 28*(1), 14–28.

Kraft, S. J., & Yairi, E. (2012). Genetic basis of stuttering: State of the art, 2011. *Folia Phoniatrica et Logopedica, 64*, 34–47.

Kramer, M., Green, D., & Guitar, B. (1987). A comparison of stutterers and nonstutterers on masking level differences and synthetic sentence identification tasks. *Journal of Communication Disorders, 20*, 379–390.

Krishnan, G., & Tiwari, S. (2013). Differential diagnosis in developmental and acquired stuttering: Do fuency-enhancing conditions dissociate the two? *Journal of Neurolinguistics, 26*, 252–257.

Kroll, R. M., De Nil, L. F., & Houle, S. (1999, November). *Towards an scientific understanding of stuttering and treatment: PET scan studies. Paper presented at the Annual Meeting of the American Speech-Language-Hearing Association*. San Francisco.

Kroll, R. M., De Nil, L. F., Kapur, S., & Houle, S. (1997). A positron emission tomography investigation of post-treatment brain activation in stutterers. In W. Hulstijn, H. F. M. Peters & P. H. H. M. van Lieshout (Eds.), *Speech production: Motor control, brain research and fluency disorders* (pp. 307–319). Elsevier.

Kroll, R. M., & Scott-Sulsky, L. (2010). The Fluency Plus Program: An integration of fluency shaping and cognitive restructuring procedures for adolescents and adults who stutter. In B. Guitar & R. J. McCauley (Eds.), *Treatment of stuttering: Established and emerging interventions* (pp. 277–311). Lippincott Williams and Wilkins.

Lagerkrantz, H. (2016). *Infant brain development: Formulation of the mind and the emergence of consciousness*. Springer.

Langevin, M., Huinck, W. J., Kully, D., Peters, H. F. M., Lomheim, H., & Tellers, M. (2006). A cross-cultural, long-term outcome evaluation of the ISTAR Comprehensive Stuttering Program across Dutch and Canadian adults who stutter. *Journal of Fluency Disorders, 31*(4), 229–256.

Langevin, M., Packman, A., & Onslow, M. (2010). Parent perceptions of the impact of stuttering on their preschoolers and themselves. *Journal of Communication Disorders, 43*(5), 407–423.

Langlois, A., Hanrahan, L. L., & Inouye, L. L. (1986). A comparison of interactions between stuttering children, nonstuttering children, and their mothers. *Journal of Fluency Disorders, 11*, 263–273.

Langlois, A., & Long, S. H. (1988). A model for teaching parents to facilitate fluent speech. *Journal of Fluency Disorders, 13*, 163–172.

Lanouette, E. B. (2011). Intervention strategies for cluttering disorders. In D. Ward & K. S. Scott (Eds.), *Cluttering: A handbook of research, intervention and education* (pp. 175–197). Psychology Press.

LaSalle, L., Ames, A., & Maguire, G. (2022). Pharmacological considerations. In P. Zebrowski, J. Anderson & E. Conture (Eds.), *Stuttering and related disorders of fluency* (4th ed.). Thieme.

LaSalle, L. R. (1999, November). *Temperament in preschoolers who stutter: A preliminary investigation. Paper presented at the Annual meeting of the American Speech-Language-Hearing Association*. San Francisco.

LaSalle, L. R., & Conture, E. G. (1995). Disfluency clusters of children who stutter: Relation of stutterings to self-repairs. *Journal of Speech and Hearing Research, 38*, 965–977.

Latterman, C., Euler, H. A., & Neumann, K. (2008). A randomized control trial to investigate the impact of the Lidcombe Program on early stuttering in German-speaking preschoolers. *Journal of Fluency Disorders, 33*, 52–65.

Lauter, J. L. (1995). Visions of speech and language: Noninvasive imaging techniques and their applications to the study of human communication. In H. Winitz (Ed.), *Current approaches to the study of language development and disorders* (pp. 277–390). York Press.

Lauter, J. L. (1997). Noninvasive brain imaging in speech motor control and stuttering: Choices and challenges. In W. Hulstijn, H. F. M. Peters & P. H. H. M. van Lieshout (Eds.), *Speech production: Motor control, brain research, and fluency disorders* (pp. 233–258). Elsevier.

Lazare, A. (1981). Current concepts in psychiatry: Conversion symptoms. *New England Journal of Medicine, 305*, 745.

Leahy, P. (2022). *The road taken: A memoir*. Simon & Schuster.

LeDoux, J. E. (2002). *Synaptic self: How our brains become who we are*. Viking.

LeDoux, J. E. (2015). *Anxious: Using the brain to understand and treat fear and anxiety*. Viking.

Lee, B. S. (1951). Artificial stutter. *Journal of Speech and Hearing Disorders, 16*, 53–55.

Lee, W.-S., Kang, C., Drayna, D., & Kornfield, S. (2011). Analysis of mannose 6-phosphate uncovering enzyme mutations associated with persistent stuttering. *Journal of Biological Chemistry, 286*, 39786–39793.

Leech, K. A., Bernstein Ratner, N., Brown, B., & Weber, C. (2017). Preliminary evidence that growth in productive language differentiates childhood stuttering persistence and recovery. *Journal of Speech Language and Hearing Research, 60*(11), 3097–3109.

Leech, K. A., Bernstein Ratner, N., Brown, B., & Weber, C. (2019). Language growth predicts stuttering persistence over and above family history and treatment experience: Response to Marcotte. *Journal of Speech Language and Hearing Research, 62*(5), 1371–1372.

Lesner, T. A., & Walden, T. A. (2018). Examining implicit and explicit attitudes toward stuttering. *Journal of Fluency Disorders, 57*, 22–36.

Levine, P. (2010). *In an unspoken voice: How the body releases tramua and restores goodness*. North Atlantic Books.

Levitin, D., & Menon, V. (2003). Musical structure is processed in "language" areas of the brain: A possible role for Brodmann Area 47 in temporal coherence. *NeuroImage, 20*(4), 2142–2152.

Lewis, M. (2000). Self-conscious emotions: Embarrassment, pride, shame and guilt. In M. Lewis & J. M. Haviland-Jones (Eds.), *Handbook of emotions* (2nd ed.). Guilford Press.

Libertus, K., & Violi, D. A. (2016). Sit to talk: Relation between motor skills and language development in infancy. *Frontiers in Psychology, 7*, 475.

Libin, N. (2019). *Five-minute mindfulness meditations for teens*. Rockridge Press.

Lidz, T. (1968). *The person: His development throughout the life cycle*. Basic Books.

Lieberman, A. (2018). Counseling issues: Addressing behavioral and emotional considerations in the treatment of communication disorders. *American Journal of Speech-Language Pathology, 27*, 13–23.

Liebetrau, R., & Daly, D. A. (1981). Auditory processing and perceptual abilities of organic and functional stutterers. *Journal of Fluency Disorders, 6*, 219–231.

Lincoln, M., & Onslow, M. (1997). Long-term outcome of an early intervention for stuttering. *American Journal of Speech-Language Pathology, 6*, 51–58.

Lindsay, J. (1989). Relationship of developmental disfluency and episodes of stuttering to the emergence of cognitive stages in children. *Journal of Fluency Disorders, 14*, 271–284.

Livingston, L. A., Flowers, Y. E., Hodor, B. A., & Ryan, B. P. (2000). The experimental analysis of interruption during conversation for three children who stutter. *Journal of Developmental and Physical Disabilities, 12*, 235–266.

Logan, K. (2020). *Fluency disorders* (2nd ed.). Plural.

Logan, K., & Conture, E. G. (1995). Length, grammatical complexity, and rate differences in stuttered and fluent conversational utterances of children who stutter. *Journal of Fluency Disorders, 20*, 35–61.

Luchsinger, R. (1944). Biological studies on monozygotic and dizigotic twins relative to size and form of the larynx. *Archiv Julius Klaus-Stiftung fur Verergungsforchung, 19*, 3–4.

Luckman, C., Wagovich, S. A., Weber, C., Brown, B., Chang, S. E., Hall, N. E., & Bernstein Ratner, N. (2020). Lexical diversity and lexical skills in children who stutter. *Journal of Fluency Disorders, 63*, 105747.

Luper, H., & Mulder, R. (1964). *Stuttering: Therapy for children*. Prentice-Hall.

Machado, L., & Cantilino, A. (2017). A systematic review of the neural correlate of positive emotion. *Brazilian Journal of Psychiatry, 39*(2), 172–179.

MacKinnon, S., Hall, S., & MacIntyre, P. (2007). Origins of the stuttering stereotype: Stereotype formation through anchoring-adjustment. *Journal of Fluency Disorders, 32*(4), 297–309.

MacPherson, M. K., & Smith, A. (2013). Influences of sentence length and syntactic complexity on the speech motor control of children who stutter. *Journal of Speech Language and Hearing Research, 56*, 89–102.

Maguire, G., LaSalle, L., Hoffmeyer, D., Nelson, M., Lochhead, J. D., Davis, K., & Yaruss, J. S. (2019). Ecopipam as a pharmacologic treatment of stuttering. *Annals of Clinical Psychiatry, 31*(3), 164–168.

Maguire, G., Nguyen, D. L., Simonson, K. C., & Kurz, T. L. (2020). The pharmacological treatment of stuttering and its neuropharmacologic basis. *Frontiers in Neuroscience, 14*, 158.

Maguire, G., Riley, G., Franklin, D., & Gumusaneli, E. (2010). The physiological basis and pharmacological treatment of stuttering. In B. Guitar & R. J. McCauley (Eds.), *Treatment of stuttering: Established and emerging interventions* (pp. 329–354). Lippincott Williams & Wilkins.

Maguire, G., Yu, B., Franklin, D., & Riley, G. (2004). Alleviating stuttering with pharmacological interventions. *Expert Opinion in Pharmacotherapy, 5*(7), 1565–1571.

Mahr, G., & Leith, W. (1992). Psychogenic stuttering of adult onset. *Journal of Speech and Hearing Research, 35*, 283–286.

Mahurin-Smith, J., & Ambrose, N. G. (2013). Breastfeeding may protect against persistent stuttering. *Journal of Communication Disorders, 46*(4), 351–360.

Malecot, A., Johnston, R., & Kizziar, P.-A. (1972). Syllabic rate and utterance length in French. *Phonetica, 26*, 235–251.

Manning, W. H., & DiLillo, A. (2018). *Clinical decision making in fluency disorders* (4th ed.). Plural Publishing.

Mansson, H. (2000). Childhood stuttering: Incidence and development. *Journal of Fluency Disorders, 25*(1), 47–57.

Market, K. E., Montague, J. C., Buffalo, M. D., & Drummond, S. A. (1990). Acquired stuttering: Descriptive data and treatment outcomes. *Journal of Fluency Disorders, 15*, 21–33.

Marshall, R. C., & Starch, S. A. (1984). Behavioral treatment of acquired stuttering. *Australian Journal of Human Communication Disorders, 12*, 87–92.

Martin, R., Haroldson, S., & Triden, K. (1984). Stuttering and speech naturalness. *Journal of Speech and Hearing Disorders, 27*, 53–58.

Maske-Cash, W., & Curlee, R. (1995). Effect of utterance length and meaningfulness on the speech initiation times of children who stutter and children who do not stutter. *Journal of Speech and Hearing Research, 38*, 18–25.

Mattes, L. J., & Omack, D. R. (1991). *Speech and language assessment for the bilingually handicapped.* Academic Communication Associates.

Matthews, S., Williams, R., & Pring, T. (1997). Parent-child interaction therapy and dysfluency: A single-case study. *European Journal of Disorders of Communication, 32*(3), 346–357.

Max, L., Guenther, F. H., Gracco, V. L., Ghosh, S. S., & Wallace, M. E. (2004). Unstable or insufficiently activated internal models and feedback-biased motor-control as sources of dysfluency: A theoretical model of stuttering. *Contemporary Issues in Communication Science and Disorders, 31*, 105–122.

McAllister, J. (2016). Behavioural, emotional and social develoment of children who stutter. *Journal of Fluency Disorders, 50*, 23–32.

McCall, G. N., & Rabuzzi, D. D. (1973). Reflex contraction of middle-ear muscles secondary to stimulation of laryngeal nerves. *Journal of Speech, Language, and Hearing Disorders, 16*, 56–61.

McCauley, R. J. (1996). Familiar strangers: Criterion-referenced measures in communication disorders. *Language, Speech, and Hearing Services in Schools, 27*, 122–131.

McClean, M. D. (1990). Neuromotor aspects of stuttering: Levels of impairment and disability. In J. Cooper (Ed.), *Research needs in stuttering: Roadblocks and future directions (ASHA Reports, 18)* (pp. *64–71*). American Speech-Language-Hearing Association.

McClean, M. D., Kroll, R. M., & Loftus, N. S. (1990). Kinematic analysis of lip closure in stutterers' fluent speech. *Journal of Speech and Hearing Research, 33*, 755–760.

McClean, M. D., & McClean, A. (1985). Case report of stuttering acquired in association with phenytoin use for post-head-injury seizures. *Journal of Fluency Disorders, 10*, 241–255.

McDearmon, J. R. (1968). Primary stuttering at the onset of stuttering: A re-examination of data. *Journal of Speech and Hearing Research, 11*, 631–637.

McDevitt, S. C., & Carey, W. B. (1978). The measurement of temperament in 3 7-year-old children. *Journal of Child Psychology and Psychiatry and Allied Disciplines, 19*, 245–253.

McDevitt, S. C., & Carey, W. B. (1995). *Behavioral style questionnaire.* TemperaMetrics.

McFarlane, S. C., & Prins, D. (1978). Neural response time of stutterers and nonstutterers in selected oral motor tasks. *Journal of Speech and Hearing Research, 21*, 768–778.

Menzies, R., O'Brian, S., Onslow, M., Packman, A., St. Clare, T., & Block, S. (2008). An experimental clinical trial of a cognitive-behavior therapy package for chronic stuttering. *Journal of Speech, Language and Hearing Research, 51*(6), 1451–1464.

Menzies, R., Onslow, M., Packman, A., & O'Brian, S. (2009). Cognitive behavior therapy for adults who stutter: A tutorial for SLPs. *Journal of Fluency Disorders, 34*, 187–200.

Merits-Patterson, R., & Reed, C. G. (1981). Disfluencies in the speech of language-delayed children. *Journal of Speech, Language and Hearing Research, 24*, 55–58.

Meyers, S. C., & Freeman, F. J. (1985a). Interruptions as a variable in stuttering and disfluency. *Journal of Speech and Hearing Research, 28*, 428–425.

Meyers, S. C., & Freeman, F. J. (1985b). Mother and child speech rate as a variable in stuttering and disfluency. *Journal of Speech and Hearing Research, 28*, 436–444.

Miles, S., & Ratner, N. B. (2001). Parental language input to children at stuttering onset. *Journal of Speech Language and Hearing Research, 44*, 1116–1130.

Milisen, R. (1938). Frequency of stuttering with anticipation of stuttering controlled. *Journal of Speech Disorders, 3*, 207–214.

Milisen, R., & Johnson, W. (1936). A comparative study of stutterers, former stutterers and normal speakers whose handedness has been changed. *Archives of Speech, 1*, 61–68.

Millard, S. K., & Davis, S. (2016). The Palin parent rating scales: Parents' perceptions of childhood stuttering and its impact. *Journal of Speech Language and Hearing Research, 59*(5), 950–963.

Millard, S. K., Edwards, S., & Cook, F. (2009). Parent-child interaction therapy: Adding to the evidence. *International Journal of Speech & Language Pathology, 11*(1), 61–76.

Millard, S. K., Nicholas, A., & Cook, F. M. (2008). Is parent-child interaction therapy effective in reducing stuttering? *Journal of Speech Language and Hearing Research, 51*, 636–650.

Millard, S. K., Zebrowski, P., & Kelman, E. (2018). Palin parent-child interaction treatment: The bigger picture. *American Journal of Speech Language Pathology, 27*(3S), 1211–1223.

Miller, B., & Guitar, B. (2009). Long-term outcomes of the Lidcombe Program for early stuttering intervention. *American Journal of Speech-Language Pathology, 18*, 42–49.

Miller, S. (1993). *Multiple measures of anxiety and psychophysiologic arousal in stutterers and nonstutterers during nonspeech and speech tasks of increasing complexity.* (Unpublished doctoral dissertation). University of Texas.

Miller, W. R., & Rollnick, S. (2012). *Motivational interviewing: Helping people change*. Guilford Press.

Mineka, S. (1985). Animal models of anxiety-based disorders: Their usefulness and limitations. In A. H. Tuma & J. Mase (Eds.), *Anxiety and the anxiety disorders*. Lawrence Erlbaum Associates.

Mineka, S., & Oehlberg, K. (2008). The relevance of recent developments in classical conditioning to understanding the etiology and maintenance of anxiety disorders. *Acta Psychologica, 127*(3), 567–580.

Minifie, F. D., & Cooker, H. S. (1964). A disfluency index. *Journal of Speech and Hearing Disorders, 29*, 189–192.

Mogenson, G., Jones, D., & Yim, C. (1980). From motivation to action: Functional interface between the limbic system and the motor system. *Progress in Neurobiology, 14*(2-3), 69–97.

Mohan, R., & Weber, C. M. (2015). Neural systems mediating processing of sound units of language distinguish recovery vs. persistence in stuttering. *Journal of Neurodevelopmental Disorders, 7*(1), 28.

Molt, L. F. (1997). *Event-related cortical potentials and language processing in stutterers. Paper presented at the 2nd World Congress on Fluency Disorders*. San Francisco, CA.

Molt, L. F., & Guilford, A. M. (1979). Auditory processing and anxiety in stutterers. *Journal of Fluency Disorders, 4*, 255–267.

Moore, W. H. (1984). Hemispheric alpha asymmetries during an electromyographic biofeedback procedure for stuttering: A single subject experimental design. *Journal of Fluency Disorders, 9*(2), 143–162.

Moore, W. H., & Haynes, W. O. (1980). Alpha hemispheric asymmetry and stuttering: Some support for a segmentation dysfunction hypothesis. *Journal of Speech and Hearing Research, 23*, 229–247.

Morgenstern, J. (1956). Socio-economic factors in stuttering. *Journal of Speech and Hearing Disorders, 21*, 25–33.

Murphy, W. P., Quesal, R. W., Reardon-Reeves, N., & Yaruss, J. S. (2013). *Minimizing bullying for children who stutter*. Stuttering Therapy Resources.

Murphy, W. P., Yaruss, J. S., & Quesal, R. W. (2007a). Enhancing treatment for school-age children who stutter I: Reducing negative reactions through desensitization and cognitive restructuring. *Journal of Fluency Disorders, 32*(2), 121–138.

Murphy, W. P., Yaruss, J. S., & Quesal, R. W. (2007b). Enhancing treatment for school-age children who stutter: II. Reducing bullying through role-playing and self-disclosure. *Journal of Fluency Disorders, 32*(2), 139–162.

Murray, F. (2001). *A stutterer's story* (2nd ed.). Stuttering Foundation of America.

My beautiful stutter (2021). *Film. Directed by Ryan Gielen. Produced by Michael Alden, Ryan Gielen et al.*

Myers, F. L. (1978). Relationship between eight physiological variables and severity of stuttering. *Journal of Fluency Disorders, 3*, 181–191.

Myers, F. L. (2002, November). *Putting cluttering on the map: Looking back/looking ahead. Paper presented at the Annual meeting of the American Speech Language and Hearing Association*. Atlanta.

Myers, F. L. (2011). Treatment of cluttering: A cognitive-behavioral approach centered on rate control. In D. Ward & K. S. Scott (Eds.), *Cluttering: A handbook of research, intervention and education* (pp. 152–174). Psychology Press.

Myers, F. L., & St. Louis, K. (1986). *Cluttering: A clinical perspective*. Singular.

Myers, F. L., & St. Louis, K. (2007). Cluttering [DVD]. Stuttering Foundation.

Namasivayam, A. K., & van Lieshout, P. (2011). Speech motor skill and stuttering. *Journal of Motor Behavior, 43*(6), 477–489.

Namasivayam, A. K., van Lieshout, P., McIlroy, W. E., & De Nil, L. F. (2009). Sensory feedback dependence hypothesis in persons who stutter. *Human Movement Science, 28*(6), 688–707.

Nandhini Devi, G., Thalamuthub, A., Valarmathic, S., Karthikeyend, N. P., & Srikumari, C. S. (2018). Genetic epidemiology of stuttering among school children in the state of Tamil Nadu, India. *Journal of Fluency Disorders, 58*, 11–21.

National Institute of Neurological Disorders and Stroke. (2011). *Mucolipidoses fact sheet*. \\http:www.ninds.nih.gov/disorders/mucolipidoses/detail_mucolipidoses.htm

Navon, D. (1984). Resources--A theoretical stone soup. *Psychological Review, 912*, 216–234.

Neef, N. E., Anwander, A., Butfering, C., Schmidt-Samoa, C., Friederici, A. D., Paulus, W., & Sommer, M. (2018). Structural connectivity of right frontal hyperactive areas scales with stuttering severity. *Brain, 141*(1), 191–204.

Neef, N. E., Primaβin, A., von Gudenberg, A. W., Dechent, P., Riedel, H. C., Paulus, W., & Sommer, M. (2021). Two cortical representations of voice control are differentially involved in speech fluency. *Brain Communications, 3*(2), 232.

Neilson, M. D. (1980). *Stuttering and the control of speech: A systems analysis approach*. (Unpublished doctoral dissertation). University of New South Wales.

Neilson, M. D., Howie, P. M., & Andrews, G. (1987). *Does foetal testosterone play a role in the aetiology of stuttering? Paper presented at the Fifth International Australasian Winter Conference on Brain Research*. Queenstown, NZ.

Neilson, M. D., & Neilson, P. D. (1987). Speech motor control and stuttering: A computational model of adaptive sensory-motor processing. *Speech Communication, 6*, 325–333.

Neilson, M. D., & Neilson, P. D. (1988). *Sensory-motor integration capacity of stutterers and nonstutterers. Paper presented at the Second Australian International Conference on Speech Science and Technology*. Sydney, Australia.

Neilson, P. D., & Neilson, M. D. (2005a). An overview of adaptive model theory: Solving the problems of redundancy, resources, and nonlinear interactions in human movement control. *Journal of Neural Engineering, 2*, S279–S312.

Neilson, P. D., & Neilson, M. D. (2005b). Motor maps and synergies. *Human Movement Science, 24*, 774–797.

Neilson, P. D., Neilson, M. D., & O'Dwyer, N. J. (1992). Adaptive model theory: Application to disorders of motor control. In J. J. Summers (Ed.), *Approaches to the study of motor control and learning*. Elsevier Science Publishers.

Neilson, P. D., Quinn, P. T., & Neilson, M. D. (1976). Auditory tracking measures of hemispheric asymmetry in normals and stutterers. *Australian Journal of Human Communication, 4*, 121–126.

Netsell, R. (1981). The acquisition of speech motor control: A perspective with direction for research. In R. Stark (Ed.), *Language behavior in infancy and early childhood*. Elsevier-North Holland.

Neumann, K., & Euler, H. A. (2010). Neuroimaging and stuttering. In B. Guitar & R. McCauley (Eds.), *Stuttering treatment: Established and emerging approaches* (pp. 355–377). Lippincott, Williams & Wilkins.

Neumann, K., Euler, H. A., Wolff von Gudenberg, A., Giraud, A.-L., Lanfermann, H., & Gall, V. (2003). The nature and treatment of stuttering as revealed by fMRI: A within- and between-group comparison. *Journal of Fluency Disorders, 28*, 381–410.

Neumann, K., Preibisch, C., Euler, H. A., Wolff von Gudenberg, A., Giraud, A.-L., & Lanfermann, H. (2005). Cortical plasticity associated with stuttering therapy. *Journal of Fluency Disorders, 30*, 23–29.

Newman, L., & Smit, A. (1989). Some effects of variations in response time latency on speech rate, interruptions, and fluency in children's speech. *Journal of Speech Language and Hearing Research, 32*, 635–644.

Nicholas, A. (2015). Solution focused brief therapy with children who stutter. *Procedia - Social and Behavioral Sciences, 193*, 209–216. 10.1016/j.sbspro.2015.03.261

Nina, G. (2019). *Stuttering interrupted: The comedian who almost didn't happen*. She Writes Press.

Nippold, M. A. (2012). Stuttering and language ability in children: Questioning the connection. *American Journal of Speech-Language Pathology, 21*, 183–196.

Nittrouer, S., Studdert-Kennedy, M., & McGowan, R. S. (1989). The emergence of phonetic segments: Evidence from the spectral structure of fricative-vowel syllables spoken by children and adults. *Journal of Speech and Hearing Research, 32*, 120–132.

Norman, R. S., Jaramillo, C. A., Eapen, B. C., Amuan, M. E., & Pugh, M. J. (2018). Acquired stuttering in veterans of the wars of Iraq and Afghanistan: The role of traumatic brain injury, post-traunmatic stress disorder, and medications. *Military Medicine, 183*(11/12), e526–e534.

Norona-Zhou, A. N., & Tung, I. (2021). Developmental patterns of emotion regulation in toddlerhood: Examining predictors of change and long-term resilience. *Infant Mental Health Journal, 42*(1), 5–20.

Ntourou, K., Anderson, J., & Wagovich, S. (2018). Executive function and childhood stuttering: Parent ratings and evidence from a behavioral task. *Journal of Fluency Disorders, 56*, 18–32.

Ntourou, K., Conture, E. G., & Lipsey, M. W. (2011). Language abilities of children who stutter: A meta-analytical review. *Journal of Speech-Language Pathology, 20*(3), 163–179.

Ntourou, K., Conture, E. G., & Walden, T. A. (2013). Emotional reactivity and regulation in pre-school age children who stutter. *Journal of Fluency Disorders, 38*(3), 260–274.

Ntourou, K., DeFranco, E., Conture, E. G., Walden, T., & Mushtaq, N. (2020). A parent-report scale of behavioral intervention: Validation and application of pre-school children who do and do not stutter. *Journal of Fluency Disorders, 63*, 1–18.

Nudelman, H. B., Herbrich, K. E., Hess, K. R., Hoyt, B. D., & Rosenfield, D. B. (1992). A model of the phonation response time of stutterers and fluent speakers to frequency-modulated tones. *Journal of the Acoustical Society of America, 92*(4), 1882–1888. (Part 1).

Nudelman, H. B., Herbrich, K. E., Hoyt, B. D., & Rosenfield, D. B. (1987). Dynamic characteristics of vocal frequency tracking in stutterers and nonstutterers. In H. F. M. Peters & W. Hulstijn (Eds.), *Speech motor dynamics in stuttering*. Springer-Verlag.

Nudelman, H. B., Herbrich, K. E., Hoyt, B. D., & Rosenfield, D. B. (1989). A neuro-science model of stuttering. *Journal of Fluency Disorders, 14*, 399–427.

Nurnberg, H. G., & Greenwald, B. (1981). Stuttering: An unusual side effect of phenothiasines. *American Journal of Psychiatry, 138*, 386–387.

O'Brian, S., Carey, S., Lowe, R., Onslow, M., Packman, A., & Cream, A. (2017). *Camperdown Program: Stuttering treatment guide*. Australian Stuttering Research Centre.

O'Brian, S., Heard, R., Onslow, M., Packman, A., & Lowe, R. (2020). Clinical trials of adult stuttering treatment: Comparison of percentage syllables stuttered with self-reported stuttering severity outcomes. *Journal of Speech Language and Hearing Research, 63*, 1387–1394.

O'Brian, S., Packman, A., & Onslow, M. (2008). Telehealth delivery of the Camperdown program for adults who stutter: A Phase I trial. *Journal of Speech, Language and Hearing Research, 51*, 184–195.

O'Brian, S., Smith, K., & Onslow, M. (2014). Webcam delivery of the Lidcombe Program for early stuttering: A Phase 1 clinical trial. *Journal of Speech Language and Hearing Research, 57*, 825–830.

Olander, L., Smith, A., & Zelaznik, H. N. (2010). Evidence that a motor timing deficit is a factor in the development of stuttering. *Journal of Speech and Hearing Research, 53*, 876–886.

Onslow, M., Andrews, C., & Costa, L. (1990a). Parental severity scaling of early stuttered speech: Four case studies. *Australian Journal of Human Communication, 18*, 47–61.

Onslow, M., Andrews, C., & Lincoln, M. (1994). A control/experimental trial of an operant treatment for early stuttering. *Journal of Speech and Hearing Research, 37*, 1244–1259.

Onslow, M., Costa, L., & Rue, S. (1990b). Direct early intervention with stuttering: Some preliminary data. *Journal of Speech and Hearing Disorders, 55*, 405–416.

Onslow, M., Harrison, E., Jones, M., & Packman, A. (2002). Beyond-clinic speech measures during the Lidcombe Program of early stuttering intervention. *ACQuiring KNowledge in Speech, Language, and Hearing, 4*, 82–85.

Onslow, M., Jones, M., O'Brian, S., Packman, A., Menzies, R., Lowe, R., & Franken, M.-C. (2018). Comparison of percentage syllables stuttered with parent-reported severity ratings as a primary outcome measure in clinical trials of early stuttering treatment. *Journal of Speech-Language Hearing Research, 61*(4), 811–819.

Onslow, M., & Kelly, E. (2020). Temperament and early stuttering intervention: Two perspectives. *Journal of Fluency Disorders, 64*, 1–8.

Onslow, M., Packman, A., & Harrison, E. (2003). *The Lidcombe program of early stuttering intervention: A clinician's guide*. Pro-Ed.

Onslow, M., Webber, M., Harrison, E., Arnott, S., Bridgeman, K., & Carey, B. (2017, December). The *Lidcombe program treatment guide*. [lidcombeprogram.org]

Ooki, S. (2005). Genetic and environmental influences on stuttering and tics in Japanese twins. *Twin Research and Human Genetics, 8*, 529–575.

Ornstein, A. F., & Manning, W. H. (1985). Self-efficacy scaling by adult stutterers. *Journal of Communication Disorders, 18*, 313–320.

Orton, S. (1927). Studies in stuttering. *Archives of Neurology and Psychiatry, 18*, 671–672.

Orton, S., & Travis, L. (1929). Studies in stuttering: IV. Studies of action currents in stuttering. *Archives of Neurology and Psychiatry, 21*, 61–68.

Oyler, M. E. (1992, November). *Self perception and sensitivity in stuttering adults. Paper presented at the Annual meeting of the American Speech-Language-Hearing Association*. San Antonio, TX.

Oyler, M. E., & Ramig, P. R. (1995, November). *Vulnerability in stuttering children. Paper presented at the Annual meeting of the American Speech-Language-Hearing Association.* Orlando, FL.

Packman, A., & Attanasio, J. (2010). *A model of the mechanisms underpinning early intervention for stuttering. Paper presented at the Annual Meeting of the American Speech-Language and Hearing Association.* Philadelphia.

Packman, A., & Attanasio, J. (2017). *Theoretical issues in stuttering* (2nd ed.). Routledge Press.

Packman, A., Code, C., & Onslow, M. (2007). On the causes of stuttering: Integrating theory with brain and behavioral research. *Journal of Neurolinguistics, 20*(5), 353–362.

Paden, E. P. (2005). Development of phonological ability: For clinicians by clinicians. In E. Yairi & N. G. Ambrose (Eds.), *Early childhood stuttering* (pp. 197–234). Pro-Ed.

Park, V., Onslow, M., Lowe, R., Jones, M., O'Brian, S., Packman, A., & Hewat, S. (2021). Psychological characteristics of early stuttering. *International Journal of Speech-Language Pathology, 23*, 622–631. 10.1080/17549507.2021.1912826

Paul, R., Norbury, C., & Goose, C. (2018). *Language disorders from infancy through adolescence: Listening, speaking, reading, writing and communicating* (5th ed.). Elsevier.

Paulesu, E., Frith, C. D., & Frackowiak, R. S. J. (1993). The neural correlates of the verbal component of working memory. *Nature, 362*, 342–345.

Pavuluri, M. N., & Passarotti, A. (2008). Neural bases of emotional processing in pediatric bipolar disorder. *Expert Review of Neurotherapeutics, 8*(9), 1381–1387.

Peacock, J. (2020). *Psychogenic stuttering: Diagnosis and treatment. Paper presented at the Michigan Speech and Hearing Association Annual Conference.*

Pearl, S. Z., & Bernthal, J. E. (1980). The effect of grammatical complexity upon disfluency behavior of nonstuttering preschool children. *Journal of Fluency Disorders, 5*, 55–68.

Peppe, S., & Wells, B. (2014). Speech prosody. In P. J. Brooks & V. Kempe (Eds.), *Encyclopdiea of language development* (pp. 584–590). Sage Publications.

Perino, M., Famularo, G., & Tarroni, P. (2000). Acquired transient stuttering during a migraine attack. *Headache, 40*, 170–172.

Perkins, W. H., Kent, R. D., & Curlee, R. F. (1991). A theory of neuropsycholinguistic function in stuttering. *Journal of Speech and Hearing Research, 34*, 734–752.

Peters, H. F. M., & Hulstijn, W. (1984). Stuttering and anxiety: The difference between stutterers and nonstutterers in verbal apprehension and physiologic arousal during the anticipation of speech and non-speech tasks. *Journal of Fluency Disorders, 9*, 67–84.

Peters, T. J., & Guitar, B. (1991). *Stuttering: An integrated approach to its nature and treatment.* Williams & Wilkins.

Pick, A. (1899). Ueber das sogenannta aphatische Stottern als Symptom verschiedenurtlich localisirter cerebraler Herdaffectionen. *Archiv fur Psychiatrie, 32*(2), 447–469.

Pierson, S. M. (2004). *Evaluating validity and reliability of the Teacher Assessment of Student Communicative Competence (TASCC) by comparing students who do and do not stutter.* (Masters thesis). University of Vermont.

Pietranton, A. A. (2012). An evidence-based practice primer: Implication and challenges for the treatment of fluency disorders. In N. Bernstein Ratner & J. Tetnowski (Eds.), *Current issues in stuttering research and practice* (pp. 47–60). Lawrence Erlbaum Associates Inc.

Pindzola, R., Jenkins, M., & Lokken, K. (1989). Speaking rates of young children. *Language, Speech, and Hearing Services in Schools, 20*, 133–138.

Platt, J., & Basili, A. (1973). Jaw tremor during stuttering block: An electromyographic study. *Journal of Communication Disorders, 6*, 102–109.

Ponsford, R., Brown, W., Marsh, J., & Travis, L. (1975). Proceedings: Evoked potential correlates of cerebral dominance for speech perception in stutterers and non-stutterers. *Electroencephalography and Clinical Neurophysiology, 39*, 434.

Pool, K. D., Devous, M. D., Freeman, F. J., Watson, B. C., & Finitzo, T. (1991). Regional cerebral blood flow in developmental stutterers. *Archives of Neurology, 48*, 509–512.

Poulos, M. G., & Webster, W. G. (1991). Family history as a basis for subgrouping people who stutter. *Journal of Speech and Hearing Research, 34*, 5–10.

Prelock, P. A., & Hutchins, T. L. (Eds.) (2019). *Essential clinical guide to communication disorders.* Springer.

Preston, K. (2013). *Out with it: How stuttering helped me find my voice.* Atria Books.

Preus, A. (1981). *Identifying subgroups of stutterers.* Universitetsforlaget.

Prins, D. (Ed.) (1991). *Theories of stuttering as event and disorder: Speech production processes.* Elsevier Science Publishers.

Prins, D. (1999). Describing the consequences of disorders: Comment on Yaruss (1998). *Journal of Speech, Language and Hearing Research, 42*, 1395–1397.

Prins, D., Mandelkorn, T., & Cerf, F. A. (1980). Principal and differential effects of haloperidol and placebo treatments upon speech disfluencies in stutterers. *Journal of Speech and Hearing Research, 23*, 614–629.

Prochaska, J. O., Velicer, W. F., Rossi, J. S., Goldstein, M. G., Marcus, B. H., Rakowski, W., & Rossi, S. R. (1994). Stages of change and decisional balance for 12 problem behaviors. *Health Psychology, 13*(1), 39.

Quader, S. E. (1977). Dysarthria: An unusual side effect of trycyclic antidepressants. *British Medical Journal, 9*, 97.

Quick: Talk fast & don't stutter. (2014, July 1). ASHA Leader. ASHA's Ad Hoc Committee on Reading Fluency for School-Age Children Who Stutter. https://doi.org/10.1044/leader.FTR2.19072014.44

Quinn, P. (1972). Stuttering, cerebral dominance, and the dichotic word test. *Medical Journal of Australia, 2*, 639–642.

Rabinowitz, A., & Chien, C. (2014). *A boy and a jaguar.* Houghton Mifflin Harcourt Books for Young Readers.

Rahman, P. (1956). *The self-concept and ideal self-concept of stutterers as compared to nonstutterers.* (Unpublished masters thesis). Brooklyn College.

Ramig, P. (1993). The impact of self-help groups on persons who stutter: A call for research. *Journal of Fluency Disorders, 18*, 351–361.

Ramig, P., & Dogde, D. (2005). *Child and adolescent stuttering treatment and activity resource guide.* Thomson Delmar Learning.

Ramos-Heinrichs, L., Mayo, L. H., & Garzon, S. (2008). Employing Latino value orientations to facilitate success in stuttering treatment. *Perspectives on Fluency and Fluency Disorders, 18*, 111–118.

Rautakoski, P., Hannus, T., Simberg, S., Sandnabba, N. K., & Santilla, P. (2012). Genetic and environmental effects on stuttering: A twin study from Finland. *Journal of Fluency Disorders, 37*, 202–210.

Raza, M., Amjad, R., Riazuddin, S., & Drayna, D. (2012). Studies in a consanguineous family reveal a novel locus for stuttering on chromosome 16q. *Human Genetics, 131*(2), 311–313.

Raza, M., Domingues, C., Webster, R., Sainz, E., Paris, E., Rahn, R., & Drayna, D. (2016). Musolipidosis types II and III and non-syndromic stuttering are associated with different varients in the same genes. *European Journal of Human Genetics, 24,* 529–534.

Raza, M., Gertz, E., Mundorff, J., Lukong, J., Kuster, J., Schaffer, A., & Drayna, D. (2013). Linkage analysis of a large African family segregating stuttering suggests polygenic inheritance. *Human Genetics, 132*(4), 385–396.

Raza, M., Mattera, R., Morell, R., Sainz, E., Rahn, R., Gutierrez, J., & Drayna, D. (2015). Association between rare variants in AP4E1, a component of intra-cellular trafficking, and persistent stuttering. *American Journal of Human Genetics, 97*(5), 715–725.

Raza, M., Riazuddin, S., & Drayna, D. (2010). Identification of an autosomal recessive stuttering locus on chromosome 3q13.2-3q13.33. *Human Genetics, 128*(4), 461–463.

Reardon-Reeves, N., & Yaruss, J. S. (2013). *School-age stuttering treatment: A practical guide.* Stuttering Treatment Resources.

Reilly, S., Onslow, M., Packman, A., Wake, M., Bavin, E., & Prior, M. (2009). Predicting stuttering onset by the age of 3: A prospective, community cohort study. *Pediatrics, 123,* 270–277.

Reilly, S., Onslow, M., Packman, A., Cini, E., Conway, L., Ukoumunne, O., Bavin, E., Prior, M., Eadie, P., Block, S., & Wake, M. (2013). Natural history of stuttering to 4 years of age: A prospective community-based study. *Pediatrics, 132*(3), 460–467.

Rentschler, G., Driver, L., & Callaway, E. (1984). The onset of stuttering following drug overdose. *Journal of Fluency Disorders, 9,* 265–284.

Riaz, N., Steinberg, S., Ahmad, J., Pluzhnikov, A., Riazuddin, S., Cox, N., & Drayna, D. (2005). Genomewide significant linkage to stuttering on chromosome 12. *American Journal of Human Genetics, 76*(4), 647–651.

Richels, C. G., & Conture, E. (2007). An indirect approach for early intervention for childhood stuttering. In E. Conture & R. Curlee (Eds.), *Stuttering and related disorders of fluency.* Thieme Medical Publishers.

Richels, C. G., & Conture, E. G. (2010). Indirect treatment of childhood stuttering: Diagnostic predictors of treatment outcome. In B. Guitar & R. J. McCauley (Eds.), *Treatment of stuttering: Established and emerging interventions* (pp. 18–55). Lippincott Williams & Wilkins.

Riley, G. (1972). A stuttering severity instrument for children and adults. *Journal of Speech and Hearing Disorders, 37,* 314–322.

Riley, G. (1994). *Stuttering severity instrument for children and adults* (3rd ed.). Pro-Ed.

Riley, G. (2009). *Stuttering Severity Instrument - 4* (4th ed.). Super Duper Publications.

Riley, G., & Riley, J. (1979). A component model for diagnosing and treating children who stutter. *Journal of Fluency Disorders, 4*(4), 279–293.

Riley, G. D., & Riley, J. (2000). A revised component model for diagnosing and treating children who stutter. *Contemporary Issues in Communication Sciences and Disorders, 27,* 188–199.

Ringo, C. C., & Dietrich, S. (1995). Neurogenic stuttering: An analysis and critique. *Journal of Medical Speech-Language Pathology, 32,* 111–122.

Ripley, A. (2005, May). How to get out alive: From hurricanes to 9/11: What the science of evacuation reveals about how humans behave in the worst of times. *Time, 165,* 58–62.

Ripley, A. (2008). *Unthinkable: Who survives when disaster strikes and why?* Crown Publishers.

Robb, M. P., Lynn, W. L., & O'Beirne, G. A. (2013). An exploration of dichotic listening among adults who stutter. *Clinical Linguistics & Phonetics, 27*(9), 681–693.

Roberts, P., & Shenker, R. (2007). Assessment and treatment of stuttering in bilingual speakers. In E. G. Conture & R. Curlee (Eds.), *Stuttering and related disorders of fluency* (3rd ed., pp. 183–210). Thieme.

Rodgers, N. H. (2022). Meet them where they're at: Maximizing adolescents' engagement in stuttering therapy. *Seminars in Speech and Language, 43*(2), 161–172.

Rodgers, N. H., Berquez, A., Hollister, J., & Zebrowski, P. (2020). Using solution-focused principles with older children who stutter and their parents to elicit perspectives of therapeutic change. *Perspectives of the ASHA Special Interest Groups, 5*(6), 1427–1440. 10.1044/2020_PERSP-20-00124

Rodgers, N. H., Gerlach, H., Paiva, A. L., Robbins, M. L., & Zebrowski, P. (2021). Applying the transtheoretical model to stuttering management among adolescents: Part II. Exploratory scale validation. *American Journal of Speech Language Pathology, 30*(6), 2510–2527.

Roessler, R., & Bolton, B. (1978). *Psychosocial adjustment to disability.* University Park Press.

Rogers, C. (1957). The necessary and sufficient conditions of therapeutic personality change. *Journal of Consulting Psychology, 21,* 95–103.

Rogers, C. (1961). *On becoming a person.* Houghton Mifflin.

Rogers, C. R. (1942). *Counseling and psychotherapy.* Riverside Press.

Rogers, C. R. (1951). *Client-centered therapy.* Houghton Mifflin.

Rogers, C. R. (1952). Communication: Its blocking and it facilitation. *ETC: A Review of General Semantics, 9*(2), 83.

Rogers, K. (2023, February 7). Crafting Biden's words with helpful shorthand: Conquering his stutter in the State of the Union. *New York Times.*

Rommel, D., Hage, P., Kalehne, P., & Johannsen, H. (2000). Development, maintenance, and recovery of childhood stuttering: Prospective longitudinal data 3 years after first contact. In K. L. Baker, L. Rustin & F. Cook (Eds.), *Proceedings of the Fifth Oxford Disfluency Conference, 7th-10th July, 1999* (pp. 168–182). Kevin L. Baker.

Rosenbek, J. C. (1984). Stuttering secondary to nervous system damage. In R. F. Curlee & W. H. Perkins (Eds.), *Nature and treatment of stuttering: New directions* (pp. 31–48). College-Hill Press.

Rosenberger, P. B. (1980). Dopaminergic systems and speech fluency. *Journal of Fluency Disorders, 5*(3), 255–267.

Rosenberry-McKibbin, C. (2018). *Multicultural students with special language needs: Practical strategies for assessment and intervention* (5th ed.). Academic Communication Associates, Inc.

Rosenfield, D., & Goodglass, H. (1980). Dichotic testing of cerebral dominance in stutterers. *Brain and Language, 11,* 170–180.

Roth, C., Aronson, A., & Davis, L. (1989). Clinical studies in psychogenic stuttering of adult onset. *Journal of Speech and Hearing Disorders, 54,* 634–646.

Roth, C., Manning, K., & Duffy, J. (2011). *Aquired stuttering in post-deployed. Paper presented at the Annual Meeting of the American Speech-Language-Hearing Association.* San Diego, CA.

Rothbart, M. K. (2011). *Becoming who we are: Temperament and personality in development*. Guilford Press.

Rothbart, M. K., Ahadi, S. A., Hershey, K. L., & Fisher, P. (2001). Investigation of temperament at three to seven years: The Children's Behavior Questionnaire. *Child Development, 72*, 1394–1408.

Rousseau, I., Packman, A., Onslow, M., Harrison, E., & Jones, M. (2007). An investigation of language and phonological development and the responsiveness of preschool age children in the Lidcombe Program. *Journal of Communication Disorders, 40*(5), 382–397.

Rubow, R., Rosenbek, J., & Schumaker, J. (1986). Stress management in the treatment of neurogenic stuttering. *Biofeedback and Self Regulation, 11*, 77–78.

Runswick-Cole, K., & Goodley, D. (2013). Resilience: A disability studies and community psychology approach. *Social and Personality Psychology Compass, 7*(2), 67–78.

Runyan, C. M., & Runyan, S. E. (1986). A Fluency Rules therapy program for young children in the public schools. *Language, Speech & Hearing Services in Schools, 17*(4), 276–284.

Rustin, L. (1991). *Parents, families, and the stuttering child*. Whurr.

Rutter, M. (1981). *Maternal deprivation reassessed*. Penguin.

Ryan, B. P. (1974). *Programmed therapy for stuttering in children and adults*. Charles C. Thomas.

Sackett, D., Straus, S., Richardson, W., Rosenberg, W., & Haynes, R. (2000). *Evidence-based medicine: How to practice and teach EBM*. Churchill Livingstone.

Santayana, G., Carey, B., & Shenker, R. (2021). No other choice: Speech-language pathologists' attitudes toward using telepractice to administer the Lidcombe Program during a pandemic. *Journal of Fluency Disorders, 70*, 105879.

Sasisekaran, J. (2014). Exploring the link between stuttering and phonology: A review and implications for treatment. *Seminars in Speech and Language, 35*(2), 95–113.

Sawyer, S. M., Azzopardi, P. S., Wickremarathne, D., & Patton, G. C. (2018). The age of adolescence. *Lancet Child & Adolescent Health, 2*(3), 223–228.

Scaler Scott, K. (2020). Cluttering symptoms in school-age children by communicative context: A preliminary investigation. *International Journal of Speech & Language Pathology, 22*, 174–183.

Scaler Scott, K. (2022). Cluttering in a school-aged child: Tackling the challenges step by step. *Seminars in Speech and Language, 43*(2), 130–146.

Scaler Scott, K., Sønsterud, H., & Reichel, I. (2022). Clutering: Etiology, symptomatology, identification, and treatment. In P. Zebrowski, J. Anderson & E. Conture (Eds.), *Stuttering and related disorders of fluency* (4th ed.). Tieme.

Scaler Scott, K., Tetnowski, J. A., Flaitz, J. R., & Yaruss, J. S. (2014). Preliminary study of disfluency in school-aged children with autism. *International Journal of Language and Communication Disorders, 49*(1), 75–89.

Scaler Scott, K., & Ward, D. (2015). Treatment techniques for children, teens, and adults with cluttering. *Procedia-Social and Behavioral Sciences, 193*, 327.

Schiavetti, N., & Metz, D. E. (1997). Stuttering and the measurement of speech naturalness. In R. F. Curlee & G. M. Siegel (Eds.), *Nature and treatment of stuttering: New directions* (2nd ed., pp. 398–412). Allyn & Bacon.

Schmahmann, J. D., & Caplan, D. (2006). Cognition, emotion and the cerebellum. *Brain, 129*(Pt. 2), 290–292.

Schwartz, M. F. (1974). The core of the stuttering block. *Journal of Speech and Hearing Disorders, 39*, 169–177.

Scott, L., & Guitar, C. (2004). Stuttering: For kids, by kids [DVD]. Stuttering Foundation.

Scott, L., & Guitar, C. (2012). Stuttering: Straight talk for teachers [DVD]. Stuttering Foundation.

Seeman, M. (1937). The significance of twin pathology for the investigation of speech disorders. *Archive gesamte Phonetik, 1*, 88–92. (Part II).

Seery, C. (2005). Differential diagnosis of stuttering for forensic purposes. *American Journal of Speech-Language Pathology, 14*, 284–297.

Segalowitz, S. J., & Brown, D. (1991). Mild head injury as a source of developmental disabilities. *Journal of Learning Disabilities, 24*(9), 551–559.

Seligman, M. E. (2013). *Positive psychology in practice*. Wiley.

Semel, E., Wiig, E., & Secord, W. (1995). *Clinical evaluation of language fundamentals - 3*. Psychological Corporation.

Senju, A., & Johnson, M. H. (2009). The eye contact effect: Mechanisms and development. *Trends in Cognitive Sciences, 13*(3), 127–134.

Shafir, R. Z. (2000). *The zen of listening: Mindful communication in the age of distraction*. Theosophical Publishing House.

Shapely, K., & Guyette, T. (2010). Review of "TOCS: Test of childhood stuttering". *Mental Measurements Yearbook, 18*, 138.

Shapiro, A. I. (1980). An electromyographic analysis of the fluent and dysfluent utterances of several types of stutterers. *Journal of Fluency Disorders, 5*, 203–231.

Shapiro, A. I., & DeCicco, B. A. (1982). The relationship between normal dysfluency and stuttering: An old question revisited. *Journal of Fluency Disorders, 7*, 109–121.

Shapiro, D. A. (1999). *Stuttering intervention: A collaborative journey to fluency freedom*. Pro-Ed.

Shapiro, D. A. (2011). *Stuttering intervention: A collaborative journey to fluency freedom* (2nd ed.). Pro-Ed.

Shaywitz, B. A., Shaywitz, S. E., Pugh, K. R., Constable, R. T., Skudlarski, P., & Fulbright, R. K. (1995). Sex differences in the functional organization of the brain for language. *Nature, 373*, 607–609.

Sheehan, J. G. (1970). *Stuttering: Research and therapy*. Harper & Row.

Sheehan, J. G. (1974). Stuttering behavior: A phonetic analysis. *Journal of Communication Disorders, 7*, 193–212.

Sheehan, J. G. (1975). Conflict theory and avoidance-reduction therapy. In J. Eisenson (Ed.), *Stuttering: A second symposium*. Harper & Row.

Sheehan, J. G., & Sheehan, V. M. (1984). Avoidance reduction therapy: A response-suppression hypothesis. In B. P. Ryan & W. H. Perkins (Eds.), *Stuttering disorders* (pp. 141–152). Thieme-Stratton.

Sherman, D. (1952). Clinical and experimental use of the Iowa scale of severity of stuttering. *Journal of Speech and Hearing Disorders, 17*, 316–320.

Shirkey, E. (1987). Forensic verification of stuttering. *Journal of Fluency Disorders, 12*, 197–203.

Shugart, Y. Y., Mundorff, J., Kilshaw, J., Doheny, K., Doan, B., & Wanyee, J. (2004). Results of a genome-wide linkage scan for stuttering. *American Journal of Medical Genetics, 124A*, 133–135.

Shulman, E. P., Smith, A. R., Silva, K., Icenogle, G., Duell, N., Chein, J., & Steinberg, L. (2016). The dual systems model: Review, reappraisal, and reaffirmation. *Developmental Cognitive Neuroscience, 17*, 103–117.

Siegel, D. J. (2010). *Mindsight: The new science of personal transformation*. Bantam.

Siegel, G. M. (2007, December). *Random observations. ASHA Leader.*

Silverman, E.-M. (1974). Word position and grammatical function in relation to preschoolers' speech disfluency. *Perceptual and Motor Skills, 39*, 267–272.

Silverman, F. H. (1988). The monster study. *Journal of Fluency Disorders, 13*, 225–231.

Simonyan, K., & Horowitz, B. (2011). Laryngeal motor cortex and control of speech in humans. *Neuroscientist, 17*(2), 197–208.

Singer, C. M., Hessling, A., Kelly, E., Singer, L., & Jones, R. M. (2020). Clinical characteristics associated with stuttering persistence: A meta-analysis. *Journal of Speech, Language and Hearing Research, 63*, 2995–3018. 10.1044/2020_JSLHR-20-00096

Singer, C. M., Otieno, S., Chang, S.-E., & Jones, R. M. (2022). Predicting persistent developmental stuttering using a cumulative risk approach. *Journal of Speech, Language and Hearing Research, 65*(1), 70–95.

Sisskin, V. (2012). Autism spectrum disorders and stuttering [DVD]. Stuttering Foundation.

Sisskin, V. (2018). Avoidance reduction therapy for stuttering (ARTS). In B. Amster & E. Klein (Eds.), *More than fluency: The social, emotional, and cognitive dimensions of stuttering*. Plural Publishing.

Sisskin, V. (2023). Disfluency-affirming therapy for young people who stutter: Unpacking ableism in the therapy room. *Language, Speech & Hearing Services in Schools, 54*(1), 114–119.

Sisskin, V., & Goldstein, B. (2022). Avoidance reduction therapy for school-aged childrn who stutter. *Seminars in Speech and Language, 43*(2), 147–160.

Skinner, E., & McKeehan, A. (1996). *Preventing stuttering in the preschool child: A video program for parents [Videotape]*. Communication Skill Builders.

Smith, A. (1989). Neural drive to muscles in stuttering. *Journal of Speech and Hearing Research, 32*, 252–264.

Smith, A. (1999). Stuttering: A unified approach to a multifactorial, dynamic disorder. In N. Bernstein Ratner & E. C. Healey (Eds.), *Stuttering research and practice: Bridging the gap*. Lawrence Erlbaum Associates.

Smith, A., Denny, M., Shaffer, L., Kelly, E., & Hirano, M. (1996). Activity of intrinsic laryngeal muscles in fluent and disfluent speech. *Journal of Speech and Hearing Research, 39*(2), 329–348.

Smith, A., & Goffman, L. (2004). Interaction of motor and language factors in the development of speech production. In B. Maasen, R. D. Kent, H. F. M. Peters, P. H. H. M. van Lieshout, & W. Hulstijn (Eds.), *Speech motor control in normal and disordered speech* (pp. 227-252). Oxford University Press.

Smith, A., Goffman, L., Sasiekaran, J., & Weber-Fox, C. (2012). Language and motor abilities of preschool children who stutter: Evidence from behavioral and kinematic indices of non-word repetition performance. *Journal of Fluency Disorders, 37*(4), 344–358.

Smith, A., & Kelly, E. (1997). Stuttering: A dynamic, multifactorial model. In R. F. Curlee & G. Siegel (Eds.), *Nature and treatment of stuttering: New directions* (2nd ed., pp. 204–217). Allyn & Bacon.

Smith, A., McCauley, R., & Guitar, B. (2000). Development of the Teacher Assessment of Student Communicative Competence (TASCC) in grades 1 through 5. *Communication Disorders Quarterly, 22*(1), 3–11.

Smith, A., Sadagopan, N., Walsh, B., & Weber-Fox, C. (2010). Phonological complexity affects speech motor dynamics in adults who stutter. *Journal of Fluency Disorders, 35*, 1–18.

Smith, A., & Weber, C. (2017). How stuttering develops: The multifactorial dynamic pathways theory. *Journal of Speech, Language and Hearing Research, 60*, 2483–2505.

Smith, K., Iverach, L., O'Brian, S., Kefalianos, E., & Reilly, S. (2014). Anxiety of children and adolescents who stutter: A review. *Journal of Fluency Disorders, 40*, 22–34.

Smits-Bandstra, S., & De Nil, L. F. (2007). Sequence skill learning in persons who stutter: Implications for cortico-striato-thalamo dysfunction. *Journal of Fluency Disorders, 32*(4), 251–278.

Snidman, N., & Kagan, J. (1994). The contribution of infant temperamental differences to the acoustic startle response. *Psychophysiology*, 31(Supplement 1), S92. (abstract).

Sommer, M., Koch, M. A., Paulus, W., Weiller, C., & Buchel, C. (2002). Disconnection of speech-relevant brain areas in persistent developmental stuttering. *Lancet, 360*, 380–383.

Sommer, M., Waltersbacher, A., Schlotmann, A., Schroder, H., & Strzelczyk, A. (2021). Prevalence and therapy rates for stuttering, cluttering and developmental disorders of speech and language: Evaluation of German health insurance data. *Frontiers in Human Neuroscience, 15*, 645292.

Sommers, R., Brady, W. A., & Moore, W. H. (1975). Dichotic ear preferences of stuttering children and adults. *Perceptual and Motor Skills, 41*, 931–938.

Sonsterud, H. (2019). The importance of the working alliance in the treatment of cluttering. *Perspectives of the ASHA Special Interest Groups, 4*, 1568–1572.

Sonsterud, H., Kirmess, M., Howells, K., Ward, D., Feragen, K. B., & Halvorson, M. S. (2019). The working alliance in stuttering treatment: A neglected variable? *International Journal of Language and Communication Disorders, 54*(4), 606–619.

Spencer, C., & Weber-Fox, C. (2014). Preschool speech articulation and nonword repetition abilities may help predict eventual recovery or persistence of stuttering. *Journal of Fluency Disorders, 41*, 32–46.

St. Louis, K. (1996). Research and opinion on cluttering: State of the art and science. *Journal of Fluency Disorders, 21*(3/4), 171–374.

St. Louis, K. (2001). *Living with stuttering: Stories, basics, resources, and hope*. Populore Publishing Company.

St. Louis, K., Myers, F. L., Bakker, K., & Raphael, L. J. (2007). Understanding and treating cluttering. In E. Conture & R. Curlee (Eds.), *Stuttering and related disorders of fluency* (3rd ed., pp. 297–322). Thieme.

St. Louis, K., Raphael, L., Myers, F., & Bakker, K. (2003). Cluttering updated. *ASHA Leader, 8*, 20–22.

St. Louis, K., & Scaler Scott, K. (n.d.). Cluttering Retrieved from www.stutteringhelp.org website.

St. Louis, K., & Schulte, K. (2011). Defining cluttering: The lowest common denominator. In D. Ward & K. Scaler Scott (Eds.), *Cluttering. A handbook of research, intervention and education* (pp. 233–253). Psychology Press.

St. Onge, K. (1963). The stuttering syndrome. *Journal of Speech and Hearing Research*, 6, 195–197.

Stager, S., Jeffries, K. J., & Braun, A. R. (2003). Common features of fluency-evoking conditions studied in stuttering subjects and controls: An H2-15-0 PET study. *Journal of Fluency Disorders, 28*(4), 319–336.

Starkweather, C. W. (1980). A multiprocess behavioral approach to stuttering therapy. *Seminars in Speech, Language and Hearing, 1*, 327–337.

Starkweather, C. W. (1985). The development of fluency in normal children. In *Stuttering therapy: Prevention and intervention with children*. Stuttering Foundation of America.

Starkweather, C. W. (1987). *Fluency and stuttering*. Prentice-Hall.

Starkweather, C. W. (1991). Stuttering: The motor-language interface. In H. F. M. Peters, W. Hulstijn & C. W. Starkweather (Eds.), *Speech motor control and fluency*. Excerpta Medica.

Starkweather, C. W. (2002). The epigenesis of stuttering. *Journal of Fluency Disorders, 27*(4), 269–288.

Starkweather, C. W., & Gottwald, S. (1990). The demands and capacities model II: Clinical application. *Journal of Fluency Disorders, 15*, 143–157.

Starkweather, C. W., Gottwald, S., & Halfond, M. H. (1990). *Stuttering prevention: A clinical method*. Prentice-Hall.

Starkweather, C. W., Hirschman, P., & Tannenbaum, R. S. (1976). Latency of vocalization onset: Stutterers versus nonstutterers. *Journal of Speech and Hearing Research, 19*, 481–492.

Starkweather, C. W., & Myers, M. (1979). Duration of subsegments within the intervocalic interval in stutterers and nonstutterers. *Journal of Fluency Disorders, 4*, 205–214.

Steinberg, L. (2014). *Age of opportunity: Lessons from the new science of adolescence*. Houghton Mifflin Harcourt.

Stephanson-Opsal, D., & Bernstein Ratner, N. (1988). Maternal speech rate modification and childhood stuttering. *Journal of Fluency Disorders, 13*, 49–56.

Stepp, C. E., & Vojtech, J. M. (2019). Speech naturalness. In J. S. Damico & M. J. Ball (Eds.), *The SAGE encyclopedia of human communication sciences and disorders*. SAGE Publications.

Sternberger, J. P. (1982). The nature of segments in the lexicon: Evidence from speech errors. *Lingua, 56*, 235–259.

Stocker, B., & Usprich, C. (1976). Stuttering in young children and level of demand. *Journal of Childhood Communication Disorders, 1*, 116–131.

Strasberg, S., Johnson, E., & Perry, T. (2016). "Stuttering" after minor head trauma. *American Journal of Emergency Medicine, 34*(3), 685.

Strong, J. C. (1977). *Dichotic speech perception: A comparison between stutterers and nonstutterers ages five to nine*. (Unpublished doctoral dissertation). Pennsylvania State University.

Studdert-Kennedy, M. (1987). The phoneme as a perceptuomotor structure. In A. Allport, D. McKay, D. Prinz & E. Scheerer (Eds.), *Language perception and production*. Academic Press.

Stuttering Foundation. (2022). *Fall newsletter*.

Subramanian, A., & Yairi, E. (2006). Identification of traits associated with stuttering. *Journal of Communication Disorders, 39*(3), 200–216.

Sudo, D., Doutake, Y., Yokota, H., & Watanabe, E. (2018). Recovery of brain abscess-induced stuttering after a neurosurgical intervention. *Case Reports*, 2018, bcr-2017223259.

Sussman, H. (2016). Why the left hemisphere is dominant for speech production: Connecting the dots. *Biolinguistics, 9*, 116–123.

Sussman, H., & MacNeilage, P. (1975). Hemispheric specialization for speech production and perception in stutterers. *Neuropsychologia, 13*, 19–26.

Tani, T., & Wada, N. (2018). Stuttering and compulsive manipulation of tools after hemorrhage in the anterior corpus collosum and cingulate gyrus: A case study. *Speech, Language and Hearing, 21*(4), 256–263.

Tanoue, Y., & Oda, S. (1989). Weaning time of children with infantile autism. *Journal of Autism and Developmental Disorders, 19*(3), 425–434.

Taylor, G. (1937). *An observational study of the nature of stuttering at onset*. (Master's thesis). State University of Iowa.

Taylor, O. (1986). *Treatment of communication disorders in culturally and linguistically diverse populations*. College-Hill Press.

Taylor, O. (1994). *Communication and communication disorders in a multicultural society*. Singular Publishing Group.

Taylor, R. M., & Morrison, L. P. (1996). *Taylor-Johnson temperament analysis manual*. Psychological Publications, Inc.

Tellis, G. (2008). Multicultural considerations in assessing and treating Hispanic Americans who stutter. *Perspectives on Fluency and Fluency Disorders, 18*, 101–110.

Tellis, G., & Tellis, C. (2003). Multicultural issues in school settings. *Seminars in Speech and Language, 24*(1), 21–26.

Tendera, A., Rispoli, M., Ambikaipakan Sethilselvan, C., & Loucksa, T. (2019). Research note: Early speech rate development: A longitudinal study. *Journal of Speech, Language and Hearing Research, 62*, 4370–4381.

Tendera, A., Wells, R., Belyk, M., Veryvoda, D., Boliek, X. A., & Beal, D. S. (2020). Motor sequence learning in children with recovered and persistent developmental stuttering: Preliminary findings. *Journal of Fluency Disorders, 66*, 105800.

The way we talk. (2015). Film. Directed by M. Turner.

Theys, C., & De Nil, L. F. (2022). Acquired stuttering: Etiology, symptomatology, identification and treatment. In P. Zebrowski, J. Anderson & E. Conture (Eds.), *Stuttering and related disorders of stuttering* (4th ed., pp. 271–186). Thieme.

Theys, C., De Nil, L. F., Thijs, V., Van Wieringen, A., & Sunaert, S. (2013). A crucial role for the cortico-striato-cortical loop in the pathogenesis of stroke-related neurogenic stuttering. *Human Brain Mapping, 34*(9), 2103–2112.

Theys, C., van Wieringen, A., & De Nil, L. F. (2008). A clinician survey of speech and non-speech characteristics of neurogenic stuttering. *Journal of Fluency Disorders, 33*(1), 1–23.

Thomas, A., & Chess, S. (1977). *Temperament and development*. Brunner/Mazel, Inc.

Thomson, K. S. (2009). *Young Charles Darwin*. Yale University Press.

Throneberg, R., & Yairi, E. (1994). Temporal dynamics of repetitions during the early stage of childhood stuttering: An acoustic study. *Journal of Speech and Hearing Research, 37*, 1067–1075.

Tichenor, S. E., & Yaruss, J. S. (2018). A phenomenological analysis of the experience of stuttering. *American Journal of Speech-Language Pathology, 27*, 1180–1194.

Tichenor, W. E., & Yaruss, J. S. (2019). Stuttering as defined by adults who stutter. *Journal of Speech, Language and Hearing Research, 62*, 4356–4369.

Till, J. A., Reich, A., Dickey, S., & Sieber, J. (1983). Phonatory and manual reaction times of stuttering and nonstuttering children. *Journal of Speech and Hearing Research, 26*, 171–180.

Tilsen, S. (2016). Selection and coordination: The articulatory basis for the emergence of phonological structure. *Journal of Phonetics, 55*, 53–77.

Toscher, M. M., & Rupp, R. R. (1978). A study of the central auditory processes in stutterers using the Synthetic Sentence Identification SSI test battery. *Journal of Speech and Hearing Research, 21*, 779–792.

Toyomura, A., Fujii, T., & Kuriki, S. (2011). Effect of external auditory pacing on the neural activity of stuttering speakers. *NeuroImage, 57*(4), 1507–1516.

Toyomura, A., Miyashiro, D., Kuriki, S., & Sowman, P. (2020). Speech-induced suppression for delayed auditory feedback in adults who do and do not stutter. *Frontiers in Human Neuroscience, 14*, 150.

Trajkovski, N., Andrews, C., Onslow, M., Packman, A., O'Brian, S., & Menzies, R. (2009). Using syllable-timed speech to treat preschool children who stutter: A multiple baseline experiment. *Journal of Fluency Disorders, 34*(1), 1–10.

Travis, L. (1925). Muscular fixation of the stutterer's voice under emotion. *Science, 62*, 207–208.

Travis, L. (1931). *Speech pathology*. Appleton-Century.

Travis, L. E., & Knott, J. R. (1937). Bilaterally recorded brain potentials from normal speakers and stutterers. *Journal of Speech Disorders, 2*, 239–241.

Trichon, M., & Raj, E. (2018). Peer support for people who stutter: History, benefits, and accessibility. In B. J. Amster & E. R. Klein (Eds.), *More than fluency: The social, emotional, and cognitive dimensions of stuttering* (pp. 187–214). Plural Publishing.

Troutman, B. (2022). How to coach parents to follow their child's lead in play. In B. Troutman (Ed.), *Attachment-informed parent coaching* (pp. 31–46). Springer International Publishing.

Tudor, M. (1939). *An experimental study of the effect of evaluative labeling on speech fluency*. (Unpublished master's thesis). University of Iowa.

Tumanova, V., Choi, D., Conture, E. G., & Walden, T. (2018). Expressed parental concern regarding childhood stuttering and the Test of Childhood Stuttering. *Journal of Communication Disorders, 72*, 86–96.

Tumanova, V., Conture, E. G., Lambert, E. W., & Walden, T. A. (2014). Speech disfluencies of preschool-age children who do and do not stutter. *Journal of Communication Disorders, 49*, 25–41.

Turgut, N., Utku, U., & Balci, K. (2002). A case of acquired stuttering resulting from left parietal infarction. *Acta Neurologica Scandinavica, 105*, 408.

Turk, A. Z., Marchoubeh, M. L., Fritsch, I., Maguire, G. A., & Sheikh-Bahaei, S. (2021). Dopamine, vocalization and astrocytes. *Brain and Language, 219*, 104970.

Turnbaugh, K. R., Guitar, B. E., & Hoffman, P. R. (1979). Speech clinicians' attribution of personality traits as a function of stuttering severity. *Journal of Speech and Hearing Research, 22*, 37–45.

Turrell, S. L., Bell, M., & Wilson, K. G. (2016). *ACT for adolescents: Treating teens and adolescents in individual and group therapy*. New Harbinger Publications.

Unicomb, R., Hewat, S., Spencer, E., & Harrison, E. (2013). Clinicians' management of young children with co-occurring stuttering and speech sound disorders. *International Journal of Speech-Language Pathology, 15*(4), 441–452.

Usler, E., & Weber-Fox, C. (2015). Neurodevelopment for syntactic processing distinguishes childhood stuttering recovery vs. persistence. *Journal of Neurodevelopmental Disorders, 7*(1), 3–4.

Utianskia, R. L., & Duffy, J. (2022). Understanding, recognizing, and managing functional speech disorders: Current thinking illustrated with case studies. *American Journal of Speech Language Pathology, 31*, 1205–1220.

van Beijsterveldt, C. E., Felsenfeld, S., & Boomsma, D. I. (2010). Bivariate genetic analyses of stuttering and nonfluency in a large sample of 5-year-old twins. *Journal of Speech Language and Hearing Research, 53*(3), 609-619.

Van Borsel, J., Maes, E., & Foulon, S. (2001). Stuttering and bilingualism: A review. *Journal of Fluency Disorders, 26*, 179–205.

Van Borsel, J., Moeyaert, J., Mostaert, C., Rosseel, R., van Loo, E., & van Renterghem, T. (2006). Prevalence of stuttering in regular and special school populations in Belgium based on teacher perceptions. *Folia Phoniatrica et Logopedica, 58*, 289–302.

van der Kolk, B. A. (2014). *The body keeps the score: Brain, mind, and body in the healing of trauma*. Penguin.

van Lieshout, P., Ben-David, B., Lipski, M., & Namasivayam, A. K. (2014). The impact of threat and cognitive stress on speech motor control in people who stutter. *Journal of Fluency Disorders, 40*, 93–109.

van Lieshout, P., Hulstijn, W., & Peters, H. F. M. (2004). Searching for the weak link in the speech production chain of people who stutter. In B. Maassen, R. D. Kent, H. F. M. Peters, P. H. H. M. van Lieshout, & W. E. Hulstijn (Eds.), *Speech motor control in normal and disordered speech* (pp. 313-356). Oxford University Press.

Van Riper, C. (1936). Study of the thoracic breathing of stutterers during expectancy and occurrence of stuttering spasm. *Journal of Speech Disorders, 1*, 61–72.

Van Riper, C. (1954). *Speech correction: Principles and methods* (3rd ed.). Prentice-Hall.

Van Riper, C. (1957). Symptomatic therapy for stuttering. In L. Travis (Ed.), *Handbook of speech* (pp. 878–896). Appleton-Century-Croft.

Van Riper, C. (1958). Experiments in stuttering therapy. In J. Eisenson (Ed.), *Stuttering: A symposium* (pp. 273–390). Harper & Row.

Van Riper, C. (1971). *The nature of stuttering*. Prentice-Hall.

Van Riper, C. (1973a). *The treatment of stuttering*. Prentice-Hall.

Van Riper, C. (1973b). Treatment of the young confirmed stutterer. In C. Van Riper (Ed.), *The treatment of stuttering* (pp. 426–451). Prentice-Hall.

Van Riper, C. (1974). A handful of nuts. *WMU Journal of Speech Therapy, 11*(2), 1–3.

Van Riper, C. (1975a). The stutterer's clinician. In J. Eisenson (Ed.), *Stuttering: A second symposium* (pp. 453–492). Harper & Row.

Van Riper, C. (1975b). Therapy in action [DVD]. Stuttering Foundation.

Van Riper, C. (1982). *The nature of stuttering* (2nd ed.). Prentice Hall.

Van Riper, C. (1982). The development of stuttering. In C. Van Riper (Ed.), *The nature of stuttering*. Prentice-Hall.

Van Riper, C. (1990). Final thoughts about stuttering. *Journal of Fluency Disorders, 15*(5/6), 317–318.

Van Riper, C., & Hull, C. J. (1955). The quantitive measurement of the effect of certain situations on stuttering. In W. Johnson & R. R. Leutenegger (Eds.), *Stuttering children and adults*. University of Minnesota Press.

Van Zaalen, Y., & Reichel, I. (2015). *Cluttering: Current views on its nature, diagnosis, and treatment*. iUniverse.

Van Zaalen, Y., & Reichel, I. (2017). Prevalance of cluttering in two European countries: A pilot study. *ASHA Perspectives, 2*(17), 42–49.

Van Zaalen, Y., Wijnen, F., & Dejonckere, P. (2011). Cluttering and learning disabilities. In D. Ward & K. S. Scott (Eds.), *Cluttering: A handbook of research, intervention and education* (pp. 100–114). Psychology Press.

Vanryckeghem, M., & Brutten, G. (1993). The Communication Attitude Test: A test-retest reliability investigation. *Journal of Fluency Disorders, 17*, 177–190.

Vanryckeghem, M., & Brutten, G. (1997). The speech-associated attitude of children who do and do not stutter and the differential effect of age. *American Journal of Speech-Language Pathology, 6*, 67–73.

Vanryckeghem, M., Hylebos, C., Brutten, G., & Peleman, M. (2001). The relationship between communication attitude and emotion of children who stutter. *Journal of Fluency Disorders, 26*(1), 1.

Vawter, V. (2013). *Paperboy*. Yearling.

Velleman, S. L. (2015). *Speech sound disorders in children*. Wolters Kluwer Health.

Veneziano, E. (2013). A Cognitive-Pragmatic Model for the change from single-word to multiword speech: A constructivist approach. *Journal of Pragmatics, 56*, 133–150.

Viswanath, N. S., Lee, H. S., & Chakraborty, R. (2004). Evidence for a minor gene influence on persistent developmental stuttering. *Human Biology, 76*, 401–412.

Vrana, S. R., Spence, E. L., & Lang, P. J. (1988). The startle probe: A new measure of emotion? *Journal of Abnormal Psychology, 97*, 487–491.

Wakaba, Y. (1998). *Research on temperament of stuttering children with early onset. Paper presented at the 2nd World Conference on Fluency Disorders*. San Francisco.

Walden, T. A., Frankel, C. B., Buhr, A. P., Johnson, K. N., Conture, E. G., & Karrass, J. M. (2012). Dual diathesis-stressor model of emotional and linguistic contributions to developmental stuttering. *Journal of Abnormal Child Psychology, 40*(4), 633–644.

Walden, T., & Lesner, T. A. (2018). Examining implicit and explicit attitudes toward stuttering. *Journal of Fluency Disorders, 57*, 22–36.

Walle, E. A., & Campos, J. J. (2014). Infant language development is related to the acquisition of walking. *Developmental Psychology, 50*(2), 336–348.

Wallen, V. (1960). A Q-technique study of the self-concepts of adolescent stutterers and nonstutterers. *Speech Monographs [Abstract], 27*, 257–258.

Walsh, B., Bostian, A., Tichenor, S. E., Brown, B., & Weber, C. (2020). Disfluency characteristics of 4 and 5 year old children who stutter and their relationship to stuttering persistence and recovery. *Journal of Speech, Language and Hearing Research, 63*(8), 2555–2566.

Walsh, B., Christ, S., & Weber, C. (2021). Exploring relationships among risk factors for persistence in childhood stuttering. *Journal of Speech Language and Hearing Research, 64*(8), 2909–2927.

Walsh, B., Mettel, K. M., & Smith, A. (2015). Speech motor planning and execution deficits in early childhood stuttering. *Journal of Neurodevelopmental Disorders, 7*(1), 27.

Walsh, B., & Smith, A. (2013). Oral electromyography activation patterns for speech are similar in preschoolers who do and do not stutter. *Journal of Speech Language and Hearing Research, 56*, 1441–1454.

Walsh, B., Usler, E., Bostain, A., Mohan, R., Gerwin, K. L., Brown, B., & Smith, A. (2018). What are predictors for persistence in childhood stuttering? *Seminars in Speech and Language, 39*(4), 299–312.

Walton, P. (2012). *Fun with fluency: For the school-age child*. Pro-Ed.

Wampold, B. E. (2015). How important are the common factors in psychotherapy? An update. *World Psychiatry, 14*, 270–277.

Ward, D. (2017). *Stuttering and cluttering: Frameworks for understanding and treatment*. Taylor and Francis.

Ward, D., Connally, E. L., Pliatsikas, C., Bretherton-Furness, J., & Watkins, K. E. (2015). Some neurological underpinnings of cluttering: Some initial findings. *Journal of Fluency Disorders, 43*, 1–16.

Ward, D., & Scott, K. S. (2011). *Cluttering: A handbook of research, intervention and education*. Psychology Press.

Waters, E. (1995). Appendix A: The attachment Q-set (version 3.0). *Monographs of the Society for Research in Child Development, 60*, 234–246.

Watkins, K., Smith, S., Davis, S., & Howell, P. (2008). Structural and functional abnormalities of the motor system in developmental stuttering. *Brain, 131*(1), 50–59.

Watkins, R. V. (2005). Language abilities of young children who stutter. In E. Yairi & N. G. Ambrose (Eds.), *Early childhood stuttering: For clinicians by clinicians* (pp. 235–251). Pro-Ed.

Watkins, R. V., Yairi, E., & Ambrose, N. G. (1999). Early childhood stuttering III: Initial status of expressive language abilities. *Journal of Speech, Language, and Hearing Research, 42*(5), 1125–1135.

Watson, B. C., & Alfonso, P. J. (1987). Physiological bases of acoustic LRT in nonstutterers, mild stutterers, and severe stutterers. *Journal of Speech and Hearing Research, 30*, 434–447.

Watson, J. B., & Kayser, H. (1994). Assessment of bilingual/bicultural children and adults who stutter. *Seminars in Speech, Language and Hearing, 15*, 149–163.

Watts, A., Eadie, P., Block, S., Mensah, F., & Reilly, S. (2014). Language ability of children with and without a history of stuttering: A longitudinal cohort study. *International Journal of Speech-Language Pathology, 17*(1), 86–95.

Weber, C. M., & Smith, A. (1990). Autonomic correlates of stuttering and speech assessed in a range of experimental tasks. *Journal of Speech and Hearing Research, 33*, 690–706.

Weber-Fox, C., Wray, A. H., & Arnold, H. S. (2013). Early childhood stuttering and electrophysiological indices of language processing. *Journal of Fluency Disorders, 38*(2), 206–221.

Webster, W. G. (1993a). Evidence in bimanual finger tapping of an attentional component to stuttering. *Behavioural Brain Research, 37*, 93–100.

Webster, W. G. (1993b). Hurried hands and tangled tongues: Implications of current research for the management of stuttering. In E. Boberg (Ed.), *Neuropsychology of stuttering* (pp. 73–111). University of Alberta Press.

Webster, W. G. (1997). Principles of human brain organization related to lateralization of language and speech motor functions in normal speakers and stutterers. In W. Hulstijn, H. F. M. Peters & P. H. H. M. van Lieshout (Eds.), *Speech production: Motor control, brain research and fluency disorders* (pp. 119–139). Elsevier.

Weiller, C., Isensee, C., Rijntjes, M., Huber, W., Muller, S., & Bier, D. (1995). Recovery from Wernicke's aphasia: A positron emission tomographic study. *Annals of Neurology, 376*, 723–732.

Weiner, A. E. (1981). A case of adult onset of stuttering. *Journal of Fluency Disorders, 6*, 181–186.

Weiss, A. L., & Zebrowski, P. M. (1992). Disfluencies in the conversations of young children who stutter: Some answers about questions. *Journal of Speech and Hearing Research, 356*, 1230–1238.

Weiss, D. A. (1964). *Cluttering.* Prentice-Hall.

Welch, J., & Byrne, J. (2001). *Jack: Straight from the gut.* Warner Books.

West, R. (1931). The phenomenology of stuttering. In R. West (Ed.), *A symposium on stuttering.* College Typing Company.

West, R., Nelson, S., & Berry, M. (1939). The heredity of stuttering. *Quarterly Journal of Speech, 25*, 23–30.

Wexler, K., & Mysack, E. (1982). Disfluency characteristics of 2-, 4- and 6-year old males. *Journal of Fluency Disorders, 7*, 37–46.

When I stutter. (2017). Film. Directed and produced by John Gomez.

Wiig, E. (2002, November). *Putting cluttering on the map: Looking back/looking ahead. Paper presented at the Annual meeting of the American Speech Language and Hearing Association.* Atlanta.

Wiig, E., Semel, E., & Secord, W. A. (2013). *Clinical evaluation of language fundamentals - 5: Screening test.* Pearson.

Wijnen, F. (1990). The development of sentence planning. *Journal of Child Language, 17*(3), 651–675.

Wilkenfeld, J. R., & Curlee, R. F. (1997). The relative effects of questions and comments on children's stuttering. *American Journal of Speech-Language Pathology, 63*, 79–89.

Williams, D., Darley, F., & Spriestersbach, D. (1978). Appraisal of rate and fluency. In F. Darley & D. Spriestersbach (Eds.), *Diagnostic methods in speech pathology* (2nd ed., pp. 256–283). Harper & Row.

Williams, D. E. (1968). A clinical success: John. In H. L. Luper (Ed.), *Stuttering: Successes and failures in therapy*. Memphis, Tennessee: Speech Foundation of America.

Williams, D. E. (1978). The problem of stuttering. In F. Darley & D. Spriestersbach (Eds.), *Diagnostic methods in speech pathology* (pp. 284–321). Harper & Row.

Williams, D. E., Silverman, F. H., & Kools, J. A. (1968). Disfluency behavior of elementary-school stutterers and nonstutterers: The adaptation effect. *Journal of Speech and Hearing Research, 11*, 622–630.

Williams, K. (2007). *Expressive vocabulary test - 2.* Pearson.

Williams, K. T. (2019). *Expressive vocabulary test [measurement instrument]* (3rd ed.). NCS Pearson.

Wilson, K. G. (2009). *Mindfulness for two: An acceptance and commitment therapy approach to mindfulness in psychotherapy.* New Harbinger Publications.

Wilson, L., Onslow, M., & Lincoln, M. (2004). Telehealth adaptation of the Lidcombe Program of early stuttering intervention: Five case studies. *American Journal of Speech Language Pathology, 13*(1), 81–92.

Wingate, M. E. (1964). Recovery from stuttering. *Journal of Speech and Hearing Disorders, 29*, 312–321.

Wingate, M. E. (1976). *Stuttering: Theory and treatment.* Irvington.

Wingate, M. E. (1983). Speaking unassisted: Comments on a paper by Andrews et al. *Journal of Speech and Hearing Disorders, 48*, 255–263.

Wingate, M. E. (1988). *The structure of stuttering: A psycholinguistic approach.* Springer-Verlag.

Winnicott, D. W. (1971). Playing and reality. Routledge.

Winslow, M., & Guitar, B. (1994). The effect of turn-taking on disfluencies: A case study. *Language, Speech, and Hearing Services in Schools, 25*, 251–257.

Wischner, G. J. (1950). Stuttering behavior and learning: A preliminary theoretical formulation. *Journal of Speech and Hearing Disorders, 15*, 324–325.

Witz, B. (2018, July 29). *Remembering a pioneer of baseball's mental side.* New York Times.

Wood, F., Stump, D., McKeehan, A., Sheldon, S., & Proctor, J. (1980). Patterns of regional cerebral blood flow during attempted reading aloud by stutterers both on and off haloperidol medication: Evidence for inadequate left frontal activation during stuttering. *Brain and Language, 9*, 141–144.

Woods, C. L., & Williams, D. E. (1976). Traits attributed to stuttering and normally fluent males. *Journal of Speech and Hearing Research, 19*, 267–278.

Woods, S., Shearsby, J., Onslow, M., & Burnham, D. (2002). Psychological impact of the Lidcombe Program of early stuttering intervention. *International Journal of Language and Communication Disorders, 37*(1), 31–40.

Woolf, G. (1967). The assessment of stuttering as struggle, avoidance, and expectancy. *British Journal of Disorders of Communication, 2*, 158–171.

World Health Organization. (1980a). *International classification of impairments, disabilities, and handicaps: A manual of classification relating to the consequences of disease.* World Health Organization.

World Health Organization. (1980b). *International classification of impairments, disabilities, and handicaps: A manual of classification relating to the consequences of disease.* World Health Organization.

World Health Organization. (2001). *The International classification of functioning, disability and health.* World Health Organization.

World Health Organization. (2007a). *International classification of functioning, disability and health: Children & youth version.* World Health Organization.

World Health Organization. (2007b). *International classification of functioning, disability and health: Children and youth version.* World Health Organization.

Wu, J., Maguire, G., Riley, G., Fallon, J., LaCasse, L., & Chin, S. (1995). A positron emission tomography [18F]deoxyglucose study of developmental stuttering. *Neuroreport, 63*, 501–505.

Wu, J. C., Maguire, G., Riley, G. D., Lee, A., Keator, D., Tang, C., & Najafi, A. (1997). Increased dopamine activity associated with stuttering. *Neuroreport, 8*, 767–770.

Wynne, M. K., & Boehmler, R. M. (1982). Central auditory function in fluent and disfluent normal speakers. *Journal of Speech and Hearing Research, 25*, 54–57.

Yairi, E. (1981). Disfluencies of normally speaking two-year old children. *Journal of Speech and Hearing Research, 24*, 490–495.

Yairi, E. (1982). Longitudinal studies of disfluencies in two-year old children. *Journal of Speech and Hearing Research, 25*, 155–160.

Yairi, E. (1983). The onset of stuttering in two- and three-year old children: A preliminary report. *Journal of Speech and Hearing Disorders, 48*, 171–178.

Yairi, E. (1997a). Early stuttering. In R. F. Curlee & G. M. Siegel (Eds.), *Nature and treatment of stuttering: New directions* (2nd ed.). Allyn & Bacon.

Yairi, E. (1997b). Home environment and parent-child interaction in childhood stuttering. In R. F. Curlee & G. M. Siegel (Eds.), *Nature and treatment of stuttering: New directions* (2nd ed., pp. 24–48). Allyn & Bacon.

Yairi, E. (2007). Subtyping stuttering. I. A review. *Journal of Fluency Disorders, 32,* 165–196.

Yairi, E., & Ambrose, N. (1992a). A longitudinal study of stuttering in children: A preliminary report. *Journal of Speech and Hearing Research, 35,* 755–760.

Yairi, E., & Ambrose, N. (1992b). Onset of stuttering in preschool children: Selected factors. *Journal of Speech and Hearing Research, 35,* 782–788.

Yairi, E., & Ambrose, N. (1996). *Disfluent speech in early childhood stuttering.* Unpublished manuscript. University of Illinois.

Yairi, E., & Ambrose, N. (1999). Early childhood stuttering I: Persistency and recovery rates. *Journal of Speech, Language, and Hearing Research, 42*(5), 1097–1112.

Yairi, E., & Ambrose, N. (2005). *Early childhood stuttering: For clinicians by clinicians.* Pro-Ed.

Yairi, E., Ambrose, N., & Cox, N. (1996a). Genetics of stuttering: A critical review. *Journal of Speech and Hearing Research, 394,* 771–784.

Yairi, E., & Ambrose, N. G. (2013). Epidemiology of stuttering: 21st century advances. *Journal of Fluency Disorders, 38*(2), 66–87.

Yairi, E., Ambrose, N. G., Paden, E., & Throneburg, R. (1996b). Predictive factors of persistence and recovery: Pathways of childhood stuttering. *Journal of Communication Disorders, 29,* 51–77.

Yairi, E., & Lewis, B. (1984). Disfluencies at the onset of stuttering. *Journal of Speech and Hearing Research, 27,* 154–159.

Yairi, E., & Seery, C. (2023). *Stuttering: Foundations and clinical applications* (3rd ed.). Plural Publishing.

Yaruss, J. S. (1998). Describing the consequences of disorders: Stuttering and the international classification of impairments, disabilities, and handicaps. *Journal of Speech, Language, and Hearing Research, 41,* 249–257.

Yaruss, J. S. (1999). Utterance length, syntactic complexity, and childhood stuttering. *Journal of Speech, Language, and Hearing Research, 422,* 329–344.

Yaruss, J. S. (2002). Facing the challenge of treating stuttering in the schools: Part 1. Selecting goals and strategies for success. *Seminars in Speech and Language, 23,* 153–159.

Yaruss, J. S. (2003). Facing the challenge of treating stuttering in schools. Part 2: Selecting goals and strategies for success. *Seminars in Speech and Language, 24*(2), 59–63.

Yaruss, J. S., Coleman, C., Beilby, J., & Herring, C. (2022). School-age children. In P. Zebrowski, J. Anderson & E. Conture (Eds.), *Stuttering and related disorders of fluency* (pp. 174–191). Thieme.

Yaruss, J. S., Coleman, C., & Quesal, R. W. (2016a). *Overall assessment of the speaker's experience of stuttering response form for school-age children 7 - 12 (OASES-S).* Stuttering Therapy Resources, Inc.

Yaruss, J. S., & Conture, E. G. (1995). Mother and child speaking rates and utterance lengths in adjacent fluent utterances: Preliminary observations. *Journal of Fluency Disorders, 20,* 257–278.

Yaruss, J. S., Newman, R. M., & Flora, T. (1999). Language and disfluency in nonstuttering children's conversational speech. *Journal of Fluency Disorders, 24,* 185–207.

Yaruss, J. S., Pelczarski, K., & Quesal, R. W. (2010). Comprehensive treatment for school-age children who stutter: Treating the entire disorder. In B. Guitar & R. J. McCauley (Eds.), *Treatment of stuttering: Established and emerging interventions* (pp. 215–244). Lippincott Williams & Wilkins.

Yaruss, J. S., & Quesal, R. W. (2006). Overall assessment of the speaker's experience of stuttering (OASES): Documenting multiple outcomes in stuttering treatment. *Journal of Fluency Disorders, 31,* 90–115.

Yaruss, J. S., & Quesal, R. W. (2016). *The Overall Assessment of the Speaker's Experience of Stuttering.* Stuttering Therapy Resources.

Yaruss, J. S., Quesal, R. W., & Coleman, C. (2016b). *Overall assessment of the speaker's experience of stuttering - Response form for teens ages 13 - 17 (OASES-T).* Stuttering Therapy Resources, Inc.

Yaruss, J. S., Quesal, R. W., & Reeves, N. (2007). Self-help and mutual aid groups as an adjunct to stuttering therapy. In E. Conture & R. Curlee (Eds.), *Stuttering and related disorders of fluency* (3rd ed., pp. 256–276). Thieme.

Yaruss, J. S., Reeves, N., & Herring, C. (2018). How speech-language pathologists can minimize bullying in children who stutter. *Seminars in Speech and Language, 39*(4), 342–355.

Young, M. A. (1961). Predicting ratings of severity of stuttering. *Journal of Speech and Hearing Disorders, Monograph Supplement, 7,* 31–54.

Young, M. A. (1981). A reanalysis of stuttering therapy: The relation between attitude change and long-term outcome. *Journal of Speech and Hearing Disorders, 46,* 221–222.

Young, M. A. (1984). Identification of stuttering and stutterers. In R. F. Curlee & W. H. Perkins (Eds.), *The nature and treatment of stuttering: New directions* (pp. 13–30). College-Hill.

Zablotsky, B., Black, L. I., Moenner, M. J., Schieve, L. A., Danielson, M. L., Bitsko, R. H., & Boyle, C. A. (2019). Prevalance and trends of developmental disabilities among children in the United States, 2009-2017. *Pediatrics, 144*(4), 10.

Zackheim, C., & Conture, E. G. (2003). Childhood stuttering and speech dysfluencies in relation to children's mean length of utterance: A preliminary study. *Journal of Fluency Disorders, 28*(2), 115–142.

Zebrowski, P. (1991). Duration of the speech disfluencies of beginning stutterers. *Journal of Speech and Hearing Research, 34(3),* 483–491.

Zebrowski, P. (2003). Developmental stuttering. *Pediatric Annals, 32*(7), 453–458.

Zebrowski, P. (2007). Treatment factors that influence therapy outcomes of children who stutter. In E. Conture & R. Curlee (Eds.), *Stuttering and related disorders of fluency* (3rd ed., pp. 23–38). Thieme.

Zebrowski, P., Anderson, J., & Conture, E. (2022). *Stuttering and related disorders of fluency* (4th ed.). Thieme.

Zebrowski, P., & Kelly, E. (2002). *Manual of stuttering intervention.* Singular.

Zebrowski, P., Rodgers, N. H., Gerlach, H., Paiva, A. L., & Robbins, M. L. (2021). Applying the transtheoretical model to stuttering management among adolescents: Part I. Scale development. *American Journal of Speech Language Pathology, 30*(6), 2492–2509.

Zebrowski, P. M., Weiss, A. L., Savelkoul, E. M., & Hammer, C. S. (1996). The effect of maternal rate reduction on the stuttering, speech rates and linguistic productions of children who stutter: Evidence from individual dyads. *Clinical Linguistics and Phonetics, 10*(3), 189–206.

Zengin-Bolatkale, H. (2016). *Cortical associates of emotional reactivity and regulation in children who stutter.* (Doctoral dissertation). Vanderbilt University.

Zengin-Bolatkale, H. (2017, November). *Cortical markers of emotion and stuttering frequency of young children. Paper presented at the Annual meeting of the American Speech-Language-Hearing Association.* Los Angeles.

Zengin-Bolatkale, H., Conture, E. G., Walden, T. A., & Jones, R. M. (2018). Sympathetic arousal as a marker of chronicity in childhood stuttering. *Developmental Neuropsychology*, *43*(2), 135–151.

Zhang, X., Sayler, K., Hartmen, S., & Belsky, J. (2021). Infant temperament, early-childhood parenting, and early adolescent development: Testing alternative models of parenting x temperament interaction. *Development and Psychopathology*, *11*(8), 1–12.

Ziegler, J. C., Perry, C., Ma-Wyatt, A., Ladner, D., & Schulte-Korne, G. (2003). Developmental dyslexia in different languages: Language-specific or universal? *Journal of Experimental Child Psychology*, *86*(3), 169–193.

Zimmerman, G. N. (1980). Articulatory dynamics of fluent utterances of stutterers and nonstutterers. *Journal of Speech and Hearing Research*, *23*, 95–107.

Zimmerman, G. N., & Knott, J. R. (1974). Slow potentials of the brain related to speech processing in normal speakers and stutterers. *Electroencephalography and Clinical Neurophysiology*, *37*, 599–607.

Zimmerman, G. N., Smith, A., & Hanley, J. M. (1981). Stuttering: In need of a unifying conceptual framework. *Journal of Speech and Hearing Research*, *24*, 25–31.

Author Index

Note: Page numbers followed by "*t*" indicate tables.

C

D

N

O

P

Subject Index

Note: Page numbers followed by "*f*" indicate figures; those followed by "*t*" indicate tables.

D

E

F

R

S